ADVANCES IN

FOOD AND NUTRITION RESEARCH

Cumulative Index: Volumes 1-45

VOLUME 46

ADVANCES IN

FOOD AND NUTRITION RESEARCH

Cumulative Index: Volumes 1-45

VOLUME 46

Edited by

STEVE L. TAYLOR

Department of Food Science and Technology

University of Nebraska

Lincoln, Nebraska

USA

ELSEVIER
ACADEMIC
PRESS

2003

Amsterdam - Boston - Heidelberg - London - New York - Oxford - Paris

San Diego - San Francisco - Singapore - Sydney - Tokyo

ELSEVIER B.V.
Sara Burgerhartstraat 25
P.O. Box 211,
1000 AE Amsterdam
The Netherlands

ELSEVIER Inc.
525 B Street,
Suite 1900
San Diego, CA 92101-4495
USA

ELSEVIER Ltd.
The Boulevard,
Langford Lane
Kidlington, Oxford OX5 1GB
UK

ELSEVIER Ltd.
84 Theobalds Road
London WC1X 8RR
UK

First edition 2003

Library of Congress Cataloging in Publication Data
A catalog record is available from the Library of Congress.

British Library Cataloguing in Publication Data
A catalogue record is available from the British Library.

ISBN: 0-12-016446-9
ISSN: 1043-4526 (Series)

∞ The paper used in this publication meets the requirements of ANSI/NISO Z39.48-1992 (Permanence of Paper).
Printed in The Netherlands.

Contents

Contents of Volumes 1–45

Volume 1

The Physiology and Chemistry of Rigor Mortis, with Special Reference to the Aging of Beef *by E.C. Bate-Smith* 1
Factors Influencing the Vitamin Content of Canned Foods *by L.E. Clifcorn* . . . 39
The Physiological Basis of Voluntary Food Intake (Appetite?) *by S. Lepkovsky* 105
Biochemical Factors Influencing the Shelf Life of Dried Whole Eggs and Means for Their Control *by H.D. Lightbody and H.L. Fevold* 149
Factors Affecting the Palatability of Poultry with Emphasis on Histological Post-mortem Changes *by B. Lowe* 203
Deterioration of Processed Potatoes *by A.F. Ross* 257
The Influence of Climate and Fertilizer Practices upon the Vitamin and Mineral Content of Vegetables *by G.F. Somers and K.O. Beeson* 291
Nonenzymatic Browning in Fruit Products *by E.R. Stadtman* 325
Microbial Inhibition by Food Preservatives *by O. Wyss* 373
High-Polymer Pectins and Their Deesterification *by G.L. Baker* 395

Volume 2

Ion Exchange Application by the Food Industry *by G.E. Felton* 1
Thermobacteriology as Applied to Food Processing *by C.R. Stumbo* 47
The Quaternary Ammonium Compounds and their Uses in the Food Industry *by C.G. Dunn* 117
The Pharmacology of DDT *by A.J. Lehman* 201
Analysis of Foods by Sensory Difference Tests *by M.M. Boggs and H.L. Hanson* 219
The Chemistry of Fruit and Vegetable Flavors *by J.G. Kirchner* 259
Histological Changes Induced in Fruits and Vegetables by Processing *by T.E. Weier and C.R. Stocking* 297
The Spoilage of Fish and Its Preservation by Chilling *by G.A. Reay and J.M. Shewan* 343
Spray Drying of Foods *by E. Seltzer and J.T. Settelmeyer* 399

Volume 3

Enzyme-Catalyzed Oxidative Browning of Fruit Products *by M.A. Joslyn and J.D. Ponting* 1
Physical and Chemical Aspects of the Production, Storage, and Utility of Dry Milk Products *by S.T. Coulter, R. Jennes and W.F. Geddes* 45
Electromagnetic Radiation Fundamentals and Their Applications in Food Technology *by B.E. Proctor and S.A. Goldblith* 119

The Pharmacological Evaluation of Antioxidants *by A.J. Lehman, O.G. Fitzhugh, A.A. Nelson and G. Woodard* 197
Salmonella Infection as a Food Industry Problem *by W.R. Hinshaw and E. McNeil* 209
Reactions between Sugars and Nitrogenous Compounds and Their Relationship to Certain Food Problems *by J.P. Danehy and W.W. Pigman* 241
Chemical and Microbial Studies on Sliced Canned Bacon *by J.A. Ulrich and H.O. Halvorson* 291
Certain Aspects of Internal Corrosion in Tin Plate Containers *by R.R. Hartwell* 327
Rationale for Studies of Consumer Food Preferences *by R.L.D. Morse* 385
Control of Microorganisms Causing Spoilage in Fruit and Vegetable Products *by M. Von Schelhorn* 429

Volume 4

Wiltshire Bacon *by N.E. Gibbons* 1
Work Methods Design and Work Simplification *by L.E. Davis* 37
Nutritional Stress Factors and Food Processing *by S. Lepkovsky* 105
The Chemistry of Chlorophyll (with Special Reference to Foods) *by S. Aronoff* 133
Reversion Problems in Edible Fats *by B.F. Daubert and P.W. O'Connell* 185
Fish Preservation in Southeast Asia *by A.G. van Veen* 209
The Effects of Heat upon the Nutritive Value of Protein *by E.E. Rice and J.F. Beuk* 233
Insects Attacking Stored Products *by A.E. Michelbacher* 281
The Use of Ascorbic Acid in Processing Foods *by J.C. Bauernfeind* 359

Volume 5

Oxidative Rancidity and Discoloration in Meat *by B.M. Watts* 1
The Chemistry of the Sugar-Sulfite Reaction and Its Relationship to Food Problems *by H. Gehman and E.M. Osman* 53
The Chemistry and Technology of the Pretreatment and Preservation of Fruit and Vegetable Products with Sulfur Dioxide and Sulfites *by M.A. Joslyn and J.B.S. Braverman* 97
Statistical Methods in Food Research *by B. Ostle and R.G. Tischer* 161
Flavonoid Compounds in Foods *by E.C. Bate-Smith* 261
The Color Problem in Foods *by G. Mackinney and C.O. Chichester* 301
Composition of Wines. I. Organic Constituents *by M.A. Amerine* 353

Volume 6

Applications of Research to Problems of Candy Manufacture *by L.F. Martin* . . 1
Bacterial Spoilage of Wines with Special Reference to California Conditions *by R.H. Vaughn* 67

Microbiological Implications in the Handling, Slaughtering, and Dressing of Meat Animals *by J.C. Ayres* 109
Microbiological Problems of Frozen Food Products *by G. Borgstrom* 163
Potato Granules, Development and Technology of Manufacture *by R.L. Olson and W.0. Harrington* 231
The Thermal Destruction of Vitamin B_1 in Foods *by K.T.H. Farrer* 257
Tunnel Dehydrators for Fruits and Vegetables *by P.W. Kilpatrick, E. Lowe and W.B. Van Arsdel* 313

Volume 7

The Profile Method of Flavor Analysis *by J.F. Caul* 1
Spoilage of Fish and Its Preservation by Chemical Agents *by Y. Tomiyasu and B. Zenitani* 41
Water Relations of Food Spoilage Microorganisms *by W.J. Scott* 83
Chlorine in Food Plant Sanitation *by W.A. Mercer and I. Somers* 129
Freeze-Drying of Food Products *by J.C. Harper and A.L. Tappel* 171
Gelatin *by B. Idson and E. Braswell* 235
Licorice *by C. Nieman* 339

Volume 8

Rheology in Food Research *by G.W. Scott Blair* 1
The Blanching Process *by F.A. Lee* 63
New Methods to Detect and Eliminate Insect-Infected Grain *by M. Milner* . . . 111
Composition of Wines. II. Inorganic Constituents *by M.A. Amerine* 133
Fermentation, Drying, and Storage of Cacao Beans *by P.A. Roelofsen* 225
Some Aspects of the Biochemistry of Apple and Pear Fruits *by A.C. Hulme* . . 297

Volume 9

Chemical Changes Associated with Aging of Meat with Emphasis on the Proteins *by J.R. Whitaker* 1
The Chemistry and Technology of the Preservation of Green Peas *by L.J. Lynch, R.S. Mitchell and D.J. Casimir* 61
Principles and Instrumentation for the Physical Measurement of Food Quality with Special Reference to Fruit and Vegetable Products *by A. Kramer and B.A. Twigg* 153
Microorganisms in Noncitrus Juices *by H. Lüthi* 221
The Chemical Constituents of Citrus Fruits *by J.F. Kefford* 285

Volume 10

Research in Food Science and Food Technology: A Status Report *by M.A. Joslyn* 1
Protein Chemistry and Food Research *by R.E. Feeney and R.M. Hill* 23
Aroma and Flavor of Japanese Soy Sauce *by T. Yokotsuka* 75
Public Health Significance of Paralytic Shellfish Poison *by E.F. McFarren, M.L. Schafer, J.E. Campbell, K.H. Lewis, E.T. Jensen and E.J. Schantz* 135
Problems of the Potato Chip Industry–Processing and Technology *by H.D. Brown* 181
Sauerkraut *by C.S. Pederson* 233
The Postharvest Biochemistry of Tropical and Subtropical Fruits *by J.B. Biale* . 293
Biochemistry and Meat Hydration *by R. Hamm* 355

Volume 11

The Chemistry of Protopectin: A Critical Review of Historical Data and Recent Developments *by M.A. Joslyn* 1
Utilization of Natural Polysaccharide Gums in the Food Industry *by M. Glicksman* 109
The Chemistry of Tea and Tea Manufacturing *by W.H. Stahl* 201
Enzymic Reactions in Foods of Low Moisture Content *by L. Acker* 263
The Action of Benzoic and Salicyclic Acids on the Metabolism of Microorganisms *by I. Bosund* 331
The Nature and Role of Fluid Consistency in Food Engineering Applications *by S.E. Charm* 355

Volume 12

Chemistry of Nonenzymic Browning. I. The Reaction Between Aldoses and Amines *by T.M. Reynolds* 1
Osmophilic Yeasts *by H. Ōnishi* 51
The Use of Carbon Dioxide in the Transport and Storage of Fruits and Vegetables *by W.H. Smith* 95
Refrigerated Transport on Shipboard *by K.C. Hales* 147
Physiology, Chemistry, and Technology of Passion Fruit *by J.S. Pruthi* 203
Utilization of Synthetic Gums in the Food Industry *by M. Glicksman* 283
Fish Sausage and Ham Industry in Japan *by E. Tanikawa* 367

Volume 13

Recent Advances in the Freeze-Drying of Food Products *by R.F. Burke and R.V. Decareau* 1
Etiological Status and Associated Studies of Pale, Soft, Exudative Porcine Musculature *by E.J. Briskey* 89

Astringency of Fruits and Fruit Products in Relation to Phenolic Content *by M.A. Joslyn and J.L. Goldstein* 179
Fundamentals of Low-Temperature Food Preservation *by O. Fennema and W.D. Powrie* 219
Minimum Growth Temperatures for Food-Poisoning, Fecal-Indicator, and Psychrophilic Microorganisms *by H.D. Michener and R.P. Elliott* 349

Volume 14

Techniques for Sensory Evaluation of Food Odors *by H. Stone, R.M. Pangborn and C.S. Ough* 1
Methods of Meat Texture Measurement Viewed from the Background of Factors Affecting Tenderness *by A.S. Szczesniak and K.W. Torgeson* 33
Chemistry of Nonenzymic Browning II *by T.M. Reynolds* 167
Unimolecular Thermal Transformations of Organic Compounds under Food Processing Conditions *by J.W. Ralls* 285
Theory and Practice of Hard-Surface Cleaning *by W.G. Jennings* 325

Volume 15

Metabolic Fate in Animals of Hindered Phenolic Antioxidants in relation to Their Safety Evaluation and Antioxidant Function *by D.E. Hathway* 1
Radiobiological Parameters in the Irradiation of Fruits and Vegetables *by R.J. Romani* 57
Food Irradiation–Physiology of Fruits as Related to Feasibility of the Technology *by E.C. Maxie and A. Abdel-Kader* 103
Ionizing Radiation for Control of Postharvest Diseases of Fruit and Vegetables *by N.F. Sommer and R.J. Fortlage* 147
Carotenoids: Properties, Occurrence, and Utilization in Foods *by B. Borenstein and R.H. Bunnell* 195
Basic Principles of Microwaves and Recent Developments *by S.A. Goldblith* . . 275
Evaporation Methods as Applied to the Food Industry *by G.D. Armerding* . . . 303

Volume 16

Processed Vegetable Protein Mixtures for Human Consumption in Developing Countries *by R. Bressani and L.G. Elias* 1
Meat Emulsions *by R.L. Saffle* 105
Food Quality as Determined by Metabolic By-Products of Microorganisms *by M.L. Fields, B.S. Richmond and R.E. Baldwin* 161
The Chemistry and Biochemistry of Cheese Ripening *by J. Schormüller* 231
Relation between Chemical Composition and Bread-Making Potentialities of Wheat Flour *by Y. Pomeranz* 335

Volume 17

Oxidation Systems in Fruits and Vegetables – Their Relation to the Quality of Preserved Products *by F. Aylward and D.R. Haisman* 1
The Utilization of Food Industries Wastes *by I. Ben-Gera and A. Kramer* 77
Tropical Fruit Technology *by N. Czyhrinciw* 153
The Chemistry and Biochemistry of Tea and Tea Manufacture *by M.A. Bokuchava and N.I. Skobeleva* 215

Volume 18

Meat Flavor *by K.O. Herz and S.S. Chang* 1
Microbial Sources of Protein *by H.E. Snyder* 85
Toxins from Fish and Other Marine Organisms *by P.J. Scheuer* 141
The Flat Sour Bacteria *by M.L. Fields* 163
Food Processing with Added Ascorbic Acid *by J.C. Bauernfeind and D.M. Pinkert* 219

Volume 19

Red and White Muscle *by R.G. Cassens and C.C. Cooper* 1
Food Browning as a Polyphenol Reaction *by A.G. Mathew and H.A.B. Parpia* . 75
The Chemistry of Dairy Powders with Reference to Baking *by J.E. Kinsella* . . 147
A Retrospective View of Sensory Analysis and Some Considerations for the Future *by D.J. Tilgner* 215
Myofibrillar Proteins of Skeletal Muscle *by E.J. Briskey and T. Fukazawa* 279

Volume 20

Aroma Recovery and Retention in Concentration and Drying of Foods *by J.L. Bomben, S. Bruin, H.A.C. Thijssen and R.L. Merson* 1
Cold Storage Design and Administration *by C.E.B. Cooper* 113
Interaction between Glycolipids and Wheat Flour Macromolecules in Breadmaking *by Y. Pomeranz* 153
Proteins of Aquatic Origin as Foods for Human Consumption *by E.R. Pariser* . 189
Heat Transfer During Freezing and Thawing of Foods *by A. Bakal and K.-I. Hayakawa* 217
Factors Affecting Tenderness During Heating of Meat *by E. Laakkonen* 257

Volume 21

Regulation of Food Intake *by S. Lepkovsky* 1

Animal Physiology and Meat Quality *by R.G. Cassens, D.N. Marple and G. Eikelenboom* . . . 71
New Concepts in Meat Processing *by R.H. Locker, C.L. Davey, P.M. Nottingham, D.R. Haughey and N.H. Law* . . . 157
Physiology and Biochemistry of Mango Fruit *by H. Subramanyam, S. Krushnamurthy and H.A.B. Parpia* . . . 223
Formation and Control of Chlorophyll and Glycoalkaloids in Tubers of *Solanum tuberosum* L. and Evaluation of Glycoalkaloid Toxicity *by S.J. Jadhav and D.K. Salunkhe* . . . 307

Volume 22

N-Nitrosamines: A Review of Chemical and Biological Properties and Their Estimation in Foodstuffs *by N.T. Crosby and R. Sawyer* . . . 1
Development of Flavor, Odor, and Pungency in Onion and Garlic *by J.R. Whitaker* 73
Clostridium botulinum and Its Importance in Fishery Products *by G. Hobbs* . . 135
Food Products Intended to Improve Nutrition in the Developing World *by S.M. Weisberg* . . . 187
Scanning Electron Microscopy in Food Science and Technology *by Y. Pomeranz* 205
Emulsion Stability and Its Relation to Foods *by G.E. Petrowski* . . . 309

Volume 23

"Warmed-Over" Flavor in Meat, Poultry, and Fish *by A.M. Pearson, J.D. Love and F.B. Shorland* . . . 1
Mathematical Methods for Estimating Proper Thermal Processes and Their Computer Implementation *by K.-I. Hayakawa* . . . 75
Abalone–An Esoteric Food *by J. Olley and S.J. Thrower* . . . 143
Wheat Germ *by S.R. Shurpalekar and P. Haridas Rao* . . . 187
Flexible Packaging for Thermoprocessed Foods *by R.A. Lampi* . . . 305

Volume 24

Sulfhydryl and Disulfide Groups in Meats *by K. Hofmann and R. Hamm* 1
Histamine (?) Toxicity from Fish Products *by S. Hudson Arnold and W.D. Brown* 113
Food Irradiation *by W.M. Urbain* . . . 155
Tea *by R.L. Wickremasinghe* . . . 229
Honey *by J.W. White, Jr.* . . . 287

Volume 25

Wine Deacidification *by R.B. Beelman and J.F. Gallander* . . . 1

Dehydrated Mashed Potatoes–Chemical and Biochemical Aspects *by D. Hadziyev and L. Steele* . . . 55
Xylitol and Oral Health *by K.K. Mäkinen* . . . 137
Metabolic and Nutritional Aspects of Xylitol *by R. Ylikahri* . . . 159
Frozen Fruits and Vegetables: Their Chemistry, Physics, and Cryobiology *by M.S. Brown* . . . 181
Byssochlamys spp. and Their Importance in Processed Fruits *by L.R. Beuchat and S.L. Rice* . . . 237

Volume 26

Single-Cell Protein: Engineering, Economics, and Utilization in Foods *by C.L. Cooney, C. Rha and S.R. Tannenbaum* . . . 1
Influence of Ante- and Postmortem Treatments upon Muscle Composition and Meat Quality *by A. Asghar and A.M. Pearson* . . . 53
Peanut Protein Ingredients: Preparation, Properties, and Food Uses *by K.R. Natarajan* . . . 215
Theories of Protein Denaturation during Frozen Storage of Fish Flesh *by S.Y.K. Shenouda* . . . 275

Volume 27

Samuel Cate Prescott *by S.A. Goldblith* . . . 1
Mechanically Deboned Red Meat *by R.A. Field* . . . 23
Mechanical Deboning of Poultry and Fish *by G.W. Froning* . . . 109
Naturally Occurring Food Toxicants: Phenolic Substances of Plant Origin Common in Foods *by V.L. Singleton* . . . 149
Technology and Flavor Chemistry of Passion Fruit Juices and Concentrates *by D.J. Casimir, J.F. Kefford and F.B. Whitfield* . . . 243
Phase Transitions of Water in Some Products of Plant Origin at Low and Superlow Temperatures *by Y. Guegov* . . . 297

Volume 28

Phytates in Legumes and Cereals *by N.R. Reddy, S.K. Sathe and D.K. Salunkhe* 1
Physical, Chemical, and Nutritional Properties of Common Bean (*Phaseolus*) Proteins *by V.C. Sgarbieri and J.R. Whitaker* . . . 93
Porcine Stress Syndromes *by G. Mitchell and J.J.A. Heffron* . . . 167
Chemical, Biochemical, Functional, and Nutritional Characteristics of Collagen in Food Systems *by A. Asghar and R.L. Henrickson* . . . 231
Food Technological Evaluation of Xylitol *by L. Hyvönen, P. Koivistoinen and F. Voirol* . . . 373

Volume 29

Cured Meat Flavor *by J.I. Gray and A.M. Pearson* 1

Chemical Aspects of the Smoking of Meat and Meat Products *by L. Tóth and K. Potthast* 87

Food Texture Perception *by C.M. Christensen* 159

Baking Quality of Wheat Flours *by F. MacRitchie* 201

Kiwifruit *by B.S. Luh and Z. Wang* 279

Volume 30

Sulfites in Foods: Uses, Analytical Methods, Residues, Fate, Exposure Assessment, Metabolism, Toxicity, and Hypersensitivity *by S.L. Taylor, N.A. Higley and R.K. Bush* 1

Maillard Reactions: Nonenzymatic Browning in Food Systems with Special Reference to the Development of Flavor *by J.P. Danehy* 77

Postharvest Changes in Fruit Cell Wall *by M.A. John and P.M. Dey* 139

Soy Sauce Biochemistry *by T. Yokotsuka* 195

New Protein Foods: A Study of a Treatise *by H.L. Wilcke, C.E. Bodwell, D.T. Hopkins and A.M. Altschul* 331

Volume 31

Carcinogen Risk Assessment *by R. Nichols Hazelwood* 1

A Review of Current Literature on *N*-Nitroso Compounds in Foods *by J.H. Hotchkiss* 53

Dietary Fiber: Chemistry, Analysis, and Properties *by R.R. Selvendran, B.J.H. Stevens and M.S. Du Pont* 117

Chocolate *by R.A. Martin, Jr.* 211

Endogenous Proteolytic Enzymes in Skeletal Muscle: Their Significance in Muscle Physiology and during Postmortem Aging Events in Carcasses *by A. Asghar and A.R. Bhatti* 343

Olive Oil: A Review *by A. Kiritsakis and P. Markakis* 453

Volume 32

A Review of Aseptic Processing *by E.L. Mitchell* 1

Convective Heat Transfer to Fluid Foods in Cans *by M.A. Rao and R.C. Anantheswaran* 39

Selenium in Foods *by G.F. Combs, Jr.* 85

Chemistry of Maillard Reactions: Recent Studies on the Browning Reaction Mechanism and the Development of Antioxidants and Mutagens *by M. Namiki* 115

Food versus Biomass Fuel: Socioeconomic and Environmental Impacts in the United States, Brazil, India, and Kenya *by D. Pimentel, A.F. Warneke, W.S. Teel, K.A. Schwab, N.J. Simcox, D.M. Ebert, K.D. Baenisch and M.R. Aaron* 185
Factors Influencing Food Selection in the American Diet *by C.I. Waslien* 239

Volume 33

Chemical and Nutritional Aspects of Folate Research: Analytical Procedures, Methods of Folate Synthesis, Stability, and Bioavailability of Dietary Folates *by J.F. Gregory III* 1
Calcium in the Diet: Food Sources, Recommended Intakes, and Nutritional Bioavailability *by D.D. Miller* 103
Dietary and Biochemical Aspects of Vitamin E *by R.S. Parker* 157
Oxidation of Polyunsaturated Fatty Acids: Mechanisms, Products, and Inhibition with Emphasis on Fish *by R.J. Hsieh and J.E. Kinsella* 233
Proteins in Whey: Chemical, Physical, and Functional Properties *by J.E. Kinsella and D.M. Whitehead* 343

Volume 34

Interfaces, Protein Films, and Foams *by S. Damodaran* 1
Stability of Food Emulsions: Physicochemical Role of Protein and Nonprotein Emulsifiers *by K.P. Das and J.E. Kinsella* 81
The Gelation of Proteins *by G.R. Ziegler and E.A. Foegeding* 203
Thermodynamic Linkage and Nonlinear Regression Analysis: A Molecular Basis for Modeling Biomacromolecular Processes *by T.F. Kumosinski* 299
Meat Mutagens *by C. Chen, A.M. Pearson and J.I. Gray* 387

Volume 35

α-Linolenic Acid: Functions and Effects on Linoleic Acid Metabolism and Eicosanoid-Mediated Reactions *by J.E. Kinsella* 1
Protein Digestibility: *In Vitro* Methods of Assessment *by H.E. Swaisgood and G.L. Catignani* 185
Protein and Enzyme Stability: Structural, Thermodynamic, and Experimental Aspects *by M.M. Kristjánsson and J.E. Kinsella* 237
Thermal Analysis of Food Proteins *by C.-Y. Ma and V.R. Harwalkar* 317

Volume 36

Physicochemical Properties of Wheat Proteins in Relation to Functionality *by F. MacRitchie* 1

Plant Food Protein Engineering *by S. Utsumi* 89
Minerals and Trace Elements in Milk *by A. Flynn* 209
Dietary Fatty Acids, Lipoproteins, and Cardiovascular Disease *by D.J. McNamara* 253

Volume 37

Food, Diet, and Gastrointestinal Immune Function *by J.J. Pestka* 1
Effect of Consumption of Lactic Cultures on Human Health *by M.E. Sanders* . 67
Defining the Role of Milkfat in Balanced Diets *by L.A. Berner* 131
Biochemistry of Cardiolipin: Sensitivity to Dietary Fatty Acids *by A. Berger, J.B. German and M.E. Gershwin* 259
Diseases and Disorders of Muscle *by A.M. Pearson and R.B. Young* 339

Volume 38

Hydrolytic and Transgalactosylic Activities of Commercial β-Galactosidase (Lactase) in Food Processing *by L.F. Pivarnik, A.G. Senecal and A.G. Rand* 1
Glass Transitions and Water-Food Structure Interactions *by L. Slade and H. Levine* 103
Corn Wet Milling: Separation Chemistry and Technology *by D.S. Jackson and D.L. Shandera, Jr.* 271

Volume 39

The Rheology of Semiliquid Foods *by G.V. Barbosa-Cánovas, L. Ma, J.L. Kokini and A. Ibarz* 1
Control of the Dehydration Process in Production of Intermediate-Moisture Meat Products: A Review *by S.F. Chang, A.M. Pearson and T.C. Huang* 71
Cheese: Physical, Biochemical, and Nutritional Aspects *by P.F. Fox, T.P. O'Connor, P.L.H. McSweeney, T.P. Guinee and N.M. O'Brien* 163
Biogenic Amines in Fish and Shellfish *by D.D. Rawles, G.J. Flick and R.E. Martin* 329

Volume 40. Mathematical Modeling in Experimental Nutrition. Vitamins, proteins, methods

Part I. Vitamin metabolism

Quantitative and Conceptual Contributions of Mathematical Modeling to Current Views on Vitamin A Metabolism, Biochemistry, and Nutrition *by M.H. Green and J. Balmer Green* 3
Mathematical Modeling in Nutrition: Constructing a Physiologic Compartmental Model of the Dynamics of β-Carotene Metabolism *by J.A. Novotny, L.A. Zech, H.C. Furr, S.R. Dueker and A.J. Clifford* 25

Experimental Approaches to the Study of β-Carotene Metabolism: Potential of a ^{13}C Tracer Approach to Modeling β-Carotene Kinetics in Humans *by J.E. Swanson, K.J. Goodman, R.S. Parker and Y.-y. Wang* 55
Modeling of Folate Metabolism *by J.F. Gregory III and K.C. Scott* 81
Molecular Biology in Nutrition Research: Modeling of Folate Metabolism *by B.-F. Lin, J.-S. Kim, J.-C. Hsu, C. Osborne, K. Lowe, T. Garrow and B. Shane* 95
Modeling Vitamin B6 Metabolism *by S.P. Coburn* 107

Part II. Protein and amino acid metabolism
Interrelationships between Metabolism of Glycogen Phosphorylase and Pyridoxal Phosphate–Implications in McArdle's Disease *by R.J. Beynon, C. Bartram, A. Flannery, R.P. Evershed, D. Leyland, P. Hopkins, V. Toescu, J. Phoenix and R.H.T. Edwards* 135
Metabolism of Normal and Met30 Transthyretin *by D. Hanes, L.A. Zech, J. Murrell and M.D. Benson* 149
Use of a Four Parameter Logistic Equation and Parameter Sharing to Evaluate Animal Responses to Graded Levels of Nitrogen or Amino Acids *by M.J. Gahl, T.D. Crenshaw, N.J. Benevenga and M.D. Finke* 157

Part III. Energy metabolism
Total Energy Expenditure of Free-Living Humans Can Be Estimated with the Doubly Labeled Water Method *by W.W. Wong* 171

Part IV. Methods for obtaining kinetic data
Microdialysis and Ultrafiltration *by E.M. Janle and P.T. Kissinger* 183
Membrane Vesicles *by P. Proulx* 197
Culture of Mammary Tissue: Glucose Transport Processes *by J.D. Turner, A. Delaquis and C. Malo* 207

Part V. Simulating complex metabolic processes
Analysis of Bioperiodicity in Physiological Responses *by L.P. Mercer and D.S. Kelley* 217
Nutrient-Response: A "Top Down" Approach to Metabolic Control *by A.R. Schulz* 227
Modeling Membrane Transport *by R.B. King* 243

Part VI. Computational aspects of modeling
Estimation and Use of Kinetic Parameter Distributions in Metabolism and Nutrition *by W.F. Beltz* 265
Essential Numerical Supports for Kinetic Modeling Software: Linear Integrators *by R.C. Boston, T. McNabb, P.C. Greif and L.A. Zech* 281
Identifiability *by J.A. Jacquez* 305
Dynamic Systems and Neural Networks: Modeling in Physiology and Medicine *by S.I. Sayegh* 323
Graph Theoretical Methods for Physiologically Based Modeling *by H. Zhang and Z. Zhang* 339

Volume 41. Starch. Basic Science to Biotechnology

Occurrence of Starch *by M.N. Sivak and J. Preiss* 1
Physicochemical Structure of the Starch Granule *by M.N. Sivak and J. Preiss* . 13
Biosynthetic Reactions of Starch Synthesis *by M.N. Sivak and J. Preiss* 33
Synthesis of the Glucosyl Donor: ADPglucose Pyrophosphorylase *by M.N. Sivak and J. Preiss* 43
Starch Synthases *by M.N. Sivak and J. Preiss* 75
Branching Enzymes *by M.N. Sivak and J. Preiss* 89
Open Questions and Hypotheses in Starch Biosynthesis *by M.N. Sivak and J. Preiss* 107
The Site of Starch Synthesis in Non photosynthetic Plant Tissues: The Amyloplast *by M.N. Sivak and J. Preiss* 115
Regulation of the Starch Synthesis Pathway: Targets for Biotechnology *by M.N. Sivak and J. Preiss* 125
Starch Accumulation in Photosynthetic Cells *by M.N. Sivak and J. Preiss* 139
Starch Degradation *by M.N. Sivak and J. Preiss* 153
Industrial Applications of Starch *by M.N. Sivak and J. Preiss* 163

Volume 42

The Role of Flavoring Substances in Food Allergy and Intolerance *by S.L. Taylor and E.S. Dormedy* 1
The Use of Amino Acid Sequence Alignments to Assess Potential Allergenicity of Proteins Used in Genetically Modified Foods *by S.M. Gendel* 45
Sequence Databases For Assessing the Potential Allergenicity of Proteins Used in Transgenic Foods *by S.M. Gendel* 63
Design of Emulsification Peptides *by D. Sheehan, K. Carey and S. O'Sullivan* . 93
X-Ray Diffraction of Food Polysaccharides *by R. Chandrasekaran* 131
Cellular Signal Transduction of Sweetener-induced Taste *by M. Naim, B.J. Striem and M. Tal* 211
Antioxidant Activity of the Labiatae *by S.L. Cuppett and C.A. Hall III* 245

Volume 43

Inulin: A Review of Nutritional and Health Implications *by L.S. Boeckner, M.I. Schnepf and B.C. Tungland* 1
Microwave Technology and Foods *by T. Ohlsson and N. Bengtsson* 65
Oriental Noodles *by G. Hou* 141
The Role of Natural Color Additives in Food Allergy *by C.D. Lucas, S.L. Taylor and J.B. Hallagan* 195
Developments in Sorghum Food Technologies *by J.R.N. Taylor and J. Dewar* . 217
Bovine Spongiform Encephalopathy – Food Safety Implications *by M.S. Brewer* 265
Microbial Attachment to Food and Food Contact Surfaces *by J.F. Frank* 319

Volume 44

Pulsed Electric Field Processing of High Acid Liquid Foods: A Review *by H.W. Yeom, K.T. McCann, C.B. Streaker and Q.H. Zhang* 1
Structure and Mechanical Properties of FAT Crystal Networks *by S.S. Narine and A.G. Marangoni* 33
Thermal Inactivation of Pathogens and Verification of Adequate Cooking in Meat and Poultry Products *by A. Orta-Ramirez and D.M. Smith* 147
Phytoestrogens in Foods *by P.A. Murphy and S. Hendrich* 195
Taste and Smell Perception in the Elderly: Effect of Medication and Disease *by S.S. Schiffman and J. Zervakis* 247
Development and Application of Multicomponent Edible Coatings and Films: A Review *by Y. Wu, C.L. Weller, F. Hamouz, S.L. Cuppett and M.I. Schnepf* 347
Buckwheat: Composition, Chemistry and Processing *by K. Ikeda* 395

Volume 45

Inositol Phosphates in Foods *by B.Q. Phillippy* 1
Pyrrolizidine Alkaloids in Foods *by R.A. Coulombe, Jr.* 61
Ultrasonic Sensors for the Food Industry *by J.N. Coupland and R. Saggin* 101
Ozone and Its Current and Future Application in the Food Industry *by J.-G. Kim, A.E. Yousef and M.A. Khadre* 167
The High Molecular Weight Subunits of Wheat Glutenin and Their Role in Determining Wheat Processing Properties *by P.R. Shewry, N.G. Halford, A.S. Tatharn, Y. Popineau, D. Lafiandra and P.S. Belton* 219

Contributors to Volumes 1–45

Aaron, M.R. *College of Agriculture and Life Sciences, Cornell University, Ithaca, New York* (**32**, 185)

Abdel-Kader, A. *Department of Horticulture, College of Agriculture, Cairo University, Cairo, Egypt* (**15**, 103)

Acker, L. *Institut für Pharmazie und Lebensmittelchemie der Universität Münster-Westfalen, Germany* (**11**, 263)

Altschul, A.M. *Departments of Medicine, and Community and Family Medicine, Georgetown University School of Medicine, Washington, DC* (**30**, 331)

Amerine, M.A. *Department of Viticulture and Enology, College of Agriculture, University of California, Davis, California* (**5**, 353; **8**, 133)

Anantheswaran, R.C. *Department of Food Science, Pennsylvania State University, University Park, Pennsylvania* (**32**, 39)

Armerding, G.D. *3477 St. Mary's Road, Lafayette, California* (**15**, 303)

Aronoff, S. *Iowa State College, Ames, Iowa* (**4**, 133)

Asghar, A. *Department of Food Science, University of Alberta, Edmonton, Alberta, Canada* (**26**, 53; **28**, 231; **31**, 343)

Aylward, F. *Department of Food Science, The University of Reading, Berkshire, England, UK* (**17**, 1)

Ayres, J.C. *Food Processing Laboratory, Iowa Agricultural Experimental Station, Iowa State College, Ames, Iowa* (**6**, 109)

Baenisch, K.D. *College of Agriculture and Life Sciences, Cornell University, Ithaca, New York* (**32**, 185)

Bakal, A. *Foster D. Snell, Inc., Hanover Road, Florham Park, New Jersey* (**20**, 217)

Baker, G.L. *University of Delaware Agricultural Experiment Station, Newark, Delaware* (**1**, 395)

Baldwin, R.E. *Food Research Laboratory, Department of Food Science and Nutrition and School of Home Economics, University of Missouri, Columbia, Missouri* (**16**, 161)

Balmer Green, J. *Nutrition Department, Pennsylvania State University, University Park, Pennsylvania* (**40**, 3)

Barbosa-Cánovas, G.V. *Biological Systems and Engineering, Washington State University, Pullman, Washington* (**39**, 1)

Bartram, C. *Department of Biochemistry and Applied Molecular Biology, UMIST, Manchester, United Kingdom* (**40**, 135)

Bate-Smith, E.C. *Low Temperature Research Station, University of Cambridge, and Department of Scientific and Industrial Research, Cambridge, England, UK* (**1**, 1; **5**, 261)

Bauernfeind, J.C. *Chemical Research Department, Hoffmann-LaRoche Inc., Nutley, New Jersey* (**4**, 359; **18**, 219)

Beelman, R.B. *Department of Food Science, The Pennsylvania State University, University Park, Pennsylvania* (**25**, 1)

Beeson, K.O. *U.S. Plant, Soil and Nutrition Laboratory, Ithaca, New York* (**1**, 291)

Belton, P.S. *School of Chemical Sciences, University of East Anglia, Norwich, UK* (**45**, 219)

Beltz, W.F. *Biocomp, San Diego, California* (**40**, 265)

Ben-Gera, I. *Food Institute, Centre for Industrial Research, Haifa, Israel* (**17**, 77)

Benevenga, N.J. *Departments of Nutritional Sciences and Meat and Animal Science, University of Wisconsin, Madison, Wisconsin* (**40**, 157)

Bengtsson, N. *Kyrkvägen 62, Mölnlycke, Sweden* (**43**, 65)

Benson, M.D. *Division of Rheumatology, Department of Medicine, Indiana University School of Medicine, Indianapolis, Indiana 46202; Rheumatology Section, Richard L. Roudebush – Veterans Affairs Medical Center, Indianapolis, Indiana* (**40**, 149)

Berger, A. *Department of Food Science and Technology, University of California, Davis, Davis, California* (**37**, 259)

Berner, L.A. *Nutrition Consultant, San Luis Obispo, California* (**37**, 131)

Beuchat, L.R. *Department of Food Science, University of Georgia Agriculture Experiment Station, Experiment, Georgia* (**25**, 237)

Beuk, J.F. *Nutrition and Biochemistry Research Division, Research Laboratories, Swift and Company, Chicago, Illinois* (**4**, 233)

Beynon, R.J. *Department of Biochemistry and Applied Molecular Biology, UMIST, Manchester, United Kingdom* (**40**, 135)

Bhatti, A.R. *Preventive Medicine Section, Defence Research Establishment, Suffield, Ralston, Alberta, Canada* (**31**, 343)

Biale, J.B. *Department of Horticultural Science, University of California, Los Angeles, California* (**10**, 293)

Bodwell, C.E. *Energy and Protein Nutrition Laboratory, Beltsville Human Nutrition Research Center, Agricultural Research Service, U.S. Department of Agriculture, Beltsville, Maryland* (**30**, 331)

Boeckner, L.S. *Panhandle Research and Extension Center, University of Nebraska, Scottsbluff, Nebraska* (**43**, 1)

Boggs, M.M. *Western Regional Research Laboratory, Albany, California* (**2**, 219)

Bokuchava, M.A. *Bakh Institute of Biochemistry, USSR Academy of Sciences, Moscow, USSR* (**17**, 215)

Bomben, J.L. *Western Regional Research Laboratory, Western Marketing and Nutrition Division, United States Department of Agriculture, Albany, California* (**20**, 1)

Borenstein, B. *Hoffmann–La Roche Inc., Nutley, New Jersey* (**15**, 195)

Borgstrom, G. *Swedish Institute for Food Preservation Research (SIK), Göteborg, Sweden* (**6**, 163)

Boston, R.C. *Clinical Studies, NBC, School of Veterinary Medicine, University of Pennsylvania, Kennett Square, Pennsylvania* (**40**, 281)

Bosund, I. *Findus Research Laboratory, Bjuv, Sweden* (**11**, 331)

Braswell, E. *Chemistry Department, Hunter College, New York, New York* (**7**, 235)

Braverman, J.B.S. *Department of Food Technology, University of California, Berkeley, California* (**5**, 97)

Bressani, R. *Institute of Nutrition of Central America and Panama (INCAP), Guatemala, Central America* (**16**, 1)

Brewer, M.S. *Department of Food Science and Human Nutrition, University of Illinois, Urbana, Illinois* (**43**, 265)

Briskey, E.J. *Campbell Institute for Food Research, Camden, New Jersey* (**13**, 89; **19**, 279)

Brown, H.D. *Potato Chip Institute International, Cleveland, Ohio, and The Ohio State University, Columbus, Ohio* (**10**, 181)

Brown, M.S. *Western Regional Research Center, Science and Education Administration, U.S. Department of Agriculture, Berkeley, California* (**25**, 181)

Brown, W.D. *Institute of Marine Resources, Department of Food Science and Technology, University of California, Davis, California* (**24**, 113)

Bruin, S. *Royal Dutch/Shell Laboratory, Amsterdam, The Netherlands* (**20**, 1)

Bunnell, R.H. *Hoffmann–La Roche Inc., Nutley, New Jersey* (**15**, 195)

Burke, R.F. *The Lummus Company, Newark, New Jersey* (**13**, 1)

Bush, R.K. *William S. Middleton Memorial Veterans Hospital, Madison, Wisconsin, and Department of Medicine, University of Wisconsin, Madison, Wisconsin* (**30**, 1)

Campbell, J.E. *Milk and Food Research Program, U.S. Department of Health, Education and Welfare, Public Health Service, Robert A. Taft Sanitary Engineering Center, Cincinnati, Ohio* (**10**, 135)

Carey, K. *Department of Biochemistry, University College, Cork, Ireland* (**42**, 93)

Casimir, D.J. *Division of Food Research, Commonwealth Scientific and Industrial Research Organization, North Ryde, New South Wales, Australia* (**9**, 61; **27**, 243)

Cassens, R.G. *Muscle Biology Laboratory, University of Wisconsin, Madison, Wisconsin* (**19**, 1; **21**, 71)

Catignani, G.L. *Department of Food Science, Southeast Dairy Foods Research Center, North Carolina State University, Raleigh, North Carolina* (**35**, 185)

Caul, J.F. *Flavor Laboratory, Arthur D. Little, Inc., Cambridge, Massachusetts* (**7**, 1)

Chandrasekaran, R. *Whistler Center for Carbohydrate Research, Purdue University, West Lafayette, Indiana* (**42**, 131)

Chang, S.F. *Department of Food Science and Technology, Pingtung Agricultural Institute, Pingtung, Taiwan, ROC* (**39**, 71)

Chang, S.S. *Department of Food Science, Rutgers, The State University, New Brunswick, New Jersey* (**18**, 1)

Charm, S.E. *Department of Nutrition, Food Science and Technology, Massachusetts Institute of Technology, Cambridge, Massachusetts* (**11**, 355)

Chen, C. *Department of Food Science and Human Nutrition, Michigan State University, East Lansing, Michigan* (**34**, 387)

Chichester, C.O. *Department of Food Technology, University of California, Berkeley, California* (**5**, 301)

Christensen, C.M. *Monell Chemical Senses Center, and School of Dental Medicine, University of Pennsylvania, Philadelphia, Pennsylvania* (**29**, 159)

Clifcorn, L.E. *Research Department, Continental Can Co., Chicago, Illinois* (**1**, 39)

Clifford, A.J. *Department of Nutrition, University of California, Davis, California* (**40**, 25)

Coburn, S.P. *Department of Biochemistry, Fort Wayne State Developmental Center, Fort Wayne, Indiana* (**40**, 107)

Combs, Jr., G.F. *Division of Nutritional Sciences, Cornell University, Ithaca, New York* (**32**, 85)

Cooney, C.L. *Department of Nutrition and Food Science, Massachusetts Institute of Technology, Cambridge, Massachusetts* (**26**, 1)

Cooper, C.C. *Muscle Biology Laboratory and Department of Meat and Animal Science, University of Wisconsin, Madison, Wisconsin* (**19**, 1)

Cooper, C.E.B. *Barnfields, Hathersage, Sheffield, England, UK* (**20**, 113)

Coulombe, Jr., R.A. *Graduate Program in Toxicology and Department of Veterinary Sciences, Utah State University, Logan, Utah* (**45**, 61)

Coulter, S.T. *Division of Dairy Husbandry, University of Minnesota, St. Paul, Minnesota* (**3**, 45)

Coupland, J.N. *Department of Food Science, Pennsylvania State University, 111 Borland Laboratory, University Park, Pennsylvania* (**45**, 101)

Crenshaw, T.D. *Departments of Nutritional Sciences and Meat and Animal Science, University of Wisconsin, Madison, Wisconsin* (**40**, 157)

Crosby, N.T. *Department of Industry, Laboratory of the Government Chemist, London, England, UK* (**22**, 1)

Cuppett, S.L. *Department of Food Science and Technology, University of Nebraska-Lincoln, Lincoln, Nebraska* (**42**, 245; **44**, 347)

Czyhrinciw, N. *Department of Chemistry and Technology, Faculty of Agronomy, University Central of Venezuela, Maracay, Venezuela* (**17**, 153)

Damodaran, S. *Department of Food Science, University of Wisconsin, Madison, Wisconsin* (**34**, 1)

Danehy, J.P. *Department of Chemistry, University of Notre Dame, Notre Dame, Indiana* (**3**, 241; **30**, 77)

Das, K.P. *Institute of Food Science, Cornell University, Ithaca, New York* (**34**, 81)

Daubert, B.F. *Koppers Company, Inc., Pittsburgh, Pennsylvania* (**4**, 185)

Davey, C.L. *Meat Industry Research Institute of New Zealand, Hamilton, New Zealand* (**21**, 157)

Davis, L.E. *College of Engineering, University of California, Berkeley, California* (**4**, 37)

Decareau, R.V. *Raytheon Company, Hooksett, New Hampshire* (**13**, 1)

Delaquis, A. *Nexia Biotechnologies, Inc., Ste. Anne de Bellevue, Quebec H9X 3V9, Canada* (**40**, 207)

Dewar, J. *CSIR, Pretoria, South Africa* (**43**, 217)

Dey, P.M. *Department of Biochemistry, Royal Holloway College, University of London, Egham Hill, Egham, Surrey TW20 0EX, England, UK* (**30**, 139)

Dormedy, E.S. *Department of Food Science and Technology, University of Nebraska-Lincoln, Lincoln, Nebraska* (**42**, 1)

Dueker, S.R. *Department of Nutrition, University of California, Davis, California* (**40**, 25)

Dunn, C.G. *Department of Food Technology, Massachusetts Institute of Technology, Cambridge, Massachusetts* (**2**, 117)

Du Pont, M.S. *AFRC Institute of Food Research, Norwich Laboratory, Colney Lane, Norwich, England, UK* (**31**, 117)

Ebert, D.M. *College of Agriculture and Life Sciences, Cornell University, Ithaca, New York* (**32**, 185)

Edwards, R.H.T. *Muscle Research Centre, Department of Medicine, University of Liverpool, Liverpool, United Kingdom* (**40**, 135)

Eikelenboom, G. *Research Institute for Animal Husbandry, "Schoonoord" Zeist, The Netherlands* (**21**, 71)

Elias, L.G. *Institute of Nutrition of Central America and Panama (INCAP), Guatemala, Central America* (**16**, 1)

Elliott, R.P. *Western Regional Research Laboratory, Western Utilization Research and Development Division, Agricultural Research Service, U.S. Department of Agriculture, Albany, California* (**13**, 349)

Evershed, R.P. *Department of Biochemistry, University of Liverpool, Liverpool, United Kingdom* (**40**, 135)

Farrer, K.T.H. *Research Laboratories, Kraft Foods Ltd., Melbourne, Australia* (**6**, 257)

Feeney, R.E. *Department of Food Science and Technology, University of California, Davis, California* (**10**, 23)

Felton, G.E. *Hawaiian Pineapple Company, Honolulu, Hawaii* (**2**, 1)

Fennema, O. *Department of Dairy and Food Industries, University of Wisconsin, Madison, Wisconsin* (**13**, 219)

Fevold, H.L. *Quartermaster Food and Container Institute for the Armed Forces, Chicago, Illinois* (**1**, 149)

Field, R.A. *Division of Animal Science, University of Wyoming, Laramie, Wyoming* (**27**, 23)

Fields, M.L. *Food Microbiology Research Laboratory, Department of Food Science and Nutrition, University of Missouri, Columbia, Missouri* (**16**, 161)

Fields, M.L. *Department of Food Science and Nutrition, University of Missouri, Columbia, Missouri* (**18**, 163)

Finke, M.D. *Departments of Nutritional Sciences and Meat and Animal Science, University of Wisconsin, Madison, Wisconsin* (**40**, 157)

Fitzhugh, O.G. *Division of Pharmacology, Food and Drug Administration, Federal Security Agency, Washington, DC* (**3**, 197)

Flannery, A. *Department of Biochemistry, University of Liverpool, Liverpool, United Kingdom* (**40**, 135)

Flick, G.J. *Department of Food Science and Technology, Virginia Polytechnic Institute and State University, Blacksburg, Virginia* (**39**, 329)

Flynn, A. *Department of Nutrition, University College, Cork, Ireland* (**36**, 209)

Foegeding, E.A. *Department of Food Science, North Carolina State University, Raleigh, North Carolina* (**34**, 203)

Fortlage, R.J. *Department of Pomology, University of California, Davis, California* (**15**, 147)

Fox, P.F. *Department of Food Chemistry, University College, Cork, Ireland* (**39**, 163)

Frank, J.F. *Center for Food Safety and Quality Enhancement, Department of Food Science and Technology, University of Georgia, Athens, Georgia* (**43**, 319)

Froning, G.W. *Department of Animal Science, University of Nebraska, Lincoln, Nebraska* (**27**, 109)

Fukazawa, T. *Department of Animal Science, Hokkaido University, Sapporo, Japan* (**19**, 279)

Furr, H.C. *Department of Nutritional Sciences, University of Connecticut, Storrs, Connecticut* (**40**, 25)

Gahl, M.J. *Farmland Industries, Inc., Kansas City, Kansas* (**40**, 157)

Gallander, J.F. *Department of Horticulture, The Ohio Agricultural Research and Development Center, Wooster, Ohio* (**25**, 1)

Garrow, T. *Department of Nutritional Studies, University of California, Berkeley, California* (**40**, 95)

Geddes, W.F. *Division of Agricultural Biochemistry, University of Minnesota, St. Paul, Minnesota* (**3**, 45)

Gehman, H. *Research Department, Chemical Division, Corn Products Refining Company, Argo, Illinois* (**5**, 53)

Gendel, S.M. *Biotechnology Studies Branch, Food and Drug Administration, National Center for Food Safety and Technology, Summit-Argo, Illinois* (**42**, 45, 63)

German, J.B. *Department of Food Science and Technology, University of California, Davis, Davis, California* (**37**, 259)

Gershwin, M.E. *Division of Rheumatology/Allergy and Clinical Immunology, University of California, Davis Medical School, Davis, California* (**37**, 259)

Gibbons, N.E. *Division of Applied Biology, National Research Council, Ottawa, Canada* (**4**, 1)

Glicksman, M. *Technical Center, General Foods Corporation, Tarrytown, New York* (**11**, 109; **12**, 283)

Goldblith, S.A. *Food Science, Massachusetts Institute of Technology, Cambridge, Massachusetts* (**3**, 119; **15**, 275; **27**, 1)

Goldstein, J.L. *Department of Nutritional Sciences, University of California, Berkeley, California* (**13**, 179)

Goodman, K.J. *Division of Nutritional Sciences, Cornell University, Ithaca, New York* (**40**, 55)

Gray, J.I. *Department of Food Science and Human Nutrition, Michigan State University, East Lansing, Michigan* (**29**, 1; **34**, 387)

Green, M.H. *Nutrition Department, Pennsylvania State University, University Park, Pennsylvania* (**40**, 3)

Gregory III, J.F. *Food Science and Human Nutrition Department, University of Florida, Gainesville, Florida* (**33**, 1; **40**, 81)

Greif, P.C. *Laboratory of Mathematical Biology, National Institutes of Helath, Bethesda, Maryland* (**40**, 281)

Guegov, Y. *Canning Research Institute, BG 4000 Plovdiv, Bulgaria* (**27**, 297)

Guinee, T.P. *National Dairy Products Research Center, Teagasc, Moorepark, Fermoy, Cork, Ireland* (**39**, 163)

Hadziyev, D. *Department of Food Science, University of Alberta, Edmonton, Alberta, Canada* (**25**, 55)

Haisman, D.R. *Unilever Research Laboratory, Colworth House, Bedford, Beds., England, UK* (**17**, 1)

Hales, K.C. *Shipowners Refrigerated Cargo Research Association, Cambridge, England, UK* (**12**, 147)

Halford, N.G. *IACR-Long Ashton Research Station, Department of Agriculture Sciences, University of Bristol, Long Ashton, Bristol, UK* (**45**, 219)

Hallagan, J.B. *International Association of Color Manufactures, Washington, DC* (**43**, 195)

Hall III, C.A. *Department of Food and Nutrition, North Dakota State University, Fargo, North Dakota* (**42**, 245)

Halvorson, H.O. *The Hormel Institute, University of Minnesota, Austin, Minnesota* (**3**, 291)

Hamm, R. *Bundesanstalt für Fleischforschung, Kulmbach, Germany* (**10**, 355; **24**, 1)

Hamouz, F. *Department of Nutritional Science and Dietetics, University of Nebraska-Lincoln, Lincoln, Nebraska* (**44**, 347)

Hanes, D. *Division of Rheumatology, Department of Medicine, Indiana University School of Medicine, Indianapolis, Indiana* (**40**, 149)

Hanson, H.L. *Western Regional Research Laboratory, Albany, California* (**2**, 219)

Haridas Rao, P. *Flour Milling and Baking Technology Discipline, Central Food Technological Research Institute, Mysore, India* (**23**, 187)

Harper, J.C. *Agricultural Engineering Department, University of California, Davis, California* (**7**, 171)

Harrington, W.0. *Western Utilization Research Branch, Agricultural Research Service, U.S. Department of Agriculture, Albany, California* (**6**, 231)

Hartwell, R.R. *General Research Laboratory, American Can Company, Maywood, Illinois* (**3**, 327)

Harwalkar, V.R. *Food Research Center, Agriculture Canada, Ottawa, Ontario, Canada* (**35**, 317)

Hathway, D.E. *Tunstall Laboratory, "Shell" Research Limited, Sittingbourne, Kent, England, UK* (**15**, 1)

Haughey, D.R. *Meat Industry Research Institute of New Zealand, Hamilton, New Zealand* (**21**, 157)

Hayakawa, K.-I. *Food Science Department, Cook College, Rutgers, The State University of New Jersey, New Brunswick, New Jersey* (**20**, 217; **23**, 75)

Heffron, J.J.A. *Department of Biochemistry, University College, Cork, Ireland* (**28**, 167)

Hendrich, S. *Department of Food Science and Human Nutrition, Iowa State University, 124 MacKay Hall, Ames, Iowa 50011-1120, USA* (**44**, 195)

Henrickson, R.L. *Oklahoma Agricultural Experiment Station, Oklahoma State University, Stillwater, Oklahoma* (**28**, 231)

Herz, K.O. *Wallerstein Laboratories, Staten Island, New York* (**18**, 1)

Higley, N.A. *International Flavors and Fragrances, Research and Development, Union Beach, New Jersey* (**30**, 1)

Hill, R.M. *Department of Biochemistry and Nutrition, College of Agriculture, University of Nebraska, Lincoln, Nebraska* (**10**, 23)

Hinshaw, W.R. *Biological Department, Chemical Corps, Camp Detrick, Frederick, Maryland* (**3**, 209)

Hobbs, G. *Ministry of Agriculture, Fisheries and Food, Torry Research Station, Aberdeen, Scotland, UK* (**22**, 135)

Hofmann, K. *Bundesanstalt für Fleischforschung, Kulmbach, Germany* (**24**, 1)

Hopkins, D.T. *Agricultural Nutritional Consultants, Inc., Cedar Rapids, Iowa* (**30**, 331)

Hopkins, P. *Department of Biochemistry and Applied Molecular Biology, UMIST, Manchester, United Kingdom* (**40**, 135)

Hotchkiss, J.H. *Institute of Food Science, Department of Food Science, Cornell University, Ithaca, New York* (**31**, 53)

Hou, G. *Wheat Marketing Center, Portland, Oregon* (**43**, 141)

Hsieh, R.J. *Campbell Institute for Research and Technology, Campbell Soup Company, Camden, New Jersey* (**33**, 233)

Hsu, J.-C. *Department of Nutritional Studies, University of California, Berkeley, California* (**40**, 95)

Huang, T.C. *Department of Food Science and Technology, Pingtung Agricultural Institute, Pingtung, Taiwan, ROC* (**39**, 71)

Hudson Arnold, S. *Institute of Marine Resources, Department of Food Science and Technology, University of California, Davis, California* (**24**, 113)

Hulme, A.C. *Ditton Laboratory, Department of Scientific and Industrial Research, Larkfield, England, UK* (**8**, 297)

Hyvönen, L. *Department of Food Chemistry and Technology, University of Helsinki, 00710 Helsinki 71, Finland* (**28**, 373)

Ibarz, A. *Food Technology, University of Lleida, Lleida, Spain* (**39**, 1)

Idson, B. *Julius Schmidt Inc., New York, New York* (**7**, 235)

Ikeda, K. *Faculty of Nutrition, Kobe Gakuin University, Nishi-ku, Kobe, Japan* (**44**, 395)

Jackson, D.S. *Department of Food Science and Technology, University of Nebraska–Linclon, Lincoln, Nebraska* (**38**, 271)

Jacquez, J.A. *Departments of Physiology and Biostatistics, University of Michigan, Ann Arbor, Michigan* (**40**, 305)

Jadhav, S.J. *Department of Food Science, University of Alberta, Edmonton, Alberta, Canada* (**21**, 307)

Janle, E.M. *Bioanalytical Systems, Inc., West Lafayette, Indiana* (**40**, 183)

Jennes, R. *Division of Dairy Husbandry, University of Minnesota, St. Paul, Minnesota* (**3**, 45)

Jennings, W.G. *Department of Food Science and Technology, University of California, Davis, California* (**14**, 325)

Jensen, E.T. *Milk and Food Program, U.S. Department of Health, Education and Welfare, Public Health Service, Washington, DC* (**10**, 135)

John, M.A. *Department of Biochemistry, University of the West Indies, Mona, Kingston 7, Jamaica* (**30**, 139)

Joslyn, M.A. *Department of Nutritional Sciences, University of California, Berkeley, California* (**3**, 1; **5**, 97; **10**, 1; **11**, 1; **13**, 179)

Kefford, J.F. *Division of Food Research, Commonwealth Scientific and Industrial Research Organization, North Ryde, New South Wales, Australia* (**9**, 285; **27**, 243)

Kelley, D.S. *Department of Consumer and Family Sciences, Western Kentucky University, Bowling Green, Kentucky 42101-3576* (**40**, 217)

Khadre, M.A. *Department of Food Science and Technology, The Ohio State University, 2015 Fyffee Road, Parker Hall, Columbus, OH* (**45**, 167)

Kilpatrick, P.W. *Western Utilization Research Branch, Agricultural Research Service, U.S. Department of Agriculture, Albany, California* (**6**, 313)

Kim, J.-G. *Department of Food Science and Technology, The Ohio State University, 2015 Fyffee Road, Parker Hall, Columbus, OH* (**45**, 167)

Kim, J.-S. *Department of Nutritional Studies, University of California, Berkeley, California* (**40**, 95)

King, R.B. *Center for Bioengineering, University of Washington, Seattle, Washington* (**40**, 243)

Kinsella, J.E. *Department of Food Science, College of Agricultural and Environmental Sciences, University of California, Davis, California* (**19**, 147; **33**, 233, 343; **34**, 81; **35**, 1, 237)

Kirchner, J.G. *United States Department of Agriculture, Laboratory of Fruit and Vegetable Chemistry, Pasadena, California* (**2**, 259)

Kiritsakis, A. *Technological Educational Institute, Thessaloniki, Greece* (**31**, 453)

Kissinger, P.T. *Bioanalytical Systems, Inc., West Lafayette, Indiana* (**40**, 183)

Koivistoinen, P. *Department of Food Chemistry and Technology, University of Helsinki, 00710 Helsinki 71, Finland* (**28**, 373)

Kokini, J.L. *Center for Advanced Foods, The State University of New Jersey, New Brunswick, New Jersey* (**39**, 1)

Kramer, A. *Department of Horticulture, College of Agriculture, University of Maryland, College Park, Maryland* (**9**, 153; **17**, 77)

Kristjánsson, M.M. *Marine Biotechnology Center, Technical University of Denmark, Lyngby, Denmark* (**35**, 237)

Krushnamurthy, S. *Central Food Technological Research Institute, Mysore, India* (**21**, 223)

Kumosinski, T.F. *Eastern Regional Research Center, Agricultural Research Service, U.S. Department of Agriculture, Philadelphia, Pennsylvania* (**34**, 299)

Laakkonen, E. *Institute of Meat Technology, University of Helsinki, Helsinki, Finland* (**20**, 257)

Lafiandra, D. *Dipartimento di Agrobiologica ed Agrochimica, Università degli Studi della Tuscia, Via San Camillo de Lellis, Viterbo, Italy* (**45**, 219)

Lampi, R.A. *Food Engineering Laboratory, U.S. Army Natick Research and Development Command, Natick, Massachusetts* (**23**, 305)

Law, N.H. *Meat Industry Research Institute of New Zealand, Hamilton, New Zealand* (**21**, 157)

Lee, F.A. *New York State Agricultural Experiment Station, Cornell University, Geneva, New York* (**8**, 63)

Lehman, A.J. *Division of Pharmacology, Food and Drug Administration, Federal Security Agency, Washington, DC* (**2**, 201; **3**, 197)

Lepkovsky, S. *Department of Poultry Husbandry, University of California, Berkeley, California* (**1**, 105; **21**, 1; **4**, 105)

Levine, H. *Nabisco, Fundamental Science Group, East Hanover, New Jersey* (**38**, 103)

Lewis, K.H. *Milk and Food Research Program, U.S. Department of Health, Education and Welfare, Public Health Service, Robert A. Taft Sanitary Engineering Center, Cincinnati, Ohio* (**10**, 135)

Leyland, D. *Department of Biochemistry, University of Liverpool, Liverpool, United Kingdom* (**40**, 135)

Lightbody, H.D. *Quartermaster Food and Container Institute for the Armed Forces, Chicago, Illinois* (**1**, 149)

Lin, B.-F. *Department of Nutritional Studies, University of California, Berkeley, California* (**40**, 95)

Locker, R.H. *Meat Industry Research Institute of New Zealand, Hamilton, New Zealand* (**21**, 157)

Love, J.D. *Food and Nutrition Department, Iowa State University, Ames, Iowa* (**23**, 1)

Lowe, B. *Iowa State College, Ames, Iowa* (**1**, 203)

Lowe, E. *Western Utilization Research Branch, Agricultural Research Service, U.S. Department of Agriculture, Albany, California* (**6**, 313)

Lowe, K. *Department of Nutritional Studies, University of California, Berkeley, California* (**40**, 95)

Lucas, C.D. *International Association of Color Manufactures, Washington, DC* (**43**, 195)

Luh, B.S. *Department of Food Science and Technology, University of California, Davis, California* (**29**, 279)

Lüthi, H. *Swiss Federal Agricultural Experiment Station, Wädenswil, Switzerland* (**9**, 221)

Lynch, L.J. *Commonwealth Scientific and Industrial Research Organization, Division of Food Preservation and Transport, Homebush, New South Wales, Autralia* (**9**, 61)

Ma, C.-Y. *Food Research Center, Agriculture Canada, Ottawa, Ontario, Canada* (**35**, 317)

Ma, L. *Biological Systems and Engineering, Washington State University, Pullman, Washington* (**39**, 1)

Mackinney, G. *Department of Food Technology, University of California, Berkeley, California* (**5**, 301)

MacRitchie, F. *CSIRO Division of Plant Industry, Grain Quality Research Laboratory, North Ryde, New South Wales, Australia* (**29**, 201; **36**, 1)

Mäkinen, K.K. *Department of Biochemistry and Biophysics, Texas A.&M. University, College Station, Texas* (**25**, 137)

Malo, C. *Membrane Transport Research Group, Department of Physiology, Faculty of Medicine, University of Montreal, Montreal, Quebec H3C 3J7, Canada* (**40**, 207)

Marangoni, A.G. *Department of Food Science, University of Guelph, Guelph, Ontario, Canada* (**44**, 33)

Markakis, P. *Department of Food Science and Human Nutrition, Michigan State University, East Lansing, Michigan* (**31**, 453)

Marple, D.N. *Department of Animal and Dairy Science, Auburn University, Auburn, Alabama* (**21**, 71)

Martin, Jr., R.A. *Hershey Foods Corporation, Technical Center, Hershey, Pennsylvania* (**31**, 211)

Martin, L.F. *Sugarcane Products Division, Southern Regional Research Laboratory, U.S. Department of Agriculture, New Orleans, Louisiana* (**6**, 1)

Martin, R.E. *National Fisheries Institute, Arlington, Virginia* (**39**, 329)

Mathew, A.G. *Central Food Technological Research Institute, Mysore, India* (**19**, 75)

Maxie, E.C. *University of California, Davis, California* (**15**, 103)

McCann, K.T. *Kellogg's Worthington Foods, Worthington, Ohio* (**44**, 1)

McFarren, E.F. *Milk and Food Research Program, U.S. Department of Health, Education and Welfare, Public Health Service, Robert A. Taft Sanitary Engineering Center, Cincinnati, Ohio* (**10**, 135)

McNabb, T. *Clinical Studies, NBC, School of Veterinary Medicine, University of Pennsylvania, Kennett Square, Pennsylvania* (**40**, 281)

McNamara, D.J. *Department of Nutrition and Food Science, University of Arizona, Tucson, Arizona* (**36**, 253)

McNeil, E. *University of Texas, Medical Branch, Department of Bacteriology, Galveston, Texas* (**3**, 209)

McSweeney, P.L.H. *Department of Food Chemistry, University College, Cork, Ireland* (**39**, 163)

Mercer, L.P. *Department of Nutrition and Food Science, University of Kentucky, Lexington, Kentucky* (**40**, 217)

Mercer, W.A. *Western Research Laboratory, National Canners Association, Berkeley, California* (**7**, 129)

Merson, R.L. *Department of Food Science and Technology, University of California, Davis, California* (**20**, 1)

Michelbacher, A.E. *Department of Entomology and Parasitology, University of California, Berkeley, California* (**4**, 281)

Michener, H.D. *Western Regional Research Laboratory, Western Utilization Research and Development Division, Agricultural Research Service, U.S. Department of Agriculture, Albany, California* (**13**, 349)

Miller, D.D. *Institute of Food Science, Cornell University, Ithaca, New York* (**33**, 103)

Milner, M. *Department of Flour and Feed Milling Industries, Kansas State College, Manhattan, Kansas* (**8**, 111)

Mitchell, E.L. *Scholle Corporation, Irvine, California* (**32**, 1)

Mitchell, G. *Department of Physiology, University of the Witwatersrand, Medical School, Johannesburg, South Africa* (**28**, 167)

Mitchell, R.S. *Commonwealth Scientific and Industrial Research Organization, Division of Food Preservation and Transport, Homebush, New South Wales, Autralia* (**9**, 61)

Morse, R.L.D. *Florida State University, Tallahassee, Florida* (**3**, 385)

Murphy, P.A. *Department of Food Science and Human Nutrition, Iowa State University, 2312 FSB, Ames, Iowa 50011-1161, USA* (**44**, 195)

Murrell, J. *Division of Rheumatology, Department of Medicine, Indiana University School of Medicine, Indianapolis, Indiana* (**40**, 149)

Naim, M. *Institute of Biochemistry, Food Science and Nutrition, Faculty of Agricultural, Food and Environmental Quality Sciences, The Hebrew University of Jerusalem, Rehovot, Israel* (**42**, 211)

Namiki, M. *Department of Food Science and Technology, Nagoya University, Nagoya, Japan* (**32**, 115)

Narine, S.S. *Department of Agricultural, Food and Nutritional Science, University of Alberta, Edmonton, Alberta, Canada* (**44**, 33)

Natarajan, K.R. *Department of Biochemistry, PSG College of Arts and Science, Coimbatore 641014, India* (**26**, 215)

Nelson, A.A. *Division of Pharmacology, Food and Drug Administration, Federal Security Agency, Washington, DC* (**3**, 197)

Nichols Hazelwood, R. *International Technology Corporation, 17461 Derian Ave., Irvine, California 92714 and University of California, Irvine University Extension Program in Toxic and Hazardous Materials, Irvine, California* (**31**, 1)

Nieman, C. *Central Institute for the Licorice Processing Industries, Amsterdam, The Netherlands* (**7**, 339)

Nottingham, P.M. *Meat Industry Research Institute of New Zealand, Hamilton, New Zealand* (**21**, 157)

Novotny, J.A. *Diet and Human Performance Laboratory, Beltsville Human Nutrition Research Center, U.S. Department of Agriculture, Beltville, Maryland* (**40**, 25)

O'Brien, N.M. *Department of Food Chemistry, University College, Cork, Ireland* (**39**, 163)

O'Connell, P.W. *Upjohn Company, Kalamazoo, Michigan* (**4**, 185)

O'Connor, T.P. *Department of Food Chemistry, University College, Cork, Ireland* (**39**, 163)

Ohlsson, T. *SIK – The Swedish Institute for Food and Biotechnology, Göteborg, Sweden* (**43**, 65)

Olley, J. *CSIRO Division of Food Research, Tasmanian Food Research Unit, Hobart, Tasmania* (**23**, 143)

Olson, R.L. *Western Utilization Research Branch, Agricultural Research Service, U.S. Department of Agriculture, Albany, California* (**6**, 231)

Ōnishi, H. *Noda Institute for Scientific Research, Noda-shi, Chibaken, Japan* (**12**, 51)

Orta-Ramirez, A. *Department of Food Science and Human Nutrition, Michigan State University, East Lansing, Michigan* (**44**, 147)

Osborne, C. *Department of Nutritional Studies, University of California, Berkeley, California* (**40**, 95)

Osman, E.M. *Department of Foods and Nutrition, Michigan State College, East Lansing, Michigan* (**5**, 53)

Ostle, B. *Montana State College, Bozeman, Montana* (**5**, 161)

O'Sullivan, S. *TEAGASC Dairy Products Research Centre, Moorepark, Fermoy, Cork, Ireland* (**42**, 93)

Ough, C.S. *Department of Viticulture and Enology, University of California, Davis, California* (**14**, 1)

Pangborn, R.M. *University of California, Davis, California* (**14**, 1)

Pariser, E.R. *The Massachusetts Institute of Technology, Cambridge, Massachusetts* (**20**, 189)

Parker, R.S. *Division of Nutritional Sciences, Cornell University, Ithaca, New York* (**33**, 157; **40**, 55)

Parpia, H.A.B. *Food and Agriculture Industries Service, Agricultural Services Division, Food and Agriculture Organization of the United Nations, Via Delle Terme Di Caracalla, Rome, Italy* (**19**, 75; **21**, 223)

Pearson, A.M. *Department of Food Science and Human Nutrition, Michigan State University, East Lansing, Michigan* (**23**, 1; **26**, 53; **29**, 1; **34**, 387)

Pearson, A.M. *Department of Animal Sciences, Oregon State University, Corvallis, Oregon* (**37**, 339; **39**, 71)

Pederson, C.S. *New York State Agricultural Experiment Station, Cornell University, Geneva, New York* (**10**, 233)

Pestka, J.J. *Department of Food Science and Human Nutrition, Michigan State University, East Lansing, Michigan* (**37**, 1)

Petrowski, G.E. *Carnation Research Laboratories, Van Nuys, California* (**22**, 309)

Phillippy, B.Q. *United States Department of Agriculture, Agricultural Research Service, Southern Regional Research Centre, New Orleans, Louisiana* (**45**, 1)

Phoenix, J. *Muscle Research Centre, Department of Medicine, University of Liverpool, United Kingdom* (**40**, 135)

Pigman, W.W. *University of Alabama, Medical-Dental Schools, Biochemistry Department, Birmingham, Alabama* (**3**, 241)

Pimentel, D. *College of Agriculture and Life Sciences, Cornell University, Ithaca, New York* (**32**, 185)

Pinkert, D.M. *Chemical Research Department, Hoffmann-LaRoche Inc., Nutley, New Jersey* (**18**, 219)

Pivarnik, L.F. *Department of Food Science and Nutrition, University of Rhode Island, Kingston, Rhode Island* (**38**, 1)

Pomeranz, Y. *U.S. Grain Marketing Research Center, Agricultural Research Service, U.S. Department of Agriculture, Manhattan, Kansas* (**16**, 335)

Pomeranz, Y. *National Barley and Malt Laboratory, United States Department of Agriculture, and Department of Agronomy, University of Wisconsin, Madison, Wisconsin* (**20**, 153)

Pomeranz, Y. *U.S. Grain Marketing Research Center, Agricultural Research Service, U.S. Department of Agriculture, Manhattan, Kansas* (**22**, 205)

Ponting, J.D. *Western Regional Research Laboratory, Bureau of Agricultural and Industrial Chemistry, U.S. Department of Agriculture, Albany, California* (**3**, 1)

Popineau, Y. *Institut National de la Recherche Agronomique, Centre de Recherches de Nantes, Laboratoire de Biochimie et de Technologie des Protéines, Nantes, France* (**45**, 219)

Potthast, K. *Institute of Chemistry and Physics, Federal Center for Meat Research, 8650 Kulmbach, Federal Republic of Germany* (**29**, 87)

Powrie, W.D. *Department of Dairy and Food Industries, University of Wisconsin, Madison, Wisconsin* (**13**, 219)

Preiss, J. *Department of Biochemistry, Michigan State University, East Lansing, Michigan* (**41**, 1, 13, 33, 43, 75, 89, 107, 115, 125, 139, 153, 163)

Proctor, B.E. *Department of Food Technology, Massachusetts Institute of Technology, Cambridge, Massachusetts* (**3**, 119)

Proulx, P. *Department of Biochemistry, Faculty of Medicine, University of Ottawa, Ottawa, Ontario K1H 8M5, Canada* (**40**, 197)

Pruthi, J.S. *Central Food Technological Research Institute, Mysore, India (Council of Scientific and Industrial Research, India)* (**12**, 203)

Ralls, J.W. *Research Foundation, National Canners Association, Berkeley, California* (**14**, 285)

Rand, A.G. *Department of Food Science and Nutrition, University of Rhode Island, Kingston, Rhode Island* (**38**, 1)

Rao, M.A. *Department of Food Science and Technology, Cornell University, Geneva, New York* (**32**, 39)

Rawles, D.D. *Department of Food Science and Technology, Virginia Polytechnic Institute and State University, Blacksburg, Virginia* (**39**, 329)

Reay, G.A. *Torry Research Station, Aberdeen, Scotland, UK* (**2**, 343)

Reddy, N.R. *Department of Food Science and Technology, Virginia Polytechnic Institute and State University, Blacksburg, Virginia* (**28**, 1)

Reynolds, T.M. *Division of Food Preservation, Commonwealth Scientific and Industrial Research Organization, North Ryde, New South Wales, Australia* (**12**, 1; **14**, 167)

Rha, C. *Department of Nutrition and Food Science, Massachusetts Institute of Technology, Cambridge, Massachusetts* (**26**, 1)

Rice, E.E. *Nutrition and Biochemistry Research Division, Research Laboratories, Swift and Company, Chicago, Illinois* (**4**, 233)

Rice, S.L. *Department of Horticulture, Food Sciences Institute, Purdue University, West Lafayette, Indiana* (**25**, 237)

Richmond, B.S. *Food Microbiology Research Laboratory, Department of Food Science and Nutrition, University of Missouri, Columbia, Missouri* (**16**, 161)

Roelofsen, P.A. *Laboratory of General and Technical Biology, Technical University, Delft, The Netherlands* (**8**, 225)

Romani, R.J. *Department of Pomology, University of California, Davis, California* (**15**, 57)

Ross, A.F. *Cornell University, Ithaca, New York* (**1**, 257)

Saffle, R.L. *Department of Food Science, University of Georgia, Athens, Georgia* (**16**, 105)

Saggin, R. *Department of Food Science, Pennsylvania State University, 111 Borland Laboratory, University Park, Pennsylvania* (**45**, 101)

Salunkhe, D.K. *Mahatma Phule Agricultural University, Rahuri, Maharashtra, India* (**21**, 307; **28**, 1)

Sanders, M.E. *Microbiology Consultant, Littleton, Colorado* (**37**, 67)

Sathe, S.K. *Department of Nutrition and Food Science, Muscle Biology Group, University of Arizona, Tucson, Arizona* (**28**, 1)

Sawyer, R. *Department of Industry, Laboratory of the Government Chemist, London, England, UK* (**22**, 1)

Sayegh, S.I. *Physics Department, Purdue University, Fort Wayne, Indiana* (**40**, 323)

Schafer, M.L. *Milk and Food Research Program, U.S. Department of Health, Education and Welfare, Public Health Service, Robert A. Taft Sanitary Engineering Center, Cincinnati, Ohio* (**10**, 135)

Schantz, E.J. *Chemistry Branch, Physical Science Division, U.S. Army Chemical Corps, Fort Detrick, Frederick, Maryland* (**10**, 135)

Scheuer, P.J. *Department of Chemistry, University of Hawaii, Honolulu, Hawaii* (**18**, 141)

Schiffman, S.S. *Department of Psychiatry, Duke University, Medical Center, Durham, NC* (**44**, 247)

Schnepf, M.I. *Department of Nutritional Science and Dietetics, University of Nebraska-Lincoln, Lincoln, Nebraska* (**43**, 1; **44**, 347)

Schormüller, J. *Institut für Lebensmittelchemie und Lebensmitteltechnologie der Technischen Universität, Berlin, Germany* (**16**, 231)

Schulz, A.R. *Department of Biochemistry and Molecular Biology, School of Medicine, Indiana University, Indianapolis, Indiana* (**40**, 227)

Schwab, K.A. *College of Agriculture and Life Sciences, Cornell University, Ithaca, New York* (**32**, 185)

Scott, K.C. *Food Science and Human Nutrition Department, University of Florida, Gainesville, Florida* (**40**, 81)

Scott, W.J. *Commonwealth Scientific and Industrial Research Organization, Division of Food Preservation and Transport, Homebush, New South Wales, Australia* (**7**, 83)

Scott Blair, G.W. *Physics Department, National Institute for Research in Dairying, University of Reading, England, UK* (**8**, 1)

Seltzer, E. *Continental Foods, Inc., Thomas J. Lipton, Inc., Hoboken, New Jersey* (**2**, 399)

Selvendran, R.R. *AFRC Institute of Food Research, Norwich Laboratory, Colney Lane, Norwich, England, UK* (**31**, 117)

Senecal, A.G. *U.S. Army Soldier Systems Command, Natick Research, Development, and Engineering Center, Natick, Massachusetts* (**38**, 1)

Settelmeyer, J.T. *Maxwell House Division, General Foods Corporation, Hoboken, New Jersey* (**2**, 399)

Sgarbieri, V.C. *Department of Food and Nutrition Planning, Faculty of Food and Agricultural Engineering, University of Campinas, Brazil* (**28**, 93)

Shandera, Jr., D.L. *Department of Food Science and Technology, University of Nebraska–Linclon, Lincoln, Nebraska* (**38**, 271)

Shane, B. *Department of Nutritional Studies, University of California, Berkeley, California* (**40**, 95)

Sheehan, D. *Department of Biochemistry, University College, Cork, Ireland* (**42**, 93)

Shenouda, S.Y.K. *General Foods Corporation, Technical Center, Tarrytown, New York* (**26**, 275)

Shewan, J.M. *Torry Research Station, Aberdeen, Scotland, UK* (**2**, 343)

Shewry, P.R. *IACR-Long Ashton Research Station, Department of Agriculture Sciences, University of Bristol, Long Ashton, Bristol, UK* (**45**, 219)

Shorland, F.B. *Department of Biochemistry, Victoria University of Wellington, Private Bag, Wellington, New Zealand* (**23**, 1)

Shurpalekar, S.R. *Flour Milling and Baking Technology Discipline, Central Food Technological Research Institute, Mysore, India* (**23**, 187)

Simcox, N.J. *College of Agriculture and Life Sciences, Cornell University, Ithaca, New York* (**32**, 185)

Singleton, V.L. *Department of Viticulture and Enology, University of California, Davis, California* (**27**, 149)

Sivak, M.N. *Department of Biochemistry, Michigan State University, East Lansing, Michigan* (**41**, 1, 13, 33, 43, 75, 89, 107, 115, 125, 139, 153, 163)

Skobeleva, N.I. *Bakh Institute of Biochemistry, USSR Academy of Sciences, Moscow, USSR* (**17**, 215)

Slade, L. *Nabisco, Fundamental Science Group, East Hanover, New Jersey* (**38**, 103)

Smith, D.M. *Department of Food Science and Toxicology, University of Idaho, Moscow, Idaho* (**44**, 147)

Smith, W.H. *Ditton Laboratory, Agricultural Research Council, Larkfield, England, UK* (**12**, 95)

Snyder, H.E. *Department of Food Technology, Iowa State University, Ames, Iowa* (**18**, 85)

Somers, G.F. *U.S. Plant, Soil and Nutrition Laboratory, Ithaca, New York* (**1**, 291)

Somers, I. *Western Research Laboratory, National Canners Association, Berkeley, California* (**7**, 129)

Sommer, N.F. *Department of Pomology, University of California, Davis, California* (**15**, 147)

Stadtman, E.R. *University of California, Berkeley, California* (**1**, 325)

Stahl, W.H. *McCormick and Company, Incorporated, Baltimore, Maryland* (**11**, 201)

Steele, L. *Department of Food Science, University of Alberta, Edmonton, Alberta, Canada* (**25**, 55)

Stevens, B.J.H. *AFRC Institute of Food Research, Norwich Laboratory, Colney Lane, Norwich, England, UK* (**31**, 117)

Stocking, C.R. *University of California, Davis, California* (**2**, 297)

Stone, H. *Stanford Research Institute, Menlo Park, California* (**14**, 1)

Streaker, C.B. *HJ Heinz Company, Pittsburgh, Pennsylvania* (**44**, 1)

Striem, B.J. *Institute of Biochemistry, Food Science and Nutrition, Faculty of Agricultural, Food and Environmental Quality Sciences, The Hebrew University of Jerusalem, Rehovot, Israel* (**42**, 211)

Stumbo, C.R. *Food Machinery and Chemical Corporation, San Jose, California* (**2**, 47)

Subramanyam, H. *Central Food Technological Research Institute, Mysore, India* (**21**, 223)

Swaisgood, H.E. *Department of Food Science, Southeast Dairy Foods Research Center, North Carolina State University, Raleigh, North Carolina* (**35**, 185)

Swanson, J.E. *Division of Nutritional Sciences, Cornell University, Ithaca, New York* (**40**, 55)

Szczesniak, A.S. *General Foods Corporation, Corporate Research Department Technical Center, Tarrytown, New York* (**14**, 33)

Tal, M. *Sigma Israel Chemicals, Rehovot, Israel* (**42**, 211)

Tanikawa, E. *Laboratory of Marine Food Technology, Faculty of Fisheries, Hokkaido University, Hakodate, Hokkaido, Japan* (**12**, 367)

Tannenbaum, S.R. *Department of Nutrition and Food Science, Massachusetts Institute of Technology, Cambridge, Massachusetts* (**26**, 1)

Tappel, A.L. *Food Technology Department, University of California, Davis, California* (**7**, 171)

Tatharn, A.S. *IACR-Long Ashton Research Station, Department of Agriculture Sciences, University of Bristol, Long Ashton, Bristol, UK* (**45**, 219)

Taylor, J.R.N. *Cereal Foods Research Unit, Department of Food Science, University of Pretoria, Pretoria, South Africa* (**43**, 217)

Taylor, S.L. *Department of Food Science and Technology, University of Nebraska-Lincoln, Lincoln, Nebraska* (**30**, 1; **42**, 1; **43**, 195)

Teel, W.S. *College of Agriculture and Life Sciences, Cornell University, Ithaca, New York* (**32**, 185)

Thijssen, H.A.C. *Eindhoven University of Technology, Eindhoven, The Netherlands* (**20**, 1)

Thrower, S.J. *CSIRO Division of Food Research, Tasmanian Food Research Unit, Hobart, Tasmania* (**23**, 143)

Tilgner, D.J. *Abrahama 1m., 3a, Sopot, Poland* (**19**, 215)

Tischer, R.G. *Iowa State College, Ames, Iowa* (**5**, 161)

Toescu, V. *Muscle Research Centre, Department of Medicine, University of Liverpool, United Kingdom* (**40**, 135)

Tomiyasu, Y. *Laboratory of Fisheries Chemistry, Kyushu University, Fukuoka, Japan* (**7**, 41)

Torgeson, K.W. *General Foods Corporation, Corporate Research Department Technical Center, Tarrytown, New York* (**14**, 33)

Tóth, L. *Institute of Food Chemistry, J.W. Goethe University, 8000 Frankfurt am Main, Federal Republic of Germany* (**29**, 87)

Tungland, B.C. *Imperial Census, Sugar Land, Texas* (**43**, 1)

Turner, J.D. *Nexia Biotechnologies, Inc., Ste. Anne de Bellevue, Quebec H9X 3V9, Canada* (**40**, 207)

Twigg, B.A. *University of Maryland, College Park, Maryland* (**9**, 153)

Ulrich, J.A. *The Hormel Institute, University of Minnesota, Austin, Minnesota* (**3**, 291)

Urbain, W.M. *10645 Welk Drive, Sun City, Arizona* (**24**, 155)

Utsumi, S. *Research Institute for Food Science, Kyoto University, Uji, Kyoto, Japan* (**36**, 89)

Van Arsdel, W.B. *Western Utilization Research Branch, Agricultural Research Service, U.S. Department of Agriculture, Albany, California* (**6**, 313)

van Veen, A.G. *University of Delft, The Netherlands Laboratory of Biochemistry* (**4**, 209)

Vaughn, R.H. *Department of Food Technology, University of California, Davis, California* (**6**, 67)

Voirol, F. *Xyrofin Ltd., 6340 Baar, Switzerland* (**28**, 373)

Von Schelhorn, M. *Institut für Lebensmitteltechnologie, Munich, Germany* (**3**, 429)

Wang, Y.-y. *Taiwan, 17 Li-Yuan, Miao-Li, Taiwan, ROC* (**40**, 55)

Wang, Z. *Wuxi Institute of Light Industry, Wuxi, Jiangsu 214004, China* (**29**, 279)

Warneke, A.F. *College of Agriculture and Life Sciences, Cornell University, Ithaca, New York* (**32**, 185)

Waslien, C.I. *Nutrition and Food Science Program, School of Health Sciences, Hunter College, City University of New York, New York, New York* (**32**, 239)

Watts, B.M. *Department of Food and Nutrition, Florida State University, Tallahassee, Florida* (**5**, 1)

Weier, T.E. *University of California, Davis, California* (**2**, 297)

Weisberg, S.M. *League for International Food Education, Washington, DC* (**22**, 187)

Weller, C.L. *Industrial Agricultural Products Center, University of Nebraska-Lincoln, Lincoln, Nebraska* (**44**, 347)

Whitaker, J.R. *Department of Food Science and Technology, University of California, Davis, California* (**22**, 73; **28**, 93; **9**, 1)

White, Jr., J.W. *Eastern Regional Research Center, Philadelphia, Pennsylvania* (**24**, 287)

Whitehead, D.M. *Institute of Food Science, Cornell University, Ithaca, New York* (**33**, 343)

Whitfield, F.B. *Division of Food Research, Commonwealth Scientific and Industrial Research Organization, North Ryde, New South Wales, Australia* (**27**, 243)

Wickremasinghe, R.L. *Tea Research Institute of Sri Lanka, St. Coombs, Talawakelle, Sri Lanka* (**24**, 229)

Wilcke, H.L. *Ralston Purina Company, St. Louis, Missouri* (**30**, 331)

Wong, W.W. *Department of Pediatrics, USDA/ARS Children's Nutrition Research Center, Baylor College of Medicine, Houston, Texas* (**40**, 171)

Woodard, G. *Division of Pharmacology, Food and Drug Administration, Federal Security Agency, Washington, DC* (**3**, 197)

Wu, Y. *The Wright Group, Airport Road 6428, P.O. Box 1365, Crowley, Lousiana* (**44**, 347)

Wyss, O. *University of Texas, Austin, Texas* (**1**, 373)

Yeom, H.W. *Department of Food Science and Technology, The Ohio State University, Columbus, Ohio* (**44**, 1)

Ylikahri, R. *Third Department of Medicine, University of Helsinki, Helsinki, Finland* (**25**, 159)

Yokotsuka, T. *Kikkoman Corporation, Noda-shi, Chiba-ken, Japan* (**10**, 75)

Yokotsuka, T. *Kikkoman Corporation, Noda-shi, Chiba-ken 278, Japan* (**30**, 195)

Young, R.B. *Department of Biological Sciences, University of Alabama in Huntsville, Huntsville, Alabama* (**37**, 339)

Yousef, A.E. *Department of Food Science and Technology, The Ohio State University, 2015 Fyffee Road, Parker Hall, Columbus, OH* (**45**, 167)

Zech, L.A. *Laboratory of Mathematical Biology, National Cancer Institute, and Molecular Disease Branch, National Heart, Lung, and Blood Institute, National Institutes of Health, Bethesda, Maryland* (**40**, 25, 149, 281)

Zenitani, B. *Department of Fisheries, Nagasaki University, Sasebo, Japan* (**7**, 41)

Zervakis, J. *Department of Psychiatry, Duke University, Medical Center, Durham, NC* (**44**, 247)

Zhang, H. *Department of Mathematical Sciences, Indiana University – Purdue University, Fort Wayne, Indiana, and Department of Biometry and Epidemiology, Medical University of South Carolina, Charleston, South Carolina* (**40**, 339)

Zhang, Q.H. *Department of Food Science and Technology, The Ohio State University, Columbus, Ohio* (**44**, 1)

Zhang, Z. *Department of Biometry and Epidemiology, Medical University of South Carolina, Charleston, South Carolina* (**40**, 339)

Cumulative Index, Volumes 1–45

a_W, *see* Water activity
Aaminaria degatata **16**, 74
Abalone **23**, 143–186
–, anatomy of **23**, 145–146
–, antiviral and antibiotic activity of **23**, 179
–, as food **23**, 146–147
–, brining of **23**, 170–171
–, by-products of **23**, 178–179
–, canning of **23**, 171–172
–, –, can liquor in **23**, 178
–, catching and handling of **23**, 166
–, chemical composition of **23**, 147–166
–, –, effects of size and season on **23**, 150–151
–, drying of **23**, 172–173
–, flavor of **23**, 174, 176–177
–, freezing of **23**, 168–170
–, gelatin and collagen in **23**, 175, 179
–, lipids of **23**, 160–162
–, names for **23**, 144
–, nucleotides of **23**, 157–160
–, odor and appearance of **23**, 177–178
–, physiology of, in air **23**, 166–168
–, pigments in **23**, 163–164
–, preservation of **23**, 168–173
–, proteins of **23**, 151–156
–, –, amino acids of **23**, 154, 155–157
–, –, properties **23**, 155
–, proximate analysis of **23**, 147–150
–, quality aspects of **23**, 174–178
–, research needs on **23**, 179
–, shell of **23**, 164, 178
–, spoilage of **23**, 164–165
–, statistics of catch of **23**, 145
–, sugar-containing compounds in **23**, 162–163
–, texture of **23**, 174
–, UV-absorbing compounds of **23**, 158
–, viscera of **23**, 178–179
–, volatile bases in **23**, 164–165
apABG, *see para*-Acetamidobenzoylglutamate
Abomasum, phospholipids in **23**, 36
Abrasion, in flexible-package leak studies **23**, 413
Abrus precatorius, glycyrrhizin and **7**, 343
Absorption (*see also* Membrane vesicle) **39**, 97–100
–, calcium, dietary requirements and **33**, 118–119
–, –, effects of complexation by ligands yielding soluble complexes **33**, 146–147
–, –, – of fiber and phytate **33**, 134–142
–, –, – of lactose, *see* Lactose effect
–, –, – of oxalic acid **33**, 142
–, –, – of protein and phosphate **33**, 143–144
–, –, – of supplements **33**, 144–147
–, –, from CCM **33**, 147
–, –, mechanisms **33**, 114–117
–, –, net absorption, calculation **33**, 121–122
–, –, net amount necessary to balance urinary losses **33**, 111
–, –, regulation **33**, 114–117
–, carbonyl **12**, 11–13
–, carcinogen risk assessment and **31**, 33, 34, 37
–, β-carotene **40**, 32, 41, 58–60, 69–70, 71
–, chocolate and, alkalization **31**, 247
–, –, cocoa bean chemistry **31**, 229
–, –, milk **31**, 255, 256
–, dietary fiber and **31**, 135, 163, 166–169
–, folates **40**, 82
–, –, age effects **33**, 68–69
–, –, altered gastrointestinal function and **33**, 67–68
–, –, conjugases and **33**, 55–56
–, –, deconjugation of dietary polyglutamyl folate **33**, 54–55
–, –, dietary components and **33**, 71–72
–, –, ethanol ingestion effects **33**, 69–70
–, –, folate-binding protein in jejunal brush border membrane **33**, 54
–, –, hepatic **33**, 54
–, –, pH dependence **33**, 53–54
–, –, pH effects **33**, 67
–, –, K_m transport values **33**, 53
–, meat mutagens **34**, 410–413
–, population kinetics **40**, 273
–, tocopherols, effects of gastric or intestinal destruction **33**, 169–170
–, –, efficiency **33**, 168–171
–, –, mechanism **33**, 168–171
–, –, via lymphatic system **33**, 168–169
Aburage **16**, 51
l-Acacatechin in cocoa **2**, 284
Acceptor molecules, effect on transgalactosylase activity **38**, 76–79
Accessory cells, in Peyer's patches **37**, 15
Accumulation, folate **40**, 101–104

Aceselfane-K, chocolate and **31**, 271
Acetaldehyde **17**, 18
–, in anaerobic metabolism **17**, 20
–, in apples **2**, 263
–, in coffee **2**, 281–282
–, in flavor deterioration **17**, 20–21
–, in frozen vegetables **17**, 5, 6
–, in oranges **2**, 264
–, in peaches **2**, 265
–, in pineapple **2**, 266–268
–, role in off-flavor development **17**, 5–6
Acetaldehyde sulfonate **5**, 108, 111
Acetals, shoyu flavor and **30**, 277–278
Acetamidation, protein stability **35**, 272–273
para-Acetamidobenzoylglutamate **40**, 86, 91
Acetate **16**, 265
–, acceleration of trimethylamine oxide reduction in fish by **2**, 370
–, chocolate and **31**, 325
Acetazolamide **44**, 302
–, for hyperkalemic periodic paralysis **37**, 386
Acetic acid **15**, 205; **16**, 185, 216
–, chocolate and **31**, 297, 324
–, –, processing **31**, 215, 216, 219, 220, 222, 223, 225
–, dietary fiber and **31**, 127, 130, 161, 180
–, effect of dilution on sourness **2**, 260
–, effect on saltiness **2**, 260
–, endogenous proteolytic enzymes and **31**, 401
–, esters, in carrot seed oil **2**, 271
–, fish spoilage and **7**, 43, 47–48, 61
–, in apples **2**, 262–263
–, in cocoa **2**, 283
–, in cocoa bean **8**, 239, 252
–, in coffee **2**, 279, 281–282
–, in grape waste **2**, 16
–, in molasses **2**, 277
–, in oranges **2**, 264
–, in peaches **2**, 265
–, in pineapple **2**, 268
–, in rye bread **2**, 276
–, in spoiling fish **2**, 370, 371
–, in strawberries **2**, 270
–, intestinal antibacterial activity **43**, 14, 15, 35
–, in wines **6**, 74, 76
–, microbial inhibition by **1**, 387
–, *N*-nitroso compounds and **31**, 68
–, olive oil and **31**, 459
Acetic esters of ethyl alcohol in strawberries **2**, 270
Acetobacter, acetylmethylcarbinol production in wines **5**, 381
–, 2,3-butylene glycol production in wines **5**, 381
–, heat destruction of **3**, 436
–, species in wine **6**, 92, 93
Acetobacter calcoaceticus **43**, 323
Acetoin flavor of vegetables **17**, 158
– of –, in food deterioration **17**, 20–21
Acetone **15**, 210
–, chocolate and **31**, 222–224, 279, 281
–, dietary fiber and **31**, 152, 159, 166
–, fat extraction by **3**, 52
–, in apples **2**, 263
–, in coffee **2**, 279, 281
–, in oranges **2**, 264
–, *N*-nitroso compounds and **31**, 60
–, solubility of DDT in **2**, 203
–, solution of quaternary ammonium compounds in **2**, 145
–, toxicity to man **2**, 212
–, treatment of protein by **3**, 51
Acetophenone, in strawberries **2**, 270
–, in tea **2**, 286
Acetylaminopolysaccharide, action of lysozyme on **1**, 377–378
Acetylation, dietary fiber and **31**, 130, 131
–, extent of in pectins **11**, 61
Acetyl-β-casein, diffusion rate to air–water interface **34**, 19
Acetylcholine, fish-spoilage and **7**, 50–51
–, in sauerkraut **10**, 269–270
Acetyl coenzyme A, in wheat germ **23**, 240
Acetylene **12**, 190
Acetylesterase, in wheat germ **23**, 241
N-Acetyl-β-D-gluocosaminidase as endpoint cooking temperature indicator **44**, 171
Acetyl groups, benzoic and salicylic acids, effects on oxidation of by micro-organisms **11**, 341–342
–, dietary fiber and **31**, 186, 187
–, in pectin **1**, 397–399
Acetylintermedine **45**, 72, 75
Acetyllycopsamine **45**, 72, 75
Acetylmethylcarbinol **16**, 195, 206, 212
Acetyl propionyl in coffee **2**, 281
2-Acetylpyrrole in Formosan black tea **2**, 288
Achras sapota, glycyrrhizin and **7**, 343
Achromobacter, effect of nitrites on **3**, 295
–, enzyme action in **2**, 369
–, growth rate of **7**, 101
–, in bacon **3**, 308, 309
–, influence of temperature on growth **2**, 359, 360

–, in fresh fish **2**, 305, 353, 354
–, in pork **3**, 293
–, trimethylamine oxide reduction by, in fish **2**, 369
Acid, action on sugars **14**, 227–230
–, aldosylamino **12**, 3
–, amino, decrease thiamine destruction **6**, 259
–, 6-amino-6-deoxy-5-hexulosonic **14**, 193–197
–, ascorbic, loss **6**, 301
–, aspartic **12**, 20
–, citric, in spoiled table wines **6**, 76
–, cleaners **14**, 348–350
–, fructoseamino **12**, 20, 22
–, galacturonic **6**, 27; **14**, 194–195
–, –, in pears **14**, 198–199
–, gluconic, in spoiled table wines **6**, 76
–, hydrosulfonic **14**, 246–248
–, hydroxy **14**, 302–303
–, in fruits **12**, 120–123
–, keto **14**, 301–302
–, ketoseamino **12**, 6–7, 9
–, lactic, formation of **6**, 71
–, –, from glycogen **6**, 123
–, –, in spoiled table wines **6**, 91
–, –, in wines **6**, 74
–, lauric, in candy production **6**, 32
–, –, replacement for cocoa butter **6**, 44
–, linoleic, in cocoa fat **6**, 39
–, malic, bacteria decomposition of **6**, 71
–, –, in wines **6**, 73
–, monochloracetic, in wines **6**, 100
–, nordihydroguaiaretic, antioxidant **6**, 13
–, oleic, elaidizing **6**, 44
–, –, in cocoa fat **6**, 39
–, pantothenic **12**, 243
–, propionic, bacteria capable of forming **6**, 81
–, –, in spoiled wines **6**, 74
–, sorbic **12**, 407–408
–, stearic, in cocoa fat **6**, 39
–, sulfonic **14**, 249–252
–, tartaric, in candy making **6**, 17
–, –, in table wines **6**, 72
–, uronic **14**, 198–199
–, –, and amines **14**, 192–199, 263–264
Acid-catalyzed decomposition, acyl hydroperoxides **33**, 278–280
Acid coagulation **39**, 165, 166
Acid-curd cheese **39**, 178–193
Acid detergent fiber, dietary fiber and **31**, 153, 180, 181
Acidex procedure, for wine deacidification **25**, 21
Acid gel formation **39**, 182–188
Acidic peptidase in wheat germ **23**, 241
Acidification **39**, 166, 174–177, 258
Acidity, changes in, in dry milk during storage **3**, 100
–, chocolate and, cocoa butter **31**, 278
–, –, conching **31**, 297
–, –, emulsifiers **31**, 282
–, –, milk **31**, 262
–, –, processing **31**, 215–217, 244, 246
–, dietary fiber and **31**, 137, 138, 141, 191
–, –, analysis **31**, 143, 148, 150, 151, 153
–, –, dicotyledonous plants **31**, 127, 130, 131, 133
–, –, intestinal bacteria **31**, 172, 175
–, –, properties **31**, 160, 164, 165
–, effect on bacterial resistance to heat **2**, 67
–, – on tin plate **3**, 337–340
–, endogenous proteolytic enzymes and, endopeptidases **31**, 360
–, –, meat technology **31**, 411
–, –, muscle physiology **31**, 372
–, –, proteinase activity **31**, 385, 386, 388
–, –, proteinase distribution **31**, 368
–, *N*-nitroso compounds and **31**, 59
–, of grapes and wines **25**, 3–10
–, olive oil and **31**, 460, 463, 473, 474
Acidolin **43**, 14
Acidophilin **43**, 14
Acidophilus milk, unfermented **37**, 86, 101
Acid phosphatase, activity, measurement **34**, 347
–, –, multivalent cation effect **34**, 348
–, –, salt extraction **34**, 346
–, cell wall isolation **34**, 345–346
–, concentration-dependent multivalent cation effects **34**, 349–350
–, EDTA treatment **34**, 346
–, function-linked binding **34**, 347
–, function-linked multivalent cation binding **34**, 354–357
–, in tea **24**, 235
–, multivalent cation, activity effect **34**, 348
–, –, combined effects **34**, 349–353
–, –, solubilized activity effects **34**, 353–354
–, test **44**, 170
–, –, endpoint cooking temperature indicator **44**, 172
–, variation with metal ions **34**, 344–357
Acids (*see also individual acids*) **17**, 177
–, age-related taste threshold **44**, 257, 259
–, contribution to meat flavor **18**, 52

Acids (*cont'd*)
–, fatty, formation in dried raw meat **11**, 303
–, fish preservation and **7**, 68
–, in citrus fruits **9**, 291–302, 307–309
–, in citrus peels **9**, 309–310
–, in fruits, effect of carbon dioxide **12**, 120–123
–, –, loss in apples **12**, 120–121
–, in honey **24**, 304–305
–, in soy sauce **10**, 83–87, 101–103
–, in tea **11**, 216–217
–, organic **14**, 229–230
–, –, in fruit juices **9**, 262–271
–, –, in passion fruits **12**, 238, 258
–, –, in tea **11**, 223–224; **17**, 243–244
–, –, use in milk beverage stabilizers **12**, 301
–, unsaturated, in off-flavor production **17**, 33
–, volatile, fish freshness and **7**, 61
Acinetobacter, attachment/detachment **43**, 332, 349
aCLs, *see* Antibodies, anti-cardiolipin
Acme spray dryer, operation of **2**, 422
Acorn starch, gelatinization temperature of **2**, 319
Acoustic impedance **45**, 117–118
Acoustic signal generator **45**, 122
Acquired immunodeficiency syndrome, gastrointestinal suppression **37**, 34
–, nutritional therapies for gastrointestinal disease **37**, 51–52
Acriflavin, inhibition of enzyme activity by **1**, 384
Acrylonitrile, chocolate and **31**, 318
Actin **9**, 4, 6, 11–12; **10**, 356–357, 389; **16**, 114; **19**, 294–300
–, F-actin **9**, 7
–, –, endogenous proteolytic enzymes and **31**, 398, 400
–, –, properties **19**, 299–300
–, F-actin, preparation of **19**, 337–343
–, endogenous proteolytic enzymes and, meat technology **31**, 394, 396, 399, 404, 407, 409, 410
–, extraction from muscle **1**, 8
–, globular (or G-actin) **9**, 7
–, isolation of **19**, 294–296
–, molecular properties and polymerization **19**, 296–299
–, molecular weight **9**, 7
–, muscle physiology **31**, 370, 371
–, myosin reaction with **19**, 300
–, polymerization of **9**, 7
–, relation to meat structure **1**, 208
–, salt effects **35**, 326
–, SH groups in **24**, 35–36
–, –, function **24**, 38–39
Actin–DNA cross-links, pyrrolizidine alkaloid antimitotic activity **45**, 90–91, 92
Actinidin, in kiwifruit, proteolytic activity **29**, 297–298
α-Actinin, endogenous proteolytic enzymes and **31**, 404, 407
–, preparation of **19**, 328–332
–, properties and structure of **19**, 306–308
Actinins, SH group role in **24**, 40
Actinomycetes, isolated from moldy cocoa beans **8**, 288
Action potential **40**, 331–332
Activation, lactase **38**, 41
–, transgalactosylase activity of lactases **38**, 82–83
Activation energies **17**, 38; **38**, 204–205
–, loss of lysine and glucose **35**, 196, 198
–, nonenzymatic browning **35**, 196–197
Activation enthalphy **17**, 38
Activation entropy **17**, 45
Active oxidation method, olive oil and **31**, 473
Actomyosin **9**, 8; **10**, 55–57, 357, 375, 376, 389, 392; **16**, 114; **19**, 300–306
–, electron microscopy of **19**, 303–306
–, endogenous proteolytic enzymes and **31**, 394, 396–398
–, enzymic and contractile activity **19**, 300–302
–, formation during rigor mortis **1**, 9
–, myofibrillar proteins **34**, 252–254
–, preparation of **19**, 345–348
–, relation to meat structure **1**, 208
–, SH group role in **24**, 39–40
–, thiol groups in **19**, 303
–, viscosity changes of **19**, 302–303
F-Actomyosin, endogenous proteolytic enzymes and **31**, 398
Acyclovir **44**, 300
Acylation, protein emulsifier modification **34**, 151–152
–, protein stability **35**, 270–271
–, whey protein modification by **33**, 418–419
Acyl coenzyme A, in wheat germ **23**, 240
Acyl composition, cardiolipin, diet effects **37**, 291–297
–, interorgan differences **37**, 291
–, interspecific differences **37**, 290
–, related factors **37**, 289
–, uniqueness **37**, 289–290
Acyl desaturases, relative activities **35**, 27–28

Acyl hydroperoxides, carbonyl compounds from, table **33**, 265
–, decomposition **33**, 270–273
–, products from homolytic thermal cleavage **33**, 272
–, volatile compounds from **33**, 273–275
Adams consistometer **32**, 48
Adaptation, water requirements and **7**, 110–111
Adaptive control **40**, 270
Addison's disease, Adrenal, glycyrrhizin and **7**, 357
–, licorice and **7**, 356–357
Additions **14**, 293–294
–, carbonyl **14**, 293–294
–, steric course **14**, 294
–, unsaturated bond **14**, 294–295
Additives, chemical **10**, 32, 65, 66–67; **13**, 288–289
Adenosine **44**, 303
Adenosine diphosphate, chelation **33**, 304–305
–, control of microsomal enzyme-associated lipid oxidation **33**, 306
–, formation during rigor mortis **1**, 5
Adenosine triphosphate (*see also* ATP) **17**, 18–20
–, breakdown in muscle **1**, 4–10
–, in phosphorylation of glucose **1**, 131
–, relation to meat structure **1**, 208
–, – to rigor in muscle **10**, 386–391, 422–423
Adenostyles alliariae (Alpendost) **45**, 76
Adenylic acid, action in muscle **1**, 4
Adenylyl cyclase cascade, involvement in sugar-taste transduction **42**, 219–223
Adherence, probiotic cultures in human intestine **37**, 74–77, 120
Adipose, *N*-nitroso compounds and **31**, 78, 80, 83
Adipose tissues (*see also* Depot fats), β-carotene **40**, 49, 61
–, food regulation **21**, 25–34
–, α-LNA conversion **35**, 74–75
–, microdialysis **40**, 194
–, tocopherol content **33**, 178–179
–, tocopherol mobilization and turnover **33**, 188
–, α-tocopherol release **33**, 188–189
ADP, endogenous proteolytic enzymes and **31**, 393, 410
ADP/ATP carrier protein, cardiolipin association **37**, 279–280
ADPGlc, *see* ADPglucose pyrophosphorylase
ADPglucose, synthesis, glycogen **41**, 125
–, –, pathway *in vivo* **41**, 34–37
–, –, role **41**, 39–40
ADPglucose pyrophosphorylase, amyloplasts **41**, 118–119
–, amyloplasts transport **41**, 119–120
–, antisense **41**, 129–130
–, cloning **41**, 59–68
–, cold storage and **41**, 136
–, genomic DNA **41**, 73–74
–, higher plant subunits **41**, 50–51
–, hydrophobic cluster analysis **41**, 68–72
–, localization **41**, 123–124, 143
–, regulation **41**, 46–47, 145–148
–, sink strength **41**, 136
–, structure-function **41**, 49–50
–, substrate binding sites **41**, 51–59
–, subunit structure **41**, 47–49
–, synthesis, pathway **41**, 43–46
–, –, regulation **41**, 131–134
–, –, role **41**, 35–38
–, transcription **41**, 72–73
Adrenalectomy, effect on rats **1**, 123
Adrenal hormones, and meat quality relationship **21**, 89–96
Adrenaline **13**, 150–152
–, and shock **13**, 144
Adrenals, vitamin A **40**, 9, 11
Adrenocortical cells, α-tocopherol binding sites **33**, 199
Adrenocorticotropin **21**, 89–90, 93
Adriamycin, cardiolipin association **37**, 287–288
Adsorbed macromolecules, structure at interface **34**, 93
Adsorption **39**, 99, 100
–, competitive, mixed emulsifier system **34**, 126–127
–, dietary fiber and **31**, 120, 142, 157, 159, 160, 163
–, diffusion-controlled, proteins **34**, 16–20
–, in food drying, aroma recovery in **20**, 34–51
–, in olfaction **14**, 20
–, proteins at fluid interfaces **34**, 1–2, 114–117
–, soil **14**, 394–396
–, water removal and **7**, 181
–, whey proteins **33**, 391–393
Aegilops cylindrica **45**, 228
Aerobacter, effect of nitrites on **3**, 295
–, enzyme action in **2**, 369
–, in fermentation **17**, 93
Aerobacter aerogenes, destruction of by X-rays **3**, 157

Aerobacter aerogenes (*cont'd*)
–, effect of lauryldimethylbenzylammonium chloride on **2**, 155
–, – of vanillic acid esters on **3**, 460
–, germicidal action of phemerol on **2**, 155
Aerobes, effect of pH on growth of **3**, 431
Aerobic bacteria in fresh fish **2**, 350, 353
– in –, cause of spoilage **2**, 369
Aerodynamics, nose **14**, 10
Aeromonas **43**, 323
Aerosol OT, action as surface-active agent **1**, 379
Aerosol OT-100, effect on tubercle bacilli **2**, 148
Affinity chromatography, polyglutamyl folates **33**, 38
Aflatoxins **16**, 33; **39**, 286–287; **45**, 198
–, B_1, aflatoxin B_1-like pyrazines produced by *Aspergillus sojae* X-1 **30**, 290–294
–, –, – by –, fluorescent compounds, identification **30**, 292
–, –, – by –, –, separation **30**, 294
–, –, – by –, nonfluorescent compounds, identification **30**, 293
–, –, – by –, –, separation **30**, 294
–, –, degradation by sulfiting agents **30**, 17
–, G_1, distinction from mold-produced compound G_3 **30**, 296
–, absence in shoyu preparation **30**, 287–289, 296–297
Africa, cheese **39**, 167
–, IM meat **39**, 79–80, 89
Aftertaste, flavor and **7**, 37
Agar, effect on germicidal activity of quarternary ammonium compounds **2**, 136
–, general properties **11**, 119–120
–, in bakery products **11**, 120–122
–, in beverages **11**, 123
–, in confectionery **11**, 122
–, in dairy products **11**, 123
–, in meat and fish products **11**, 122–123
–, in meringues **12**, 304
–, in miscellaneous foods **11**, 124
–, nutrient **12**, 60, 110
–, salt **12**, 60
–, viscosity **11**, 118
Agar-agar in inhibition of corrosion **3**, 342
Agar cup-plate test for germicidal action of quaternary ammonium compounds **2**, 161
Agarose, molecular shapes and interactions **42**, 184–185
Age **14**, 56
–, and food attitudes **32**, 246–250
–, and food preference **32**, 242, 253–254
–, and meal patterns **32**, 250–253
–, and senses of taste and smell **32**, 245–246
–, effects, calcium absorption **33**, 117–118
–, –, folate bioavailability **33**, 68–69
–, –, surface rheology of whey protein interfacial films **33**, 394
–, –, vitamin E status **33**, 190–191
–, effects on fat composition **23**, 32–33
Agene-treated flour, nutritional stress factor in **4**, 114
Agene treatment of flour **10**, 32
Ageusia (*see also* Taste perception) **44**, 249
–, elderly people **44**, 256
Agglomeration **38**, 209–210
Aggregation, protein digestibility **35**, 189
Aging **14**, 58
–, and meat quality **26**, 140–142
–, biochemistry of **26**, 140–141
–, bovine muscle **14**, 60
–, changes **31**, 395–403
–, chemical change **14**, 59–62
–, Δ^6-desaturase, regulation **35**, 46
–, effect of starch **12**, 418
–, effects on muscle function **37**, 368–369
–, endogenous proteolytic enzymes and **31**, 345, 394, 395, 412, 413
–, enzymology **31**, 403–411
–, fish sausage and ham **12**, 418–420
–, numbers of bacteria **12**, 419
–, of meat, artificial **9**, 37–46
–, –, effect on meat flavor **18**, 9–14
–, –, SH groups and **24**, 55–58
–, of post-mortem muscle **20**, 268–277
–, oxygen penetration of casing **12**, 420
–, research needs **37**, 407
–, technology of **26**, 141–142
–, temperature **12**, 418
Agitated processing **32**, 60–74
Agitators, power consumption of **11**, 424–425
Aglycones **17**, 29
–, in flavonols **17**, 227
–, specificity of transgalactosylase reaction **38**, 81
Agmatine, in putrid abalone **23**, 166
Agrobacterium tumefaciens **41**, 126
Agrobacterium tumefaciens-mediated transformation system **36**, 164
Agrobacterium tumefaciens transformation vector **45**, 254
Agroforestry **32**, 204, 205
AIDS, carcinogen risk assessment and **31**, 19, 44
–, *see* Acquired immunodeficiency syndrome
Air, entrained **14**, 416–417

–, occluded **14**, 417–419
–, removal of, from thermoprocessed-food packaging **23**, 369–375
Air broom for product accumulation control in spray dryer **2**, 493
Air classification, of wheat germ **23**, 201–204
Air density, effect on terminal velocity in spray-drying **2**, 465–467
Air drying, IM meat **39**, 102, 144
Air pollution **32**, 188, 223–224
–, carcinogen risk assessment and **31**, 38–41
Air–water interface **34**, 9–10
–, acetyl-β-casein diffusion rate **34**, 19
–, fatty acid and alkanol molecules **34**, 11–12
–, free energy of adsorption **34**, 10
–, methylene group adsorption **34**, 11
–, protein, adsorption **34**, 11–13
–, –, desorption **34**, 52
Alanine, acceleration of trimethylamine oxide reduction by **2**, 369
–, effect on dried egg **1**, 172
–, – on egg albumen **3**, 274
–, in browning reaction **32**, 123–126, 131–133
β-Alanine in relation to microbial inhibition **1**, 387
Alaskan butter-clam industry **10**, 136, 141–142, 145, 146, 163
Albacore **39**, 339
Albumen, gelatin clarification and **7**, 248
Albumin (*see also* Bovine serum albumin) **16**, 353
–, endogenous proteolytic enzymes and **31**, 362, 375
–, foaming of solutions **6**, 21
–, HMW, genetic control **36**, 35–36
–, –, wheat proteins **36**, 26–27
–, in candy production **6**, 20
–, modifications of sugar properties produced by **6**, 53
–, serum, blood proteins **34**, 259–260
–, wheat proteins **36**, 28
–, –, genetic control **36**, 36–37
Albuterol sulfate **44**, 301
Alcaptonuria **37**, 397
Alcohol dehydrogenase, in wheat germ **23**, 240
–, of tea **24**, 235–236
Alcoholic beverages, sulfite occurrence formation by yeast, control of **30**, 6–7
–, – by –, limitations **30**, 6
–, – by –, residual SO_2 **30**, 7
Alcoholic fermentation **17**, 196–199
Alcohol-insoluble residues (AIR), dietary fiber and, intestinal bacteria **31**, 175, 178, 183, 186
–, properties **31**, 160, 166
Alcoholism **40**, 84–85, 91
Alcohols, adsorption kinetics **34**, 30–31
–, as food preservatives **1**, 386, 388
–, carcinogen risk assessment and **31**, 17, 19, 22, 41
–, chocolate and **31**, 268, 269, 271, 297
–, concentration in wines **6**, 84
–, contribution to meat flavor **18**, 52–53
–, dietary fiber and **31**, 139
–, effect on fababean protein thermal characteristics **35**, 334
–, ethyl alcohol in wine **5**, 359
–, fat extraction from dry milk by **3**, 52
–, from fruits **17**, 94
–, from molasses **17**, 125
–, furfuryl, isolation from heated milk **3**, 99
–, gel rigidity, and **7**, 297
–, glycerol content of wines **5**, 376
–, glycerol in wines **5**, 372, 373
–, glycerol ratios in wines **5**, 378
–, higher alcohols in wines **5**, 367
–, in *Allium* **22**, 100–103
–, in California table wines **6**, 82
–, in fruit juices **9**, 259–262
–, in solution of CPCl **2**, 153
–, in soy sauce **10**, 82
–, in tea **2**, 286
–, in wines **5**, 358; **8**, 137, 145, 148
–, –, content **5**, 371
–, mechanism of formation **5**, 370
–, methyl alcohol **5**, 366
–, –, in wines **5**, 368
–, *N*-nitroso compounds and **31**, 56
–, –, fundamentals **31**, 61, 63
–, –, nitrite/nitrate addition **31**, 87
–, –, processing **31**, 91
–, olive oil and **31**, 466, 470, 477
–, percentage, in apple oil **2**, 264
–, –, in celery seed oil **2**, 271
–, –, in orange peel oil **2**, 264
–, production of **17**, 20–21, 93, 125, 126
–, –, in cocoa bean pulp **8**, 245
–, shoyu flavor and **30**, 265–266
–, source of alcohol in wines **5**, 367, 374
–, – of glycerol in wines **5**, 379
–, sulfated **14**, 352
–, tolerance by wine spoilage bacteria **6**, 91
–, treatment of dry-milk protein by **3**, 51
–, yield **5**, 364

Aldehydes, as food preservatives **1**, 386, 388–389
–, binding to unprocessed whey proteins **33**, 411
–, chocolate and **31**, 234, 235, 251, 266, 297
–, compound **12**, 296
–, formation **12**, 38–39
–, – in tea **11**, 220
–, formation of **17**, 240–241
–, from Maillard browning **18**, 63
–, in *Allium* **22**, 100–103
–, in dough during fermentation and baking **30**, 100–102
–, in smoke condensate, effect on color formation **29**, 137–139
–, in tea aroma **17**, 239
–, α-lactalbumin binding **33**, 415
–, *N*-nitroso compounds and **31**, 56
–, percentage, in apple oil **2**, 264
–, –, in bread **2**, 276
–, –, in cherries **2**, 264
–, –, in maple syrup **2**, 277
–, –, in parsley oil **2**, 274
–, shoyu flavor and **30**, 267–268
Aldesleukin **44**, 293
Aldolase, as endpoint cooking temperature indicator **44**, 171
–, in wheat germ **23**, 241
Aldosamines **14**, 207–208
Aldoses, and amines **14**, 262–263
–, and proteins **14**, 211–221
–, browning reactions with amines, Amadori rearrangement **30**, 82, 87–88
–, – with –, glycosamine formation **30**, 87
Aldosylamines **12**, 3–5; **14**, 169–177
Aleurone concentrate **17**, 115
Aleurone layer, analysis **31**, 150
–, dietary fiber and **31**, 190
–, intestinal bacteria **31**, 183, 189
–, monocotyledonous plants **31**, 136, 137
Aleutian disease **37**, 399–400
Alfalfa, dehydrated, palatability of **1**, 124
–, dietary fiber and **31**, 170, 171
–, nutritional stress factor in **4**, 110, 112–113
–, phosphorus content of, effect of fertilizers on **1**, 313
Alfalfa phytoestrogens **44**, 197, 203
–, coumestans **44**, 211
–, isoflavones **44**, 203, 207
Alfalfa sprouts, ozone treatment **45**, 196
Algae **16**, 16, 24, 73
–, amino acid composition of **18**, 109
–, as feed additives **30**, 345
–, as sources of protein **18**, 116–128
–, carotenoids in **15**, 208
–, nutritional value **18**, 124–128
–, poisonous **10**, 137
–, propagation conditions **18**, 118–124
–, toxicity of **18**, 124–125, 157
–, useful species for **18**, 117–118
Algin, immobilization of lactases **38**, 43
Alginate gels, ultrasonic analysis **45**, 152
Alginates, general applications in foods **11**, 138–139
–, in artificial cherries **11**, 156
–, in bakery toppings and fillings **11**, 151
–, in beverages **11**, 152–154
–, in canned fish **11**, 149
–, in chocolate milk **11**, 147
–, in confectionery **11**, 154
–, in dairy products **11**, 147
–, in dessert gels **11**, 139–144
–, in dietetic foods **11**, 154
–, in dough products **11**, 155
–, in fining beer **11**, 153
–, in fish and meat preservation **11**, 148–150
–, in frozen fish **11**, 148
–, in fruit drinks **11**, 152
–, in guacamole spread **11**, 156
–, in ice cream stabilization **11**, 145
–, in icings and toppings **11**, 151
–, in jellies and pie fillings **11**, 152
–, in macaroni and spaghetti **11**, 157
–, in meat-like items **11**, 153
–, in milk puddings **11**, 144–145
–, in miscellaneous foods **11**, 153, 157
–, in processed cheese **11**, 147
–, in salad dressing **11**, 154
–, in synthetic potato chips **11**, 155
–, in synthetic sausage casings **11**, 150
–, in water ices and sherbets **11**, 147
–, in whipped cream **11**, 147
–, in wine clarification **11**, 153
–, on meats as a preservative **11**, 149
–, specialized food applications **11**, 155–157
–, typical food applications **11**, 140–141
–, viscosity **11**, 118
Alginic acid, molecular shapes and interactions **42**, 172–175
Alicyclobacillus acidocaldarius **45**, 197
Alien genes, incorporation, in wheat proteins **36**, 70–73
Alimentary absorption **15**, 9
–, micellar formation in **15**, 32
Alipal **16**, 119
Aliphatic amino acids, thermal stability role **35**, 258–259, 261
Aliphatic indices, proteins **35**, 258, 260

Alkalies, in sugar **14**, 230
–, mild **14**, 348
–, strong **14**, 347–348
Alkaline proteases, endogenous proteolytic enzymes and **31**, 353–355, 388–391, 410, 411
Alkalinity, endogenous proteolytic enzymes and **31**, 367, 385, 411
Alkalization, chocolate and **31**, 213, 246–249, 307, 330
Alkaloids, in tea **17**, 234–236
Alkanes, ultrasonic phase transition monitoring **45**, 141
Alkanols, abnormalities in apparent diffusion coefficient **34**, 29
Alkenyldemethylethylammonium bromide, inhibitor of **2**, 166
Alkylamines **14**, 203–204
–, reaction with dehydroascorbic acid **32**, 146
Alkylarylpyridinium chloride, inhibitors of **2**, 166
Alkylation, endogenous proteolytic enzymes and **31**, 382
–, *N*-nitroso compounds and **31**, 55
–, reductive, protein emulsifier modification **34**, 158
Alkyl chain, length effect of ester group **34**, 153
Alkylcyclopentadiones, shoyu flavor and **30**, 277–278
Alkylcysteines, in *Allium* **22**, 77
–, –, biosynthesis **22**, 85–89
Alkylcysteine sulfoxides, in *Allium* **22**, 77–79
–, –, biosynthesis **22**, 85–89
Alkyldimethylbenzylammonium chloride, chemical structure of **2**, 120, 124, 126, 146–147
–, effect of blood serum on germicidal action of **2**, 148, 183
–, – of pH on germicidal activity of **2**, 133, 147–149
–, – of temperature on germicidal activity of **2**, 135, 136
–, effect on bacterial count of milk **2**, 178
–, inactivator of tetanus toxin **2**, 183
–, inhibitors of **2**, 166
–, tests for **2**, 168
–, tests for toxicity of **2**, 130
–, use as rinse for dishes **2**, 179
–, use in dairy industry **2**, 176
Alkyldimethyl 3,4-dichlorobenzylammonium chlorides, corrosive effect of **2**, 175
–, germicidal action of **2**, 149
–, structure of **2**, 120, 149
Alkyl nitrites, *N*-nitroso compounds and **31**, 61
Alkylperoxy radicals **15**, 3
Alkylphenols, formation during shoyu production **30**, 278–279
Alkyl sulfates, abnormalities in apparent diffusion coefficient **34**, 29
Alkyltrimethylammonium bromide, structure of **2**, 122
Alkyltrimethylammonium chloride, structure of **2**, 122
Allantoin, determination by ion exchanges **2**, 38
Allergenicity, proteins, *see* Amino acid sequence alignments, allergenicity potential assessment
Allergens **41**, 32
–, detection and avoidance **37**, 46
–, food, characterization and identification **37**, 40–42
–, research needs **37**, 54
Allergies, food, *see* Food allergies *and* Food intolerance
Allicin **44**, 321
–, as major flavor component in garlic **22**, 94, 95
–, in garlic oil **2**, 272
–, isolation of, from garlic **22**, 74
–, structure of **22**, 91
Alliin, discovery of **22**, 90
Alliinase, discovery of **22**, 74, 91
–, enzymatic activity **22**, 92, 93, 99, 121–122
–, in flavor development **22**, 118–122
–, substrates for **22**, 120
Alliin in garlic oil **2**, 272
Allium, alcohols and aldehydes in **22**, 100–103
–, alkylcysteines in **22**, 77
–, alkylcysteine sulfoxides in **22**, 77–79
–, –, biosynthesis **22**, 90
–, alliinase in, role in flavor development **22**, 118–122
–, glutamyl peptidases in, role in flavor development **22**, 122–123
–, γ-glutamyl peptides in **22**, 79–83
–, pungency, flavor and aroma of **22**, 73–133
–, –, –, enzyme role in **22**, 116–124
–, –, –, measurement **22**, 114–116
–, –, –, research needs on **22**, 125–126
–, sulfur compounds in **22**, 74–83
–, –, biosynthesis **22**, 83–90
–, –, in crushed *Allium* **22**, 90–114
Allium scorodoprasum L. constituents of volatile oil **2**, 273

Allolactose, in yogurts **38**, 84
–, production, *Kluyveromyces lactis* β-galactosidase velocity **38**, 65, 70
–, –, potassium and magnesium effects **38**, 82
Allopurinol **44**, 314
S-Allyl-L-cysteine sulfoxide, as odor-principle in garlic **22**, 91
Allyl-propyl disulfide in garlic **2**, 272
Allyl sulfide, in garlic **2**, 272
–, in onion oil **2**, 273
Allylthiocyanate in onion oil **2**, 273
Almond paste, in candies **6**, 45
Almonds **16**, 16
–, composition of **6**, 46
–, leuco-anthocyanins **5**, 288
–, used by the candy industry **6**, 3
Alpendost (*Adenostyles alliariae*) **45**, 76
–, α-gliadins **45**, 222
–, α-trinositol (inositol(1,2,6)trisphosphate) **45**, 28, 40
Alpha hydroysulfonic acid **5**, 104
–, combined with glucose **5**, 110
Alpha radiation **15**, 71
Alprazolam **44**, 310
Alternaria citri **15**, 177
–, germination of **7**, 95
Aluminosilicates, gel type of **2**, 4
–, structure of **2**, 3
Aluminum, effect on low-ester pectins **1**, 414
–, in prevention of corrosion **3**, 343
–, – of –, oxide with coffee infusion **3**, 178, 180
–, in wines **8**, 138, 139, 172
–, salts, effect on pectin viscosity **1**, 406
–, –, gelatin clarification and **7**, 248
–, –, use in pectin extraction **1**, 400, 405
–, use in spray dryers **2**, 490
Aluminum–inositol phosphate interactions **45**, 32, 36
Alzheimer's disease, smell/taste perception changes **44**, 280–282
Amadori, products **12**, 5–11, 17
–, –, from simple alkylamines **12**, 7
–, –, open chain form **12**, 11
–, –, ring form **12**, 10
–, rearrangement **12**, 4–6, 15–16
–, –, nonaromatic amines **12**, 5
–, –, primary aromatic amines **12**, 5
Amadori compounds **35**, 190–191, 194
–, shoyu oxidative browning during storage and **30**, 254–255
Amadori rearrangement **14**, 193–197, 261; **32**, 120, 121, 122–123, 126, 132–137
Amberlite IR-1, cation exchanger **2**, 5
Amberlite IR-4, adsorption of acidic amino acid by **2**, 34
–, biological tests on **2**, 32
–, saturation by hydrogen sulfide **2**, 38
–, use in grape industry **2**, 16
Amberlite IR-100, removal of calcium from milk by **2**, 24
–, use in grape industry **2**, 16
Amberlite IRC-50, use in fractionating basic amino acids **2**, 35
Amberlite XE-43, biological tests on **2**, 32
Amebicides, taste sensation effects **44**, 286
Amelioration, wine deacidification by **25**, 13–16
American Cancer Society, carcinogen risk assessment and **31**, 13, 39
American Can Company Research Department **32**, 3
Americas, cheese **39**, 167
–, IM meat **39**, 80–83
Ames test **32**, 156
–, 2-amino-3,4-dimethylimidazo[4,5-*f*]-quinoline **34**, 406
–, carcinogen risk assessment and **31**, 28
Amidation, whey protein modification by **33**, 419–420
Amide bond, endogenous proteolytic enzymes and **31**, 344
Amide nitrogen in fruit products, relation to browning **1**, 352
Amides, fundamentals **31**, 58–60, 66
–, indirect contamination **31**, 95
–, in flour gluten, effect on baking **29**, 265–267
–, in tea **11**, 218–219
–, nitrite/nitrate addition **31**, 76
–, *N*-nitroso compounds and **31**, 97
–, sulfonated **14**, 353
Amiloride **44**, 303
–, sweet-taste transduction **42**, 229–230
Amine formation in spoiling fish **2**, 368, 370
Amine oxidase, fish spoilage and **7**, 47
Amines **16**, 246, 278
–, and aldoses **14**, 169–192
–, and uronic acids **14**, 192–199
–, aromatic **14**, 202
–, as nitrosamine precursors **22**, 11–12
–, biogenic (*see also* Biogenic amines), meat mutagen modulation **34**, 433
–, chocolate and **31**, 234
–, fish spoilage and **7**, 43, 46–47
–, D-glucuronolactone **14**, 197–198
–, keloses **14**, 199–210
–, –, products **14**, 202–207

–, *N*-nitroso compounds and **31**, 54, 55, 97
–, –, fundamentals **31**, 59, 60, 62, 66
–, –, indirect contamination **31**, 94, 95
–, –, nitrite/nitrate addition **31**, 78, 82, 83, 87
–, –, processing **31**, 89–91, 93
–, *N*-oxides **14**, 304
–, primary **14**, 179–180
–, properties as anion exchangers **2**, 7–8
–, secondary **14**, 181–183, 206–207
Amino acid composition, effect on functional properties of whey proteins **33**, 367
–, of abalone **23**, 154–157
–, of foodstuffs **4**, 241
–, –, imbalance as stress factor **4**, 119
–, whey proteins from bovine milk, table **33**, 350
Amino acids (*see also* Biogenic amines) **12**, 3–4, 6, 39; **14**, 309–310
–, addition to dough, aroma and **30**, 101–102
–, adsorption by ion exchangers **2**, 34
–, age-related taste thresholds **44**, 257, 260
–, alkaline deamination of **3**, 253–254
–, analysis, reactive lysine measurement **35**, 193–194
–, and ketoses **14**, 204–206
–, apolar, effect on whey protein gels **33**, 389
–, as feed additives **30**, 344–345
–, availability decrease in Maillard reaction **30**, 121
–, browning reactions **32**, 119–150, 168
–, – with sugars **30**, 89
–, – with –, volatiles and aromas **30**, 91, 92–93
–, cereal enrichment by **30**, 355
–, cheese **39**, 227, 231–234
–, chocolate and, cocoa bean chemistry **31**, 226, 231–233, 235, 236
–, –, conching **31**, 297, 298
–, –, milk **31**, 263
–, –, milk crumb **31**, 286
–, –, processing **31**, 223, 224, 238, 239
–, –, sweeteners **31**, 269
–, –, *Theobroma cacao* L. **31**, 327
–, citric, in roasted cocoa **8**, 260
–, close packing **35**, 265
–, containing selenium **32**, 88–89
–, contribution to meat flavor **18**, 40–42
–, dietary fiber and **31**, 167, 186
–, digestibility **35**, 212
–, dose–response **40**, 157–160, 162–166
–, effect of cathode rays on **3**, 167–174
–, effect on browning in dehydrated potatoes **1**, 262, 273–275, 277–278, 285
–, – on egg white **3**, 273–274
–, endogenous proteolytic enzymes and **31**, 344, 412
–, endopeptidases **31**, 354, 355, 357, 360, 361
–, essential **17**, 102–103
–, –, racemization and cross-linking **35**, 208
–, essentiality in diet of rat **4**, 239
–, exchanges, mesophilic and thermophilic proteins **35**, 259, 261
–, exopeptidases **31**, 347, 348
–, fatty, in unroasted cocoa **8**, 279
–, fish **39**, 336–346
–, flavors from products of sugar reactions with **19**, 197
–, free **12**, 267–268; **14**, 122
–, – in cocoa beans, fermentation and **30**, 94, 95
–, – in –, roasting and **30**, 95, 96–97
–, gelatin and **7**, 261–265
–, gelatin manufacture and **7**, 240–241
–, hydration capacity **28**, 290–293
–, hydrophilicity/hydrophobicity **42**, 100–102
–, IM meat **39**, 136–137
–, in apple leaves **8**, 370
–, in apples **8**, 300, 303
–, in cereals **16**, 8
–, in cheese **16**, 233, 240, 259, 303
–, in cocoa cotyledons **8**, 263
–, in corn by-products **17**, 118
–, in fruits **17**, 183
–, in honey **24**, 308–312
–, in legumes **16**, 9
–, in milk powders **3**, 64
–, –, flavor related to **19**, 195–197
–, in nuts **16**, 16
–, in oilseed proteins **30**, 360, 361–362, 363
–, in oil seeds **16**, 13
–, in palm kernels **16**, 16
–, in peanuts **16**, 52
–, in pears **8**, 300
–, in peas, loss in processing **9**, 71
–, –, relation to maturity **9**, 70–71
–, in plants, winter hardiness and **25**, 205–206
–, in potatoes **10**, 191–192
–, in soybeans **16**, 44
–, in soy sauce **10**, 79, 80–81
–, in tea **11**, 218–219; **17**, 236–241
–, in wheat flour **16**, 346, 359ff, 395
–, in wheat germ **23**, 203, 216–220
–, meat technology **31**, 410
–, metabolism, enzymes of **17**, 22–23
–, microwave effects **43**, 92
–, muscle physiology **31**, 372, 374, 375, 377, 378, 382

Amino acids (*cont'd*)
–, neutral **12**, 6
–, *N*-nitroso compounds and **31**, 55
–, of tea **24**, 240–241
–, organic, in apples and pears **8**, 300, 320, 322
–, oxalic, in roasted cocoa **8**, 260
–, oxidation of **17**, 29, 31
–, polygalacturonic, in apples **8**, 336
–, preferential hydration of proteins **35**, 293
–, primary sequences of β-lactoglobulin B **33**, 351
–, products of **19**, 200
–, proteinase activity **31**, 385–387, 389, 391
–, protein quality improvement **40**, 161–162
–, protein stability, composition **35**, 266–269
–, protein value, relation to **16**, 25, 34
–, *o*-quinone complexing with, in enzymic browning **19**, 98–102
–, reactions with dehydroascorbic acid **32**, 143–146
–, – with sulfites **30**, 23–24
–, reaction with aldehyde groups **3**, 97
–, – with fructose **3**, 249
–, – with glucose **3**, 249, 265
–, – with *N*-glycosyl **3**, 262
–, – with maltose **3**, 249
–, – with sugar **3**, 246
–, relative radio sensitivities of **3**, 175
–, residues **14**, 213–215
–, –, racemization and cross-linking reactions **35**, 201–202
–, sequence alignments, algorithms **42**, 46
–, –, allergenicity potential **42**, 64–65
–, –, assessment **42**, 45–91
–, –, BLAST, with transgene proteins **42**, 56–57, 59
–, –, databases **42**, 47–48, 59, 63–91
–, –, –, food allergen sequences **42**, 69–74
–, –, –, nonfood allergen sequences **42**, 75–84
–, –, –, number of accessions **42**, 67
–, –, –, summary **42**, 88
–, –, –, wheat gluten sequences **42**, 85–87
–, –, extending local alignments **42**, 57–59
–, –, FASTA **42**, 50, 52–53, 59–60
–, –, –, with transgene proteins **42**, 53–56
–, –, methods **42**, 47–50, 65–67
–, –, Needleman and Wunsch algorithm **42**, 50–51
–, –, –, positive control sequence construction **42**, 48
–, side chains, inductive constants **35**, 202–203
–, Strecker degradation of mechanism **19**, 199
–, substitution **40**, 150
–, sulfur-containing in flour gluten, effect on baking **29**, 267–268
–, thermal conversion to flavor compounds **19**, 201
–, transgene test sequences **42**, 48–50
–, uronic, from pectin **8**, 233
α-Amino acids, *N*-nitroso compounds and **31**, 76
Amino acid sequences, dystrophin gene **37**, 357
β-Aminobenzoic acid content of canned pineapple **1**, 82
para-Aminobenzoylglutamate **40**, 86, 91
γ-Aminobutyric acid, agonist and uptake blockers, for epilepsy **37**, 372
2-Amino-3,4-dimethylimidazo[4,5-*f*]quinoline **32**, 158, 159–161, 169; **34**, 400, 402–403
–, absorption and excretion **34**, 412
–, toxicology **34**, 405–408
2-Amino-3,8-dimethylimidazo[4,5-*f*]-quinoxaline, formation **34**, 416
–, toxicology **34**, 405–408
Amino groups, acylation, protein emulsifiers **34**, 151
2-Amino-3-methylimidazo[4,5-*f*]quinoline **32**, 158, 159–161, 169; **34**, 400, 402
–, absorption and excretion **34**, 412
–, fat content and formation **34**, 419
–, formation **34**, 416
–, toxicology **34**, 405–408
2-Amino-3-methylimidazo[4,5-*f*]quinoxaline **34**, 402–403
2-Amino-1-methyl-6-phenylimidazo[4,5-*b*]-pyridine **34**, 402–403
Amino nitrogen, content, in soy sauce **10**, 79
–, fish spoilage and **7**, 49
–, in browning reaction **3**, 103
–, –, decrease in **3**, 104
–, in fruit products, changes during browning **1**, 351–353
Aminopeptidases, endogenous proteolytic enzymes and **31**, 345, 412
–, endopeptidases **31**, 356
–, meat technology **31**, 410
–, skeletal muscles **31**, 346, 347, 352
Aminopropyl derivative, enzyme immobilization **35**, 222
Aminopyrene demethylase **15**, 37
Aminopyridine, treatment of oranges with **3**, 464
δ-Amino valeric acid, fish spoilage and **7**, 45

Amiodarone **44**, 303, 320
Amitriptyline **44**, 310, 312, 323
Amlodipine **44**, 303
Ammonia **14**, 202–203
–, chocolate and **31**, 218, 234
–, dietary fiber and **31**, 173
–, fish freshness and **7**, 48–49, 59
–, formation, in coffee gases **2**, 280
–, –, in dogfish **2**, 381
–, –, in spoiling fish **2**, 370, 371, 376, 379
–, –, in tea **11**, 220
–, for treating oranges **12**, 185
–, gelatin manufacture and **7**, 241
–, in protein spoilage **16**, 168, 279
–, refrigerant in ships **12**, 149, 165
–, shark flesh and **7**, 53
–, treatment of citrus fruits with **3**, 465
–, use in demethylation of pectin **1**, 411
Ammonium **14**, 353–354
Ammonium alginate, calculated vs. experimental center-line temperatures **11**, 421
–, calculated vs. experimental heat transfer **11**, 419
–, flow constants for **11**, 387
–, shear rate relations with shear stress **11**, 373, 375, 376, 377
Ammonium chloride, licorice candy and **7**, 349
Ammonium oxalate, effect on adhesive properties of pea coats **2**, 315
–, treatment of potatoes with **2**, 315
Ammonium salts, solubility **34**, 309
Amorphous food **39**, 117
Amoxapine **44**, 310
AMP deaminase, in abalone **23**, 158
Amphetamine **44**, 313, 323
Amphiphilicity, graphical representations **42**, 99–102
Amphotericin B **44**, 289
Ampicillin **44**, 289
Amplitude, flavor profile and **7**, 13–15
Amygdala **44**, 255
Amyl acetate in bananas **2**, 271
Amyl alcohol, in apples **2**, 263
–, in cocoa **2**, 283
–, in oranges **2**, 264
α-Amylase **41**, 157–158
–, as time–temperature integrator **44**, 180–181
–, composition **28**, 142–144
–, dietary fiber and, analysis **31**, 142–145
–, distribution **28**, 142
–, in wheat flour, effect on baking **29**, 205–206
–, Lys acylation **35**, 270
–, medical importance **28**, 144
–, nutritional significance **28**, 144
–, occurrence in beans **28**, 141
–, physicochemical properties **28**, 142–144
–, physiological importance **28**, 142
–, properties **31**, 154, 169, 170
–, protein inhibitors of **28**, 141–144
–, stabilizing effect of polyols **35**, 293
–, thermal stability **35**, 254, 247–248
β-Amylase **41**, 157
Amylases **16**, 428
–, chocolate and **31**, 248
–, conservation **41**, 102–103
–, dietary fiber and **31**, 143, 152, 170, 171
–, in eggs **1**, 183
–, in honey **24**, 321–324
–, in wheat germ **23**, 210–211, 239
–, mechanisms **41**, 159–160
–, of *Byssochlamys* spp. **25**, 267
–, starch degradation **41**, 153–154
Amyl butyrate in cocoa **2**, 283
Amyl isovalerate in bananas **2**, 271
Amylograph, Brabender **41**, 167
Amyloidosis **40**, 150–155
Amyloid protein (*see also* Transthyretin metabolism) **40**, 150
α-Amylolysis **41**, 156
Amylopectin, branching enzymes **41**, 95
–, *Chlamydomonas reinhardtii* **41**, 85–86
–, granule bound synthases **41**, 79
–, granules **41**, 13, 16, 20–23
–, molecular shapes and interactions **42**, 161
–, molecular weight **9**, 66
–, molecule size **41**, 164
–, orientation **41**, 28
–, SSS in **41**, 76–77
–, structure **6**, 34; **41**, 23–25
Amyloplasts, biosynthesis, analysis **41**, 116–117
–, –, characterization **41**, 115–116
–, carbon transport **41**, 119–124
–, cell fractionation **41**, 117–119
Amylose, branching enzymes **41**, 93–95
–, *Chlamydomonas reinhardtii* **41**, 85–86
–, dietary fiber and **31**, 143, 170
–, granules **41**, 13, 16, 20–23
–, molecular shapes and interactions **42**, 156–168
–, –, amylopectin **42**, 161
–, –, A-amylose **42**, 157–160
–, –, B-amylose **42**, 160–163

Amylose, molecular shapes and interactions (*cont'd*)
–, –, V-amylose **42**, 161–165
–, –, derivatives **42**, 165, 167–168
–, –, KOH–amylose complex **42**, 165–166
–, molecular weight **9**, 66
–, molecule size **41**, 164
–, orientation **41**, 28
–, processing **41**, 169–170
–, structure of **6**, 34
Amylotylic enzymes **41**, 135–136
β-Amyrin, glycyrrhetic acid and **7**, 363–365
Anabaena sp., toxicity of **18**, 124–125
Anaerobe bacteria, cause of early spoilage in fish **2**, 369
–, effect of medium on heat resistance of **2**, 66–67
–, effect on canned foods **2**, 79–80
–, in fresh fish **2**, 351
–, thermal death time curve for **2**, 36, 79, 88
–, thermal resistance of **2**, 36, 79, 80, 81, 94, 97–99
–, thermal resistance of spores in canned peas **2**, 71
Anaerobic glycolysis **17**, 20
Analgesic–antipyretic agents, smell sensation effects **44**, 320
–, taste sensation effects **44**, 294–297
Analphylactoid reactions **42**, 10–11
Analyses of foods by sensory differences **2**, 220–254
– of – by –, accuracy of tests **2**, 227
– of – by –, – of –, cooking effects on **2**, 229
– of – by –, – of –, effect of quality of foods on **2**, 230
– of – by –, – of –, need for standards in **2**, 231–232
– of – by –, chemical and physical tests as supplements **2**, 249–251
– of – by –, conditions of testing **2**, 244
– of – by –, – of –, effects of environment on judging **2**, 244
– of – by –, – of –, – of sample size **2**, 245
– of – by –, – of –, – of temperature **2**, 246
– of – by –, – of –, – of utensils on judging **2**, 244
– of – by –, judges, variation in sensory ability of **2**, 234–244
– of – by –, methods of analyzing differences **2**, 222
– of – by –, – of –, dilution tests **2**, 224–225
– of – by –, – of –, paired and triangle tests **2**, 222–224
– of – by –, – of –, ranking tests **2**, 227
– of – by –, – of –, scoring tests **2**, 225–226
Analyte recovery **40**, 187–190
Anaphylactic reactions **43**, 199
–, annatto extract **43**, 207, 208
–, carmine **43**, 203, 204, 205–206
–, saffron **43**, 211
Anaphylactic shock **42**, 5
Anaphylactoid reactions **43**, 201
–, to sulfites **30**, 47, 58
Anchovy **39**, 340
Andersen's disease **37**, 377
Anemasterol, olive oil and **31**, 467
Anesthetics, smell sensation effects **44**, 320
–, taste sensation effects **44**, 287
Aneuploidization **34**, 390
Angel cake, freeze-dried egg albumen and **7**, 225
Angiosarcoma, carcinogen risk assessment and **31**, 41, 47
Anhydrosecoisolariciresinol **44**, 199
Aniline, combination with *o*-quinones **3**, 19
–, effect of ion size on adsorption of **2**, 11–12
–, effect on browning in orange juice **1**, 354
Animal bioassays, protein digestibility **35**, 211–213
Animal fats, ascorbic acid protection of **18**, 244–247
–, composition of **23**, 20–37
Animal feeds **17**, 79
–, apple pomace **17**, 94
–, brewery wastes **17**, 130
–, citrus molasses **17**, 90–91, 124–125
–, citrus pulp **17**, 90–93
–, corn **17**, 81, 120
–, cottonseed **17**, 109
–, from mangoes **17**, 194
–, pineapple bran **17**, 95–96
–, safflower meal **17**, 112
Animal flesh model, manufacturing process **30**, 359–360
–, meat product partial replacement by, oilseed high-protein residues **30**, 358–359
–, –, soy flour or protein **30**, 359–360
Animal husbandry, effect on milkfat composition modifications **37**, 233–235
Animal products, effect of heating on nutritive value of protein in **4**, 262–267
–, inositol phosphate content **45**, 26–27
Animals, cardiolipin **37**, 264
–, dietary fat effects on cancer risk **37**, 219–224
–, household, *Salmonella* infection in **3**, 227
–, invertebrate seafoods, farming, clams **30**, 350–351

–, –, –, lobsters **30**, 351
–, –, –, mussels **30**, 351
–, –, –, oysters **30**, 350
–, –, –, shrimps **30**, 351
–, land, feed additives, algae **30**, 345
–, –, –, amino acids **30**, 344–345
–, –, –, animal waste **30**, 346
–, –, –, cellulosic waste **30**, 345–346
–, –, –, micro-organisms **30**, 345
–, –, marketing, dairy products **30**, 347–348
–, –, –, food service industry and **30**, 348–349
–, –, –, meat products **30**, 346–347
–, –, –, poultry and eggs **30**, 347
–, –, production, future for industrialized countries **30**, 352–354
–, –, –, goal for year 2000 **30**, 342
–, –, –, land resources for **30**, 340, 341
–, –, –, nonruminants **30**, 343–344
–, –, –, poultry **30**, 344
–, –, –, ruminants **30**, 342–343
–, –, –, technology **30**, 340
–, marine, farming **30**, 350
–, –, fish, catch from oceans **30**, 349
–, –, preservation technique **30**, 351–352
–, marketing **30**, 351–352
–, phosphatidylglycerol **37**, 263
Animal species, relation to water-holding capacity of meat **10**, 379
Animal waste products **17**, 132–135
Anion binding, soy isolate **34**, 308–310
Anion exchange, wine deacidification by **25**, 24
Anion exchangers, adsorbability of **2**, 10, 11
–, commercial types of **2**, 7
–, in adsorption of amino acids **2**, 34
–, in grape industry **2**, 15–18
–, in pineapple industry **2**, 18–20
–, in sugar beet industry **2**, 6
–, in treating ulcers **2**, 8
–, reaction of typical **2**, 8
–, use in apple industry **2**, 15
Anionic azo dyes, reactive lysine measurement **35**, 194
Anise oil, licorice candy and **7**, 349
Annatto **15**, 246, 258
Annatto extract **43**, 196, 207
–, adverse reactions **43**, 202, 207–209, 213
–, –, anaphylactic **43**, 207, 208
–, –, asthma **43**, 208
Anosmia (*see also* Smell perception) **14**, 21; **44**, 249
Anoxia **15**, 120
Anserine, role in histamine toxicity **24**, 141–142
Antacids, antifolate effects **33**, 71
Ante-mortem treatment and muscle composition **26**, 94–129
–, influence of climatological stressors **26**, 127–128
–, – of electrical stimulation **26**, 128–129
–, – of exercise **26**, 128
–, – of genetics **26**, 95–96
–, – of hormones **26**, 120–125
–, – of –, adrenal **26**, 122
–, – of –, pituitary **26**, 120–121
–, – of –, sex **26**, 123–125
–, – of –, thyroid **26**, 121–122
–, – of ions **26**, 127
–, – of lathyrogens **26**, 126–127
–, – of nutrition **26**, 100–120
–, – of proteolytic enzymes **26**, 125–126
–, – of sex **26**, 96–98
Anthocyanidins, in grapes **8**, 264
–, leucoanthocyanidin as precursor of food browning **19**, 129–130
Anthocyanins **5**, 263, 283; **15**, 132
–, bleaching by SO_2 **5**, 104
–, chocolate and **31**, 221, 222, 229, 326
–, decoloration by peroxidase **17**, 18
–, in apples and pears **8**, 359
–, in corrosion **17**, 202
–, in edible fruits **5**, 284
–, in food browning **19**, 80
–, in strawberries **5**, 328
–, in tropical fruit **17**, 174
–, olive oil and **31**, 479
–, reactions with sulfites **30**, 26
–, structures of **19**, 79
Anthocyan pigments in corrosion **3**, 341–342
Anthoxanthins **5**, 285
Antiarrhythmic/antifibrillatory agents, smell sensation effects **44**, 320–321
–, taste sensation effects **44**, 302–307
Antiarthritic agents, taste sensation effects **44**, 294–297
Antiasthmatic drugs, taste sensation effects **44**, 301–302
Antibacterial agents in eggs **10**, 36
Antibiotic activity, in abalone **23**, 179
Antibiotics, effect on flat sour bacteria spores **18**, 184–186
–, fish preservation and **7**, 70
–, β-lactam, in foods **37**, 43
–, possible use as food preservatives **1**, 385
–, scanning electron microscopic studies of effects of **22**, 249–250

Antibiotics (*cont'd*)
–, used in meat **6**, 150
Antibodies, anti-cardiolipin, discovery **37**, 304
–, –, endothelial cell binding **37**, 307–308
–, –, in absence of well-defined disease **37**, 306
–, –, in systemic lupus erythematosus **37**, 305
–, –, in thrombosis **37**, 304–305
–, –, in various diseases **37**, 306–307
–, –, lupus anticoagulant levels **37**, 308–309
–, –, noncardiolipin antigens directed against **37**, 310–312
–, –, platelet binding **37**, 307
–, –, red blood cell binding **37**, 308
–, –, splenic B and T cell binding **37**, 309–310
–, antinuclear, in systemic lupus erythematosus **37**, 400
–, endogenous proteolytic enzymes and **31**, 360, 369
Anticaking agent, gaseous ozone treatment **45**, 179–180, 198
Anticancer activity, inositol phosphates **45**, 37, 38–39
Anticholesteremic/antilipidemic agents, smell sensation effects **44**, 320
–, taste sensation effects **44**, 287–288
Anticoagulants, taste sensation effects **44**, 287–288
Antienzymes, inhibition by **1**, 385
Antiepileptic agents, taste sensation effects **44**, 310–313
Antifoam "A" **15**, 355
Antifolates, dietary **33**, 78–80
–, ethanol **33**, 69–71
–, therapeutic drugs **33**, 70–71
Antigens, carcinogen risk assessment and **31**, 45
–, food, detection and avoidance **37**, 46
–, orally presented **37**, 22
–, uptake in gut, via intestinal cells **37**, 12–14
–, – in –, via Peyer's patch **37**, 14–15
Antihelmintics, taste sensation effects **44**, 286
Antihemophilic factor **44**, 315
Antihistamines, taste sensation effects **44**, 288–289
Antihypertensive agents, buckwheat **44**, 408
–, smell sensation effects **44**, 320–321
Anti-inflammatory agents, smell sensation effects **44**, 321
–, taste sensation effects **44**, 294–297
Anti-inflammatory drugs, for rheumatoid arthritis **37**, 399
Anti-inflammatory effects, short-term fasting **37**, 52
Antimicrobial agents, smell sensation effects **44**, 321–322
–, taste sensation effects **44**, 289–293
Antimicrobials, production by lactic acid bacteria **37**, 77–78
Antimutagenesis **32**, 165–166
Antinuclear antibodies, in systemic lupus erythematosus **37**, 400
Anti-nutritional factors, *see* Toxicity
Antioxidant activity, *see* Labiatae
Antioxidants **5**, 3, 24; **15**, 3, 5, 25, 35, 50, 257; **17**, 27, 31
–, acute toxicity of **3**, 200–201
–, anticancer activity **45**, 39
–, ascorbic acid **33**, 310
–, as preventatives of "warmed-over" flavor **23**, 57–58
–, butylated hydroxyanisole **6**, 13; **33**, 309–310
–, butylated hydroxytoluene **33**, 309–310
–, carcinogen risk assessment and **31**, 22, 24
–, chronic toxicity of **3**, 202–204
–, classification **5**, 24; **33**, 309
–, effect of heat on **3**, 204
–, effects on IQ-like compound formation during frying **34**, 435
–, flavonoids **33**, 311–314
–, for color protection **5**, 27
–, for dehydrated mashed potatoes **25**, 117–122
–, in browning reaction **32**, 123, 150–156, 169
–, inhibition of warmed-over flavor in cooked meat **29**, 44–46
–, inhibitory effects on fish gill 12-lipoxygenase, table **33**, 308
–, inositol phosphates **45**, 28, 29
–, in prolonging storage life of dry whole milk **3**, 95, 96
–, mode of action on fat **5**, 24, 25
–, modulation of meat mutagens **34**, 427
–, multicomponent edible film carriage **44**, 384
–, naturally occurring **17**, 59; **33**, 310
–, *N*-nitroso compounds and **31**, 64, 73, 81
–, olive oil and **31**, 469, 472
–, oriental noodles **43**, 160
–, ozone interactions **45**, 177
–, pharmacological evaluation of **3**, 197–208
–, phytoestrogens **44**, 225–226
–, propyl gallate **6**, 12

–, requirements of chemicals for use as **3**, 198–199
–, structure and activity relationship **32**, 153–155
–, tocopherols **33**, 310
–, use in food processing **32**, 155–156
–, use on meats **5**, 26
Antioxidant status **40**, 58
Anti-Parkinson's disease drugs, taste sensation effects **44**, 309–310
Antiplasticization, by sugars **38**, 156–159
Antirheumatic agents, taste sensation effects **44**, 294–297
Antisense **41**, 129–130
Antiseptics, taste sensation effects **44**, 298
Antispasmodics, taste sensation effects **44**, 298
Antithrombin III **44**, 315
Antithyroid agents, smell sensation effects **44**, 322
–, taste sensation effects **44**, 298–299
Antitrypsin in egg albumen **1**, 127, 169
Antiulcerative agents, taste sensation effects **44**, 299–300
Antiviral activity, of abalone **23**, 179
Antiviral agents, taste sensation effects **44**, 300
AP-2 (adaptor protein 2) **45**, 25, 30, 38
AP-3 (adaptor protein 3) **45**, 30
APE, *see* Atom percentage excess
Apical kernels **41**, 38–39
Apiginein **44**, 197
Apiol in parsley **2**, 273
APIZYM enzyme system **44**, 170
Aplysin, as marine toxin **18**, 157
β-Apo-8′-carotenal **15**, 211, 246, 251
Apoenzyme, of enzymes **17**, 34
Apois americana Medicus **44**, 202
Apolipoprotein IV, energy-minimized structures **42**, 109–111
Apolipoproteins, dietary fat type and source effects **37**, 154–159
–, in MUFA-rich vs. low-fat diets **37**, 174, 189
–, *n*-3 polyunsaturated fatty acid effects **37**, 178–179
–, serum, butter effects **37**, 166–169
Apophyllite, volume per oxygen atom in **2**, 3
Apoproteins, plasma lipoproteins **36**, 258
Apoptotic pathways, taste bud cells **44**, 251
Apparent kinetic parameters, desaturase enzymes **35**, 31–32
Apparent viscosity **39**, 5–6, 25, 274
–, role in fluid consistency **11**, 373
Appellation d'Origine Contrôlée **39**, 236
Appetite, as indication of nutritional need in humans **1**, 107–111
–, causes of **21**, 9–14
–, cessation of **21**, 15–17
–, decrease, caused by thiamine deficiency **1**, 117
–, depressants, adaptation to **1**, 128–129
–, –, counteraction by nutrients **1**, 127–128
–, –, destruction of physical and chemical means **1**, 127
–, –, effect of amino acids on **1**, 115–116
–, effect of deleterious compounds on **1**, 124
–, – of endocrines on **1**, 122–124
–, – of fat-soluble vitamins on **1**, 119
–, – of fats on **1**, 118–119
–, – of minerals on **1**, 119–122
–, – of proteins on **1**, 113–115
–, – of water-soluble vitamins on **1**, 116–118
, factors affecting **21**, 10–17
–, hormonal relationships **21**, 11–12, 14, 23–24, 27–34
–, influence of brain centers on **1**, 136
–, – of caloric output on **1**, 129
–, – of enzymes on **1**, 131
–, – of flavor on **1**, 135
–, – of gastro-intestinal tract on **1**, 134
–, – of growth on **1**, 130
–, – of internal environment on **1**, 130
–, – of taste mechanism on **1**, 137
–, – of tissue irritability on **1**, 133
–, physiological basis for **1**, 107–141
–, psychological *vs.* physiological factors affecting **1**, 141
–, sensory stimulus **21**, 35–43
Apple cider, pulsed electric field (PEF) processing, flavor **44**, 21
–, shelf-life **44**, 16
Apple industry, use of ion exchangers in **2**, 15
Apple marc, preparation for pectin extraction **11**, 17–21
Apples **16**, 208, 213
–, action of growth substances on **8**, 381
–, alcohol concentration in **2**, 263
–, anthocyanins **5**, 284
–, ascorbic acid content **4**, 380
–, ascorbic acid oxidase in **3**, 16
–, Australian **3**, 16
–, Ben Davis, oil in **2**, 262–263
–, biochemistry of **8**, 297
–, brown heart **12**, 111–112, 181
–, canned, use of ascorbic acid in **4**, 367
–, color changes in **3**, 2–6, 8, 11

Apples (*cont'd*)
–, composition of **8**, 300
–, compounds in **2**, 262–263
–, corrosion by **3**, 338, 341
–, crab, distillation of **2**, 263
–, dehydrated **6**, 316
–, dicotyledonous plants **31**, 126–129
–, dietary fiber and, analysis **31**, 146, 148, 150
–, distillation and saponification of **2**, 262–263
–, dried, chemical changes during browning in **1**, 347–351
–, –, color changes during browning in **1**, 328
–, –, effect of temperature on browning in **1**, 330, 333–334
–, –, influence of oxygen on deterioration of **1**, 342, 344, 345
–, –, minimizing browning in **1**, 365
–, –, rate of browning in **1**, 335
–, –, use of SO_2 **5**, 141
–, effect of ozone **3**, 466
–, – of salts and inhibitors **3**, 30
–, – of temperature **3**, 17
–, – of –, on subjective scoring **2**, 248
–, flavonoids **5**, 280
–, flavor constituents of **8**, 380
–, freezing breakdown **12**, 181
–, frozen **5**, 112
–, –, retarding enzymic browning in **3**, 31
–, gas storage of **3**, 468
–, glycosides of quercetin **5**, 281
–, humidity in storage of **3**, 468
–, immature, jelly units of pectin from **1**, 402
–, inhibition of browning in **3**, 30
–, – of polyphenolase in **3**, 20
–, intestinal bacteria **31**, 172, 175, 176, 183
–, juice, ascorbic acid loss during bottling **1**, 63–64
–, –, browning of **5**, 54
–, –, canned, ascorbic acid content **4**, 375
–, –, chemical changes during browning in **1**, 349–350
–, –, color changes during browning in **1**, 329
–, –, combination of sulfur dioxide **5**, 79
–, –, concentrate **3**, 453
–, –, –, sorption isotherms for **3**, 454
–, –, destruction of wine yeast in **3**, 436
–, –, effect of cathode rays on **3**, 176
–, –, – of sonic vibration on **3**, 131
–, –, flavor/vitamin C content retention **44**, 20–21
–, –, fruit washing water-related disease outbreaks **45**, 169, 195
–, –, increase of pH value in **3**, 24
–, –, microbial inactivation **44**, 13–14
–, –, pectin in **1**, 398
–, –, preservation of **3**, 442
–, –, pulsed electric field (PEF) processing **44**, 26, 27
–, –, reduction of pH value in **3**, 24
–, –, shelf-life **44**, 16
–, –, use of ascorbic acid in **4**, 369, 375–379, 381
–, leuco-anthocyanins **5**, 288
–, marine transport **12**, 179–182
–, –, handling **12**, 182
–, –, temperature **12**, 179–181
–, market surveys on **3**, 413
–, mineral elements in **8**, 369
–, Newtown **3**, 27
–, nitrogen content of **8**, 299
–, oil in **2**, 263
–, oxidizing enzymes in **8**, 354
–, ozone treatment **45**, 192, 195
–, –, of washing water **45**, 190
–, pectin, deesterification of **1**, 411
–, –, demethylation of **1**, 409–412
–, pectinate, changes in gels made from **1**, 420
–, peels, quercetin in **3**, 12
–, phenolase in **3**, 27
–, pH experiments on **3**, 25, 29
–, –, value of **3**, 432
–, polyphenols and enzymic browning in **19**, 114–115
–, preparation for bakers' use **5**, 128, 146
–, preparation of polyphenolase from **3**, 8, 9
–, preservation of pomace **5**, 147
–, problems in subjective scoring of **2**, 241, 243
–, properties **31**, 157–160, 164, 166
–, pulp, pectin in **1**, 400–401
–, radiowave treatment of **3**, 144
–, removal of tissue gases from **3**, 36, 37
–, respiration in **3**, 17
–, skins, toughness of **8**, 43
–, Springdale, hydrolysis of **2**, 262–263
–, storage diseases in **3**, 17
–, sulfiting **5**, 132
–, treatment for storage rots in **3**, 464
–, vitamin content of **8**, 360
–, Yellow Newtown **3**, 5
Applesauce, calculated vs. experimental center-line temperatures **11**, 421
–, calculated vs. experimental heat transfer **11**, 419
–, flow constants for **11**, 387

–, pumping system for **11**, 407
–, shear rate relations with shear stress **11**, 375
Apple wastes **17**, 94–95
–, pomace, as animal feed **17**, 94
Apricots **15**, 223
–, browning in **3**, 26
–, canned, nutrients in **1**, 43, 46–49
–, –, use of ascorbic acid in **4**, 367
–, –, vitamin retention in **1**, 82
–, cathode ray irradiation of **3**, 182
–, concentrate, minimizing browning in **1**, 365
–, darkening of stored fractions of **2**, 36
–, dried, chemical changes during browning in **1**, 347–348, 351–352
–, –, color change in **5**, 88
–, –, effect of temperature on browning of **1**, 329–330, 334
–, –, enzymic changes in **11**, 289, 290
–, –, influence of oxygen on deterioration of **1**, 342–345
–, –, inhibition of browning **5**, 129
–, –, minimizing browning in **1**, 360–365
–, –, rate of browning in **1**, 335
–, –, restoration of color **5**, 104
–, –, resulfuring with liquid SO_2 **5**, 133
–, –, storage **5**, 103
–, –, storage deterioration **5**, 142
–, –, use of SO_2 **5**, 141
–, effect of salts and inhibitors **3**, 30–31
–, – of sound waves on enzymes of **3**, 36
–, – of temperature on "oxidase" **3**, 28
–, – of – on peroxidase **3**, 28–29
–, – of – on phenolase **3**, 28–29
–, enzyme preparation of **3**, 7
–, freeze-dried **12**, 20
–, frozen, retarding enzymic browning in **3**, 30
–, inhibition of phenolase in **3**, 30
–, melanoidin in **3**, 263
–, nectar, canned, ascorbic acid content **4**, 375
–, peroxidase reaction in **3**, 10
–, pH experiments on **3**, 24, 25
–, polyphenols and enzymic browning in **19**, 119
–, removal of gases from **3**, 36–37
–, Royal variety **3**, 7, 29
–, syrup, chemical changes during browning in **1**, 357–358
–, –, minimizing browning in **1**, 366
–, –, rate of browning **5**, 54
–, tannin extract from **3**, 12
–, test for "organic peroxide" in **3**, 31
–, thiamine retention or storage **6**, 297, 304
Apyrase, in wheat germ **23**, 240, 241
Aquatic food proteins (*see also* Fishery products) **20**, 189–216
–, consumer preference and demand for **20**, 196–197
–, forms of consumption of **20**, 195–196
–, future prospections of **20**, 197–210
–, husbanding of **20**, 199–201
–, increasing biomass for **20**, 204–207
–, new processes and products from **20**, 201–210
–, problems of acceptance of **20**, 210
–, species utilization for **20**, 200–201
Araban, content in pectins **11**, 73–80
Arabidopsis Escherichia coli phytase transgenic expression **45**, 34
–, phytate (inositol hexakisphosphate) synthetic pathway **45**, 8
Arabidopsis thaliana, as starch model **41**, 10
–, branching enzymes **41**, 100
Arabinans, dicotyledonous plants **31**, 130, 131, 135
–, dietary fiber and **31**, 148
–, intestinal bacteria **31**, 172, 175, 176
–, molecular shapes and interactions **42**, 198–201
Arabinogalactan, in coffee beans, disappearance during roasting **30**, 110
–, in primary plant cell wall **30**, 145
Arabinogalactins, analysis **31**, 146, 148
–, dicotyledonous plants **31**, 130–132, 135
–, dietary fiber and **31**, 172, 176
Arabinose, chocolate and **31**, 272
–, dietary fiber and, dicotyledonous plants **31**, 126, 132
–, –, intestinal bacteria **31**, 123, 137, 148, 172, 175, 177, 181, 185, 187, 188
–, effect on dried egg **1**, 172
–, in pectins **1**, 397–399; **11**, 76
–, –, effect on pectin viscosity **11**, 77
–, salt requirement and **7**, 112
α-L-Arabinosidase, in ripening fruits, cell wall softening and **30**, 178
Arabinoxylans, analysis **31**, 148, 150
–, dicotyledonous plants **31**, 126, 129
–, dietary fiber and **31**, 122, 191
–, intestinal bacteria **31**, 172, 185, 187, 189
–, monocotyledonous plants **31**, 136, 137
Arabitol, D- **12**, 77
Arachidonate, autoxidation, mechanism **33**, 247

Arachidonate (*cont'd*)
–, carbonyl compounds generated from, table **33**, 265
–, di-, tri-, and tetrahydroxy derivatives, formation from hydroperoxide precursors **33**, 248
Arachidonic acid, autoxidation **33**, 247–248
–, concentration **35**, 12–13
–, dietary linoleic acid **35**, 89–90
–, dietary α-LNA effects, animals **35**, 86–88
–, –, humans **35**, 83–84
–, eicosanoid metabolites, inflammation **35**, 139
–, hydroperoxide, trihydroxy derivative formation **33**, 271
–, inhibition and inflammation **35**, 140–141
–, lipoxygenase-catalyzed oxidation and generation of oxidative flavor compounds **33**, 300
–, metabolism, α-LNA and *n*-3 PUFA effects **35**, 88–89
–, oxygenation **35**, 94–95
–, regulation of concentration **35**, 156–157
–, release and phospholipases **35**, 93–94
–, tissue, dietary α-LNA effects **35**, 89–90
Architecture, naval **12**, 151–152
–, –, theoretical cargo density **12**, 151
Area under concentration–time curve **40**, 50–52, 60, 70
Area under moment curve **40**, 50–52
Arg content, thermostable proteins **35**, 266–268
Argentarina **16**, 71
Arginine **16**, 247
–, adsorption by using resinous exchanger **2**, 38
–, endogenous proteolytic enzymes and **31**, 350, 410
–, fish spoilage and **7**, 45
–, gelatin manufacture and **7**, 241
–, gel formation and **7**, 308
–, in fruit products, relationship to browning **1**, 353
–, separation from other amino acids **2**, 34
Argon, ozone combined sanitization procedures **45**, 201
Aridin **10**, 37
Aroma (*see also* Flavor), compounds important for **20**, 4
–, definition of **7**, 11
–, development of **17**, 274
–, flavor profile and **7**, 10
–, of cheese **16**, 268ff; **39**, 206, 237
–, of IM meat **39**, 131, 132
–, of tea **11**, 228–231; **17**, 233, 248
–, processes for **20**, 7–38
–, recovery and retention of, in food drying **20**, 1–111
Aromatic compounds, bicyclic, in curing smoke **29**, 134
–, monocyclic, non-phenolic in curing smoke **29**, 132, 134
–, polycyclic hydrocarbons, *see* Polycyclic aromatic hydrocarbons (PAH)
Aromatic substances, in tea **17**, 248–255
Arrhenius behavior, compared to WLF behavior **38**, 188–200
Arrhenius equation **17**, 35; **25**, 188; **35**, 343
–, explicit reference temperature **38**, 207
–, integrated form of **25**, 189
Arrhenius kinetics, contrast with WLF kinetics **38**, 204–212
Arrhenius plots **38**, 205–206
–, thermal denaturation, proteolytic enzymes **35**, 255–256
Arrhenius relaxation behavior **38**, 193
Arrowroot starch, distinguishing from sago starch **2**, 320
–, gelatinization temperature of **2**, 319
Arsenic, counteraction of selenium poisoning by **1**, 128
–, in milk **36**, 238
–, in wines **8**, 135, 137, 173
–, use of ion exchangers for removal from apple products **2**, 15
Arsenic compounds, inhibition of enzymes by **1**, 382
Arthrochalasis multiplex congenita **37**, 392
Arthropods, *Salmonella* in **3**, 228, 229
Artichokes, canned, use of ascorbic acid in **4**, 371
–, effect of blanching on **1**, 66
–, production of syrup from **2**, 29–30
Artificial sweeteners, chocolate and **31**, 269–271
Arum esculentum, starch gelatinization temperature of **2**, 319
Arum maculatum, starch gelatinization temperature of **2**, 319
Arylamidases, endogenous proteolytic enzymes and, exopeptidases **31**, 346, 347, 350–352
–, meat technology **31**, 411
–, proteinase activity **31**, 385, 388
Asbestos, carcinogen risk assessment and epidemiology **31**, 39, 40
–, statistics **31**, 13, 15, 16
Ascomycetes **15**, 167

Ascorbate, effect on folate retention **33**, 49–50
–, – on "warmed-over" flavor **23**, 55
–, *N*-nitroso compounds and **31**, 62, 80, 81, 84
Ascorbate oxidase, inhibition by sulfiting agents **30**, 11
Ascorbate oxidation **15**, 68
Ascorbic acid (*see also* Vitamin C) **14**, 232–234; **15**, 77, 124
–, accumulation of **17**, 231
–, addition to foods **18**, 219–315
–, – to –, as a nutrient **18**, 222–238
–, – to –, bread and flour **18**, 272–277
–, – to –, butter **18**, 292–294
–, – to –, cabbage products **18**, 237
–, – to –, carbonated beverages **18**, 232–234
–, – to –, cheese **18**, 294–295
–, – to –, dairy products **18**, 287–295
–, – to –, fish **18**, 256–266
–, – to –, fruit juices and fruit drinks **18**, 223–226, 253–254
–, – to –, juice and drink processing precautions **18**, 227–232
–, – to –, methods **18**, 221–222
–, – to –, milk products **18**, 234–236, 291–292
–, – to –, potato products **18**, 236–237
–, – to –, vegetable juice **18**, 227
–, – to –, vegetables **18**, 255–256
–, – to –, yogurt **18**, 294
–, adsorption by anion exchanger treatment of orange juice **2**, 30
–, and selenium uptake **32**, 107
–, as additive to fruit juices **9**, 256–257
–, as flour and dough improver **4**, 406–407
–, as meat color stabilizer **18**, 266–272
–, as a nutrient **4**, 361–364
–, as oxygen acceptor in beer processing **18**, 277–282
–, as plant and tree sprays **18**, 295–296
–, as reducing agent in wine **18**, 283–287
–, as substrate **17**, 16
–, as synergist in fat protection **18**, 241–248
–, chemistry of **4**, 364–366
–, chlorine and **7**, 165
–, content of apples and pears **8**, 362
–, – of turnip green leaves **5**, 184
–, destruction of **3**, 142; **5**, 269; **17**, 4–5, 17
–, dicarbonyls produced by oxidation of **19**, 193
–, effect of cathode rays on **3**, 170–174
–, – of X-rays on **3**, 158
–, effect on enzyme-catalyzed oxidation in frozen fruits **4**, 381–388
–, – on flavor and nutritive value of juices **4**, 371–381
–, erythorbic acid vs. **18**, 297–304
–, FDA standards for **18**, 298
–, federal and military specifications for use of **18**, 300
–, freeze-dried beef and **7**, 211
–, freeze-dried lemon juice and **7**, 228
–, freeze-dried peas and **7**, 229
–, fruit browning protection by **18**, 249–255
–, in browning reaction **3**, 31, 33; **32**, 142–143
–, inhibition of fish lipid oxidation **33**, 310
–, – of oxidative losses to reduced folates **33**, 15
–, – of warmed-over flavor development in cooked meat **29**, 41, 44
–, in kiwifruit juice during vinification **29**, 303–305
–, in lipid deterioration in dry milk products **3**, 93
–, in meat curing, color stabilization **29**, 14
–, –, flavor and odor improvement **29**, 15
–, –, *N*-nitrosamine formation blocking **29**, 14–15, 59–60
–, in milk **3**, 75
–, in passion fruit **12**, 212–213, 228, 243–244, 249, 255–257, 263
–, in processed foods, history **4**, 359–361
–, in tallowiness in dry milk products **3**, 95
–, in tea **17**, 218
–, in wine **5**, 457
–, long-chain acetals, inhibition of *N*-nitrosamine formation in cured meat **29**, 60
–, loss, due to carbon dioxide **12**, 121–122
–, –, during blanching of vegetables **8**, 76, 89
–, –, in frozen foods **17**, 4–5
–, *N*-nitroso compounds and **31**, 62, 63, 73, 81
–, oxidase activity **3**, 16
–, oxidation of **5**, 103; **17**, 13
–, –, pH **3**, 28
–, –, reactions **18**, 242–243
–, protection by citric acid and SO_2 **5**, 87
–, reactions **18**, 238–241
–, – with sulfites **30**, 24
–, reaction with O_2 in sealed containers **4**, 366–367
–, regulations concerning use of **18**, 296–302
–, retention of in blanched foods **3**, 136
–, stability in food products **18**, 228–231

Ascorbic acid (*cont'd*)
–, synergistic action in preventing fat oxidation **4**, 388–389
–, test for **2**, 334–335
–, α-tocopherol interactions **33**, 211–212
–, use in controlling oxidized flavor in beverages **4**, 403–406
–, – in freezing of fruit **3**, 26, 31
–, – in improving nutritive value of miscellaneous products **4**, 407–408
–, – in lard **5**, 29
–, – in meats **5**, 25, 27
–, – in minimizing meat discoloration and rancidity **4**, 392–394
–, – in preventing oxidative browning **4**, 367–371
–, – in preventing rusting and rancidity in frozen fish **4**, 390–392
–, – in processed foods **4**, 359–431
–, – in retarding oxidized flavor in dairy products **4**, 395–403
Ascorbic acid content, effect of pH on stability of **1**, 301
–, foods, effect of heat sterilization on **1**, 89
–, fruit products, effect of oxygen on loss of **1**, 337, 310–341, 345
–, –, – of temperature on browning reactions **1**, 327, 337, 348–351, 356, 358
–, –, – of – on loss of **1**, 330–334
–, –, loss of in relation to browning **1**, 330–332, 348–351, 362
–, fruits, effect of raw product handling **1**, 82
–, –, – of storage **1**, 65, 90–97
–, influence of climate on **1**, 295–299
–, – of light on **1**, 299–303, 318
–, juices, effect of canning **1**, 52–63
–, –, tin vs. glass **1**, 98–100
–, loss in potatoes during drying **1**, 261, 266
–, methods of determining **1**, 292–294
–, of canned foods **1**, 41, 43, 60
–, oxidase in apple juice **1**, 82
–, plants, effect of fertilizers on **1**, 307–310
–, –, – of rainfall on **1**, 304–305
–, –, – of temperature on **1**, 303–304
–, sampling methods for **1**, 294–295
–, vegetables, effect of blanching on **1**, 67–79
–, –, – of storage **1**, 65, 90–97
Ascorbic acid oxidase **16**, 432
–, in wheat germ **23**, 241
Ascorbyl palmitate, effect on mortality of rats **3**, 205
–, inhibition of *N*-nitrosamine formation in cured meat **29**, 60
–, pathologic effects of **3**, 207
Ascospores, of *Byssochlamys* spp. **25**, 252–264
Aseptic processing **32**, 1–37
–, definition **32**, 2
–, packaging systems **32**, 27–30
–, sterilizing agents **32**, 25–27
Ash, in cow's milk **2**, 21
–, in peas **9**, 76–78
–, loss during blanching **8**, 68
–, removal from corn sugar liquor **2**, 30
Asia, fish **39**, 345–346
–, IM meat, *see* China, Indonesia, Malaysia
Asian immigrant, food selection by **32**, 261–262
Asparagine, endogenous proteolytic enzymes and **31**, 355
–, in fruit products, relation to browning **1**, 353–354
–, licorice root and **7**, 343
Asparagus, canned, nutrients in **1**, 43, 46–50
–, –, thiamine content of **1**, 66
–, crude lipid from **8**, 100
–, effect of storage on vitamin content of **1**, 65
–, inulin content **43**, 9
–, loss of carotene during blanching **8**, 72
–, – of –, of thiamine during blanching **8**, 74
–, nonenzymatic browning in **19**, 127
–, pH of **3**, 432
–, tannin **5**, 289
–, thiamine loss **6**, 286, 296
–, tissues in stem of **2**, 303
–, B vitamins in **1**, 42, 44, 45
–, waste **17**, 85–86
Aspartame, carcinogen risk assessment and **31**, 24
–, chocolate and **31**, 270, 271, 275
Aspartate, endogenous proteolytic enzymes and **31**, 345, 381, 383, 406
L-Aspartate-2-oxoglutarate aminotransferase as endpoint cooking temperature indicator **44**, 171
Aspartate proteinases, endogenous proteolytic enzymes and **31**, 360–362
Aspartic acid, endogenous proteolytic enzymes and **31**, 352, 360
–, in fruit products, relation to browning **1**, 352–353
–, –, – to microbial inhibition **1**, 387
Aspartic acid–proline sequence **35**, 207
L-Aspartyl residues, extent of racemization in commercial foods **35**, 205–206
Aspergillus **44**, 213
–, M4-1, compound G_3 production **30**, 296

–, aflatoxin nonproducers **30**, 287–289
–, classification **30**, 289
–, germination of **7**, 95, 96
–, growth rate of **7**, 98
–, heat resistance of **3**, 456
–, in bacon **3**, 298
–, water requirements **7**, 115
–, –, light and **7**, 110
–, –, nutrition and **7**, 107–108
–, –, pH and **7**, 109
–, –, stability of **7**, 110
–, –, temperature and **7**, 109
Aspergillus fonsecaeus, lactase **38**, 59
Aspergillus fumigatus, phytase transgenic expression **45**, 34
Aspergillus glaucus, humidity conditions for **3**, 451
–, survival of at low temperatures **3**, 446
Aspergillus niger **45**, 11, 12, 36
–, effect of pH on thermal death point of **3**, 438
–, – of vanillic acid esters on **3**, 460
–, inhibition of **3**, 444
–, lactase, potential application in HTST pasteurization of milk **38**, 89
–, lethal effect of acetic acid on **3**, 458
–, lethal temperature **3**, 437
–, phytase **45**, 20
–, product inhibition **38**, 9–10
–, saccharide production and temperature **38**, 70–71
–, transgalactosylase products **38**, 79–80
Aspergillus oniki, 1784 strain, isocoumarin and related compounds from **30**, 295
Aspergillus oryzae, food fermentation **30**, 201, 220
–, immobilized enzyme system, column reactor using **38**, 47, 49
–, koji making **30**, 222
–, lactase, temperature effects **38**, 34–35
–, saccharide production and temperature **38**, 70–71
–, transgalactosylase products **38**, 79–80
Aspergillus repens, humidity conditions for **3**, 45
–, sterilization of **3**, 134
Aspergillus sojae **10**, 76, 108, 113
–, food fermentation **30**, 201, 220
–, koji making **30**, 222, 227
–, production of mycotoxins differing from aflatoxins **30**, 297
–, proteases produced by **30**, 221
–, strain X-1, aflatoxin B_1-like pyrazine production **30**, 290–294
–, strains no. 48 and X816, degradation of shoyu koji **30**, 236
–, –, enzyme activities in shoyu koji **30**, 236
Aspergillus sydowi, mycelium of, effect of in diet of rats **1**, 125–127
Aspirin, antifolate effects **33**, 71
Assay methods, transgalactosylic activity **38**, 64–69
Astaxanthin **15**, 241
Asteraceae (Compositae), pyrrolizidine alkaloids **45**, 65
Asterosaponins, as marine toxins **18**, 157
Asthma, 1981 American Academy of Allergy and Immunology reports **30**, 50
–, Australian group report **30**, 50–52
–, blockage by cromoglycate **30**, 50
–, FEV_1 decrease **30**, 48–49, 53, 55–57, 60
–, history **30**, 47–50
–, La Jolla group reports **30**, 52–55
–, latest reports **30**, 55–57
–, metabisulfite capsules and **30**, 50–53, 56–57
–, protection by cyanocobalamin **30**, 54
–, reaction to sulfites **30**, 2–3, 47–57
–, sulfite-induced **42**, 12–13
–, sulfite oxidase depression and **30**, 54
Asthmatic reactions, annatto extract **43**, 208
–, carmine **43**, 206–207
Astringency, analytical assay **13**, 191–195
–, –, colorimetric **13**, 192
–, –, permanganate reduction **13**, 191
–, cheese **39**, 240–241
–, drugs **13**, 194–195
–, fruits **13**, 195–209
–, –, apples and cider **13**, 196–198
–, –, bananas **13**, 202, 206–208
–, –, binding hypothesis **13**, 206–207
–, –, cherries **13**, 197
–, –, grapes **13**, 195, 197
–, –, peaches **13**, 199–200, 207
–, –, pears **13**, 201
–, –, persimmons **13**, 197–198
Asymmetrin, from *Byssochlamys* spp. **25**, 276–277
Atabrine, inhibition of enzymes by **1**, 384
Atherogenesis, *n*-3 PUFAs **36**, 327–328
Atherosclerosis, MUFAs **36**, 303–304
Atmosphere, as SO_2 source **30**, 32
Atomic absorption spectrophotometry, for detecting selenium **32**, 87
Atomic force microscopy, fat crystal networks **44**, 66–75
Atomization, effect of speeds on bulk density **2**, 471–474

Atomization (*cont'd*)
–, rules for fluids by pressure spray nozzles **2**, 446
–, theory of in spray-drying **2**, 439–445
Atom percentage excess **40**, 67, 68, 71–72
Atovaquone **44**, 289
ATP (*see also* Adenosine triphosphate), endogenous proteolytic enzymes and, endopeptidases **31**, 354, 355, 357, 361
–, in abalone **23**, 157–158
–, in muscle contraction **9**, 6, 11–13, 14–26
–, in muscle relaxation **9**, 26–28
–, meat technology **31**, 393, 394, 396–398, 402, 410
ATPase, F_1F_0, association with cardiolipin **37**, 279
–, assay, in myofibrillar proteins **19**, 323
–, Na^+/K^+, association with cardiolipin **37**, 277–279
ATP-dependent protease factor I **31**, 380
Atractiline, detection of **7**, 348
–, licorice extract and **7**, 347–348
Atrophic myopathies **37**, 363–364
Attraction forces, electrostatic **14**, 370
–, potential energies in colloidal suspensions **11**, 368
–, Van der Waals **14**, 369–370
Attractive hydrophobic potential **34**, 32
Attractor, strange **40**, 327
AUC, *see* Area under concentration–time curve
Auger filler, for thermoprocessed food **23**, 367–368
AUMC, *see* Area under moment curve
Auranofin **44**, 294
Aureobasidium pullulans (de By) **15**, 173
Aureomycin, fish preservation and **7**, 70
Aurothioglucose **44**, 294
Australian buckwheat products **44**, 415
Autocatalysis **41**, 140
Autoimmunity, myasthenia gravis **37**, 367
–, nutritional therapies **37**, 52
–, research needs **37**, 55
–, role of gut immune system **37**, 33
–, suppression by oral tolerance induction **37**, 50–51
Autolysis, chocolate and **31**, 215, 221
–, endogenous proteolytic enzymes and **31**, 345, 356, 358, 359, 413
–, fish spoilage and **7**, 43
Automatic cleaning, *see* Cleaning
Automation, cleaning **14**, 420–430
Automobile, fuel use **32**, 203–204
Autophagocytosis, endogenous proteolytic enzymes and **31**, 377, 378, 389
Autoxidation **15**, 3
–, arachidonic acid **33**, 247–248
–, docosahexaenoate **33**, 250
–, docosahexaenoic acid **33**, 248–250
–, eicosapentaenoic acid **33**, 248–250
–, linoleic acid **33**, 242–243
–, linolenic acid **33**, 243–246
–, lipids **33**, 239–249
–, oleate **33**, 241
–, oleic acid **33**, 241–242
–, olive oil and **31**, 471, 473
Auxins (*see also* Growth regulators) **15**, 85, 128
–, chocolate and **31**, 322
–, dietary fiber and **31**, 128
–, enzyme activation **30**, 160
–, in plant cell elongation **30**, 157–160
–, lag period **30**, 157
–, mechanism of action, pea epicotyl **30**, 157–159
Available chlorine, definition of **7**, 141–14
Avenin **36**, 124
Avicel **12**, 290–294
Avidin in egg albumen, destruction by heat **1**, 127
Avocado **10**, 297, 298, 300, 304–305, 307, 308, 311–313, 317, 318–319, 322, 330, 338
–, effect of sound waves on enzymes of **3**, 36
–, inositol phosphate content **45**, 23
–, oil, reversion problems in **4**, 201
–, relationship of carbon dioxide to ripening in **3**, 17
Avoidance diet **42**, 6
Avoset process **32**, 4–5
Away-from-home meals **32**, 251–253
Axial-annular flow reactor **38**, 45–46
Axial rotation, and heat transfer **32**, 69–70
Azathioprine **44**, 293
Azide, inhibition of enzymes by **1**, 384
Azochloramide **7**, 156
–, therapeutic action of **2**, 141
Azo dyes **15**, 255
Azoreductase, fecal, lactic culture effects **37**, 99–101
Azotobacter, competitive inhibition of enzyme of **1**, 384
Aztreonam **44**, 289

B cells, linoleic acid effects **35**, 101
B lymphocytes, characterization **37**, 8
–, splenic, aCLs binding **37**, 309–310

Babassu, lauric fats in **6**, 32
Babcock Gardner conche, chocolate and **31**, 300
Bacillus **45**, 186, 198
–, attachment **43**, 334
–, –, S layers **43**, 323
–, growth rate of **7**, 101–103, 105
–, in bacon **3**, 308
–, in fresh fish **2**, 350, 353
–, in pork **3**, 293
Bacillus acidurans, use of thermal resistance values in canned foods **2**, 81
Bacillus aertryke, action of cathode rays on **3**, 163
Bacillus amyloliquefaciens α-amylase **44**, 181, 182
Bacillus anthracis, germicidal action of CPCl on **2**, 153
Bacillus brevis, extraction of tyrocidine from **1**, 378
Bacillus cereus **13**, 355; **45**, 186
–, effect of pH on thermal death point of **3**, 438
–, effect on amino acids **3**, 305
–, lethal temperature of **3**, 437
Bacillus circulans, β-galactosidase from **38**, 86, 89
Bacillus coagulans (*see also* Flat sour bacteria), as thermal processing target **23**, 77
–, characteristics of **18**, 172
–, classification of **18**, 168–169
–, comparative morphology of **18**, 170–171
–, in flat sour spoilage **18**, 164–208
–, –, of tomato juice **18**, 187–188
–, nutrient requirements of **18**, 195
Bacillus coli, destruction of by cathode rays **3**, 163
Bacillus licheniformis α-amylase **44**, 180–181
Bacillus mesentericus, effect of cathode rays on **3**, 164
–, – of pH on thermal death point of **3**, 438
–, lethal temperature of **3**, 437
Bacillus metiens, use for germicidal tests of quaternary compounds **2**, 161
Bacillus mycoides, effect of vanillic acid esters on **3**, 460
Bacillus prodigiosus, action of cathode rays on **3**, 163
Bacillus saccharolyticus, growth of in jams **3**, 450
Bacillus stearothermophilus (*see also* Flat sour bacteria) **45**, 186, 187
–, characteristics of **18**, 172
–, classification of **18**, 169
–, destruction of by ultraviolet light **3**, 151
–, in flat sour spoilage **18**, 164–208
–, lactase **38**, 58
–, nutrient requirements of **18**, 195
–, spores of **18**, 197–203
–, –, amino acid composition **18**, 200–203
Bacillus subtilis **13**, 355; **45**, 187, 199, 202
–, destruction of **3**, 130
–, –, by cathode rays **3**, 163, 164
–, –, in protein decomposition **3**, 304
–, effect of pH on germicides for **2**, 133
–, germicidal action of ADBACl on **2**, 148, 149
–, – of CPCl on **2**, 153
–, phytase **45**, 12
–, variations in thermal resistance of **2**, 66
Bacillus subtilis α-amylase **44**, 182
Bacillus thermoacidurans, heat destruction of **3**, 437, 441, 442
–, in flat sour spoilage **18**, 166
Baclofen **44**, 309
Bacon, antioxidants, use of **5**, 26
–, brightness **5**, 18
–, Canadian Wiltshire **3**, 298
–, canned sliced, dehydration of **3**, 317–321
–, –, differences between dehydrated and nondehydrated **3**, 318
–, –, preservation of **3**, 317–321
–, carcass quality **4**, 19–20
–, changes in microbial population of during processing **3**, 293–295
–, color data **3**, 314, 315
–, –, analysis of variance **5**, 195
–, cooling prior to cure **4**, 8–9
–, curing **4**, 9–14
–, dehydrated, chemical changes in during storage **3**, 320
–, –, microbial and organoleptic changes in during storage **3**, 320
–, –, weight losses in **3**, 318
–, discoloration in **3**, 315, 316
–, effect of postslaughter treatment on quality of **4**, 8–19
–, – of preslaughter treatment on quality of **4**, 5–8
–, – of smoking on bacteria in **3**, 300–801
–, factors influencing color in **4**, 25–27
–, factors influencing flavor of **4**, 20–25
–, factors influencing microbiological condition of **4**, 27–29
–, flavor, nitrite effect **29**, 24–26
–, free fatty acids in **3**, 313
–, liquid smoke-treated, phenol composition **29**, 144

Bacon (*cont'd*)
–, loss of thiamine on processing **6**, 276
–, materials and methods in study of **3**, 295–303
–, maturation **4**, 14–15
–, microbial contamination in **3**, 292–293
–, nitrogen ratios in **3**, 306, 307
–, *N*-nitroso compounds and **31**, 73–84, 86, 99
–, proteolytic changes in during storage **3**, 303–308
–, rancidity in **3**, 309–314
–, slime production in **3**, 308–309
–, smoked, chemical changes in during storage **3**, 301–303
–, storage **4**, 15–19
–, –, souring in **3**, 308
–, –, taints in **3**, 308
–, Wiltshire **4**, 1–35
–, –, bacteria in **3**, 294
–, –, effect of position during curing **3**, 299
–, –, thawing and curing procedure **5**, 194
Bacteria (*see also specific bacteria and* Contamination, Fermentation, Microbial control, Micro-organisms, Ripening) **15**, 291
–, acetic acid, sulfite effects **30**, 11
–, amino acid composition **18**, 109
–, as cause of spoilage in fish **2**, 346–348
–, as sources of protein **18**, 88–116
–, – of –, nutritional value **18**, 107–116
–, – of –, propagation methods **18**, 91–107
–, – of –, useful species **18**, 90–91
–, carcinogen risk assessment and **31**, 15, 25, 28
–, carotenoids in **15**, 208
–, chlorine and **7**, 133–141
–, chocolate and **31**, 217, 218, 268
–, –, milk **31**, 256
–, –, processing **31**, 244, 246
–, –, sweeteners **31**, 268
–, death during thermal process **2**, 62
–, destruction of by ultraviolet light **3**, 149
–, dietary fiber and **31**, 120, 139, 140, 191
–, –, analysis **31**, 142, 150, 151, 153
–, –, degradation **31**, 187–190
–, –, fermentation **31**, 173–186
–, –, properties **31**, 154–157, 164–166, 171–173
–, effect of cation and anion agents on **2**, 132
–, – of delayed spore germination on thermal processes **2**, 104
–, – of growing medium on **2**, 66
–, – of heated suspension medium on **2**, 67
–, – of location in container on survival **2**, 91–96
–, effects in sugar beet industry **2**, 26
–, endogenous proteolytic enzymes and **31**, 362
–, fish freshness and **7**, 44, 63–64, 72
–, flat sour type, *see* Flat sour bacteria
–, flora of fresh and spoiled fish **2**, 348, 356
–, formula for death rate of **2**, 63
–, formula for heat destruction of **3**, 434
–, freezing death of **6**, 170
–, gelatin testing and **7**, 250
–, growth factor for, in wine **6**, 85
–, halophilic **12**, 68
–, heat destruction of in fruits and vegetables **3**, 433–443
–, histamine-forming bacteria **39**, 331–336
–, increase during spoilage **2**, 356, 378
–, in fermenting cocoa, acetic acid **8**, 234, 245, 252
–, influence of salts and nonelectrolytes **12**, 58–59
–, – of temperature and pH **2**, 358–361
–, in frozen eggs **6**, 194
–, inhibition by nitrite and nitrate during meat curing **29**, 13–14, 46–48
–, in meat animals **6**, 112
–, in noncitrous fruit juices **9**, 223–228
–, –, acetic acid bacteria **9**, 225
–, –, effects on malic acid **9**, 264–267
–, –, lactic acid bacteria **9**, 225–227
–, –, other bacteria **9**, 227–228
–, in soy sauce mash **10**, 115, 121
–, intestinal, effect on appetite **1**, 134–135
–, in wines **6**, 70, 90, 92, 97, 99
–, koji contamination, shoyu preparation **30**, 224–225
–, lactic acid bacteria (lactobacilli) **8**, 234; **39**, 164–165, 174–175
–, –, antibotulinal activity in cured meat **29**, 55–56
–, –, in California wines **6**, 95
–, –, metabolism during mash fermentation **30**, 231
–, –, peptidases **39**, 215, 216–218
–, –, proteolysis **39**, 211
–, –, sulfite effects **30**, 11
–, nitrite/nitrate addition **31**, 81, 82, 84, 85
–, *N*-nitroso compounds and, fundamentals **31**, 64
–, –, indirect contamination **31**, 94, 96, 97
–, non-sporeforming **8**, 235
–, –, thermal death curves for **3**, 440

–, nonstarter lactic acid bacteria **39**, 198, 199, 211, 219–220, 230
–, –, future research **39**, 295
–, –, quality **39**, 250–251
–, –, temperature **39**, 256–257
–, olive oil and **31**, 461, 471
–, on frozen fish **6**, 190
–, on frozen meat **6**, 188
–, on frozen poultry **6**, 192
–, pathogenic, on refrigerated beef **6**, 138
–, –, survival time, in frozen strawberries **6**, 166
–, penetration into flexible packaging **23**, 315–317
–, putrefactive, effect of pH on growth of **3**, 431
–, role in tooth decay **25**, 138
–, route of attack in fish **2**, 357–358
–, shark spoilage and **7**, 53–54
–, slime-forming on meat **6**, 140
–, spore-forming **8**, 235
–, starter bacteria **39**, 196, 201, 203, 215–225, 250
–, –, modified **39**, 258–259
–, survival of, in frozen sucrose solutions **6**, 167
–, tests for fish spoilage by **2**, 383
–, thermal resistance in foods **2**, 65–88
–, thermotolerant **12**, 397–401
–, –, in factory and equipment **12**, 399–401
–, –, in raw materials **12**, 396–399
–, –, in starch **12**, 398
–, vinegar, in spoiled table wines **6**, 76, 92
–, water requirements of **7**, 101–106
–, –, growth rate and **7**, 101–105
–, –, halophiles and **7**, 111–113
–, wine spoilage caused by **6**, 75
Bacterial agents, gastroenteritis-producing **37**, 35–37
–, ingested, immunostimulatory properties **37**, 49–50
Bacterial cell envelope **43**, 321–323
–, capsules **43**, 321–322
–, fimbriae (pili) **43**, 322
–, S layers **43**, 323
–, outer membrane polymers **43**, 322–323
–, response to environmental change **43**, 324
–, surface active polymers **43**, 321, 322–323
Bacterial diarrheal diseases **37**, 23–24
Bacterial endotoxins, role in histamine toxicity **24**, 145–146
Bacterial growth, in milk **10**, 52
Bacterial toxins, irradiation effects on **24**, 186
Bactericidal activity of tea polyphenols **17**, 218
Bacteriocin, production by lactic acid bacteria **37**, 77–78
Bacteriostasis, effect of pH on **1**, 380–381
Bacterium fluorescens, effect on amino acids **3**, 305
Bacteroides **43**, 12, 13
–, dietary fiber and **31**, 174, 177, 178, 181, 183, 187
–, inulin substrate **43**, 18
Bagasse, definition of **17**, 123–124
Bag filters for spray dryers **2**, 481–484
Bag-in-box containers **32**, 22, 33–34
Bag-in-box packaging **32**, 20–23
Baicalein, lipoxygenase inhibition **33**, 318
Bakal and Hayakawa's method, for study of heat conduction problems **20**, 230–234
Baked goods, for improved world nutrition **22**, 191–193
Baker's yeast, uptake of benzoic acid as function of pH **11**, 335–336
Bakery products, agar in **11**, 120–122
–, carrageenan in **11**, 132–133
–, dairy powders added to **19**, 151
–, flexible packaging for **23**, 327
–, guar gum in **11**, 168
–, gum arabic in **11**, 173
–, gum kuraya in **11**, 188
–, gums in **11**, 114–115
–, gum tragacanth in **11**, 185
–, locust bean gum in **11**, 165
–, retorting system for **23**, 391
–, wheat germ use in **23**, 273–281
Baking (*see also* Bread, Breadmaking, Dough) **15**, 292
–, dairy powders used in **19**, 147–213
–, thermal effects of **19**, 181
–, wheat flour quality for **29**, 201–271
–, –, approaches to research **29**, 214–216
–, –, evaluation **29**, 204–216
–, –, limiting variables **29**, 204–206
Baking by electronic heat **3**, 138–142
Baking products **41**, 165
Baking test, bread **29**, 206–211
–, cake and cookies **29**, 211
–, small-scale rapid, Residue Protein test **29**, 213–214
–, –, SDS–Sedimentation test **29**, 213–214
Ball, C. Olin **32**, 2–4
Balsam of Peru, contact sensitivity **42**, 24–26
Bamifylline **44**, 314
Bananas **10**, 298, 304, 305, 308, 309–311, 317, 323, 325, 330

Bananas (*cont'd*)
–, dietary fiber and **31**, 158, 159, 170
–, effect of carbon dioxide **12**, 100–101
–, flavor of **17**, 176
–, pH of **3**, 432
–, purée, calculated vs. experimental center-line temperatures **11**, 421
–, –, calculated vs. experimental heat transfer **11**, 419
–, –, flow constants for **11**, 387
–, –, shear rate relations with shear stress **11**, 376
–, refrigerated on ships **12**, 165, 188–191
–, relationship of carbon dioxide to ripening of **3**, 17
–, usage of **17**, 104–105
–, volatile constituents of **2**, 6, 271
Bande **39**, 80
Barium, in wine **8**, 137
Barium chloride, microbial mutations caused by **1**, 376
Barium salts, effect on potato tissue **2**, 315
Barley, ascorbic acid oxidase in **3**, 16
–, dietary fiber and **31**, 136–138, 150, 189
–, inositol phosphate degradation during processing **45**, 21
–, leuco-anthocyanin **5**, 288
–, malting **45**, 22
–, *N*-nitroso compounds and **31**, 89, 91
–, phosphorus content of, effect of fertilizers on **1**, 313
–, phytases **45**, 9
–, prolamins **36**, 95
–, reduced phytate gene mutations **45**, 34
Barley malt flour, enzymatic hydrolysis in **11**, 312
–, phospholipid-hydrolytic activity in **11**, 305
–, sorption isotherms for **11**, 305, 307, 312
Barley starch, gelatinization temperature of **2**, 319
Barnhill spray dryer, operation of **2**, 403
Barracouta, aerobic bacterial flora of **2**, 350
Base-pair mutations **34**, 390
Bases, volatile, estimation of **7**, 59–61 195
Basic-tastes test **7**, 15–16
Basidiomycetes **15**, 167
Basolateral membrane **40**, 198–200
Basturma **39**, 74–75
Batter, carrageenan in **11**, 133
Bauermeister conche, chocolate and **31**, 305, 306
Bax **44**, 251
Bayesian estimation **40**, 269–270
Beach–Russ pump **15**, 316
Bean (*Phaseolus*) protein, amino acid composition **28**, 102–105
–, amino acids, biological availability **28**, 111–112
–, biological value **28**, 106–109
–, body membrane proteins **28**, 98–99
–, Bowman–Birk soybean trypsin inhibitor **28**, 135
–, chemical properties, influence of storage and processing on **28**, 144–148
–, chymotrypsin **28**, 138
–, composition **28**, 99–102
–, digestibility **28**, 109–111
–, digestive enzyme inhibitors **28**, 128–144
–, –, binding **28**, 130
–, –, composition **28**, 130
–, –, inhibitors of α-amylase **28**, 141–144
–, –, – of –, composition **28**, 142–144
–, –, – of –, distribution **28**, 142
–, –, – of –, medical importance **28**, 144
–, –, – of –, nutritional significance **28**, 144
–, –, – of –, physicochemical properties **28**, 142–144
–, –, – of –, physiological importance **28**, 142
–, –, – of protease **28**, 128–141
–, –, – of –, distribution in plants **28**, 133
–, –, – of –, medical importance **28**, 139–141
–, –, – of –, nomenclature **28**, 129–133
–, –, – of –, occurrence **28**, 129–133
–, –, – of –, physicochemical properties **28**, 134–139
–, –, – of –, –, significance in plants **28**, 133
–, –, – of trypsin **28**, 131–133
–, –, – of –, amino acid sequence **28**, 134
–, –, – of –, biosynthesis of crypsinogen, effect on **28**, 140
–, –, molecular weight **28**, 130
–, isolates, composition **28**, 105–106
–, lectins in, medical importance **28**, 123–128
–, –, nutritional importance **28**, 123–128
–, –, nutritional properties, influence of storage and processing on **28**, 144–148
–, –, physicochemical properties **28**, 115–123
–, protease inhibitors, composition **28**, 134–139
–, research needs **28**, 148–151
–, seeds, lectins from **28**, 122
–, storage **28**, 96–98
–, –, biosynthesis of **28**, 95
–, –, identification **28**, 96–98
–, –, quantitation **28**, 96–98
–, trypsin inhibitors from **28**, 131
Beans (*see also separate species*) **16**, 66
–, baked, canned, nutrients in **1**, 43, 46–50

–, canned, effect of calcium chloride on **2**, 315
–, canned green, corrosion characteristics of **3**, 336
–, changes in unblanched frozen **8**, 98
–, cocoa, curing of **8**, 226
–, –, fermentation of **8**, 227, 230
–, –, sundrying of **8**, 228
–, dicotyledonous plants **31**, 127–129, 132, 133, 135
–, dietary fiber and, analysis **31**, 146, 153
–, dried, vitamin content **5**, 204
–, dry, insects infesting **4**, 306, 308, 322, 324
–, effect of copper on **3**, 355
–, gelatinization of starch in **2**, 323
–, green, ascorbic acid content of, effect of season on **1**, 295
–, –, canned, nutrients in **1**, 43, 46–50
–, –, carotene content of processed **5**, 225
–, –, effect of blanching on vitamins in **1**, 68, 72–73, 79, 81
–, –, – of storage on vitamin content of **1**, 65
–, –, frozen **6**, 175, 179
–, –, loss of nutrients during blanching of **8**, 66
–, –, B vitamins in **1**, 42, 44, 45
–, green cut, loss of thiamine on processing **6**, 286
–, inspection of **8**, 121
–, intestinal bacteria **31**, 181
–, leucoplasts in **2**, 306
–, lima, effects of blanching, decrease in bacterial content **6**, 184
–, –, – of –, loss of ascorbic acid **8**, 76 89
–, –, – of –, – of niacin **8**, 75
–, –, – of –, – of nutrients **8**, 66
–, –, – of –, – of riboflavin **8**, 75
–, –, – of –, – of thiamine **8**, 74
–, navy, autiamylase in **1**, 126
–, –, effect of heat on nutritive value **4**, 247
–, nutritional stress factor in **4**, 112–113
–, pH value of **3**, 432
–, phytic acid content, effect of cooking and canning **28**, 46–47
–, plants, ascorbic acid content of, effect of light on **1**, 299
–, properties **31**, 159, 161, 163, 164, 166, 170
–, runner, leuco-anthocyanins **5**, 288
–, snap, canned, use of ascorbic acid in **4**, 368
–, –, crude lipid from **8**, 100
–, –, loss of thiamine on processing **6**, 286
–, soaking **28**, 66–67
–, string, changes in chlorophyll during blanching of **8**, 81
–, thiamine destruction in **6**, 258, 286, 296
–, thiamine retention on storage **6**, 297
–, F value for industrial processing of **2**, 102
Becker's muscular dystrophy **37**, 351–359
Beclomethasone dipropionate **44**, 301, 321
Beef **14**, 56; **16**, 24; **39**, 75, 80, 81–82, 83
–, acid formation in, post mortem **1**, 3–8
–, aging and storing **1**, 21–33
–, bacteria in refrigerated **6**, 138
–, canned, correlation coefficients between quality factors **5**, 243
–, –, moisture content and processing temperature **5**, 237
–, chilled, appearance **12**, 173
–, –, carbon dioxide **12**, 172–173
–, –, ozone **12**, 172–173
–, –, ultraviolet light **12**, 172
–, –, weight loss **12**, 173–174
–, control of mold and bacteria on **1**, 18–21
–, cooked, creatinine production **34**, 415–416
–, "dark-cutting" **1**, 17
–, effects of freezing on **1**, 31, 33
–, enzymes in relation to rigor mortis **1**, 21
–, factors influencing color of **1**, 16–18
–, factors influencing tenderness of **1**, 24–33
–, fat rancidity in **5**, 4, 5; **6**, 142
–, fats and mutagen formation **34**, 418–419
–, fatty acid content **5**, 6; **23**, 23
–, flavor of, *see* Meat flavor
–, freeze-dried **7**, 204
–, –, commercial aspects of **7**, 216–218
–, –, deterioration of **7**, 211–214
–, –, gas-flow and **7**, 191–195
–, –, history of **7**, 207–208
–, –, papain and **7**, 211
–, –, preparation of **7**, 208–209
–, –, properties of **7**, 209–211
–, –, rehydration of **7**, 210, 214
–, –, storage of **7**, 214–216
–, freezing of **9**, 24–25
–, fried, mutagens **34**, 413
–, frozen, effect of storage on biological value of protein in **4**, 270
–, –, optimum carriage temperature **12**, 169–170
–, grain **14**, 49
–, ground trimmings **6**, 146
–, hypoxanthine constant **14**, 60–61
–, pH of **1**, 15–16
–, prepared in temperate zones **6**, 115
–, processing **21**, 187–193, 195, 203–206

Beef (*cont'd*)
–, refrigerated on ships **12**, 147–148, 150–151, 160, 168–174
–, rigor mortis in **1**, 3–21
–, shear testing **14**, 77
–, slaughter of **6**, 124
–, slime on fresh **6**, 145, 147
–, tenderness of **9**, 28–29
–, –, effect of salt on **9**, 32–35
–, thiamine loss in **6**, 275, 276, 283
Beef broth, flavor studies on **19**, 233–234
Beef muscle, rigor in **9**, 20
Beer, alginates in fining **11**, 153
–, background solution for calibration curves **8**, 136
–, carrageenan in stabilization **11**, 137
–, determination of total SO_2 **5**, 122
–, effect of sample size on judging **2**, 245
–, – of temperature on judging **2**, 247
–, fundamentals **31**, 70, 71, 74
–, licorice and **7**, 351
–, nitrite/nitrate addition **31**, 86–89, 91
–, *N*-nitroso compounds and **31**, 98
–, processing, ascorbic acid as oxygen acceptor in **18**, 277–282
–, radio-frequency pasteurization of **3**, 133
–, ropiness of **6**, 82
–, selecting judges for scoring of **2**, 236
–, sodium in **8**, 196
–, turbidity, cause and prevention **19**, 131
–, use of ascorbic acid in **4**, 403–405
Beet pulp, composition of **17**, 123–124
Beet root, β-gliadins **45**, 222
–, inositol phosphate content **45**, 23
–, red pigment betanin **5**, 277, 284
Beets, canned, nutrients in **1**, 43, 46–50
–, corrosiveness of **3**, 341
–, decrease in bacterial content during blanching **6**, 184
–, dehydrated, loss of thiamine on processing **6**, 287, 300
–, in children's diet **1**, 109
–, lignified fibers in **2**, 304
–, pectin, deesterification of **1**, 411
–, polyphenols and enzyme browning in **19**, 121–122
Belladonna, licorice and **7**, 354
Benazepril **44**, 303
Bentonite suspensions, heat transfer in **2**, 89, 93, 96, 100
Benzaldehyde, in cherries **2**, 264
–, in manufactured tea **2**, 286, 287
–, in molasses **2**, 277
–, in raspberries **2**, 269
Benzamphetamine **44**, 313
Benzene, carcinogen risk assessment and **31**, 7
–, effect on solubility of **2**, 205
–, epidemiology **31**, 39, 40
–, fat extraction by **3**, 52
–, laboratory data **31**, 29, 30, 33, 35
–, solubility of DDT in **2**, 203
–, statistics **31**, 15
Benzene ring compounds, contribution to meat flavor **18**, 54
Benzidine in temperature experiment with enzymes **3**, 28
Benzoates, fish preservation and **7**, 67–68
Benzocaine **44**, 287
Benzoic acid, action on metabolism of micro-organisms **11**, 331–353
–, derivatives of **3**, 459
–, effect on cell-free enzymes **11**, 347
–, – on micro-organism assimilatory processes **11**, 343–347
–, – on micro-organism oxidation, of TCA-cycle intermediates **11**, 342–343
–, – on –, of the acetyl group **11**, 341–342
–, – on oxidative phosphorylation in isolated mitochondria **11**, 347
–, – on processes of intact cells **11**, 339–347
–, – on *Pseudomonas fluorescens* adaptation from acetate to succinate **11**, 346–347
–, – on *Pseudomonas fluorescens* oxidation of acetate **11**, 344
–, – on *Saccharomyces cerevisiae* **11**, 334–336
–, in food preservation **3**, 458
–, in Formosan black tea oil **2**, 287
–, inhibition of cell-free enzymes **11**, 348
–, in raspberries **2**, 269
–, in strawberries **2**, 270
–, metabolic pathways in micro-organisms **11**, 338
–, relation between biological activity and water solubility **11**, 336
–, rendered nontoxic in body **1**, 127
–, research needs on metabolic inhibition in micro-organisms **11**, 349–451
–, uderobial inhibition by **1**, 398, 390
–, uptake by baker's yeast as function of pH **11**, 335–336
–, – by *Proteus vulgaris* as function of pH **11**, 335
–, with other preservatives **3**, 459, 460
Benzo[*a*]pyrene, in curing smoke **29**, 92, 135, 140–141, 147–149

–, smoked meat product contamination **29**, 147–149
Benzoquinone, inactivation of enzyme by **3**, 19
–, oxidation of catechol to **3**, 18, 20
Benzoxaprofen **44**, 294
Benzoxazin-3-ones **14**, 312–313
Benzyl alcohol in manufactured tea **2**, 286, 288
Benzyl benzoate, solubility of DDT in **2**, 203
Benzyl cyanide in peppergrass **2**, 275
Benzylethyl alcohol, in manufactured tea **2**, 286
Benzyl isothiocyanate in mushroom oil **2**, 277
Benzyl-*a*-oxysulfide in coffee **2**, 281
Bepridil **44**, 315
Beriberi, caused by eating white bread **1**, 110–111
–, prevention of, with toddy yeast **1**, 107
Berries **15**, 171, 225
–, corrosion characteristics of **3**, 336
–, frozen **6**, 169
–, –, micro-organisms in **6**, 209
–, –, sources of infection of **6**, 182
–, microbial development on **6**, 180
Betaine, separation from sugar beet molasses **2**, 35
Beta radiation (*see also* Cathode rays) **3**, 129; **15**, 71
Betaxolol **44**, 303
Betony (*Pedicularis*) **45**, 77
Better Process Control School **32**, 14
Beverages, agar in **11**, 123
–, alginates in **11**, 152–154
–, ascorbic acid addition to **18**, 232–234
–, guar gum in **11**, 169
–, gum arabic in **11**, 175
–, gums in **11**, 114
–, high-protein type, for developing countries **22**, 195
–, licorice and **7**, 351
–, sampling of **7**, 24–25
–, use of ascorbic acid in **4**, 403–406
BHA, *see* 2-*tert*-Butyl-4-methoxyphenol
BHT, *see* 3,5-Di-*tert*-butyl-4-hydroxytoluene
Biaxial extension **39**, 16–17, 58, 59
Bifidobacteria **43**, 12
–, bacteriocidal substances production **43**, 14
–, effects on, cancer-related fecal enzyme levels **37**, 99–101
–, –, cancer suppression **37**, 99–103
–, –, *Candida*-related diseases **37**, 92
–, –, cholesterol reduction **37**, 97–98
–, –, immune response **37**, 109–110
–, exogenous/endogenous modifiers **43**, 13
–, fecal recovery **37**, 72–74
–, impact of antibiotics **43**, 13
–, intestinal anticarcinogenic activity **43**, 35, 36, 38
–, intestinal microflora **43**, 10, 11
–, –, beneficial health effects **43**, 12, 13
–, inulin fermentation products **43**, 23
–, lactase production **43**, 15
–, optimum pH **43**, 15
–, prebiotics **43**, 16
–, –, carbohydrate substrates **43**, 20
–, –, dose–response relations **43**, 21
–, –, inulin substrate **43**, 18, 20, 21, 22
–, probiotics **43**, 15, 34
–, role in lactose intolerance alleviation **37**, 83–84
–, vitamins production **43**, 15, 34
Bifidobacterium, dietary fiber and **31**, 174–177, 181
–, growth promoters **38**, 95
Bifidobacterium angulatum **43**, 18
Bifidobacterium bifidum **43**, 18, 20
–, antibacterial activity **43**, 14
Bifidobacterium breve **43**, 20
Bifidobacterium cuniculi **43**, 20
Bifidobacterium infantis **43**, 18, 20
Bifidobacterium longum **43**, 18, 38
Bifidobacterium minimum **43**, 20
Bifidobacterium pseudolongum **43**, 18
Bifidobacterium thermophilum **43**, 20
Bifunctional reagents, enzyme stability **35**, 274–275
Bilayers, phospholipid, α-tocopherol effects **33**, 215–216
Bile **15**, 34
–, carcinogen risk assessment and **31**, 22, 23
–, distribution of DDT in **2**, 210
–, α-tocopherol metabolites in **33**, 199–201
Bile salt binding characteristics, dietary fiber and **31**, 159–163, 168
Bilichromes, in abalone shell **23**, 164
Biltong **39**, 79–80, 89, 124
Binders **16**, 138
Binding of meat emulsions **16**, 131
Bingham plastic behavior **39**, 6
Bingham plastic flowing in tubes **11**, 413
Bioassays, for folate bioavailability **33**, 58–61
Bioavailability, calcium **36**, 215–216
–, –, definition **33**, 119–120
–, –, diet effects on urinary excretion **33**, 120
–, –, effects of, fiber and phytate **33**, 134–142
–, –, –, oxalic acid **33**, 142

Bioavailability, calcium, effects of (*cont'd*)
–, –, –, protein and phosphates **33**, 143–144
–, –, –, supplements **33**, 144–147
–, –, lactose effect **33**, 124–125
–, –, –, in animals **33**, 125–126
–, –, –, in elderly subjects **33**, 134
–, –, –, in human infants **33**, 132–134
–, –, –, in humans **33**, 128–132
–, –, measurement **33**, 120–121
–, –, –, animal models **33**, 124
–, –, –, balance methods **33**, 121–122
–, –, –, isotopic tracer techniques **33**, 122–123
–, folates, absorption **33**, 53–57
–, –, aging effects **33**, 68–69
–, –, assessment methods, bioassays with animals and humans **33**, 58–61
–, –, –, isotopic methods **33**, 61–64
–, –, deconjugation **33**, 54–55
–, –, dietary antifolates **33**, 78–80
–, –, dietary components and **33**, 71–80
–, –, endogenous, in various foods, table **33**, 72
–, –, ethanol effects **33**, 69–71
–, –, folate-binding protein role in jejunal brush border membranes **33**, 54
–, –, gastrointestinal functions and **33**, 67–68
–, –, hepatic uptake and secretion **33**, 54
–, –, in legumes **33**, 74
–, –, in milk **33**, 75–76
–, –, in orange juice **33**, 74–75
–, –, intestinal conjugases **33**, 55–56
–, –, in vegetables **33**, 75
–, –, *in vivo* turnover kinetics **33**, 57–58
–, –, in yeast **33**, 73–74
–, –, nutrient interactions **33**, 79–80
–, –, pH dependence **33**, 53–54
–, –, K_m transport values **33**, 53
–, iron **36**, 223–224
–, Malliard reaction effect **35**, 200–201
–, manganese **36**, 231
–, minerals and trace elements **36**, 239
–, monoglutamyl folates, inherent availability **33**, 65–66
–, polyglutamyl folates, inherent availability **33**, 64–65
–, tocopherols, diet composition effects **33**, 171–173
–, –, fiber effects **33**, 171–173
–, –, pectin effects **33**, 171–172
–, –, wheat bran effects **33**, 172–173
–, zinc **36**, 227–228
Biochanin A **44**, 197
–, sources **44**, 203, 207
Biochemical systems theory **40**, 233, 236–238
Biofilm glycocalyx, bacterial slimes **43**, 323
–, formation **43**, 348
–, sanitizer resistance **43**, 347
Bioflavonoid, as drugs **27**, 174–181
Biogas, for smallholders **32**, 209–211
–, production **32**, 206–209
–, toxic products of **32**, 224
Biogenic amines, cheese **39**, 290–292
–, fish and shellfish (*see also names of amines and names of fish*) **39**, 329–365
–, –, amine detoxification **39**, 330–331
–, –, amine formation, nonvolatile **39**, 330
–, –, amine occurrence **39**, 336–346
–, –, –, finfish **39**, 336–344
–, –, –, seafood products **39**, 346
–, –, –, shellfish **39**, 344–345
–, –, analytical techniques **39**, 353–358
–, –, background information **39**, 330
–, –, chromatography **39**, 336, 339, 340, 341, 353–356
–, –, –, electrophoresis **39**, 357–358
–, –, –, enzymic tests **39**, 356–357
–, –, decarboxylase-forming bacteria **39**, 331–336
–, –, definition **39**, 330
–, –, ecosystem **39**, 336
–, –, flavor **39**, 349
–, –, freshness indicator **39**, 348–351
–, –, limits **39**, 351–352
–, –, quality control **39**, 351–352
–, –, quality index **39**, 350
–, –, scombrotoxicosis **39**, 337, 346–348
Biological rhythm, *see* Bioperiodicity
Biological value, of proteins **4**, 238–240
–, –, using humans **4**, 244
–, of tea **17**, 278–279
–, racemization and cross-linking effects **35**, 208–211
Biomacromolecular processes, variation **34**, 299–301
Biomass, for aquatic food development, increasing of **20**, 204–207
Biomass energy, use **32**, 189, 191
Biomass harvesting, and productivity **32**, 225–226
Bioperiodicity **40**, 217–226
–, categories **40**, 219–220
–, characterization **40**, 218–220
–, food intake, weight gain **40**, 220–226
–, human subject **40**, 225
Biopolymeric material **39**, 48–53
Biopsies, muscle **37**, 345, 405

Biosynthesis, ADPglucose **41**, 34–37
–, alternative pathways **41**, 37–38
–, amyloplasts **41**, 115–116
–, CAM plants **41**, 150–152
–, complete pathway **41**, 111–113
–, enzymes, limiting **41**, 134–135
–, *glg* C and **41**, 131–134
–, immunocytochemical studies **41**, 116–117
–, in fruit, of ascorbic acid **10**, 345–346
–, –, of ethylene **10**, 343–345
–, –, of fatty acids **10**, 346
–, –, of pectin **10**, 346
–, leaves **41**, 148
–, manipulation **41**, 135–136
–, microscopy **41**, 116–117
–, rate **41**, 38–39
–, seed storage proteins **36**, 123–125
–, studies **41**, 33–34
Biotechnology, role in plant proteins **36**, 91
BIOTEST **45**, 138
Biotester, for flexible packaging **23**, 316, 411
Biotin, content of apples and pears **8**, 368
–, deficiency **1**, 118
–, –, in canned foods **1**, 42, 44–45, 47
Bird–Carreau model **39**, 37–39, 49–52, 54
Birefringence **41**, 27–28
Bisabolen in carrot seed oil **2**, 271
Biscuitmaking, seed storage proteins **36**, 133
Biscuits **15**, 292
–, nutritious, for developing countries **22**, 193–194
–, wheat germ use in **23**, 284
Bishop spray dryer, operation of **2**, 410
Bis(monoacylglycero)phosphate degradation **37**, 274–275
–, distribution **37**, 262
–, synthesis **37**, 262, 264
Bismuth compounds, inhibition of enzymes by **1**, 382
Bisoprolol **44**, 303
Bisulfites **14**, 255–259, 267
–, addition products **5**, 104
–, as browning inhibitors **3**, 273
–, inhibition of browning in potatoes by **1**, 261
Biting devices **14**, 86–95
–, "KT" **14**, 92–93
Bitolterol mesylate **44**, 301, 322
Bitterness, cheese **39**, 239–240
–, differentiation of substances in oats **11**, 295–297
–, fish **39**, 349
–, inhibition in oats **11**, 297–298
Bitter taste, age-related threshold **44**, 257, 259
Bixin **15**, 246
Black beans **32**, 212–214
–, inositol phosphate degradation during processing **45**, 21, 22
Blackberries (*Rubus fruticosus*) **15**, 225; **44**, 207, 211
–, canned, nutrients in **1**, 43, 46–49
–, canned with sulfur **3**, 353
–, effect of acidity on **3**, 338
–, – of freezing temperatures on microorganisms in **3**, 448
–, pH of **3**, 432
–, storage of **3**, 468
–, sulfiting **5**, 145
Blackberry wine, detection of grape wine in **5**, 357
Black tea, aroma development in **24**, 256–257
–, carotenes in **24**, 257
–, fatty acids in **24**, 259–260
–, fermentation of **24**, 253–260
–, firing of **24**, 260–261
–, grading of **24**, 261
–, organoleptic properties of **24**, 263–265
–, preconditioning of **24**, 252
–, rolling of **24**, 252–253
–, storage of **24**, 267–268
–, volatile constituents of **24**, 250–251
–, withering of **24**, 252
Bladder cancer, carcinogen risk assessment and **31**, 15, 16, 22
Blakeslea trispora **15**, 212
Blanching **15**, 240, 289
–, carotene degradation in carrot tissue by **2**, 328
–, changes in chromoplasts during **2**, 328–330
–, displacement of intercellular air during **2**, 330–333
–, effect on chlorophyll **17**, 5
–, – on vitamins in vegetables **1**, 68–82
–, efficiency of **17**, 3–4
–, electronic, effect on vitamin losses **1**, 81
–, of foods **3**, 136, 137
–, of fruits and vegetables **17**, 3
–, steam vs. water **1**, 67–82
BLAST, with transgene proteins **42**, 56–57, 59
Blazing star (*Liatris punctata*) **45**, 77
Bleaching, olive oil and **31**, 463
Blend, flavor and **7**, 36
Bleomycin **44**, 289
Blood, bacteria count of **6**, 188
–, calcium effects **36**, 218

Blood (*cont'd*)
–, distribution of DDT in **2**, 210, 212
–, effect of ascorbic acid on color of **4**, 393
–, flow constants for **11**, 387
Blood pressure, glycyrrhizin and **7**, 355
–, *n*-3 PUFA effects **35**, 138
Blood proteins, definition and classification **34**, 259
–, plasma proteins **34**, 260–261
–, serum albumin **34**, 259–260
Blood serum, effect on germicidal action of ADBACl **2**, 148
–, – on quaternary ammonium salts **2**, 136, 150
Blueberries (*Vaccinium corymbosum*) **15**, 225; **44**, 211
–, anaerobic mold in **3**, 438
–, canned, nutrients in **1**, 43, 46–49
–, –, *penicillium* in **3**, 443
–, citric acid as corrosion inhibitor in **3**, 342
–, corrosiveness of in enameled cans **3**, 374
–, effect of freezing temperatures on micro-organisms in **3**, 448
Bluebottle fly, toxicity of DDT to **2**, 208
Blue cheese, contamination **39**, 288
–, flavor **39**, 206, 208
–, lipolysis **39**, 201, 205, 206–207, 208
–, peptides **39**, 231
–, proteinases **39**, 223, 224
–, proteolysis **39**, 226
–, salting **39**, 177
–, texture **39**, 254
–, ultrafiltration **39**, 194
Blue mold, *see Penicillium italicum*
Boais-Frias **32**, 214
Body weight, set point **21**, 25–34
Bologna **39**, 81–82
–, ascorbic acid use in **18**, 268
Boltzmann constant **17**, 38
Boltzmann superposition principle **39**, 10–12
Bond breaking **14**, 289–291
–, electrophilic **14**, 290–291
–, homolytic **14**, 289
–, nuclophilic **14**, 290
–, reagent **14**, 289–290
Bone, freeze-drying and **7**, 217, 219
–, phytoestrogen health protective effects **44**, 227–229
Bonita, spoilage of **7**, 50
Boraginaceae, pyrrolizidine alkaloids **45**, 65
Borate, interference with phosphate metabolism by **1**, 386, 388
Boric acid, interference with phosphate metabolism by **1**, 388
l-Borneol in strawberries **2**, 270
Boron, content of apples and pears **8**, 371
–, deficiencies attributed to **8**, 377
–, effect on vitamins in plants **1**, 308
–, in milk **36**, 238
–, in plants, effect on absorption of other elements **1**, 314
–, in wines **8**, 137, 141
Bostwick consistometer **32**, 48
Botryosphaeria ribis **15**, 177
Botrytis, effect of carbon dioxide **12**, 109
–, innoculated fruit **12**, 106
Botrytis cinerea **15**, 167, 172; **45**, 181, 191
–, effect of oxygen on **3**, 468
–, – of temperature on **3**, 468
Botulinum toxin, effects on gastrointestinal immunity **37**, 35
Botulism, from fishery products **22**, 135–185
–, occurrence and control of **22**, 5–6
Bound moisture **39**, 98
Bovine albumin, reaction with acetaldehyde **3**, 276
–, – with glucose **3**, 275–276
Bovine casein, as function of calcium ion concentration **34**, 317, 320
–, association constants **34**, 321–322
–, at 1°C **34**, 312, 314–315
–, at 37°C **34**, 312–314
–, calcium binding site classes **34**, 323–324
–, cation effect at 1°C **34**, 317, 319, 321
–, electrolyte effects on salting-out **34**, 315–316
–, parameter *n* **34**, 322–323
–, phosphate group effect **34**, 316–320
–, procedures **34**, 311
–, resolubilization **34**, 324
–, salt-induced solubility profiles **34**, 310–325
–, P-serine and structures **34**, 323–324
–, theory **34**, 311
Bovine Catalase test **44**, 170
–, endpoint cooking temperature indicator **44**, 171–172
Bovine isocitrate dehydrogenase, Dixon plot **34**, 358
–, enzyme–substrate interactions **34**, 361–362
–, inhibition by citrate **34**, 357–360
–, interpretation **34**, 360–362
–, linked-function analysis **34**, 360–361
–, variation with precursor **34**, 357–362
Bovine prion protein gene (PrP) **43**, 266
Bovine serum albumin, adsorption and temperature **34**, 119–120
–, adsorption kinetics **34**, 114–116
–, flavor binding **33**, 412–413

–, foam volume increase rate **34**, 61
–, intermediates, adsorption kinetics **34**, 30–31
–, –, apparent diffusion coefficients **34**, 27–29
–, –, conformational properties **34**, 27
–, load and concentration **34**, 117–118
–, π–a plots **34**, 57–58
–, rate of collapse of foams **34**, 61–62
–, salt effect on adsorption density **34**, 119
–, structure **33**, 357
–, thermodynamic and binding constants, table **33**, 414
–, time to surface pressures **34**, 18
Bovine spongiform encephalopathy **43**, 265–308
–, cattle by-products **43**, 296–299
–, –, gelatin **43**, 298–299, 303, 305
–, –, tallow **43**, 296–297, 303, 305
–, characteristics **43**, 266–271
–, clinical signs **43**, 267
–, diagnostic tests **43**, 299–301
–, EC control measures **43**, 302, 303
–, incidence in non-UK countries **43**, 267
–, – in UK **43**, 266, 267, 268, 269
–, infected feed as primary cause **43**, 267–268
–, –, feeding practices changes **43**, 272
–, –, mechanism of CNS infection **43**, 269
–, –, rendering practices changes **43**, 270, 271, 297
–, infective tissues **43**, 269–270
–, new variant Creutzfeldt–Jakob disease (vCJD) link **43**, 289–290, 292–293
–, oral transmission route **43**, 268
–, origins **43**, 270–271
–, prions (disease-causing agent) **43**, 272–275
–, –, inactivation **43**, 295–296
–, –, infectivity **43**, 294–295
–, –, strains **43**, 288–289
–, related prion diseases **43**, 275–285
–, surveillance **43**, 299–301, 306
–, UK control measures **43**, 301–304
–, USA preventive measures **43**, 304–307
–, vertical transmission **43**, 268–269
–, World Health Organization recommendations **43**, 305
Bowel, dietary fiber and **31**, 141, 191
Bowen spray dryer, air sweeper in **2**, 493
–, high inlet gas temperature in **2**, 474
–, operation of **2**, 411–413, 435
Bowman–Birk soybean trypsin inhibitor, amino acid sequence **28**, 135
Box-counting dimension **44**, 86–88
Boxfishes, pahutoxin from **18**, 152
Brabender amylograph **41**, 167
Bradyrhizobium japonicum **44**, 200
Bragg Peak **15**, 75
Brain, lipids, *n*-3 PUFA deprivation **35**, 121
–, α-LNA conversion **35**, 74–78
–, neural network model **40**, 333–334
–, of meat animals **6**, 133
–, vitamin B6 **40**, 112
Brain tissue, distribution of DDT in **2**, 210
–, α-tocopherol turnover **33**, 187
Bran, analysis **31**, 150, 152, 153
–, cereal, effect on calcium absorption **33**, 138–139
–, dietary fiber and **31**, 120, 127, 133, 136, 138
–, intestinal bacteria **31**, 172, 174, 178, 179, 182–185, 187–189
–, of wheat kernel **23**, 193–194
–, phytic acid content **28**, 14
–, properties **31**, 158, 160, 165, 168, 170, 171
–, wheat, effect on, calcium absorption **33**, 137–138
–, –, tocopherol bioavailability **33**, 172–173
Branching enzymes, assay **41**, 89, 91–92
–, characterization **41**, 89
–, genes **41**, 95–98
–, mode of action **41**, 93–95
–, C_4 plants **41**, 150
–, purification **41**, 92–93
–, structure-function **41**, 101–103
Branching-linkage assay **41**, 91–92
Brandy, production of **17**, 94
Brazil, annual agricultural and forestry harvest **32**, 193
–, annual biomass production **32**, 192
–, biomass energy used **32**, 191
–, biomass resources **32**, 190–194
–, ethanol production **32**, 202–204, 211–215
–, forest utilization **32**, 194
–, gross national product **32**, 189
–, IM meat **39**, 82
–, land distribution by use **32**, 190
–, soil erosion in **32**, 216–221
Brazil nuts **16**, 72
–, leuco-anthocyanins **5**, 288
Bread (*see also* Dough *and* Wheat flour) **14**, 239–240; **15**, 289; **16**, 335ff
–, aldehydes during fermentation and baking **30**, 100–102
–, aroma, effects of amino acids and sugars **30**, 101–102
–, ascorbic acid addition to **18**, 272–277
–, as mouth rinse in flavor judgments **2**, 248
–, baking, amino acid changes during **19**, 197

Bread, baking (*cont'd*)
–, –, enzymes in **16**, 428
–, baking canned **6**, 269
–, baking tests **29**, 206–211
–, Boston brown **3**, 134
–, bromates in **16**, 371
–, canned, spoilage of **7**, 121–122
–, carbohydrates **16**, 382ff
–, crumb, internal structure of **8**, 121
–, dough **8**, 15
–, –, freezing storage of **6**, 197
–, –, thiamine in **6**, 266
–, –, use of ascorbic acid in **4**, 406–407
–, "dough softening factor" in **3**, 81, 82
–, effect of preparation on nutritive value of protein **4**, 247
–, enzymic changes in **11**, 291–292
–, flavor chemistry of **19**, 198–202
–, heat treatment of skim milk in **3**, 80–83
–, lipids **16**, 397ff, 410ff
–, loaf volume, depression in **3**, 81
–, –, effect of lipids in flours **29**, 251–258
–, loss of thiamine in **6**, 264, 265, 271, 296
–, manufactured from radar-treated flour **3**, 135
–, microbial inhibition in by propionic acid **1**, 387
–, milk powder use in making of **19**, 149–152
–, odor producing factors in **2**, 276
–, packaged, sterilization of **3**, 134
–, phytic acid content **28**, 15
–, proteins **16**, 343ff
–, quality **16**, 340ff, 357, 386ff
–, quality related milk proteins in **19**, 170–181
–, shortening effect on **16**, 414
–, staling **8**, 30; **16**, 387
–, sulfur amino acid role in **19**, 179–180
–, testing **16**, 337ff
–, ultrasonic texture sensing **45**, 146, 147
–, volatiles, identification **30**, 101
Breadfruit, anatomy of **17**, 170
Breadmaking (*see also* Glutenin high-molecular-weight subunits), effect of wheat flour composition proteins **29**, 246–251
–, – of –, starch **29**, 262
–, – of –, water solubles **29**, 261
–, glycolipid–wheat flour interaction with, in baking **20**, 153–188
–, –, in protein-enriched bread **20**, 178–184
–, –, mechanism **20**, 166–167
–, –, practical implications **20**, 175–178
–, inositol phosphates degradation **45**, 16, 20
–, phytic acid destruction and **28**, 55–60
–, seed storage proteins **36**, 131–133
Break-point approach, *see* Linear system *and* Rectilinear approach
Break-point chlorination, definition of **7**, 143–145
Breast cancer, carcinogen risk assessment and **31**, 15, 17, 20, 22
–, effects of lactic cultures **37**, 106–107
Breast feeding, effects on gastrointestinal immune system **37**, 45
Breast milk, fatty acid composition **35**, 153–154
–, lipids **35**, 62–64
Breeding, wheat for flour baking quality **29**, 211–213
Brevibacterium epidermidis **44**, 213
Brewery wastes **17**, 128–131
–, as animal feeds **17**, 130
Brewing, scanning electron microscopy of **22**, 278–281
Brewing industry, use of quaternary ammonium compounds in **2**, 175
Brick cheese **39**, 287
Brie cheese **39**, 199, 200, 224, 288
Brightness-discrimination test **35**, 124–125
Brik Pak filler **32**, 17
Brine **12**, 149, 161, 165–167; **15**, 305, 355
–, fish preservation and **7**, 68
Brix/acid ratio **9**, 289, 291, 295, 297, 307
Broad beans **16**, 9, 67
Broccoli, calcium content of, effect of limestone on **1**, 310
–, changes in unblanched, frozen **8**, 97
–, decrease in bacterial content by blanching **6**, 184
–, frozen **6**, 176
–, loss of ascorbic acid during blanching of **8**, 89
–, ozone treatment **45**, 192
Bromates, effects on wheat germ **23**, 278
–, in bread **16**, 371
Bromelin, in pineapple **17**, 188
Bromide, in wines **8**, 142
Bromine, as oxidizing agent for cation exchangers **2**, 6
Bromoacetate, inhibition of enzymes by **1**, 382
Bromophenol blue color test for quaternary ammonium compounds **2**, 167
Bronchodilators, smell sensation effects **44**, 322
–, taste sensation effects **44**, 301–302
Brown core **15**, 179
Brown heart **12**, 124

Browning **14**, 267–268; **39**, 128–129, 132, 134, 135, 141, 275
–, bisulfites as inhibitors of **3**, 273
–, carbonyl-amine, freeze-dried beef and **7**, 213, 214
–, –, freeze-dried fruits and **7**, 224
–, chemical manifestations of **3**, 103
–, dependence on system water content **12**, 44
–, effect of pH on **3**, 273
–, enzymatic **17**, 18–19
–, –, inhibition by sulfiting agents, ascorbate oxidase and **30**, 11
–, fields for further study **12**, 45–46
–, flavors, odors **14**, 235–244
–, freeze-dried lemon juice and **7**, 228
–, gelatin color and **7**, 247
–, increase with pH **12**, 45
–, – with temperature **12**, 44
–, in dried egg white **3**, 273
–, in foods (*see also* Food browning) **10**, 10, 30–31, 43, 54, 60–61, 87, 117, 191–193
–, in frozen fruits **17**, 4
–, in fruit products **1**, 325–369
–, –, chemical changes during **1**, 346–360
–, –, color measurement of **1**, 328–329
–, –, factors influencing color development during **1**, 329–346
–, –, inhibition of **1**, 360–369
–, –, reaction, active aldehyde theory of **1**, 327
–, –, –, ascorbic acid theory of **1**, 327
–, –, –, Maillard theory of **1**, 327, 351, 354
–, in fruits (*see also* Fruit) **12**, 45
–, inhibition **14**, 245–262
–, inhibitors, meat mutagens and **34**, 423
–, in milk products **3**, 99, 100
–, in shoyu, during brewing **30**, 244–251
–, –, during storage **30**, 252–257
–, in xylose and glycine solution, shoyu addition and **30**, 248
–, lipoxygenase and **30**, 11
–, mutagenicity in model system sugar–ammonia **30**, 122
–, *N*-nitroso compounds and **31**, 55, 56
–, nonamino **14**, 227–234, 265–266
–, nonenzymatic (*see also* Maillard reactions) **12**, 1–52; **14**, 167–283
–, –, activation energies **35**, 196–197
–, –, cathode ray experiments with **3**, 180–184
–, –, inhibition by sulfiting agents **30**, 9–10
–, –, – by –, sulfite–carbonyl reaction products **30**, 9, 22–23
–, nutrient loss, limited **30**, 120–122
–, –, lipid peroxidation and **30**, 121
–, –, lysine and **30**, 120–121
–, –, protein digestibility and **30**, 121
–, –, total amino acids **30**, 121
–, oxidative, freeze-dried beef and **7**, 213
–, polyphenoloxidase and **30**, 10
–, quinone–sulfite complexes **30**, 10
–, rate **12**, 44–45
–, reaction (*see* also Maillard browning), antioxidants from
–, –, discovery
–, –, final stage
–, –, initial stage
–, –, intermediate stage
–, –, mechanisms
–, –, mutagen formation
–, –, nonsugar
–, sulfite–carbonyl reaction products **30**, 22–23
–, temperature coefficients in **3**, 102
–, variation with amino acids **12**, 45
Brown rot **15**, 173
Brucella abortus, germicidal action of CPCl on **2**, 152
–, in milk **2**, 82
Brucella maletensis in milk **2**, 82
Brucella suis in milk **2**, 82
Brush border **41**, 158
Brush border membrane **40**, 197–199, 200–204
Brushes (or rakes) in spray dryer **2**, 492
Brusine, effect of ion size on adsorption of **2**, 11–12
Brussel sprouts, blanching of **8**, 85
–, chlorination **45**, 188
–, effect of blanching on **1**, 68
–, loss of thiamine on processing **6**, 287
–, pH of **3**, 432
BS integrator, *see* Bulirsch Stoer integrator
Btl gene **41**, 120
Buckwheat **44**, 395–419
–, allergy **44**, 408–409
–, breeding programmes **44**, 397
–, component studies **44**, 409–410
–, culture of utilization **44**, 399–400
–, flour composition **44**, 402–408
–, –, carbohydrate **44**, 405–406
–, –, dietary fiber **44**, 406
–, –, enzymes/enzyme inhibitors **44**, 405
–, –, lipid **44**, 406–407
–, –, minerals **44**, 407–408
–, –, protein **44**, 403–405
–, –, rutin **44**, 408

Buckwheat, flour composition (*cont'd*)
–, –, vitamins **44**, 408
–, flour fractions **44**, 402, 416–417
–, fluorescent dye found in **1**, 125
–, mechanical properties of products **44**, 416–417
–, milling **44**, 402
–, molecular basis of palatability **44**, 416–418
–, nutritional stress factor in **4**, 111–113
–, processing **44**, 410–416
–, –, China **44**, 413 414
–, –, Europe **44**, 414–415
–, –, groats **44**, 413, 414
–, –, Japan **44**, 412–413, 417
–, –, Korea **44**, 414
–, –, noodle technology **44**, 410–411
–, –, North America **44**, 415–416
–, –, Russia **44**, 414–415
–, quality characteristics **44**, 398
–, research approaches **44**, 418–419
–, storage-related changes **44**, 417–418
–, taxonomic/phylogenetic studies **44**, 397
–, varieties **44**, 396–398
–, worldwide cultivation **44**, 398–399
–, worldwide names **44**, 401–402
Buckwheat starch, gelatinization temperature of **2**, 319
Budding, chocolate and **31**, 323
Buffering capacity **39**, 175–176
Buflovak spray dryer, operation of **2**, 402–403
Bulbs **15**, 179
Bulgarican **43**, 14
Bulirsch Stoer integrator **40**, 290, 297, 299–303
Bulk density control in spray-drying **2**, 471–477
Bulk pack **32**, 10–13, 21, 33–34
Bulk tank **32**, 13–14, 23
Bundle sheath **41**, 150
Buspirone **44**, 310, 323
n-Butanol in apples **2**, 263
Butorphanol **44**, 294
Butter **16**, 196, 198ff
–, ascorbic acid as antioxidant for **18**, 292–294
–, bacterial count in freezing storage **6**, 193
–, blending and mixing of **8**, 13
–, cocoa (*see* also Cocoa butter)
–, –, composition of
–, DDT in **2**, 212, 214
–, effect of quality on sensory tests **2**, 230
–, effects on serum lipoproteins and apolipoproteins **37**, 166–170
–, flavor in candies **6**, 31
–, flavor studies on **19**, 234
–, in diets **1**, 109
–, off-flavors and **7**, 25
–, spreadability of **8**, 16
–, theory of the working of **8**, 11
–, vector tests on **8**, 23
Butter creams, butter in **6**, 20
–, stability of fats in **6**, 13
Butterfat, as source of dietary fat **37**, 168–169
–, chocolate and **31**, 311
–, lactones and methyl ketones in **19**, 191
Buttermilk, in muffins **6**, 272
Buttermilk powder (BMP), amino acids **19**, 158
–, composition of **19**, 154
–, lipids in **19**, 187
–, minerals and salts in **19**, 194
–, production and utilization of **19**, 150
–, vitamins in **19**, 192
Butter oil, fishy flavors in **4**, 191
–, oxidation of in milk **3**, 71
Butterscotch, stability of fats in **6**, 12
Butyl alcohol, in black tea **2**, 288
N-Butyl alcohol, solubility of DDT in **2**, 203
Butylamine, effect on browning in orange juice **1**, 354
Butylated hydroxyanisole (BHA), as antioxidant **33**, 309–310
–, inhibition of lipoxygenase **33**, 307
–, *N*-nitroso compounds and **31**, 64, 81
–, pathologic effects of **3**, 207
–, toxicity of as an antioxidant **3**, 201
Butylated hydroxytoluene (BHT), inhibition of lipoxygenase **33**, 307
–, *N*-nitroso compounds and **31**, 64, 81
Butyl-catechol, 4-tertiary, in respiration of plant tissues **3**, 14
Butyl crotonyl mustard oil sulfide in radish **2**, 274
2-*tert*-Butyl-4-methoxyphenol **15**, 5, 11, 22, 40
3-*tert*-Butyl-4-methoxyphenol **15**, 5, 11, 22, 40
Butyraldehyde in Formosan black tea oil **2**, 287
Butyric acid **16**, 185
–, esters in parsley seed oil **2**, 274
–, fish spoilage and **7**, 48
–, in carrot seed oil **2**, 271
–, in decomposing salmon **2**, 371
–, in tea leaves **2**, 285, 287
–, microbial inhibition by **1**, 387
Butyric acid bacteria, effect of pH on growth of **3**, 431

Butyric esters of ethyl alcohol in strawberries **2**, 260
Byssochlamic acid, from *Byssochlamys* spp. **25**, 267–272
Byssochlamys **25**, 237–288
–, ascospores of **25**, 252–264
–, –, activation **25**, 255–256
–, –, germination **25**, 256–258
–, –, inactivitation **25**, 258–264
–, –, production **25**, 252–253
–, classification and nomenclature of **25**, 238–243
–, detection and enumeration of **25**, 277–280
–, distribution and sources of contamination from **25**, 242–244
–, enzymes of **25**, 264–267
–, growth of, control **25**, 248–252
–, –, factors affecting **25**, 246–248
–, imperfect state of **25**, 240–242
–, in processed fruits **25**, 237–288
–, metabolic activities of **25**, 252–277
–, mycotoxins of **25**, 267–277
–, occurrence of **25**, 244–245
–, perfect state of **25**, 238–240
–, research needs on **25**, 280–281
–, spoilage from **25**, 242–252
Byssochlamys fulva, growth inhibition by SO_2 **5**, 125, 126
–, heat resistance of **3**, 436
Byssotoxin A, from *Byssochlamys* spp. **25**, 276–277

β-C metabolism, *see* β-Carotene metabolism
C_4 plants **41**, 148–150
Ca^{2+}, intracellular, imaging following stimulation by sweeteners **42**, 225, 227
CAAT box **36**, 97
Cabbage, analysis for SO_2 **5**, 119
–, ascorbic acid content of, effect of blanching on **1**, 77
–, –, – of fertilizers on **1**, 309
–, –, – of season and location on **1**, 295–297
–, ascorbic acid in **10**, 235–236
–, blanching of **2**, 333
–, –, changes during **8**, 87
–, chemical constituents in **10**, 269–273
–, chlorination **45**, 188
–, chloroplasts in **2**, 306
–, decrease in bacterial content by blanching **6**, 184
–, dehydrated, thiamine loss in **6**, 300
–, dehydration of **3**, 143
–, dicotyledonous plants **31**, 126, 127, 129, 130, 132, 133
–, dietary fiber and **31**, 146, 166
–, dried, enzymic changes in **11**, 287
–, gelatinization of starch in **2**, 323
–, inositol phosphate content **45**, 23
–, intestinal bacteria **31**, 178, 186
–, lignification in **2**, 304
–, loss of thiamine on processing **6**, 287
–, minor vitamins in **10**, 239–240
–, nutritional stress factor in **4**, 112–113
–, parenchyma cells in **2**, 304
–, pH of red **3**, 432
–, – of Savoy **3**, 432
–, – of White **3**, 432
–, potash in soil effects on **10**, 265–266
–, products, ascorbic acid addition to **18**, 237
–, puree, thiamine destruction **6**, 292
–, sulfiting **5**, 142
–, sulfur compounds in **10**, 266–269
CACA box, 7S globulins **36**, 105
Cacao, *see* Cocoa
Cachana (*Liatris punctata*) **45**, 77
Cachexia, carcinogen risk assessment and **31**, 24
Cadaverine, cheese **39**, 234
–, fish **39**, 337–345, 349–356, 358
–, fish spoilage and **7**, 46
–, in putrid abalone **23**, 166
Cadinene in peaches **2**, 265
Cadmium, in wine **8**, 174
Cadmium–inositol phosphate interactions **45**, 32
Caffeic acids, inhibition of soybean lipoxygenase **33**, 317
–, olive oil and **31**, 467
Caffeine, effects of **17**, 234–235
–, in cocoa beans and nibs **6**, 38
–, in coffee **2**, 279
–, –, loss of **3**, 177
–, in tea **2**, 286; **11**, 217–218; **17**, 234
–, in tea plant **11**, 232
–, structure **17**, 234
–, synthesis **17**, 236
Cake mixes, enzymic changes in **11**, 290–291
–, radar cooking of **3**, 140
Cakes **15**, 260
–, baking tests **29**, 211
–, crumbliness of **8**, 35
–, internal structure of **8**, 121
–, quality, effect of lipids in wheat flours **29**, 260–261
–, wheat germ use in **23**, 284
Caking **38**, 209–210

Calandria pans **15**, 324
Calcification, abnormal, collagen and elastin **37**, 401
Calcitonin **44**, 315
Calcium **16**, 233, 252
–, absorption, *see* Calcium absorption
–, amount required for gelation of low-solids gels **1**, 416–420
–, balance, *see* Calcium balance
–, binding, α-lactalbumin **33**, 354–356
–, bioavailability, *see* Calcium bioavailability
–, chocolate and **31**, 257, 270, 284
–, concentrations in intra- and extracellular fluids **33**, 112–114
–, cytosolic free concentrations **33**, 112
–, decreased absorption of in rickets **1**, 132
–, deficiency **1**, 120
–, dietary fiber and, components **31**, 120, 140
–, –, dicotyledonous plants **31**, 129, 131
–, –, properties **31**, 155, 158, 164
–, dietary sources **36**, 214
–, effect of blanching on **8**, 66
–, effects on β-lactoglobulin gels **33**, 388
–, – on low-ester pectins **1**, 415
–, – on thermal denaturation behavior of whey proteins **33**, 379–381
–, – on whey protein foams **33**, 401
–, endogenous proteolytic enzymes and **31**, 347, 357
–, –, endopeptidases **31**, 353, 354, 360, 362
–, –, meat technology **31**, 396, 397, 400, 403, 408, 409
–, –, muscle physiology **31**, 377, 379–381
–, –, nonmuscle cathepsins **31**, 365
–, –, proteinase activity **31**, 386, 391
–, homeostasis **33**, 112–114
–, in mechanically deboned red meat **27**, 84–86
–, in milk **36**, 213–218
–, in muscle chemistry **9**, 26–28
–, inositol phosphate effects **45**, 27, 29, 30–31
–, inositol(1,4,5)PU3u signaling **45**, 27–28
–, intake, by parathyroidectomized rats **1**, 123
–, –, long term **33**, 112
–, –, milk avoidance and **38**, 4
–, –, table of **33**, 106
–, –, within groups **33**, 105–106
–, in wines **8**, 135, 137, 138, 139, 174
–, ion exchange in chemical reactions with **2**, 10
–, pigs fed diet deficient in **1**, 111
–, plasma concentrations **33**, 112–114
–, Recommended Dietary Allowance **33**, 105–106, 108–112
–, removal from milk **2**, 21–24
–, – from sugar beet juice **2**, 27
–, sequestration **39**, 263–265, 270
–, structural distribution **36**, 213
–, sulfate, added to musts **8**, 158
Calcium absorption **36**, 216–217
–, dietary requirements and **33**, 118–119
–, during development **33**, 115–116
–, effects of, cereals **33**, 136–139
–, –, complexation by ligands yielding soluble complexes **33**, 146–147
–, –, fruit and vegetable fiber **33**, 139–141
–, –, protein and phosphates **33**, 143–144
–, –, purified fibers **33**, 141–142
–, –, supplements **33**, 144–147
–, from CCM **33**, 147
–, impairment **45**, 32, 35
–, inulin/fructooligosaccharide effects **43**, 32, 33, 34, 43
–, mechanisms **33**, 114–117
–, net absorption, calculation **33**, 121–122
–, net amount to balance urinary losses **33**, 111
–, regulation **33**, 114–117
Calcium-activated factor **31**, 357
Calcium-activated neutral proteinase **31**, 412–414
–, endopeptidases **31**, 357–360
–, meat technology **31**, 403, 404, 407–409
–, muscle physiology **31**, 379, 380, 382
–, proteinase activity **31**, 390
–, proteinase distribution **31**, 369
Calcium balance, definition **33**, 108, 121
–, excretion and **33**, 108
–, in males **33**, 111
–, in perimenopausal women **33**, 110–111
–, measurement of calcium bioavailability with **33**, 121–122
–, measurements **33**, 108
Calcium bioavailability **36**, 215–216
–, definition **33**, 119–120
–, diet effects on urinary excretion **33**, 120
–, effects of, fiber and phytate **33**, 134–142
–, –, oxalic acid **33**, 142
–, –, protein and phosphates **33**, 143–144
–, –, supplements **33**, 144–147
–, lactose effect **33**, 124–125
–, –, in animals **33**, 125–126
–, –, in elderly subjects **33**, 134
–, –, in human infants **33**, 132–134
–, –, in humans **33**, 128–132
–, measurement **33**, 120–121

–, –, animal models **33**, 124
–, –, balance methods **33**, 121–122
–, –, isotopic labeling of foods **33**, 123–124
–, –, isotopic tracer techniques **33**, 122–123
Calcium carbonate, for molding hard creams **6**, 36
Calcium chloride, effect of treating potatoes with **1**, 272
–, effect on canned foods **2**, 315–316
–, freeze-dried fruits and **7**, 224
–, gelatin manufacture and **7**, 240
Calcium content, of apples and pears **8**, 371, 386
–, of canned foods **1**, 44, 48
–, of plants, effect of fertilizers on **1**, 310–314, 318–319
–, of various foods, table **33**, 106–107
Calcium ion, intracellular, in malignant hyperexia **37**, 386–387
–, role in protein stability **35**, 254
Calcium lactate in diet of rats **1**, 112
Calcium malate in apple juice **2**, 15
Calcium pectate, molecular shapes and interactions **42**, 169–172
Calcium salts, effect of removal from potato tuber **2**, 316
–, water solubility and calcium content, table **33**, 145
Calcium sulfate, in inhibition of can corrosion **3**, 343
Caldolysin, thermal stability **35**, 255
Calf **14**, 40
Calipers, use in flexible-package seal defect detection **23**, 409
Callus **41**, 128
Callus culture, chocolate and **31**, 320–328
Calmodulin, endogenous proteolytic enzymes and **31**, 379
Caloric output, relationship to appetite **1**, 129–130
Calories, carcinogen risk assessment and **31**, 20, 22
–, chocolate and **31**, 267, 268, 272–274
Calorimetry, differential scanning **41**, 167–168
–, indirect **40**, 171, 172, 178–179
–, room **40**, 171, 172
Camas lily (*Camassia quamash*) **43**, 40
Camembert cheese, contamination **39**, 287, 288
–, lactate **39**, 198, 199, 200
–, proteinases **39**, 224
–, ripening **39**, 255
–, texture **39**, 254
–, ultrafiltration **39**, 194
Camera **14**, 6–7, 11
Ca^{2+}/Mg^{2+} ATPase, *n*-3 PUFA effects **35**, 129–131
Camosine, role in histamine toxicity **24**, 141–142
cAMP, as second messenger in sweet-taste transduction **42**, 223
–, Δ^6-desaturase, regulation effects **35**, 44–45
Campesterol, olive oil and **31**, 467, 473
CAM plants **41**, 150–152
Campylobacter **45**, 193
–, foodborne illness **44**, 152, 162
Campylobacter coli **44**, 162
Campylobacter fetus **44**, 162
Campylobacter jejuni **44**, 162
Can, heating food in **32**, 40–42
–, surface roughness in **32**, 74
Canada, ascorbic acid regulations for food in **18**, 297–302
Cancer (*see also specific cancers*) **40**, 57
–, dietary fiber and **31**, 190
–, epidemiological studies **34**, 388–389
–, intestinal tract **37**, 24–25
–, *N*-nitroso compounds and **31**, 100
–, *n*-3 PUFA effects **35**, 143–146
–, risk factors, breast cancer **37**, 211–212
–, –, colon cancer **37**, 212–213
–, –, milk- and dairy product-related, animal studies **37**, 219–223
–, –, research needs **37**, 237
–, suppression, effects of lactic cultures **37**, 99–107, 119–120
Cancer patients, flavor-enhanced food preferences **44**, 330
–, learned food aversions **44**, 280
–, smell/taste perception changes **44**, 275–280
Cancer-protective effects, lignans **44**, 230–231
–, phytoestrogens **44**, 229–232
–, soy bean isoflavones **44**, 229–230
Candida, as sources of protein **18**, 90–116
Candida albicans, germicidal action of CPCl on **2**, 152
Candidal vaginitis, effects of *Lactobacillus acidophilus* cultures **37**, 112–114
Candida utilis, nutritional analyses **18**, 108
Candida versatilis, salt-tolerant, in mash **30**, 230, 232
Candied products, desulfiting **5**, 127
Candies, from kiwifruit peeled slices **29**, 306–307
Candy, chemical composition of **6**, 10

Candy (*cont'd*)
–, color **6**, 8
–, insects infesting **4**, 307
–, made from fruit juices **6**, 28
–, manufacture **6**, 1
–, physical properties **6**, 6
–, production methods **6**, 48
–, rheology of **8**, 36
–, sugar **8**, 36
–, toffee **8**, 37
Canned foods, chlorine and **7**, 131–133
–, mineral composition of **1**, 44, 48
–, preservation of **7**, 121–122
–, use of ascorbic acid in **4**, 367–371
Canned fruit, ascorbic acid addition to **18**, 254–255
Canned meat products, reprocessing **34**, 422
Canning **15**, 239
–, effect on vitamin content **1**, 52–89
–, filling operations **45**, 130
–, kiwifruit, effect on chemical composition **29**, 294, 299
–, –, technique **29**, 299–300
–, meat mutagens formation **34**, 422–423
–, of abalone **23**, 171–172
–, phytate degradation **45**, 16
Canning operations, materials added in **3**, 350–352
–, sterilization developments in **3**, 440–441
–, variations produced by **3**, 345–350
Cans, comparison with flexible packages **23**, 402
Cantaloupes, ascorbic acid content of, effect of nitrogen on **1**, 309
–, –, – of sunlight on **1**, 302
Canthaxanthin **15**, 210, 246, 253; **43**, 210
–, adverse reactions **43**, 210–211
Capacola **39**, 79
Capillary, IM meat drying **39**, 104
Capillary chromatography, inositol phosphates **45**, 6
Capillary condensation, in muscle fiber **10**, 359, 362
Capillary membrane (*see also* Membrane transport *and* Membrane vesicle) **40**, 184
Capillary-strengthening effect, *see* Vitamin P
Capillary system, of muscle **19**, 12–13
Capillary tube geometry **39**, 24–26
Capillary zone electrophoresis, phytoestrogens **44**, 202
Caproaldehyde, in apples **2**, 263
–, in Formosan black tea **2**, 287
Caproic acid, in apples **2**, 262, 263
–, in parsnip seed oil **2**, 274
–, in raspberries **2**, 269
–, in strawberries **2**, 270
–, in tea leaves **2**, 285, 287
Caprylic acid, effect on cell membrane **1**, 387
–, in apples **2**, 263
–, in black tea oil **2**, 297
–, in orange peel oil **2**, 265
–, –, esters of **2**, 265
–, in peaches **2**, 265
Capsaicin, age-related taste threshold **44**, 257–260
Capsanthin **15**, 246
Capsorubin **15**, 246
Capsules, bacterial **43**, 321–322
–, gelatin and **7**, 326
Captopril **44**, 304
Caramelan, product of sugar decomposition **6**, 16
Caramel coloring agent **43**, 196
Caramelization, chocolate and, milk **31**, 253, 255, 257, 260
–, milk crumb **31**, 284, 287, 288, 290
Caramels, chemical composition and properties of **6**, 10
–, drying **6**, 7
–, ingredients in **6**, 29
–, stability of fats in **6**, 12
Caraway, monterpenes **42**, 250
Carbamazepine **44**, 310
Carbenicillin **44**, 289
Carbimazole **44**, 298, 322
Carbohydrate metabolism **41**, 144–145
–, effect on appetite **1**, 131, 132
Carbohydrate nutrition **39**, 278
Carbohydrates **12**, 119; **14**, 215–218
–, chlorine and **7**, 153
–, chocolate and **31**, 247, 326
–, collagen, interactions with **28**, 260–261
–, contribution to meat flavor **18**, 38–39
–, decomposition **16**, 203
–, dietary fiber and, analysis **31**, 143, 145, 146, 148, 149, 152, 153
–, –, components **31**, 124, 125
–, –, dicotyledonous plants **31**, 126, 129, 132–135
–, –, intestinal bacteria **31**, 180, 183, 186, 188
–, –, monocotyledonous plants **31**, 136, 138
–, –, properties **31**, 169
–, effect on calcium absorption **33**, 130–131
–, glass transition temperature **38**, 148–149
–, halophilic bacteria and **7**, 113
–, in bread **16**, 382ff
–, in cheese **16**, 250

–, in citrus juices, pectic substances **9**, 303–304
–, –, sugars **9**, 302–303
–, in citrus pulps and peels **9**, 304–307
–, in cocoa beans **6**, 38; **8**, 262
–, in dough **16**, 421
–, in fruits **17**, 182–183
–, in honey **24**, 299–304
–, in milk powders **19**, 183–187
–, in passion fruit **12**, 236–237, 258, 267
–, in plants, winter hardiness and **25**, 204–205
–, in soy sauce **10**, 82
–, in tea **17**, 231–233
–, in wheat germ **23**, 204, 230–232
–, in wine **6**, 86
–, licorice root and **7**, 342–343
–, loss in blanching of vegetables **8**, 71
–, low-molecular-weight, disparity **38**, 229
–, –, C'_g values **38**, 167–168
–, olive oil and **31**, 463
–, radiation effects on **24**, 174
–, role in lactobacilli adherence **37**, 76
–, solute-specific subzero glass transition temperature **38**, 139
Carbohydrate–water systems, kinetically metastable, WLF behavior **38**, 189
Carbon **14**, 287–289
–, chocolate and **31**, 254
–, *N*-nitroso compounds and **31**, 65
Carbonated beverages, ascorbic acid addition to **18**, 232–234
Carbon bisulfide, use in infrared chemical analysis **3**, 147
Carbon dioxide **14**, 234; **16**, 265
–, added to air **12**, 130–132
–, – to –, by dry ice **12**, 131–132
–, and functional disorders **12**, 111–116
–, chilled beef on ships **12**, 172–173
–, control of fruit ripening **12**, 96
–, delay of fungal rotting **12**, 109–111
–, effects in supernormal concentrations **12**, 98–109
–, – in –, apple **12**, 99
–, – in –, apricot **12**, 99–100
–, – in –, banana **12**, 100–101
–, – in –, blackberry **12**, 101
–, – in –, black currant **12**, 101
–, – in –, cherry **12**, 102
–, – in –, grape **12**, 103
–, – in –, limits of safe treatment **12**, 98–99
–, – in –, peach **12**, 103
–, – in –, pear **12**, 103
–, – in –, plum **12**, 104–105
–, – in –, raspberry **12**, 105
–, – in –, strawberry **12**, 105
–, – in –, vegetables **12**, 108
–, efficiency **12**, 110
–, energy expenditure **40**, 173–175, 177–178
–, equilibria in milk powder **3**, 60
–, evolution **12**, 37–38
–, fish preservation and **7**, 70–71
–, formation during browning in fruit products **1**, 344–345, 346–948, 350–352, 356, 358, 360
–, formation in tea **11**, 220
–, influence on post-harvest physiology **12**, 116–127
–, inhibiting effect on germination **3**, 444–445
–, in irradiated fruits **15**, 68
–, in packaging of milk products **3**, 86, 88
–, in sparkling wines **8**, 136
–, in spoiled table wines **6**, 76
–, in spoiling fish **2**, 370
–, in wines **6**, 71; **8**, 143
–, ozone combined sanitization procedures **45**, 201–202
–, packaging dehydrated potatoes in **1**, 271–272
–, production in dehydrated potatoes **1**, 276–276
–, – in dry milk products **3**, 100 101, 102
–, – in passion fruits **12**, 226
–, relationship to ripening in fruit **3**, 17
–, transport and storage **12**, 95–146
–, use in processing fruit juices **9**, 250–251
–, water requirements and **7**, 110
Carbon dioxide–oxygen mixtures >50% **12**, 124
Carbon monoxide, as inhibitor **17**, 53
–, freeze-dried beef and **7**, 212
–, inhibition of enzyme activity by **1**, 384
Carbon suboxide, use in detecting amino groups **1**, 383
Carbon tetrachloride **15**, 38
–, solubility of DDT in **2**, 203
Carbon-13 tracer **40**, 64–75, 171–172
Carbon transport **41**, 119–124
Carbonyl-amine reactions **35**, 189–201
–, chemistry **35**, 189–191
–, Maillard reaction, factors affecting degree **35**, 195–199
–, –, protein digestibility and biological availability **35**, 200–201
–, reactive lysine measurement methods **35**, 192–195
Carbonyl compounds, formation in onion **22**, 101

Carbonyl compounds (*cont'd*)
–, freeze-dried beef and **7**, 213
–, from acyl hydroperoxides, table **33**, 265
–, volatile flavor compounds from lipid oxidation, of biological tissue, table **33**, 274
–, – from –, of fish tissues, table **33**, 275
Carbonyls (*see also individual carbonyls*), contribution to meat flavor **18**, 39–40, 53–54
–, in peas **17**, 6
–, in potato products **25**, 105
–, production of **17**, 29
–, reactions with sulfites **30**, 9, 22–23
–, unsaturated, in peas **17**, 32
Carboplatin **44**, 293
Carbopol **12**, 340–349
–, applications **12**, 344–346
–, –, cosmetics **12**, 345–346
–, –, pharmaceuticals **12**, 344–345
–, background **12**, 340–342
–, –, neutralized resin **12**, 341
–, properties **12**, 342–344
–, –, aging **12**, 343
–, –, compatibility **12**, 343
–, –, effect of pH **12**, 342
–, –, toxicology **12**, 343
Carboxyhemoglobin **7**, 212
Carboxylesterase, cardiolipin association **37**, 287
Carboxyl groups, dietary fiber and **31**, 163–165
–, endogenous proteolytic enzymes and **31**, 361
–, esterification of by epoxides **1**, 383
–, in pectin **1**, 398
Carboxylic acids **16**, 253, 259ff
–, in melanin formation **3**, 23
–, in rye bread **2**, 276
–, *N*-nitroso compounds and **31**, 83, 84
Carboxyl proteinases, endogenous proteolytic enzymes and **31**, 352
Carboxymethylcellulose, dietary fiber and **31**, 158, 161, 167, 191
–, solution viscosity, instrumental readings **29**, 183
–, –, perceived **29**, 183
Carboxymethylhydroxyethylcellulose **12**, 331–332
Carboxypeptidases, endogenous proteolytic enzymes and **31**, 345, 412
–, endopeptidases **31**, 362
–, meat technology **31**, 411
–, skeletal muscles **31**, 346–348, 350–352
Carcass, composition **14**, 55
–, cooling **21**, 137–138, 158–159
–, grade **14**, 52–55
–, measurements **14**, 111–112
–, tenderness **14**, 54
Carcinogens, dietary fiber and **31**, 173
–, intestinal microflora metabolism **43**, 13, 35, 36
–, nitrosamines as **22**, 27–32
–, *N*-nitroso compounds and **31**, 54, 98, 100
–, –, fundamentals **31**, 64, 66, 72
–, –, nitrite/nitrate addition **31**, 74
–, –, processing **31**, 91
–, risk assessment **31**, 2–4, 41, 42
–, –, early approaches **31**, 7, 8
–, –, epidemiology, air pollution **31**, 39
–, –, –, estimates **31**, 39, 40
–, –, –, testing hypothesis **31**, 38
–, –, IARC approach **31**, 10–12
–, –, individual **31**, 5, 6
–, –, laboratory data **31**, 34–38
–, –, –, animals **31**, 24–26
–, –, –, dose conversions **31**, 33, 34
–, –, –, dose–response data **31**, 29–33
–, –, –, long-term bioassays **31**, 26–28
–, –, –, short-term tests **31**, 28, 29
–, –, National Academy of Sciences report **31**, 8, 9
–, –, problems **31**, 9, 10
–, –, rare events **31**, 4, 5
–, –, regulatory effects **31**, 6, 7
–, –, research needs **31**, 42, 43
–, –, –, epidemiology **31**, 47, 48
–, –, –, exposures **31**, 45–47
–, –, –, immune system **31**, 44, 45
–, –, –, model systems **31**, 43, 44
–, –, statistics **31**, 13, 14
–, –, –, causes **31**, 14–17
–, –, –, diet **31**, 23, 24
–, –, –, food **31**, 20–23
–, –, –, industrial exposure **31**, 19, 20
–, –, –, proportion **31**, 17–19
–, –, –, specific agents **31**, 12, 13
–, xylitol as possible **25**, 173–174
Carcinomas, connective tissue **37**, 404–405
–, *N*-nitroso compounds and **31**, 64
Cardiac muscle, effects of DDT on **2**, 207
Cardiolipin, acyl changes, effects of, development **37**, 297
–, –, –, ethanol administration **37**, 297
–, –, –, external temperature **37**, 299
–, –, –, hyperthyroidism **37**, 297–298
–, –, –, malignancy **37**, 298–299
–, –, –, membrane fluidity **37**, 299
–, acyl composition **37**, 289–290

–, –, factors affecting **37**, 289
–, –, interspecific differences **37**, 290
–, –, uniqueness **37**, 289–290
–, acyl-specific derivatives, chemical synthesis **37**, 314–317
–, adriamycin association **37**, 287–288
–, analogs, binding to aCLs **37**, 310–312
–, anti-cardiolipin antibodies, discovery **37**, 304
–, –, endothelial cell binding **37**, 307–308
–, –, in absence of well-defined disease **37**, 306
–, –, in systemic lupus erythematosus **37**, 305
–, –, in thrombosis **37**, 304–305
–, –, in various diseases **37**, 306–307
–, –, lupus anticoagulant levels **37**, 308–309
–, –, noncardiolipin antigens directed against **37**, 310–312
–, –, platelet binding **37**, 307
–, –, red blood cell binding **37**, 308
–, –, splenic B and T cell binding **37**, 309–310
–, cholesterol interaction **37**, 271
–, chromatographic separation **37**, 317–318
–, conformation in biomembranes **37**, 270–274
–, degradation **37**, 274–275
–, diet effects, on acyl composition **37**, 291–297
–, –, on quantity **37**, 300
–, distribution, asymmetric **37**, 270–274
–, enzyme associations, ADP/ATP carrier protein **37**, 279–280
–, –, F_1F_0 ATPase **37**, 279
–, –, carboxylesterase **37**, 287
–, –, carnitine/acyl carnitine translocase **37**, 282–283
–, –, carnitine palmitoyl-transferase **37**, 282–283
–, –, cytochrome *c* oxidase **37**, 277–279
–, –, DNA polymerase **37**, 286
–, –, glutamate dehydrogenase **37**, 285–286
–, –, α-glycerol-phosphate dehydrogenase **37**, 283
–, –, Na^+/K^+ ATPase **37**, 277–279
–, –, NADH ubiquinone oxidoreductase **37**, 286
–, –, phosphate carrier protein **37**, 280–281
–, –, phospholipase A_2 **37**, 284–285
–, –, protein kinase C **37**, 285
–, –, various enzymes **37**, 286–287
–, fatty acids, positional distribution **37**, 290
–, hex II formation **37**, 271–273
–, in animals **37**, 264
–, in micro-organisms **37**, 263
–, in mitochondrial protein importation and translocation **37**, 275–277
–, in plants **37**, 263–264
–, ionophore **37**, 273–274
–, oxidation **37**, 275
–, reactive epitope **37**, 312–314
–, space-filling models **37**, 271
–, steroidogenicity **37**, 271
–, structure of **23**, 6
–, synthesis, acyl-specific **37**, 266–267
–, –, intracellular location **37**, 267–270
–, –, pathway **37**, 265–266
Cardiopulmonary toxicity, pyrrolizidine alkaloids **45**, 80–81
Cardiovascular disease **40**, 57–58
–, dietary fat saturation and **36**, 261–263
–, dietary fatty acids **36**, 331–333
–, plasma lipoproteins **36**, 260–261
Cardiovascular protective effects, phytoestrogens **44**, 232–234
Cargoes, dairy **12**, 177–179
–, –, butter **12**, 177–178
–, –, cheese **12**, 178
–, –, eggs **12**, 178–179
–, frozen packaged foods **12**, 179
–, fruits, apples **12**, 179–182
–, –, apricots **12**, 182
–, –, bananas **12**, 188–191
–, –, grapes **12**, 183
–, –, peaches **12**, 183
–, –, pears **12**, 183–184
–, –, pineapples **12**, 191
–, –, plums **12**, 184
–, meats, beef **12**, 168–174
–, –, fish **12**, 176–177
–, –, mutton and lamb **12**, 174–175
–, –, offal **12**, 175
–, –, pork and bacon **12**, 175
–, –, poultry **12**, 175
–, –, rabbit **12**, 175–176
–, –, whale **12**, 176
–, shipboard **12**, 168–192
–, vegetables **12**, 192
–, –, potatoes **12**, 192
Caries **39**, 283–285
Carle and Montanari conche, chocolate and **31**, 301
Carmelization **19**, 184
Carmine **43**, 202
–, adverse reactions **43**, 202, 203–207, 213
–, –, anaphylactic **43**, 203, 204, 205–206
–, –, asthma **43**, 206–207
Carmustine **44**, 293

Carnitine, in abalone **23**, 165
Carnitine/acyl carnitine translocase, cardiolipin association **37**, 282–283
Carnitine deficiency, effects in muscle **37**, 381–382
Carnitine palmitoyl-transferase, cardiolipin association **37**, 282–283
–, deficiency effects in muscle **37**, 382
Carnosic acid, conversion to rosmanol **42**, 259, 261
Carnosol, conversion to rosmanol **42**, 260
Carotenase in eggs **1**, 183
Carotene, effect of blanching on **2**, 330, 331
–, – of cathode rays on **3**, 170, 171
–, loss during blanching of vegetables **8**, 72
–, retention, during blanching of vegetables **1**, 67–68
–, –, in blanched foods **3**, 136
–, ultraviolet measurement on **3**, 153
α-Carotene **15**, 246
β-Carotene **15**, 126, 205, 209, 241; **43**, 196, 210
–, adverse reactions **43**, 210–211
–, carcinogen risk assessment and **31**, 21, 24
–, in abalone **23**, 165
–, metabolism (*see also* Retinol, Retinol-binding protein, Retinyl ester, Vitamin A metabolism) **40**, 25–54, 55–79
–, –, absorption **40**, 32, 41, 58–60, 69–70, 71
–, –, adipose tissue **40**, 49, 61
–, –, animal model limitations **40**, 61–62
–, –, antioxidant status **40**, 58
–, –, background information **40**, 26–29, 56
–, –, bioconversion **40**, 59–60
–, –, biological effects **40**, 57–58
–, –, cancer **40**, 57
–, –, cardiovascular disease **40**, 57–58
–, –, catabolic rate **40**, 61
–, –, chylomicrons **40**, 32, 37, 41, 62–63, 69, 71
–, –, compartmental modeling **40**, 26–54
–, –, –, behavior predicted **40**, 43–50
–, –, –, construction **40**, 32–35
–, –, –, empirical descriptions **40**, 45, 50–52
–, –, –, final version **40**, 41, 43
–, –, –, iteration **40**, 35–43
–, –, –, materials, methods, constraints **40**, 29–32
–, –, –, statistical evaluation **40**, 40–43
–, –, –, unobservable behavior **40**, 46–50
–, –, dietary factors **40**, 59, 60
–, –, distribution **40**, 69–70
–, –, enterocyte **40**, 36–37, 38–39
–, –, gastrointestinal delay **40**, 36–37
–, –, human subject **40**, 29–32, 62–67
–, –, immune function **40**, 58
–, –, organs **40**, 33, 49
–, –, –, liver **40**, 38–40, 46–48, 60, 69, 71
–, –, tracer methods **40**, 26, 30–31, 42–43, 63–75
–, –, –, carbon-13 **40**, 64–75
–, –, –, dosage **40**, 65
–, –, –, GC-C-IRMS analysis **40**, 66–71, 73–74
–, –, –, nontracer versus **40**, 62–64
–, –, –, plasma analysis **40**, 65–66
–, –, –, utility **40**, 64, 70–75
–, –, transport **40**, 60–61
–, –, vitamin A conversion **40**, 49–50, 59
–, olive oil and **31**, 466, 467, 472
–, oxidation of **17**, 6, 28–30
–, quenching of singlet oxygen **33**, 303
–, reactions with sulfites **30**, 25
γ-Carotene **15**, 126, 206
ζ-Carotene **15**, 206
Carotene content, apples and pears **8**, 368, 379, 380
–, canned foods **1**, 41–44, 47, 50
–, effect of storage on **1**, 92–96, 97
–, fresh vegetables, effect of storage on **1**, 65
–, peaches, effect of heat sterilization on **1**, 89
–, plants, effect of climate on **1**, 305–306
–, –, – of fertilizers on **1**, 308–309
–, spinach **8**, 104
Carotenoids (*see also* β-Carotene, metabolism) **14**, 307–308; **15**, 125, 132, 202; **40**, 59–61; **43**, 210
–, adverse reactions **43**, 210–211
–, biosynthesis **15**, 204, 210, 262
–, color **15**, 218
–, commercial synthesis **15**, 210, 263
–, function **15**, 208, 262
–, in fruits **17**, 190
–, in passion fruit juice **27**, 277–281
–, in tea **17**, 241; **24**, 246
–, microbial synthesis **15**, 210
–, nomenclature **15**, 196
–, occurrence in animals **15**, 260
–, – in fruit **15**, 217, 225
–, – in vegetables **15**, 226, 234
–, odors from **17**, 33
–, pigments, in tropical fruits **17**, 174
–, properties **15**, 202, 231, 239, 254
–, – in storage **15**, 241
–, – in toxicology **15**, 212
Carotol in carrot seed oil **2**, 271

Carrageenan, effect on other polymers **11**, 126
–, in antibiotic ice **11**, 133
–, in artificial protein fibers **11**, 135
–, in bakery products **11**, 132–133
–, in bakery toppings **11**, 133
–, in beer stabilization **11**, 137
–, in breading and batter mixes **11**, 133
–, in candies **11**, 137
–, in canned meat and fish **11**, 134
–, in cheese products **11**, 130
–, in dessert gels **11**, 125–128
–, in dietetic foods **11**, 136
–, in dough products **11**, 132
–, in fountain toppings **11**, 136
–, in fruit products **11**, 137
–, in ice cream stabilization **11**, 131
–, in ice pop stabilization **11**, 132
–, in meat, fish, and poultry **11**, 133–135
–, in milk stabilization **11**, 129–130
–, in miscellaneous foods **11**, 137
–, in protective food coatings **11**, 134
–, in puddings and pie fillings **11**, 128–129
–, in relishes **11**, 135
–, in salad dressings **11**, 135
–, in sauces **11**, 135
–, molecular shapes and interactions **42**, 180–184
–, properties **11**, 124–125
–, typical food applications **11**, 127
–, viscosity **11**, 118
Carrier-mediated transport **40**, 251–257, 261–262
Carrots **15**, 226
–, analyses for SO_2 **5**, 119
–, blanching of **2**, 332; **8**, 65
–, canned, nutrients content of **1**, 43, 46–50
–, carotene content of, effect of nitrogen on **1**, 809
–, –, – of season on **1**, 306
–, –, – of temperature on **1**, 306
–, carotenoid pigments in **2**, 306, 328–329
–, decrease in bacterial content by blanching **6**, 184
–, dietary fiber and **31**, 129, 146, 148
–, dried, enzymic changes in **11**, 288
–, effect of steaming on pectic substances of **2**, 311
–, gelatinization temperature of starch in **2**, 323
–, in children's diet **1**, 109
–, inositol phosphate content **45**, 23
–, intestinal bacteria **31**, 172, 178, 183
–, lignified fibers in **2**, 304
–, loss of ascorbic acid during **8**, 89
–, – of thiamine **6**, 287, 295
–, nutrient content of, effect of blanching on **1**, 67, 77
–, oil constituents in leaf of **2**, 271
–, – in seed oil **2**, 271
–, parenchyma tissue in **2**, 304
–, pH value of **3**, 432
–, properties **31**, 157, 158, 166
–, puree, thiamine destruction **6**, 292
–, radio frequency experiments on **3**, 143
–, sulfiting **5**, 142
–, B vitamin in **1**, 42, 44, 45
Carrots and peas, F value for industrial processing of **2**, 102
Cartenoids, in passion fruits **12**, 238–239
Carvacrol **42**, 249–250
Carver–Greenfield process **15**, 349
Caryopsis, definition **41**, 1–2
–, development **41**, 7
Case hardening **39**, 109
Casein (*see also* Bovine casein) **16**, 237, 289, 299; **39**, 165, 169–173, 175–176; **40**, 231–232, 238–240
–, amino acid compositions of **19**, 157
–, browning reaction with glucose **30**, 89–90
–, calcium-induced micelle stability **34**, 325–334
–, –, κ-casein effect **34**, 328–331, 333
–, –, colloidal stability test **34**, 325–326
–, –, interpretation **34**, 331, 333–334
–, –, micelle precipitation **34**, 331–332
–, –, model colloids **34**, 328–332
–, –, theory **34**, 326–328
–, chocolate and **31**, 254, 255, 259
–, composition and distribution of **19**, 155
–, disappearance in ripening cheddar cheese **34**, 363–366
–, effect on solubility **3**, 67, 79
–, effects of heat treatment on nutritive value **4**, 247, 251
–, effects on whey protein thermal characteristics **35**, 332–333
–, fresh acid-curd cheese **39**, 178, 182–184
–, heat effects on **19**, 163–165
–, hydration **39**, 270
–, in diet of rats **1**, 112, 114
–, in insolubilization **3**, 101
–, in milk **10**, 45–46, 48
–, isoelectric, moisture–vapor pressure curves for **3**, 57
–, β-lactoglobulin interaction with **19**, 168–170
–, meat mutagen modulation **34**, 434

Casein (*cont'd*)
–, precipitation of **3**, 83
–, proteolysis **39**, 212–214, 219–230
–, quality of cheese and **34**, 376
–, reaction on sulfhydryls **3**, 75
–, reaction with glucose **3**, 275, 276–277
–, role in breadmaking **19**, 176–177
–, salt variation of micelle clotting via rennin **34**, 334–337
–, self-association **34**, 271
–, stable emulsions **34**, 140
–, structure and chemical properties of **19**, 160–161
–, time-dependent changes in cheddar cheese **34**, 369, 371–375
–, ultrasonic micelle particle sizing **45**, 150
–, use in spray-drying **2**, 496
–, vitamins in **19**, 192
αS1-Casein **42**, 9494
–, energy-minimized structures **42**, 109–111
β-Casein, adsorption behavior in presence of chaotropic and kosmotropic salts **34**, 48–50
–, adsorption isotherms **34**, 48–50
–, configurations **34**, 58
–, diffusion rate to air–water interface **34**, 19
–, foam volume increase rate **34**, 61
–, molecular properties **34**, 23–24
–, rate of collapse of foams **34**, 61–62
–, π–a relationship **34**, 40–41, 57–58
–, steady-state surface concentration, salt effect **34**, 49, 51
–, steady-state surface pressure, salt effect **34**, 49, 51
κ-Casein, calcium-induced insolubility effect **34**, 328–330, 333
–, effect on salting-out and salting-in **34**, 330–331
para-Casein **39**, 264, 265–267
Caseinates **38**, 37
–, calcium, moisture–vapor pressure curves for **3**, 57, 58
–, effect of heat on **3**, 53, 55
–, sodium, moisture–vapor pressure curves for **3**, 57
Caseinate salts, production of **2**, 24
Casein-lipid films **44**, 372–373
Caseoglutines **16**, 235
Casings, for meat emulsions **16**, 152
–, –, edible collagen casings **16**, 154
–, –, natural **16**, 152
–, –, removal **16**, 144, 154ff
–, –, synthetic **16**, 153
–, ham, boiling and cooling **12**, 389
–, –, fish **12**, 388–389, 391
–, –, sealing **12**, 388
–, sausage, fish **12**, 384–389
–, –, kinds of **12**, 386–389
–, –, sizes **12**, 385
–, –, stuffing **12**, 384–386
Cassava **41**, 99
Cassava starch **43**, 231
Cassette mutagenesis **36**, 174
Casson model **39**, 34, 46
Castellija rhexifolia **45**, 77
Castellija sp. (Indian paint brush) **45**, 77
Castor bean, nutritional stress factor in **4**, 110, 112–113
Castor bean meal **17**, 107
Catabolic rate, β-carotene **40**, 61
–, folate **40**, 88–89, 90
–, vitamin A **40**, 7, 13
Catalase **16**, 432; **17**, 10
–, biological role **10**, 7–8
–, effect of temperature **17**, 42–43
–, estimation, fish freshness and **7**, 64
–, in eggs **1**, 183
–, in food deterioration **17**, 18
–, inhibition of oxidative losses to reduced folates **33**, 15
–, in honey **24**, 329–330
–, in respiration of fruits **3**, 17
–, in wheat germ **23**, 239–240
–, oxidation mechanisms **17**, 16–17
–, regeneration **17**, 56–57
–, removal of hydrogen peroxide with **33**, 303
Catalase content of peas, effect of blanching on **1**, 69
Catalysis, endogenous proteolytic enzymes and **31**, 344, 349, 352
–, enzymic **17**, 9
–, metallic **17**, 7–8, 27
–, *N*-nitroso compounds and, fundamentals **31**, 59–64
–, –, indirect contamination **31**, 96
–, nonenzymic **17**, 4
–, olive oil and **31**, 470, 473
Catalysts, for lipid oxidation **23**, 40–45
Catechin-gallate in green tea **2**, 284, 285
Catechins, condensation of **17**, 268–271
–, in cocoa **2**, 284
–, in fermentation **17**, 265
–, in food browning **19**, 77–78
–, in tea **11**, 210–214; **17**, 217, 221, 258, 276, 278
–, protection against Strontium-90 **17**, 218–219
–, reaction with amino acids **17**, 240
–, structure of **17**, 222–223; **19**, 77

–, synthesis **17**, 225–227, 244
–, Vitamin P activity **17**, 218
Catecholamine, in porcine stress syndrome **28**, 187–189
Catecholase, *see* Oxidase, *o*-diphenol *and* Polyphenol oxidase
Catecholase activity, of food polyphenoloxidases **19**, 90–91
Catechol compounds, effect on mortality of rats **3**, 206
–, experiments with in respiration of plant tissues **3**, 14, 15
–, oxidation of in browning **3**, 18, 20–21
–, pathologic effects of **3**, 207
–, precipitation of in plant tissues **3**, 11
–, separation of in plant tissues **3**, 3
–, test for determining enzyme inactivation in fruit **3**, 30
–, toxicity of as an antioxidant **3**, 201, 206
Catechols, inhibition of lipoxygenase **33**, 307
–, structure, role in lipoxygenase inhibition **33**, 317–318
Cathepsin D **39**, 214–215
Cathepsin in relation to aging of poultry meat **1**, 210
Cathepsins (*see also* Enzymes, proteolytic)
–, endogenous proteolytic enzymes and **31**, 412, 413
–, endopeptidases **31**, 355–357, 361, 362
–, exopeptidases **31**, 347, 348, 350, 351
–, meat technology **31**, 403, 404, 406, 407, 410
–, muscle physiology **31**, 375, 380–383
–, proteinase activity **31**, 384–392
–, proteinase distribution **31**, 368, 369
–, serine proteinases **31**, 364, 365
–, thiol proteinases **31**, 365, 366
–, unclassified proteinases **31**, 366
Cathode rays, data on penetration of **3**, 130
–, dosage for bacteria destruction **3**, 164
–, effect of, on coffee **3**, 176–180
–, –, on enzymes **3**, 174–176
–, –, on packaging materials **3**, 187
–, –, on pharmaceuticals **3**, 187
–, –, on vitamins **3**, 167–174
–, equipment for **3**, 160–162
–, explanation of **3**, 129
–, germicidal action of **3**, 163–167
–, in fish spoilage **3**, 184–187
–, in nonenzymic browning **3**, 180–184
–, in study of chemical reactions **3**, 180–187
–, toxicity of materials irradiated by **3**, 187
–, use of **3**, 160–189
Cathodoluminescence, in scanning electron microscopy **22**, 216, 219
Cation exchange, wine deacidification by **25**, 24
Cation exchange capacity, dietary fiber and **31**, 164–166
Cation exchangers, aluminosilicates **2**, 34
–, chemical structure **2**, 5
–, commercial type of **2**, 7
–, effect of concentration on **2**, 10
–, removal of pectase by **2**, 37
–, resinous cation exchangers **2**, 4
–, separation of amino acids by **2**, 34
–, sulfonated coals **2**, 4
–, titration curve for **2**, 5
–, types of **2**, 3
–, use as catalyst **2**, 36
–, use in apple industry **2**, 15
–, – in determination of copper in milk **2**, 38
–, – in grape industry **2**, 15–18
–, – in pineapple industry **2**, 18–20
–, – in preparation of organic acids from salts **2**, 35, 36
–, – in sugar beet industry **2**, 6
Cations, endogenous proteolytic enzymes and, endopeptidases **31**, 354
–, exopeptidases **31**, 346
–, meat technology **31**, 395, 398, 408, 409
–, of quaternary ammonium compounds **2**, 119, 124
–, –, effect of pH on activity of **2**, 133–134
–, –, method of determining concentration of **2**, 168
–, –, therapeutic action of **2**, 143
Catol 2, film formation of **2**, 144
–, therapeutic action of **2**, 143
Cats, toxicity of DDT to **2**, 208
Catsup, color specifications for **5**, 321
Cattle, digestive process of **6**, 116
–, skinning **6**, 152
–, slaughter of **6**, 125
Cauliflower, effect of blanching **1**, 66
–, – of –, decrease in bacterial content **6**, 184
–, frozen **6**, 176
–, loss of thiamine **6**, 287
–, nonenzymatic food browning in **19**, 126–127
–, ozone treatment **45**, 192
–, pH of **3**, 432
Cauliflower mosaic virus S25 **41**, 128
Caustic soda, gelatin manufacture and **7**, 239, 240
Cavitation **15**, 348

Cavity magnetron, use in heat-treating foods **3**, 125, 126
Cavity perturbation, dielectric properties measurement **43**, 79, 80, 82
CBCCDS integrator **40**, 297, 299–303
CCM salt, calcium absorption from **33**, 147
cDNA (*see also* Complementary DNA), cloning **36**, 140–142
–, –, factors affecting **36**, 139
–, –, procedure **36**, 135
–, –, seed storage proteins **36**, 139–142
–, screening of libraries **36**, 143
–, synthesis **36**, 140–142
Cecina **39**, 82–83
Ceepryn, medical application of **2**, 181
–, structure of **2**, 123
–, therapeutic action of **2**, 143
–, toxicity of **2**, 130
Cefamandole **44**, 289
Cefpodoxime **44**, 290
Ceftriaxone **44**, 290
Cefuroxime **44**, 290
Celery, chloroplasts in parenchyma cells in **2**, 305
–, dietary fiber and **31**, 158, 183
–, inositol phosphate content **45**, 23
–, volatile constituents of **2**, 271
Celiac disease **37**, 29–30; **42**, 9; **43**, 197, 198
Celite, meat mutagen modulation **34**, 434
Cell cultures, muscle, research needs **37**, 407
–, sulfite cytogenicity **30**, 47
Cell fractionation **41**, 117–119
Cell growth, during kiwifruit growth and ripening **29**, 288–289
Cell-mediated allergies **42**, 8–9
Cell-mediated immunity, effects of lactic cultures **37**, 107–110
–, gut **37**, 19–21
Cellobiose, effect on calcium absorption **33**, 127
Cells, benzoic and salicylic acids effects on processes of **11**, 339–347
–, parenchyma **13**, 306–311
Cellular adhesion, processing techniques affecting **2**, 310–316
Cellulose **15**, 81, 118; **41**, 158
–, action of intestinal bacteria on **1**, 135
–, alpha **12**, 290
–, biosynthesis, model **30**, 165
–, chocolate and **31**, 247
–, derivatives **12**, 287–289
–, dietary fiber and **31**, 118, 191
–, –, analysis **31**, 148, 150, 153
–, –, components **31**, 120, 122, 123, 139
–, –, dicotyledonous plants **31**, 126–128, 133, 135
–, –, intestinal bacteria **31**, 176, 178–181, 185, 187
–, –, monocotyledonous plants **31**, 136–138
–, –, properties **31**, 158, 170, 171
–, effect on, calcium absorption **33**, 141
–, ester formation between pectins and **11**, 66–70
–, in cocoa beans and nibs **6**, 38
–, in fruits **17**, 182
–, microcrystalline **12**, 290–294
–, molecular shapes and interactions **42**, 148–153
–, monocrystalline **12**, 290–294
–, –, applications **12**, 291–294, 296
–, –, dry form **12**, 292–293
–, –, gel-based products **12**, 293–294
–, –, properties **12**, 291
–, plant cell wall, binding to, glucurono-arabinoxylan **30**, 151
–, –, xyloglucans **30**, 150–151
–, pyrolysis, phenol production **29**, 123
–, structure and content **30**, 147
–, tocopherol bioavailability **33**, 173
α-Cellulose, dietary fiber and, dicotyledonous plants **31**, 124, 127, 130, 132, 133
–, intestinal bacteria **31**, 180
–, properties **31**, 158, 162
Cellulose film, chocolate and **31**, 318, 320
Cellulose waste, for ruminant feed **30**, 345–346
Cell wall **15**, 80
–, biosynthesis **30**, 162–165
–, chemical breakdown, by endoglucanase **30**, 161–162
–, –, by endopolygalacturonase **30**, 160–161
–, growth **30**, 156–160
–, –, auxin effect **30**, 157–160
–, –, enzymes, activation by auxin **30**, 160
–, –, event sequences, two models **30**, 157, 159–160
–, –, pH and **30**, 160
–, modified, cellulose fiber layers **30**, 164
–, –, enzymatic actions, explanations **30**, 167–168
–, –, growth mechanism **30**, 165–167
–, –, –, pH and **30**, 166–167
–, –, pectin layers **30**, 164
–, Monro's **30**, 154–155
–, –, appraisal **30**, 156
–, –, for lupin hypocotyl **30**, 155
–, plant, appraisal **30**, 154–156
–, –, endoglucanase use and **30**, 162

–, –, endopolygalacturonase use and **30**, 160–161
–, –, for sycamore callus cells **30**, 153
–, –, models, Albersheim's **30**, 152–153
Cell wall material **12**, 119–120
–, dietary fiber and **31**, 119, 133, 138
–, intestinal bacteria **31**, 172, 176, 179, 181, 183, 185
–, properties **31**, 161–163, 165, 166
Center-line temperatures, calculated vs. experimental, for ammonium alginate **11**, 421
–, –, for banana purée **11**, 421
–, for applesauce **11**, 421
Centrifugal atomizers, effect of frictional air on **2**, 461
–, methods of feeding **2**, 459–460
–, power consumption comparison **2**, 464
–, stress on **2**, 459
–, types and uses **2**, 454–458
–, use of high speed motors on **2**, 460
Centrifugation, creaming measurement **34**, 175
–, dietary fiber and **31**, 145, 157, 159
–, of fruit juices **9**, 247
–, of olive oil **31**, 462, 463, 469, 475
Centrifuges, for aroma recovery in freeze concentration **20**, 44
Cephalin content, of dried eggs **1**, 175–178
–, of egg yolk **1**, 151
Ceramide, biosynthesis of **23**, 17
–, structure of **23**, 16
Ceratonia, licorice extract and **7**, 348
Cercospora **12**, 100, 191
Cereal grains **16**, 6ff
–, consumption **16**, 7
–, degradation during processing **45**, 16, 21–22
–, digestibility **16**, 75
–, inositol phosphates **45**, 5–6
–, ozone treatment **45**, 198
–, production **16**, 7
–, proteins **16**, 7, 19
–, pyrrolizidine alkaloids contamination **45**, 68, 69–70
–, radurization of **24**, 194–196
–, scanning electron microscopy of **22**, 259–274
–, –, processing studies **22**, 275–278
Cereal–legume model, enrichment with, amino acids **30**, 355
–, –, protein **30**, 356
–, nutritive value improvement **30**, 357
Cereal products, insects infesting **4**, 307, 311, 313, 316–324, 326–330, 339–346
Cereals, amylase inhibitor in **1**, 385
–, analysis **31**, 143, 146, 148–151
–, biosynthesis **36**, 124
–, bran, effect on calcium absorption **33**, 138–139
–, breakfast, internal structure of **8**, 121
–, –, thiamine loss **6**, 269
–, classification **36**, 93, 95–96
–, components **31**, 120, 122, 140
–, consensus sequence **36**, 97
–, dicotyledonous plants **31**, 126
–, dietary fiber and **31**, 119, 135–138, 190, 191
–, enzymatic changes in **11**, 274–278
–, fiber, effect on calcium bioavailability **33**, 136–139
–, foods, sanitary status of **8**, 111
–, gene structure **36**, 96–100
–, human food **6**, 231
–, in diets **1**, 110
–, in preparation of fish paste **4**, 217, 219, 221, 224
–, intestinal bacteria **31**, 171, 172, 177, 178, 182, 184, 186–188
–, milled products, enzymatic changes during storage **11**, 280–285
–, nutritional stress factors in **4**, 111–113
–, phytase activity in **28**, 21–23, 63
–, phytic acid phosphorus content **28**, 10–13
–, products, contamination of **8**, 126
–, prolamin structure and conformation **36**, 100–103
–, properties **31**, 155, 157, 160, 165, 169
–, protective effect on thiamine **6**, 261
–, protein contents **36**, 92–93
–, souring **11**, 301–302
–, storage of, scanning electron microscopic studies of **22**, 242–245
–, storage proteins **36**, 93, 95–103
–, sugar-coated, moisture sorption curves **35**, 349
–, thiamine loss in **6**, 264, 274
–, wheat germ supplementation of **23**, 284–285
Cerebrosides, structure of **23**, 16, 17
Cervelat **39**, 78
Cervical cancer, carcinogen risk assessment and **31**, 22
Cetamium, therapeutic action of **2**, 143, 151
Cetavlon, medical applications of **2**, 182, 183
–, structure of **2**, 121, 150
–, toxicity of **2**, 130

Cetyldimethylbenzylammonium chloride, germicidal effects of **2**, 135
–, structure of **2**, 120
Cetyldimethylethylammonium bromide, bactericidal powers of **2**, 135
–, structure of **2**, 122
–, toxicity of **2**, 131
Cetylpyridinium chloride, compatibility of **2**, 133
–, effect of pH on germicidal power **2**, 134, 135
–, effect on influenza virus **2**, 138
–, film formation of **2**, 144
–, germicidal action **2**, 151–152, 183
–, inhibitors of **2**, 166
–, medical applications **2**, 181
–, structure of **2**, 123, 124, 151
–, toxicity of **2**, 130, 131, 153–154
Cetyltrimethylammonium bromide, action as surface-active agent **1**, 379
–, effect of sodium sulfate on **2**, 136
–, germicidal action of **2**, 150, 183
–, medical application of **2**, 181–182
–, structure of **2**, 121, 124, 150
–, therapeutic action of **2**, 143
–, toxicity of **2**, 130, 131
Cetyltrimethylammonium iodide, therapeutic action of **2**, 143
CFR, *see* Code of Federal Regulations
Chains, for product accumulation control in spray dryer **2**, 493
Chain scission, polymers in shear **36**, 15
Challenge tests **42**, 32, 34–35
Chao-mai, *see* Buckwheat
Chaos **40**, 324–326
Chaotropes **35**, 296
Chaotropic salts **34**, 47–48
Character notes, flavor profile and **7**, 12
Chard (*see also* Spinach beet), carotene content of processed **5**, 225
–, total folate content, table **33**, 40
Charged groups, frequency, wheat proteins **36**, 8
Charqui **39**, 82
CHD, *see* Coronary heart disease
Cheddar cheese, amino acids **39**, 231
–, casein components, time-dependent changes **34**, 369, 371–375
–, citrate **39**, 201
–, contamination **39**, 289
–, dental caries **39**, 285
–, extraction and sodium dodecyl sulfate gel electrophoresis **34**, 366–368
–, flavor **39**, 209, 235, 241–245
–, α_{s1}-I fragment **34**, 375
–, lactate **39**, 198, 199
–, lipolysis **39**, 201, 205, 208, 209
–, nonlinear regression analysis **34**, 369–376
–, NSLAB **39**, 211, 219–220
–, peptides **39**, 226, 227, 237
–, polyacrylamide gel electrophoresis **34**, 363
–, protein analysis **34**, 366
–, protein extraction **34**, 363–366
–, quality **39**, 250–251, 252
–, ripening **34**, 362–376; **39**, 255, 256
–, salting **39**, 177, 178
–, sample preparation **34**, 362–363
–, SDS-PAGE analysis **34**, 368–369
–, texture **39**, 176, 254
–, theory **34**, 363–366
–, ultrafiltration **39**, 194
–, volatile compounds **39**, 238
Cheese (*see also names of cheeses*) **39**, 163–328
–, acid gel formation **39**, 182–188
–, acidification **39**, 166, 174–177, 258
–, analytical techniques, chromatography **39**, 210, 237–238, 243–247, 354–355
–, –, electrophoresis **39**, 210, 226, 230–231, 242–243
–, –, mass spectrometry **39**, 227, 231, 238
–, background material **39**, 164–168
–, –, consumption **39**, 166, 179
–, –, history **39**, 164–165
–, –, manufacturing **39**, 166, 168
–, –, production **39**, 165–166, 260
–, bacterial growth-time variation **34**, 376–382
–, –, materials and methods **34**, 377
–, –, pH dependence of *Clostridium botulinum* JTD-IV **34**, 377–378, 380
–, –, – of toxin synthesis **34**, 381–382
–, –, theory **34**, 377
–, ball hardness test for **8**, 17
–, cheddar, experiments on **8**, 52
–, cheshire, experiments on **8**, 52
–, composition **39**, 180
–, curd tension of milk for **8**, 19
–, fatty acids and **7**, 27–28
–, flavor **39**, 232, 233, 235–254
–, –, analytical methods **39**, 236–254
–, –, astringency **39**, 240–241
–, –, bitterness **39**, 239–240
–, –, defects **39**, 236, 239–242
–, –, development **39**, 166, 168, 169
–, –, emulsifying salts **39**, 272
–, –, fatty acid catabolism **39**, 206, 208–209
–, –, fruitiness **39**, 241

–, –, quality factors **39**, 246–254
–, –, varietal comparisons **39**, 242–246
–, future research **39**, 293–296
–, grading scheme **39**, 252, 295–296
–, image **39**, 292–293
–, milk constituents **39**, 168–169
–, milk conversion to curd **39**, 164–165, 166, 169–195
–, – to –, fresh acid-curd varieties **39**, 178–193
–, – to –, rennet addition **39**, 188
–, – to –, rennet coagulation **39**, 169–178, 249–250
–, – to –, ultrafiltration **39**, 193–195
–, *N*-nitroso compounds and **31**, 70, 71, 85, 86
–, nonvolatile compounds **39**, 236–237
–, nutrition **39**, 277–283
–, –, carbohydrate **39**, 278
–, –, fat and cholesterol **39**, 278–280
–, –, minerals **39**, 280, 282–283
–, –, protein **39**, 277
–, –, vitamins **39**, 280–281
–, organoleptic judging of **2**, 240
–, pH, milk conversion **39**, 165, 172, 175–176, 178, 182–183
–, –, processed cheese **39**, 265, 270, 276
–, –, quality **39**, 251–252
–, –, texture **39**, 254
–, processed **34**, 376
–, processed products **39**, 259–277
–, –, blend ingredients **39**, 272–276
–, –, classification **39**, 261
–, –, cooling **39**, 266–267
–, –, emulsifying salts **39**, 263, 267–272
–, –, manufacturing **39**, 262–266
–, –, structure formation **39**, 266–267
–, –, texture **39**, 272–277
–, psychorheology of **8**, 46
–, quality attributes (*see also* Cheese, flavor *and* Cheese, texture) **39**, 184–193
–, –, gelation **39**, 186–188, 191–193
–, –, rheology **39**, 186
–, –, sensory characteristics **39**, 186
–, –, syneresis **39**, 174, 185–186, 190–191
–, quality factors **39**, 246–254
–, quasi-properties of **8**, 10
–, ripening **16**, 231ff; **39**, 166, 178, 195–234
–, –, accelerated **39**, 255–259
–, –, acids in **16**, 259ff, 270
–, –, agents **39**, 196–197, 210–211
–, –, amino acids **16**, 240ff; **39**, 227, 231–234
–, –, aroma **16**, 268ff
–, –, assessment **39**, 209–210
–, –, carbohydrates in **16**, 250ff
–, –, carbon dioxide fixation in **16**, 265ff
–, –, carboxylic acids in **16**, 253
–, –, casein in **16**, 237
–, –, characterization **39**, 226–232
–, –, citrate metabolism **39**, 200–201
–, –, contamination **39**, 286–288
–, –, decomposition products **16**, 233
–, –, enzymes **16**, 233, 255, 281, 287ff
–, –, fermentation **16**, 311ff
–, –, flavor **16**, 239, 247, 257, 268ff
–, –, glycolysis **39**, 196, 198–201, 255
–, –, lactose metabolism **39**, 174–177, 198–200
–, –, lipolysis **39**, 201–209, 255
–, –, micro-organisms **16**, 232
–, –, nitrogen in **16**, 235
–, –, peptides in **16**, 239, 270
–, –, proteinases **39**, 211–225, 257–258
–, –, proteolysis **39**, 176–177, 209–234, 236, 255
–, –, respiration **16**, 311ff
–, –, temperature **39**, 253–254, 256–257
–, –, varietal comparisons **39**, 242–246
–, –, vitamins in **16**, 279ff
–, ripening period for **8**, 12
–, safety **39**, 283–292
–, –, additives **39**, 283
–, –, biogenic amines **39**, 290–292
–, –, dental caries **39**, 283–285
–, –, mycotoxins **39**, 285–290
–, salting **39**, 166, 177–178
–, slurries **39**, 259
–, technology **39**, 166, 168
–, –, ultrafiltration **39**, 193–195
–, texture **39**, 168, 169, 254–255
–, –, flavor perception **39**, 236
–, –, milk-curd conversion **39**, 176
–, –, processed products **39**, 272–277
–, –, processing factors **39**, 188–190
–, thiamine in **6**, 261, 262, 293, 304
–, –, in processed **6**, 298
–, ultrasonic texture sensing **45**, 146, 147
–, ultrasonic velocity changes during melting **45**, 142
–, vector tests on **8**, 23
–, volatile compounds **39**, 237–239, 244–246
–, X-ray aging of **3**, 160
Cheese base **39**, 274
Cheese manufacturing **10**, 49–50, 53
Cheese products, alginates in **11**, 147
–, carrageenan in **11**, 130
–, guar gum in **11**, 168
–, locust bean gum in **11**, 163

Cheesman–Kirby apparatus **14**, 11
Chelating **14**, 355–358
Chelating agents, as preventatives of "warmed-over" flavor **23**, 57–58
–, effects on thermal denaturation behavior of whey proteins **33**, 379–381
–, inhibition of warmed-over flavor in cooked meat **29**, 44–45
Chelation, dietary fiber and **31**, 129, 140, 148, 164
Chemesthesis, taste perception relationship **44**, 253
Chemical indicators of food quality **16**, 161ff, 164
Chemical Industry of Toxicology, carcinogen risk assessment and **31**, 25, 47
Chemically interesterified (CIE) lard **44**, 38
–, rheological analysis **44**, 57
Chemically interesterified (CIE) milkfat, fractal dimensions **44**, 56, 57
–, macroscopic hardness indicators **44**, 38–41, 57
–, rheological analysis **44**, 56–57
–, scanning electron microscopy **44**, 61, 63, 64
Chemically interesterified (CIE) palmoil **44**, 38
–, rheological analysis **44**, 57
Chemical modification, of whey proteins **33**, 417–422
–, protein thermal behavior effects **35**, 329–331
Chemicals, foodborne, immunotoxicity **37**, 41–43
–, research needs **37**, 54–55
Chemical synthesis, acyl-specific cardiolipin derivatives **37**, 314–317
Chemical time–temperature integrators **44**, 182–183
Chemoprevention, rosemary and carnosol **42**, 266
Chemotherapy, smell/taste perception changes **44**, 275, 277, 278, 279, 293–294
Cherimoya **10**, 307, 308
Cherries, artificial, alginates in **11**, 156
–, "barrelling," 143 **5**, 144
–, brining **5**, 143, 144
–, canned, corrosiveness **3**, 336
–, –, –, of black **3**, 340
–, –, –, of Royal Anne **3**, 340, 346, 347
–, –, –, of white **3**, 338
–, –, nutrients in **1**, 43, 46–49
–, –, vitamin retention in **1**, 82
–, combined SO_2 **5**, 139
–, composition and distillation of **2**, 264
–, dehydration of **5**, 142
–, desulfiting **5**, 127
–, effect of copper on **3**, 364
–, inhibition of corrosion in by citric acid **3**, 342
–, iodine in wrapping for **3**, 465
–, Maraschino **5**, 98
–, –, in candies **6**, 45
–, micro-organisms in frozen **6**, 179
–, pH of **3**, 432
–, processing of **3**, 349
–, sweet, canned, use of ascorbic acid in **4**, 367
–, test for "organic peroxide" in **3**, 31
–, with sulfur, Bing **3**, 352
–, –, Royal Anne **3**, 352, 353
Cherry juice, canned, use of ascorbic acid in **4**, 377–378
–, combined SO_2 **5**, 139
Cheshire cheese **39**, 176, 254
Chestnuts, leuco-anthrocyanins **5**, 288
Chestnut starch, gelatinization temperature of **2**, 319
Chewiness **14**, 134–135
Chewing (*see also* Mastication), role in nutrition **21**, 17–18
Chicken **15**, 260; **39**, 75
–, chow-mein, frozen **6**, 199
–, fatty acid **5**, 6
–, fatty acids in fat of **23**, 23
–, flavor studies on **19**, 233
–, freeze-drying of **7**, 220–221
–, home frozen creamed **6**, 207
–, à la king, bacterial count of frozen **6**, 200
–, loss of thiamine in cooking **6**, 280
–, *Salmonella* in eviscerated **6**, 193
–, thiamine retention in frozen **6**, 294
–, toxicity of DDT on **2**, 208
Chicken embryo method of testing quaternary ammonium compound **2**, 165
Chicken muscle, rigor in **9**, 21
Chickpea phytoestrogens **44**, 197
–, isoflavones **44**, 203
Chickpeas **16**, 9
–, inositol phosphate degradation during malting **45**, 22
Chicory (*see also Cichorium intybus*), effect of blanching on **1**, 66
Child–Satorius shear **14**, 67
Chili, color range for **5**, 320
Chilling injury, in fruit **10**, 318, 319
China, IM meat, production problems **39**, 90

–, –, traditional methods **39**, 75–77, 119, 123–124
–, soil erosion in **32**, 217
Chinese buckwheat products **44**, 413–414, 416
Chinese millet, phytate content **45**, 13
Chinese raw noodles (*see also* Oriental noodles) **43**, 148, 156, 168, 181
–, quality evaluation **43**, 171, 173, 175
Chinese tallownut **16**, 72
Chinese wet noodles (*see also* Oriental noodles) **43**, 148, 160, 162
–, quality evaluation **43**, 171, 175, 176
Chips potato, bubbles in **10**, 183–186, 187
–, fat content **10**, 181, 185, 188–189, 194
–, frying equipment **10**, 208–210
–, histological characteristics **10**, 184–185
–, low-fat **10**, 200–201
–, nutritional values **10**, 200
–, oxidation control **10**, 196–197, 199
–, packaging **10**, 211–212
–, preheating **10**, 185–186
–, problems in the industry **10**, 224–226
–, quality control **10**, 213–215
–, related products **10**, 215–218
–, salting **10**, 210–211
–, shipping **10**, 212–213
–, temperature in processing **10**, 186–187
Chi-square analysis of sensory differences tests **2**, 222, 236
Chitosan-lipid edible films **44**, 358
Chives (*see also Allium*), γ-glutamyl peptides in **22**, 80–82
Chlamydomonas reinhardtii, as starch model **41**, 11
–, mutants **41**, 85–87
Chloracetic acid, microbial inhibition by **1**, 386, 389
Chloramine T **7**, 130
–, fish preservation and **7**, 67
–, germicidal agent in **7**, 135–136
–, nitrogenous compounds and **7**, 156
–, plant chlorination and **7**, 147
Chloramines, chlorine demand and **7**, 142–143
Chlorbenzoate, microbial inhibition by **1**, 386
Chlordan **15**, 38
Chlordiazepoxide **44**, 310
Chlorella **16**, 73
–, as sources of protein **18**, 117–128
Chlorella 7-11-05, gross composition of **18**, 125
Chlorhexidine digluconate **44**, 301
Chloride, endogenous proteolytic enzymes and **31**, 350
–, in milk **36**, 212–213
–, in wines **8**, 150
–, *N*-nitroso compounds and **31**, 60
–, polyvinyl **12**, 156
Chlorination, can-cooling and **7**, 158–159
–, effectiveness, factors affecting **7**, 147–158
–, food quality and **7**, 162–165
–, in-plant **7**, 158
Chlorine, as oxidizing agent for cation exchangers **2**, 6
–, bacterial resistance to **7**, 156–158
–, chloramine formation and **7**, 133–134
–, deficiency **1**, 121
–, –, interference with cell membrane by **1**, 377
–, demand, definition of **7**, 142
–, detergents and **7**, 140
–, dioxide sanitization **45**, 188, 189
–, discovery of **7**, 130
–, dosage, definition of **7**, 142
–, early uses of **7**, 130
–, effect on bacteria **2**, 108
–, – on flat sour bacteria spores **18**, 186–187
–, fish preservation and **7**, 65–67
–, gaseous, properties of **7**, 145
–, germicidal activity of **7**, 133–141
–, large scale application of **7**, 158–160
–, liquid, plant chlorination and **7**, 145–146
–, mist sterilization **32**, 20
–, plant sanitation and **7**, 141–165
–, sanitization **45**, 169–170, 188–189
–, –, ozone combined procedures **45**, 200–201
–, sanitizers **14**, 434–439
Chlormezanone **44**, 309
Chlorobenzoic acid as a food preservative **3**, 462
Chloroform, solubility of DDT in **2**, 203
Chlorogenic acid, in coffee **2**, 280
–, –, content **3**, 153, 177
–, in food browning **19**, 81
–, in green coffee beans **30**, 110
–, inhibition of soybean lipoxygenase **33**, 317
–, in sunflower seeds, food discoloration **30**, 376
–, reaction with *o*-diphenol oxidase **17**, 11
–, structure of **3**, 13; **19**, 80
Chlorophyll **15**, 133
–, analytical methods and criteria of purity for **4**, 155–174
–, as a deodorizer **4**, 175
–, by-products from **4**, 174–179

Chlorophyll (*cont'd*)
–, changes during blanching of vegetables **8**, 81
–, chemistry **4**, 138–150
–, –, in relation to food problems **4**, 134–184
–, control of formation in potato **21**, 331–342
–, conversion to pheophytin **5**, 104
–, degradation of **17**, 14, 31–32
–, disappearance of **5**, 326
–, distribution and biosynthesis in potato **21**, 310–316
–, effect of blanching **17**, 5
–, extraction and isolation of **4**, 150–155
–, in apples and pears **8**, 379
–, in fruits **17**, 174
–, in kiwifruit after storage and canning **29**, 295
–, in peas, changes in processing **9**, 74–76
–, –, conversion to pheophytins **9**, 75–76
–, in potato, factors affecting formation **21**, 316–331
–, in tea **17**, 241–243; **24**, 245–246
–, odors from **17**, 33
–, olive oil and **31**, 460, 466, 469, 472, 474
–, retention in frozen vegetables **17**, 4–5
–, use in medicine **4**, 175–178
Chlorophyllase **17**, 22
–, in tea **24**, 235
Chlorophyll compounds, nomenclature **4**, 135–133
Chlorophyll metabolism in animals **4**, 178–179
Chloroplasts, ADPGlc PPase **41**, 145–148
–, as transporting organelle **41**, 143–144
–, characterization **41**, 115
–, function in parenchyma vegetable cells **2**, 306
–, phosphoglucose isomerase mutants **41**, 146
–, starch degradation outside **41**, 156–157
–, starch in **2**, 316–317
Chlorosis in peas **9**, 74
Chlorpheniramine **44**, 288
Chlorphenols, destruction of bacterial membrane by **1**, 386
Chlortetracycline **16**, 180
Chocolate **31**, 213–215, 329, 330
–, alkalization **31**, 247–249
–, bitterness **5**, 274
–, bloom **6**, 14
–, bulking agents **31**, 272–274
–, bulk sweeteners **31**, 274, 275
–, –, amino acid **31**, 269
–, –, corn syrup solids **31**, 265, 266
–, –, dextrose **31**, 266, 267
–, –, fructose **31**, 267
–, –, polyhydric alcohols **31**, 268, 269
–, –, sorbose **31**, 267, 268
–, candies **6**, 30, 37
–, cocoa bean chemistry, changes **31**, 219–222
–, –, flavor **31**, 234–237
–, –, flavor precursors **31**, 231–233
–, –, grinding **31**, 241–243
–, –, quality **31**, 225–231
–, –, roasting **31**, 237–241, 243–246
–, cocoa butter **31**, 249, 250, 275–277
–, –, composition **31**, 250, 251
–, –, deodorization **31**, 251–253
–, conching **31**, 296, 299–308
–, –, physicochemical reactions **31**, 296, 297
–, –, processing **31**, 297–299
–, confectionary fats **31**, 277–281
–, creams, stability of fats in **6**, 12
–, emulsifiers **31**, 281–284
–, fermentation, chemical changes **31**, 221–225
–, –, methods **31**, 215–217
–, –, microbiology **31**, 217–219
–, flavor and aroma of **8**, 226, 278
–, flavor studies on **19**, 232–233
–, high-intensity sweeteners, artificial **31**, 269–271
–, –, natural **31**, 271, 272
–, made from cocoa **8**, 283
–, milk **6**, 44; **31**, 253–255
–, –, condensed **31**, 256, 257
–, –, crumb **31**, 284–291
–, –, dried **31**, 258–261
–, –, lactose **31**, 255, 256
–, milk-derived ingredients, fat **31**, 263, 264
–, –, lactose **31**, 263
–, –, whey **31**, 261–263
–, packaging **31**, 313, 314, 320
–, –, evaluation **31**, 319, 320
–, –, materials **31**, 318, 319
–, –, requirements **31**, 314–317
–, physical properties **6**, 39
–, refining **31**, 291–296
–, sugar **31**, 264, 265
–, tempering **31**, 308–313
–, tests on **8**, 25
–, *Theobroma cacao* L. **31**, 320–322, 328
–, –, embryonic axis growth **31**, 326, 327
–, –, flushing **31**, 327
–, –, lipid metabolism **31**, 324, 325
–, –, plant pathology **31**, 328
–, –, secondary metabolism **31**, 325, 326
–, –, shoot organogenesis **31**, 322

–, –, somatic embryogenesis **31**, 322–324
–, types of candy **6**, 2
Chocolate coatings, application of rheology to **11**, 394–399
–, calculating thickness for horizontal surfaces **11**, 397–399
–, calculating thickness for vertical surfaces **11**, 396
Cholera toxin, effects on gastrointestinal immunity **37**, 35
Cholesterol (*see also* Lipoproteins) **15**, 33; **39**, 278–280; **40**, 57–58
–, biosynthesis of **23**, 18
–, carcinogen risk assessment and **31**, 22, 23
–, cardiolipin interaction **37**, 271
–, content, in mechanically deboned fish **27**, 117–119
–, –, in mechanically deboned poultry **27**, 117–119
–, content in dairy products **37**, 150–152
–, dietary fiber and **31**, 159, 163, 168, 169
–, in milkfat **37**, 150
–, lactic acid bacteria effects **37**, 92–98, 120
–, *N*-nitroso compounds and **31**, 73
–, olive oil and **31**, 477
–, serum levels, fat quality and dietary cholesterol effects **37**, 160–161
–, structure of **23**, 18, 19
Cholesterol esters, fatty acid changes **35**, 56–58
Cholesterol-lowering effects, soy protein/soy isoflavones **44**, 232–234
–, Tartary buckwheat **44**, 409
Cholesteryl ester transfer protein **37**, 193
Cholestyramine **44**, 287
Choline, in pastes **11**, 300
–, *N*-nitroso compounds and **31**, 78
Choline deficiency **1**, 118
–, in fruit products, relationship to browning **1**, 353
Choline magnesium trisilicate **44**, 295
Choline phosphoglycerides, fatty acid concentrations **35**, 62
Cholinesterase **15**, 292
–, in eggs **1**, 183
–, inhibitors, effects on myasthenic muscle **37**, 367
Chondroitin sulfuric acid, gelatin and **7**, 272
Chondrus crispus **16**, 74
Chopped meat **39**, 94
–, effect of chopping on “warmed-over” flavor **23**, 53
Chorizos **39**, 110
Chow-mein, bacterial count of frozen **6**, 199
Chromanoxyl radical, formation **33**, 208
–, regeneration by **33**, 211–212
–, α-tocopherol, ascorbic acid quenching **33**, 211
Chromatid, carcinogen risk assessment and **31**, 28
Chromatographic separation, in flavor chemistry **9**, 211
Chromatography, cardiolipin separation **37**, 317–318
–, cheese **39**, 210, 237–238, 243–247, 354–355
–, fish **39**, 336, 339, 340, 341, 353–356
–, gas–liquid **14**, 18–20, 22, 235, 238; **17**, 6, 253–254
–, GC-C-IRMS **40**, 66–70, 71, 73–74, 177
–, HPLC **40**, 29, 60, 66, 72, 74
–, in fruit analysis **10**, 309, 312, 327, 335
–, meat **39**, 354
–, –, endpoint temperature monitoring **44**, 175
–, of aldehydes **17**, 253
–, of amino acids **17**, 239
–, of carbohydrates **17**, 231
–, of flavonols **17**, 228–229
–, paper, of tea catechins **17**, 221–223
–, –, use in analysis of fruit juices **9**, 269
–, partition, of tea tannins **17**, 221
–, thermal conductivity **14**, 23–24
Chromic acid, as oxidizing agent for cation exchange **2**, 6
Chromium, carcinogen risk assessment and **31**, 40, 46
–, in milk **36**, 237
–, tolerance of in wine **8**, 138
Chromium–inositol phosphate interactions **45**, 36
Chromogens, relationship of to browning **3**, 3, 4, 6, 12, 13, 24
Chromoplasts in parenchyma vegetable cells **2**, 306
– in –, carotenoid pigments in **2**, 328
– in –, changes induced by blanching **2**, 328–330
Chromosomal engineering **36**, 75–76
Chromosomal structure, wheat **36**, 30–32
Chromosome aberration assays **34**, 396
Chromosome mutations **34**, 390
Chromosomes, carcinogen risk assessment and **31**, 25, 28
Chronic wasting disease (CWD) of mule deer/rocky mountain elk **43**, 277–278, 296
Chronobiologic rhythm (*see also* Bioperiodicity) **40**, 218

Chronobiology (*see also* Bioperiodicity) **40**, 224–226
Chu Berman integrator **40**, 290–292
Chuka-men (*see also* Oriental noodles) **43**, 148
–, quality evaluation **43**, 171, 177
Chylomicrons **36**, 258
–, β-carotene **40**, 32, 37, 41, 62–63, 69, 71
–, levels, fat quantity and **36**, 306
–, metabolism, PUFA **36**, 273–275, 318–319
–, role in tocopherol transport **33**, 183–184
–, vitamin A **40**, 4, 16
Chymosin **39**, 170–172, 177, 211–213, 249–250
–, casein micelle coagulation **34**, 335–336
Chymotrypsin, dietary fiber and **31**, 170, 171
–, endogenous proteolytic enzymes and **31**, 345
–, –, endopeptidases **31**, 353, 354
–, –, muscle physiology **31**, 379
–, –, nonmuscle cathepsins **31**, 364
–, –, proteinase activity **31**, 391
–, inhibitors, in Leguminosae **28**, 138
α-Chymotrypsin, amino group alkylation **35**, 270–271
Chymotrypsinogen, alcohol concentration dependence **35**, 291–292
Cichorium endivia **43**, 10
Cichorium intybus (chicory) **43**, 6, 7–8, 48
–, cultivation **43**, 9–10
–, inulin **43**, 3, 5, 6
–, –, production **43**, 9, 10
Cider, biochemical work on **8**, 298
–, blending for astringency **5**, 273
–, fruit washing water-related disease outbreaks **45**, 169, 195
–, pasteurization recommendations **45**, 195
Cigarettes, nitrosamines in smoke of **22**, 53–55
Ciguatera poisoning **10**, 138
–, toxins causing **18**, 143–147
Ciguatoxin, composition and properties of **18**, 145–146
Cinnamic acid, in strawberries **2**, 270
–, microbial inhibition by **1**, 386
Cinnamic acid derivatives, in food browning **19**, 81
Cinnamon, flavor and **30**, 78
Ciprofloxacin **44**, 290, 321
Circadian rhythm (*see also* Bioperiodicity) **40**, 219
Circle design, for retort packaging **23**, 342
Circular dichroism measurements, emulsification peptides **42**, 116, 118, 120–121
Circumvallate papillae **44**, 251, 252, 253
Cirrhosis, etiology and treatment **37**, 403–404
Cisplatin **44**, 293
Citral **15**, 210
–, in oranges **2**, 264, 265
–, in peaches **2**, 265
Citrate **39**, 200–201, 267–269
–, bovine isocitrate dehydrogenase inhibition **34**, 357–360
–, inhibition of enzymes by **1**, 384
β-Citraurin **15**, 223
Citric acid, addition to milk **2**, 21
–, as a corrosion inhibitor **3**, 338, 339, 342
–, –, in prevention of discoloration in fruit **3**, 26
–, chocolate and **31**, 220, 272
–, effect on browning in fruit products **1**, 358, 367
–, – on saltiness **2**, 260
–, fish preservation and **7**, 68
–, freeze-dried citrus juice and **7**, 228
–, in fruit juices **9**, 269–270
–, in fruits **17**, 177–179
–, method of recovery from pineapple waste **2**, 18–20
–, olive oil and **31**, 459, 461
–, use of cation exchanger to increase yield from sugar **2**, 37
Citron, bleaching **5**, 98
–, brining **5**, 144
Citronellol in black tea oil **2**, 287
Citrulline, determination by ion exchanger **2**, 38
Citrus, loss of thiamine in **6**, 296
–, terminology **5**, 290, 291
Citrus brown rot, *see Phytophthora*
Citrus fruits (*see also* Grapefruit, Lemon, Lime, Orange) **15**, 176, 218
–, by-products of **17**, 89–94
–, –, composition **17**, 91
–, –, origin **17**, 90
–, components **9**, 287, 289
–, composition of, factors affecting **9**, 292–302
–, –, variability **9**, 291–292
–, distribution **9**, 293
–, effect of humidity on spray-drying of **2**, 498
–, flavonoid compounds **5**, 289
–, ion exchange treatment on peel of **2**, 30
–, juice **15**, 218, 350

–, varieties **9**, 287, 288
Citrus juices, darkening of **5**, 87
–, freeze-drying of **7**, 226
–, oxidation of ascorbic acid in **5**, 103
–, preservative action of sulfurous acid on **5**, 62
–, sulfiting **5**, 134
–, sulfur dioxide, combining power of **5**, 83, 135
Citrus pectin, effect on calcium absorption **33**, 141
Citrus peel, bleaching **5**, 98
Citrus products, aseptic processing **32**, 32–33
Citrus pulp, nutritional properties **17**, 90
Citrus seed meal, composition **17**, 91–92
CL, *see* Cardiolipin
Cladosporium, in beef **12**, 169
–, survival of at low temperatures **3**, 446
Cladosporium herbarum **15**, 173, 176
Clams, saxitoxin from **18**, 155
Clarithromycin **44**, 290
Clastogenesis **34**, 390
Clavulanate **44**, 293, 322
Clay, adsorbability of **2**, 11
–, use in synthetic aluminosilicates **2**, 4
Cleaning, automatic **15**, 344
–, hard surface **14**, 325–458
–, in place **14**, 420–430
–, sonic, ultrasonic **15**, 348
Cleavage, endogenous proteolytic enzymes and **31**, 344
–, –, endopeptidases **31**, 352, 356, 357, 360
–, –, exopeptidases **31**, 346, 350
–, –, meat technology **31**, 396, 397, 406, 409, 411
–, *N*-nitroso compounds and **31**, 68
Cleiomycin, effect on flat sour bacteria spores **18**, 185
Clidinium bromide **44**, 299
Climacteric, artificially induced **12**, 111
–, eating-ripeness **10**, 298
–, in bananas **12**, 188–189
–, in fruit maturation, color changes in **10**, 298, 311
–, in passion fruit **12**, 224–227
–, mitochondrial oxidations in **10**, 337–340
–, nonclimacteric fruits **10**, 298–299, 313–315
Climate, effect on irradiated fruits **15**, 122
Clindamycin **44**, 290
Clinical examinations, for muscle diseases and disorders **37**, 343
Clofazimine **44**, 290
Clofibrate **44**, 288
Clomipramine **44**, 310, 323
Clonidine **44**, 304
Clostridia, in bacon **3**, 308
–, in fresh fish **2**, 349, 351
–, in pork **3**, 293
–, *N*-nitroso compounds and **31**, 85
Clostridium, S layers **43**, 323
Clostridium botulinum **13**, 354, 357; **22**, 135–185
–, as thermal processing target **23**, 77
–, canned foods and **7**, 121
–, classification and nomenclature of **22**, 142–146
–, effect of location in container on survival **2**, 91–92, 96–99
–, – of sodium chloride on **3**, 293, 295
–, factors affecting heat resistance of **2**, 36, 66, 76–81
–, germination and growth of, factors affecting **22**, 154–157
–, glycerol and pyruvate effect on growth **34**, 378–379
–, growth rate of **7**, 105
–, heat resistance of **3**, 436
–, incidence and distribution of **22**, 137–142
–, in fishery products **22**, 135–185
–, in frozen foods **6**, 202
–, inhibition **22**, 157–160
–, –, in cured meat, by fumarate esters **29**, 52
–, inhibition in cured meat, by lactic acid-producing bacteria **29**, 55–56
–, – in –, by nitrate **29**, 13–14
–, – in –, by nitrite **29**, 13–14, 46–48
–, – in –, by radiation **29**, 52, 55
–, – in –, by sodium hypophospite **29**, 52
–, – in –, by sorbic acid **29**, 49–52
–, in vegetables **6**, 185
–, isolated from fresh fish **2**, 351
–, isolation and identification of **22**, 146–151
–, JTD-IV, pH dependence of growth **34**, 377–378, 380
–, lowest growth temperatures **13**, 355–356
–, *N*-nitroso compounds and **31**, 73, 81
–, pH dependence of toxin synthesis **34**, 381–382
–, spores, thermal inactivation **44**, 181, 182
–, thermal death time of **3**, 435, 441
–, toxin formation by **6**, 210
–, toxins from, factors affecting **22**, 154–157
–, –, properties **22**, 151–153
–, type A **13**, 356–357
–, type B **13**, 354, 356–357, 381–382
–, type C **13**, 354, 356–357, 381–382
–, type D **13**, 356

Clostridium botulinum (*cont'd*)
–, type E **13**, 354, 356, 381
Clostridium capitovalis, isolated from fresh fish **2**, 351
Clostridium difficile infection, inulin supplements **43**, 18
Clostridium pasteuranum, use of thermal resistance values in canned foods **2**, 81
Clostridium perfringens **13**, 353–355
–, germicidal effect of CPCl on **2**, 153
Clostridium putrificum, effect of sodium nitrite on **3**, 295
–, isolated from fresh fish **2**, 351
Clostridium sporogenes, concentration in food processing **2**, 73
–, effect of sodium nitrite on **3**, 295
–, germicidal action of CPCl on **2**, 153
–, heat resistance of **3**, 437
–, in meat, inhibition by nitrite and nitrate during curing **29**, 13–14
–, isolated from fresh fish **2**, 351
–, thermal death time curve **2**, 51
Clostridium tetani, germicidal action of CPCl on **2**, 153
–, isolated from fresh fish **2**, 351
Clostridium thermocellum detachment **43**, 350
Clostridium welchii, germicidal action of ADBACl on **2**, 148
Cloud point, of emulsifiers **22**, 324–325
Clove, flavor and **30**, 78
Clover, effect on meat flavor **23**, 38
Clover phytoestrogens **44**, 197
–, coumestans **44**, 211
–, isoflavones **44**, 203, 207
–, lignans **44**, 207
Clozapine **44**, 311
Clupeoid poisoning, occurrence of **18**, 154
Coagulation **34**, 130, 207; **39**, 165, 166
–, future research **39**, 293–294
–, rennet action **39**, 169–178, 197, 249–250, 293
–, test **44**, 170
Coalescence **34**, 135–145
–, as function of droplet size **34**, 140–141
–, – of protein load at oil/water interface **34**, 143, 147
–, correlation of stability with surface viscosity and elasticity **34**, 139–140
–, first-order kinetics **34**, 137
–, maximum absorption effect on rate constants **34**, 140, 142
–, maximum adsorption and droplet size **34**, 142–143
–, measurement **34**, 176–181
–, –, Coulter counting **34**, 177
–, –, emulsion stability diagram **34**, 180
–, –, hexane extraction method **34**, 179–180
–, –, microscopy **34**, 176–177
–, –, oiling-off test **34**, 180
–, –, turbidity **34**, 177–179
–, –, viscosity method **34**, 180–181
–, pH effects **34**, 136
–, processing effects **34**, 143–144, 147
–, rate variation with zeta potential **34**, 138
–, small surface-active molecule additives **34**, 144–145
–, surface hydrophobicity **34**, 143
–, surfactants versus protein-stabilized **34**, 138
–, variation of average size parameter **34**, 140, 144
Coatings, edible **12**, 327
–, ethylcellulose **12**, 330–331
Coatomer **45**, 30
Coaxial open-ended probe, dielectric properties measurement **43**, 80, 81, 82
Coaxial viscometers, narrow-gap **11**, 374–377
Cobalt, in milk **36**, 237
–, in plants, deficiency **1**, 121
–, –, effect of fertilizers on **1**, 314
–, in wines **8**, 137
Cobalt–inositol phosphate interactions **45**, 36
Cobaltous chloride, meat mutagen modulation **34**, 433
Cocaine **44**, 320
Cochineal (*see also* Carmine) **43**, 196
Cockroach, toxicity of DDT on **2**, 208
Cocoa, constituents of oil of **2**, 283–284
–, cotyledon **8**, 249
–, curing, fermentation and drying of **8**, 226
–, fermentation **5**, 295
–, flavor and aroma of **8**, 226, 278
–, insects in **8**, 288
–, nibs, composition of **6**, 38
–, organisms found in **8**, 231
–, polyphenols and enzymic browning in **19**, 112–114
–, types **5**, 294
Cocoa beans, chemistry, flavor **31**, 234–237
–, –, flavor precursors **31**, 231–233
–, –, quality **31**, 225–231
–, composition of **6**, 37
–, fermentation **30**, 93–95
–, –, free amino acid increase **30**, 94, 95
–, –, sucrose conversion to fructose and glucose **30**, 94
–, ground **6**, 37

–, harvest **17**, 106
–, processing **31**, 237–241
–, roasting **30**, 95–97
–, –, free and peptide-bound amino acid destruction, individual **30**, 95, 96
–, –, –, total **30**, 97
–, –, glucose and fructose decrease **30**, 97
–, volatiles **30**, 97–100
, , aroma reconstitution failure **30**, 98
Cocoa butter, cocoa bean chemistry **31**, 225, 229–231, 249, 250
–, composition **31**, 250, 251
–, conching **31**, 297, 300, 301, 303
–, confectionary fats **31**, 277, 278
–, deodorization **31**, 251–253
–, emulsifiers **31**, 282
–, equivalents **31**, 279–281
–, in candies **6**, 29, 37
–, milk **31**, 257, 258, 263
–, milk crumb **31**, 289, 291
–, packaging **31**, 324
–, properties of **6**, 40
–, refining **31**, 292
–, stability of **6**, 14
–, sweeteners **31**, 275
–, tempering **31**, 308, 309, 311–313
–, *Theobroma cacao* L. (*see also under* Chocolate) **31**, 329
Cocoa fat, composition of **6**, 39
–, effect of lecithin upon **6**, 41
Cocoa products, composition of **6**, 37
–, used by the candy industry **6**, 3
Cocoa solids, in candies **6**, 29
Coconut, extraction of **17**, 111
–, impulse process **17**, 112
–, in candies **6**, 47
–, lauric fats in **6**, 32
–, preservation with SO_2 **5**, 146
–, proteins of **17**, 111–112
–, usage **17**, 110–112
–, used by the candy industry **6**, 3
Coconut meal **17**, 111
–, diets containing, effect on animal depot fats **23**, 25
Coconut oil **16**, 15; **17**, 111
–, replacement for cocoa butter **6**, 44
Cod, aerobic bacterial flora of **2**, 350–353
–, Atlantic, aerobic bacterial flora of **2**, 353
–, bacterial attack on **2**, 357, 358
–, bacterial flora of **6**, 191
–, formation of dimethylamine in stored **2**, 371
–, North Sea, comparison of aerobic bacterial flora in fresh and spoiling **2**, 354
–, Norwegian, aerobic bacterial flora of **2**, 350
–, organoleptic spoilage of **2**, 377
–, pH value of **2**, 363, 381
–, rigor mortis in **2**, 366
–, tests for quality of **2**, 380
–, trimethylamine oxide reduction in **2**, 369, 376
Codeine **44**, 323
Code of Federal Regulations (CFR), sulfiting agents in food processing **30**, 4, 5
Codfish **13**, 283, 287
Codling, comparison of aerobic bacterial flora in fresh and spoiling **2**, 353, 354
Cod liver oil, effect of feeding on palatability of poultry meat **1**, 219–220
–, in diet of rats **1**, 112
Coefficient, stress **39**, 13, 23
Coefficient of viscosity **39**, 4–5
Coefficients, activity **17**, 38
–, temperature **17**, 35
Coefficients of digestibility, fats **35**, 20–21
Coenzymes **17**, 18–20, 34
–, Coenzyme A **17**, 25
Coffee **14**, 241
–, blended for aroma **8**, 284
–, carcinogen risk assessment and **31**, 22
–, causes of staleness in **2**, 277–279
–, chlorogenic acid content **30**, 110
–, constituents of gases of **2**, 279
–, effect of cathode rays on **3**, 176–180
–, – of temperature on scoring of **2**, 247
–, – of time of day on scoring of **2**, 243
–, flavor improvement in **3**, 153
–, flavor studies on **19**, 233
–, freeze-drying of **7**, 231
–, kahweal in **2**, 281–282
–, Maillard reactions **30**, 110–111
–, oxidation-induction periods of fat extracts from **2**, 277–278
–, patents **30**, 111
–, photomicrographs of spray-dried **2**, 514
–, precursors of aroma in **8**, 279
–, roasting **3**, 138; **8**, 280
–, –, arabinogalactan disappearance **30**, 110
–, –, sucrose pyrolysis **30**, 110
–, soluble extracts prepared by freeze-concentration, flavor of **19**, 236
–, spherical formation during spray-drying **2**, 473
–, spray dryers for **2**, 410, 420
–, use of Pangborn collector in spray-drying **2**, 484
–, – of standards for sensory tests of **2**, 231

Coffee (*cont'd*)
–, volatiles, identification **30**, 109, 110
Coffee lignans **44**, 207
Coffee whiteners **34**, 165–166
Coffeol compound in coffee **2**, 283
Colaminoformylmethyl, germicidal action of **2**, 156
–, *N*(higher acyl esters of colaminoformylmethyl) pyridinium chloride, structure of **2**, 123, 124, 155
–, toxicity of **2**, 156
Colchicine **44**, 295
Cold dehydration, microencapsulation by **34**, 166–167
Cold hardiness, of plants, development **25**, 202–209
Cold shortening, carcass suspension **26**, 138–139
–, electrical stimulation **26**, 139–140
–, hide-on electrical stimulation **26**, 140
Cold storage, classification of **20**, 114–115
–, compressors for **20**, 138–144
–, condensers for **20**, 144–145
–, design considerations of **20**, 113–152
–, –, for industrial agricultural projects **20**, 123
–, –, for lower temperatures **20**, 123–124
–, –, levels in **20**, 124–125
–, economic factors in **20**, 115–116
–, fans for **20**, 146–150
–, financial feasibility of, factors in **20**, 119–121
–, for frozen foods **20**, 116–117
–, for fruit precooling **20**, 118–119
–, –, specialized designs in **20**, 125–128
–, in treatment of fruit juices **9**, 252–254
–, preliminary assessments for **20**, 114–116
–, refrigeration plants, design of **20**, 128–150
Collagen **10**, 57, 58–59, 433; **14**, 41
–, abnormal calcification **37**, 401
–, aged cows **14**, 41–42
–, amide groups of **7**, 241, 253–254, 273
–, amino acid composition of **7**, 264
–, amino acid content **9**, 9
–, amino acids, functional role **28**, 250–251
–, and meat quality **26**, 83–84
–, biological value **28**, 319–320
–, carbohydrates, interactions with **28**, 260–261
–, catabolism **28**, 272–274
–, cementing substance and **7**, 260
–, characterization **14**, 116–117, 119–120
–, chemistry **28**, 240–250
–, –, amino acid composition **28**, 241–244
–, –, amino acid sequences **28**, 247–250
–, –, –, nonhelical regions **28**, 250
–, –, –, triple-helical regions **28**, 249–250
–, –, molecular organization **28**, 245–246
–, composition **28**, 274–287
–, –, ante-mortem factors **28**, 275–284
–, –, –, caloric and nitrogen intake **28**, 275–276
–, –, –, chronological age **28**, 281–284
–, –, –, hormones **28**, 277–279
–, –, –, lathyrism **28**, 280
–, –, –, sex **28**, 275
–, –, –, thiolism **28**, 281
–, –, –, vitamins and minerals **28**, 276–277
–, –, post-mortem factors **28**, 284–287
–, –, –, aging **28**, 284
–, –, –, –, heating **28**, 285–286
–, –, –, –, lysosomal enzymes **28**, 285
–, composition and structure of **20**, 264–266
–, contracted, gelatin and **7**, 287
–, cross-linking reactions **28**, 257
–, deficient synthesis in Ehlers–Danlos syndrome **37**, 392–393
–, definition **9**, 8
–, dermatosparactic **37**, 389–390
–, digestibility **28**, 318–319
–, DLVO theory, diagrammatic presentation **28**, 302
–, edible fibrous, production of **28**, 322–326
–, effect of bases **28**, 299–300
–, – of strong acids **28**, 297–299
–, – of swelling **28**, 306–309
–, – of various salts **28**, 300–306
–, – of weak acids **28**, 297–299
–, emulsifying capacity **28**, 309–311
–, endogenous proteolytic enzymes and **31**, 412
–, endopeptidases **31**, 362, 363
–, ester links in **7**, 254–255
–, foaming **28**, 311–312
–, food-grade, production of **28**, 325
–, food systems, use in **28**, 328–331
–, food uses **28**, 322–331
–, fortification methods **28**, 320–322
–, fractionation of **7**, 258–260
–, functional properties **28**, 287–332
–, –, amino acids, hydration capacity **28**, 290–293
–, –, protein structural forces **28**, 294
–, –, water binding **28**, 288–306
–, function in tissues **28**, 266–267
–, gelatin, use as **28**, 327–328
–, gelatin and **7**, 236, 237, 252–261
–, genetic types **28**, 233–238

–, guanidyl groups of **7**, 255
–, heating **14**, 63
–, hydrogen bonding in **7**, 255
–, hydroxylysine cross-linking reactions **28**, 258
–, identification of types **28**, 238–240
–, immunochemistry of **28**, 266
–, in abalone **23**, 175, 179
–, in bologna sausage emulsion **28**, 328–331
–, in hepatic fibrosis **37**, 404
–, in muscle tissue, heating effects on **20**, 285–292, 311–312
–, in poultry meat **1**, 211
–, in skin **28**, 323
–, interchain cross-linkages **28**, 251–260
–, –, biosynthesis on polyribosomes **28**, 267–269
–, –, – on –, glycosylation of hydroxylysine **28**, 270–272
–, –, – on –, hydroxylation of proline **28**, 269–270
–, –, covalent bonds **28**, 255–260
–, –, hydrogen bond **28**, 252–254
–, –, hydrophobic bonds **28**, 254–255
–, –, ionic bonds **28**, 255
–, –, metabolism **28**, 267–272
–, ionic groups of **7**, 263
–, meat technology **31**, 401–403, 406, 411
–, metabolism disorders **37**, 391
–, microcrystalline, production of **28**, 326–327
–, morphology **28**, 233
–, muscle physiology **31**, 371, 372, 374
–, *N*-nitroso compounds and **31**, 76
–, nonmuscle cathepsins **31**, 366
–, nutritional aspects **28**, 312–322
–, organization, gelatin and **7**, 253–260
–, peptide hydrolase action **28**, 273
–, physiological function of **9**, 8
–, polysaccharides in **9**, 9
–, polysaccharides of connective tissue and **28**, 261–265
–, products, salient features **28**, 324
–, properties **7**, 250–252; **9**, 8–9
–, protein quality assays **28**, 313–318
–, –, biological value **28**, 314
–, –, chemical (amino acid) score assays **28**, 316–318
–, –, digestibility **28**, 314
–, –, net protein ratio **28**, 315
–, –, net protein utilization **28**, 315
–, –, protein efficiency ratio **28**, 314–315
–, –, relative nutritive value **28**, 315
–, research needs **28**, 331–332
–, salt and hydrogen interaction **28**, 308–309
–, terminal amino acids and **7**, 266
–, thermal stability **35**, 326
–, titration curve of **7**, 278
–, viscoelasticity **28**, 312
Collagenase, activity of, in aging meat **20**, 275–276
–, endogenous proteolytic enzymes and **31**, 362, 406
Collagen triple helix **34**, 219
Collards, calcium content of, effect of limestone on **1**, 310
Collastromin, *see* Collagen
Collenchyma cells in vegetable tissues, composition and shape of **2**, 304
– in –, desirability in foods **2**, 306
Collision theory **17**, 38
Colloidal gels **44**, 45–54
–, elastic properties **44**, 48–54
–, fractal nature **44**, 45–47
–, scaling relationships **44**, 49–54
Colloidal stability test **34**, 325–326
Colloidal suspensions, potential energies of attraction and repulsion forces **11**, 368
–, ratios of hydrodynamic to dry specific volumes **11**, 366
–, role in fluid consistency **11**, 366
Colloid mills **16**, 128
Colombia, Incaparina use in **22**, 197–198
Colon, analysis **31**, 142, 150, 151, 153
–, dietary fiber and **31**, 119, 138, 139, 191
–, intestinal bacteria **31**, 173–176, 178, 182, 185, 186
–, properties **31**, 154–157, 164, 165, 170
Colon cancer, bifidobacteria effects **37**, 105
–, carcinogen risk assessment and **31**, 16, 22, 29
–, dietary fiber and **31**, 176
–, inulin inhibitory effect **43**, 34–39
Color **15**, 241
–, effect of vessel on judging beverages **2**, 241
–, freeze-dried foods **13**, 79–80
–, IM meat **39**, 127–130
–, in meat **10**, 401–402
–, lighting necessary for judging food **2**, 244
–, of foods, assessment of **19**, 254–259
–, of fruit **15**, 126
–, perception **9**, 159–161
–, –, standards of illumination **9**, 159
–, synthetic **15**, 253
Color additives, food labeling regulations **43**, 197
–, natural **43**, 196

Color additives, natural (*cont'd*)
–, –, adverse reactions **43**, 202–213
–, oriental noodles **43**, 162
–, safety standards **43**, 196
–, synthetic **43**, 196
Colorants **15**, 246
Color chemistry, of muscle **26**, 88–90
Color development **14**, 118–120, 125–128
–, effects on **14**, 211–212
Colorectal cancer, carcinogen risk assessment and **31**, 13, 17
–, dietary fiber and **31**, 173
Colorimetry **9**, 162–165
Colostrum **10**, 47
–, effects on gastrointestinal immune system **37**, 45
Coltsfoot (*Tussilago farfara*) **45**, 76, 91
Combined available chlorine, definition of **7**, 143
Comfrey (*Symphytum*) **45**, 74–76, 91
Commelina communis, phytate (inositol hexakisphosphate) synthetic pathway **45**, 8
Comminuted meat systems, thermal scanning rheological analysis **35**, 352, 354–355
Common beans **16**, 9, 67
Common buckwheat (*Fagopyrum esculentum*) **44**, 396, 397
Common mucosal immune system **37**, 21
Commutator, differential equation **40**, 329–330
Compartment, definition **40**, 13
Compartmental modeling, β-carotene **40**, 26–54
–, dynamic systems **40**, 333
–, folate **40**, 100–101
–, graph theory **40**, 340–341, 348–351
–, identifiability **40**, 306, 307, 309–310, 312
–, membrane transport **40**, 244
–, parameters **40**, 34, 40–43
–, population kinetics **40**, 267
–, transthyretin **40**, 152–154
–, vitamin A **40**, 9–21
Competitive binding methods, alternative approach to **33**, 25–26
–, differences between procedures **33**, 23
–, for folate determination **33**, 22–26
–, plasma and red cell folate measurement **33**, 24
–, problems and limitations **33**, 24–25
–, selectivity of assay **33**, 23
Competitive colonization, by probiotic microbes **37**, 91
Complementary DNA (*see also* cDNA *and* Genetic transfection) **40**, 96, 99, 101
Complex viscosity **39**, 23
Compliance, creep test **39**, 20
Compositae (Asteraceae), inulin **43**, 3, 9
–, pyrrolizidine alkaloids **45**, 65
Composite breadmaking flours **43**, 229
–, applications **43**, 231
–, chemical additives (dough improvers) **43**, 230
–, emulsifiers **43**, 230
–, mechanical dough development (Chorleywood) process **43**, 229–230
Composition, analysis **35**, 339
–, chemical, of passion fruit **12**, 214–220
–, date of picking **12**, 215
–, fruit size **12**, 215, 219
–, juice content after storage **12**, 227
–, variations, plant-to-plant **12**, 215, 219
–, –, regional and orchard **12**, 219
–, –, seasonal and yearly **12**, 219–220
–, variety **12**, 214–217
Composition/functionality relationships **36**, 44
Compound C_3, from *Aspergillus* M4-1, distinction from aflatoxin G_1 **30**, 296
Compounds, carbonyl (*see also Carbonyl compounds*), formation **12**, 36–37
–, –, N, assimilation by yeasts **12**, 69
–, –, yeast-static **12**, 85
Compressibility measurements, polymer hydration analysis **45**, 151–152
Compression, effect on nonfat dry milk solids and dry whole milk **3**, 89
Compression devices **14**, 97–99
Compressive stress **39**, 7–8
Compressors, for cold-storage facilities **20**, 138–144
Computational modeling, *see* Dynamic system, Graph theory, Identifiability problem, Kinetic parameter distribution, Linear integrator, Neural network
Computerized tomography, for muscle cross-sectional area **37**, 346
–, research needs **37**, 405–406
Computers, programs for **23**, 110–138
–, use in thermal process estimation **23**, 91–97
Conalbumin **1**, 150; **10**, 35, 42
Concentrated solution/melt theory **39**, 37–41
Concentrates, preservation of **7**, 120
Concentration, chlorination and **7**, 149–151
–, kinetic modeling **39**, 141
Concentration-dependent self-association phenomenon, folates **33**, 6

Concentration processes, in food drying, aroma retention in **20**, 38–64
–, –, cost of **20**, 87–90
Concentration–time curve **40**, 50–52, 60, 70
Concentric cylinder geometry **39**, 31–33
Conching, chocolate and **31**, 296, 330
–, emulsifiers **31**, 282
–, milk **31**, 253, 257
–, physicochemical reactions **31**, 296, 297
–, processing **31**, 297–299
–, refining **31**, 292, 295
–, sweeteners **31**, 267, 268
–, types **31**, 299–308
Condensation, water removal and **7**, 178–180
Condensers **15**, 321
–, Byer type **15**, 322
–, for cold storage facilities **20**, 144–145
Condensing in the manufacture of dried milk **3**, 83
Conditional identifiability **40**, 314
Conductance, membrane **40**, 248–249, 252–257, 331–332
–, specific **14**, 113
Conduction, heating, freeze-drying and **7**, 182
Conductivities, thermal, of foods **13**, 281–283
Cone-and-plate viscometers **11**, 377
Cone-plate geometry **39**, 27–28
Confectionery, agar in **11**, 122
–, alginates in **11**, 154
–, carrageenan in **11**, 137
–, gum arabic in **11**, 172
–, gums in **11**, 116
–, gum tragacanth in **11**, 185
–, products, milk powders used in, list **19**, 151
Confectionery fats, chocolate and **31**, 277–281
Confocal laser scanning microscopy, fat crystal networks **44**, 38, 63–67
–, microbial attachment to foods **43**, 354–357
b-Conglycinin **36**, 114
–, subunits **36**, 125
Conjugases, enzyme efficiency in folate analysis **33**, 18–19
Connectin, endogenous proteolytic enzymes and **31**, 371, 372, 400, 401, 408
Connective tissue **9**, 3
–, chemical composition of **20**, 264–267
–, collagen in **9**, 8–9
–, diseases (*see also specific diseases*), acquired disorders **37**, 401–405
–, –, genetic **37**, 389–401
–, –, nutritional **37**, 387–389
–, –, research needs **37**, 408–469
–, glycosaminoglycans associated with **28**, 261–262
–, ground substance of **9**, 10
–, in meat, heating effects on **20**, 285–292
–, in muscle **19**, 4
–, meat tenderness and **20**, 267
–, mucopolysaccharides associated with **9**, 10; **28**, 261–262
–, proteins, endogenous proteolytic enzymes and **31**, 395, 401, 402, 412
Connectivity, identifiability **40**, 306, 315
–, modeling **40**, 27, 32, 43
Conoxacin **44**, 290
CONSAM software **40**, 6, 9, 21, 32, 274, 290
Consistency **32**, 48
–, determining fundamental constants **11**, 373–393
–, elements of **11**, 357–358
–, influence of in filtration **11**, 429–432
–, in fluid foods **11**, 371–373
–, sliding friction as element of **11**, 357
–, viscous friction as element of **11**, 358
Consistency index **32**, 47; **39**, 6, 56
Consistometers **14**, 99–100; **32**, 48
Constants, Boltzmann **17**, 38
–, equilibrium **17**, 38
–, Planck's **17**, 38
Constipation, effects of lactic cultures **37**, 110–111
Constitutive models, rheology **39**, 33–44, 62
Consumer surveys **3**, 387–412
Contact dermatitis, spices **42**, 29
Contact sensitivities **42**, 9–10, 24–26
Containers, chlorination of **7**, 161–162
–, refrigerated **12**, 167
Contaminants, in foods **37**, 41–43
Contamination, bacterial, after processing **12**, 402–403
–, biogenic amines **39**, 290–292, 330–358
–, casein precipitation **39**, 184
–, control **39**, 119–121
–, in equipment **12**, 399–400
–, mycotoxisis **39**, 285–290
–, pet food production **39**, 85
–, process improvement **39**, 89–90
–, quality factor **39**, 248–249
–, sources **39**, 164
–, synergistic stabilization **39**, 149
–, traditional production **39**, 75, 77, 78, 80, 82
Continental Can Company, flexible packaging by durability of **23**, 401–402

Continuity, equation of **32**, 42
Continuous stirred tank reactors, lactase immobilization **38**, 18–19
Contractile process of muscle **19**, 313–314
Contractile proteins, endogenous proteolytic enzymes and **31**, 395–398
Contraction, of muscle fibers **20**, 262–263
Contraction and expansion losses, in determining pumping requirements **11**, 409–412
Control equipment, in evaporators **15**, 348
Controlled atmosphere storage, mango fruits **21**, 278–280
–, potato **21**, 340
Control of micro-organisms causing spoilage in fruit and vegetable products **3**, 429–482
Control systems, freeze-drying **13**, 63–67
–, Leybold's tempamatic **13**, 27, 65–67
–, –, VPR techniques **13**, 66–67
–, platen techniques **13**, 63–64
–, pressure **13**, 64–65
Convective heat transfer, *see* Heat transfer, convective
Conway diffusion method, of determining ammonia nitrogen in soy sauce **10**, 79–80
Cookies, absence of polymerization and glutenins and gliadins **38**, 224
–, baking tests **29**, 211
–, glass transition **38**, 185
–, nutritious, for developing countries **22**, 193–194
–, quality, effect of lipids in wheat flours **29**, 259–260
–, ultrasonic texture sensing **45**, 146
Cooking (*see also* Processing) **14**, 62–64; **15**, 241
–, by electronic heat **3**, 138–142
–, effects on meat quality **20**, 300–303
–, folate stability during **33**, 47–51
–, meat mutagens, formation (*see also* Beef) **34**, 420–422
–, meat/poultry products, *see* Thermal processing
–, microwave **15**, 290
–, vacuum **15**, 309
Cooling curve, curvilinear portion of **23**, 81
Cooling treatments, meat quality relationship **21**, 137–138
Copper, content, apples and pears **8**, 371
–, –, plants, effect of fertilizers on **1**, 314
–, –, –, effect on ascorbic acid, in canned grape-fruit juice **1**, 55
–, –, –, – on –, in tomato juice **1**, 61, 62
–, deficiency of, in apples and pears **8**, 378
–, determination in milk **2**, 38
–, effect on tallowiness in dry milk **3**, 95
–, fish lipid oxidation **33**, 289–290
–, gelatin color and **7**, 247
–, hepatotoxic synergism with pyrrolizidine alkaloids **45**, 79
–, in brandy **8**, 177
–, in browning **3**, 99, 100
–, in cocoa beans **8**, 258
–, in food canning **3**, 355
–, in milk **10**, 47, 51; **36**, 228–229
–, in wines **8**, 135, 136, 139, 176
–, olive oil and **31**, 473
–, peroxidation, alteration with EDTA chelation **33**, 304–305
–, phytate (inositol hexakisphosphate) interactions **45**, 32, 35–36, 40
–, phytic acid and bioavailability **28**, 41–42
–, role in polyphenoloxidase activity **19**, 91–94
Copper ion, inhibition of enzymes by **1**, 382
Copper salts, effect on pectins **1**, 400, 406, 414
Copra, from coconuts **17**, 110
Coprophagy caused by phosphorus deficiency **1**, 119
Core flush, *see* Brown core
Cori–Forbes disease **37**, 377
Corn **15**, 228, 235; **16**, 6
–, blanching of **3**, 136
–, bran/flour phytate content **45**, 16
–, by-products **17**, 117
–, carotene content of **1**, 306
–, changes in unblanched frozen **8**, 98
–, chemical components **38**, 271–272
–, correlation of quality of raw, frozen, canned **5**, 244
–, corrosion characteristics of **3**, 336
–, crude lipid from **8**, 100
–, cut, losses during blanching of **8**, 88
–, dietary fiber and **31**, 184, 185
–, effect of storage on biological value of protein in **4**, 268–269
–, gluten feed **17**, 117–120
–, gluten meal **40**, 160
–, inositol phosphate degradation during processing **45**, 21
–, insect species infesting **8**, 111
–, inspection of **8**, 121
–, loaves, thiamine in **6**, 274
–, loss of thiamine on processing **6**, 287
–, moisture content **5**, 217, 219
–, nutritional stress factor in **4**, 111–113
–, "pellagragenic" factor in **1**, 125

–, percentage sulfur content from methionine, cystine **5**, 229
–, production, and erosion **32**, 218
–, –, and ethanol production **32**, 197–201
–, quality protein maize **38**, 274
–, structure **38**, 273–278
–, –, caryopsis **38**, 274
–, –, endosperm **38**, 275–277
–, –, enzymatic degradation **38**, 291–292
–, –, germ **38**, 277–278
–, –, protein bodies **38**, 275, 277
–, –, seed coat **38**, 274–275
–, –, steeping agent effects **38**, 283–286
–, sweet, canned, consistency, analysis of variance **5**, 208
–, –, –, nutrients in **1**, 43, 46–50
–, –, pH value of **3**, 432
–, –, B vitamin in **1**, 42, 44, 45
–, titration and temperature values in moisture determination **5**, 215
–, types used **38**, 273
–, F value for industrial processing of **2**, 102
–, varieties and crosses, analysis of variance of puncture tests **5**, 201–203
–, wet milling **38**, 271–297
–, –, biochemical effects **38**, 287
–, –, cleaning **38**, 278
–, –, industry scale **38**, 273
–, –, kernel degradation **38**, 283–286
–, –, laboratory versus commercial milling **38**, 288–290
–, –, lactic acid role **38**, 281–282
–, –, milling and final processing **38**, 287–288
–, –, nonstarch by-products **38**, 296
–, –, process flow **38**, 272
–, –, products, derived from starch **38**, 292–295
–, –, –, modified starches **38**, 293–294
–, –, –, native starches **38**, 292–293
–, –, –, using fermentation or enzymatic technologies **38**, 294–295
–, –, research to improve **38**, 290–292
–, –, steeping **38**, 278–280
–, –, steepwater absorption **38**, 280–281
–, –, sulfur dioxide role **38**, 282–283, 285–286
–, –, temperature role **38**, 286–287
Corn flour, protein digestibility **35**, 201
Corning process, hydrolysis of lactose **38**, 47, 51
Corn oil, reversion problems in **4**, 201
Corn starch, aging of gels of **6**, 12
–, effect of sonic vibration on **3**, 131
–, expansion of lamellae of **2**, 319
–, gelatinization temperature of **2**, 319
–, used by the candy industry **6**, 3
–, viscosity curve of **2**, 320
Corn sweeteners **38**, 294–295
Corn syrup, chocolate and **31**, 263, 265, 266, 274, 275
–, composition and properties of **6**, 19
–, in canning **5**, 146
–, in ice cream mix **3**, 91
–, proportions of **6**, 11
–, spray-drying **2**, 499
–, –, effect of humidity **2**, 424
Corn zein-lipid films, applications **44**, 381
–, water barrier properties **44**, 375–376
Corn zein protein composite films **44**, 382
Coronary heart disease, genetic factors **37**, 192–194
–, link with dietary fatty acids **37**, 153–154
–, risk factors, milk- and dairy product-related **37**, 203–206
–, –, research needs **37**, 237
Correlation coefficients, flour quality parameters **36**, 54–55
Corrosion **14**, 443–449; **15**, 346
–, by food acids **3**, 337–340
–, –, in canning operations **3**, 344–350
–, –, inhibitors of **3**, 342–344
–, –, measurements of **3**, 344
–, –, miscellaneous factors concerning in foods **3**, 342
–, –, studies of in tin plate **3**, 376
–, –, tests in tin plate **3**, 366–371
–, concentration cell **14**, 447–449
–, galvanic **14**, 447
–, in cans **17**, 201–212
–, prevention **14**, 449
Corticoid hormones, and meat quality **21**, 90–95
Corticosteroids, glycyrrhetic acid and **7**, 366
Cortisol, effects on cardiolipin content **37**, 300
Corynebacterium diptheriae, germicidal action of CPCl on **2**, 152
Cosinor method **40**, 221
Cosmid vectors, gene cloning **36**, 139
Cost, drying **39**, 102
–, energy **39**, 143–147
–, refrigeration **39**, 74
Cost analysis, bases for **20**, 86
Cottage cheese **39**, 178, 201
–, contamination **39**, 292
–, heat treatment of skim milk for **3**, 80
–, sludge formation **39**, 184
–, syneresis **39**, 190, 191

Cottage cheese (*cont'd*)
–, treatment of by cathode rays **3**, 165
Cottonseed **15**, 288; **16**, 11, 60ff
–, effect of dielectric heating on **3**, 144
–, – of heat treatment on nutritive value **4**, 247, 254–262
–, glandless **17**, 109–110
–, globoid composition **28**, 9
–, nutritional stress factor in **4**, 110, 112–113
–, oleic and linolenic fats in **6**, 32
–, products from **17**, 108–110
–, proteins, nutritive value **17**, 110
–, usages **17**, 78–79
Cottonseed meal, effect of storage on biological value of protein in **4**, 269
–, effect on chicks **1**, 124
–, – on pigs **1**, 124
Cottonseed oil, color of **5**, 321
–, reversion problems in **4**, 192–193, 198, 202
–, solubility of DDT in **2**, 203
–, use in ranking sensory difference test on judging of **2**, 227
Cotyledon, chocolate and, processing **31**, 217, 222, 237
–, –, *Theobroma cacao* L. **31**, 322, 323, 325, 326
–, dietary fiber and **31**, 120, 128, 135, 148, 154
Couette cylinder geometry **39**, 31
Coughwort (*Tussilago farfara*) **45**, 76
Coulter counter **34**, 171–172
–, coalescence measurement **34**, 177
p-Coumaric acid, dietary fiber and **31**, 124, 138, 139, 189
Coumarin **5**, 263; **15**, 38
Coumestans **44**, 196, 197
–, analytical methods **44**, 201
–, bioavailability/metabolism **44**, 221
–, chemistry **44**, 198
–, sources **44**, 211–212, 214
Coumestrol **44**, 198, 199, 221
–, anticancer activity **44**, 232
–, antioxidant activity **44**, 225
–, estrogen receptor interactions **44**, 222, 223
–, *in vitro* effects **44**, 223
–, *in vivo* estrogenic effects **44**, 224–225
–, sources **44**, 211–212
Counterpressure, for package air removal **23**, 372–373
Covariate, population kinetics **40**, 272–273
Cow, germicidal action of Phemerol on **2**, 155, 182
–, secretion of DDT in milk of **2**, 211
–, storage of DDT in **2**, 211
–, toxicity of cetyltrimethylammonium bromide to **2**, 131, 176
–, use of quaternary ammonium compounds on **2**, 175, 182
Cowpea flour, protein digestibility **35**, 201
Cow's milk, calcium content **36**, 214
–, chromium concentration **36**, 237
–, cobalt concentration **36**, 237
–, copper concentration **36**, 228–229
–, fluoride content **36**, 238
–, iodine content **36**, 234–236
–, iron content **36**, 221–224
–, magnesium content **36**, 219
–, manganese in **36**, 230
–, minerals and trace elements **36**, 211–212, 239
–, molybdenum content **36**, 236
–, phosphorus content **36**, 220
–, protein intolerance **37**, 30–31
–, zinc concentration **36**, 227–228
Crab **39**, 350, 351
Crabmeat decomposition **16**, 172
Crackers, as mouth rinse in flavor judgments **2**, 248
–, glass transition **38**, 185
–, nutritious, for developing countries **22**, 193–194
Cranberries (*Vaccinium oxycoccos*) **15**, 225
–, dried, chemical changes during browning in **1**, 347–348
–, –, influence of oxygen on deterioration of **1**, 344–345
–, –, measurement of color changes during browning in **1**, 328
–, effect on corrosion **3**, 338
–, lignans **44**, 211
–, pH value of **3**, 432
Cranberry juice, canned, ascorbic acid content **4**, 375
–, –, use of ascorbic acid in **4**, 369, 375–376
–, chemical changes during browning in **1**, 349–350
–, electrical conductivity influence **44**, 22–23
–, measurement of color changes during browning in **1**, 328
–, microbial inactivation **44**, 14–15
–, pulsed electric field (PEF) processing, flavor/color impact **44**, 21, 22
–, shelf-life **44**, 16
Crassostrea gigas **10**, 145
Cream **16**, 196, 198ff
–, bacterial content during freezing storage **6**, 197

–, consistency of **8**, 38
–, crystallized **6**, 36
–, effect of spray nozzles on drying of **2**, 453
–, homogenization equipment for **2**, 463
–, use of ascorbic acid in **4**, 402
–, – of Swenson dryer for **2**, 420
–, whipped, alginates in **11**, 147
Cream cheese **39**, 187, 190, 193
Creaming **34**, 130–133; **39**, 273, 276–277
–, measurement **34**, 174–175
–, pH effect **34**, 131–132
–, protein concentration effect **34**, 131–132
–, rate, dependence on dispersed phase volume fraction **34**, 133
–, –, emulsion droplet size and **34**, 131
–, –, Stokes equation **34**, 130
–, –, xanthan gum and **34**, 133–135
–, stabilities of phosphorylated and native β-lactoglobulin **34**, 154–155
Creatine, formation during rigor mortis **1**, 3
–, IQ-like compound formation role **34**, 414–417
Creatine and creatinine, in abalone **23**, 165
Creatine kinase, serum levels **37**, 344
Creatine phosphate, breakdown during rigor mortis **1**, 3, 10
Creatine phosphotransferase as endpoint cooking temperature indicator **44**, 171
Creatinine, excretion index for muscle mass **37**, 350
–, IQ-like compound formation role **34**, 414–417
–, ultrafiltration **40**, 192–193
Creatinine phosphate, endogenous proteolytic enzymes and **31**, 394
Creep test **39**, 20, 43, 56–57
Creolin, concentration to destroy staphylococci **2**, 135
Cresol, inhibition of oxidation of **3**, 20
–, in respiration of plant tissues **3**, 15
Cresolase, *see* Oxidase, *o*-diphenol
Cresolase activity, of food polyphenoloxidases **19**, 88–90
Cresol in Formosan black tea oil **2**, 286, 287
Creutzfeldt–Jakob disease **43**, 281–283
–, genetic predisposition **43**, 287
–, human risk **43**, 292–294
–, iatrogenic acquisition **43**, 282, 283
–, inherited form **43**, 281, 282
–, –, prion precursor protein (PrP) gene mutations **43**, 282
–, new variant (vCJD) **43**, 283–284, 289–290, 292–293
–, sporadic cases **43**, 280, 281, 292, 307
Critical control point **39**, 151
Critical micelle concentration, of emulsifiers **22**, 322–323
Critical moisture content **39**, 105–106
Critical opalescence **34**, 209
Crocin **43**, 211
–, oxidation of **17**, 16, 30
Crohn's disease **37**, 31–32
Cromoglycate, sulfite-induced asthma and **30**, 50
Cromolyn sodium **44**, 301
Crop residue, as fuel **32**, 205–206
Cross equation **39**, 34, 46
Cross-linking (*see also* Racemization and cross-linking) **41**, 168
Cross sections, muscle **37**, 346
Crotalaria **45**, 80
–, contamination of staple foods **45**, 69, 70
–, prevention **45**, 91
Crotalaria fulva **45**, 74, 91
Crown rot (*Phytophtora* sp.), kiwifruit killing **29**, 285
Crustaceans **15**, 238; **39**, 345
Cryobiopsy **21**, 108
Cryoday unit **15**, 285
Cryostabilization **38**, 162–163, 165–166
Cryostabilizers, food proteins as **35**, 345–348
Cryptococcus hominus, germicidal action of ADBACl on **2**, 147
Cryptococcus neoformans, germicidal action of CPCl on **2**, 152
Cryptosporidium parvum **45**, 169, 189
Crystallization **13**, 244–259; **39**, 117–118, 135
–, control of, baked products **12**, 302–305
–, –, confectionery **12**, 307–308
–, –, dairy products **12**, 297–302
–, extracellular **13**, 257–258
–, growth **13**, 226, 260, 267–268
–, –, heat removal rate **13**, 247–252
–, –, temperature **13**, 247
–, intracellular **13**, 257–259
–, –, freezing rate **13**, 258–259
–, kinetics **38**, 210–212
–, recrystallization **13**, 253–257
–, time, WLF- versus Arrhenius-type temperature dependence **38**, 181–182
–, tissue in cellular suspension **13**, 257–259
Crystallizers, for aroma recovery in freeze concentration **20**, 40–43
Crystoplasm **13**, 309
CTAB, structure of **2**, 121, 150
–, toxicity of **2**, 130
Cubed meat **39**, 75

Cucumbers, ascorbic acid content of, effect of fertilizers on **1**, 309
–, composition of oils of **2**, 275–276
–, dietary fiber and **31**, 158
–, effect of plasmolysis on **2**, 308
–, ozone/carbon dioxide mixed gas treatment **45**, 202
–, treatment of by radio waves **3**, 144
Cumin, monterpenes **42**, 250
Curcumin, *see* Turmeric/curcumin
Curd **39**, 169–195
–, buffering capacity **39**, 175–176
–, fresh acid-curd varieties **39**, 178–193
–, rennet coagulation **39**, 169–178
–, rennet inactivation **39**, 197
–, syneresis **39**, 174
–, ultrafiltration **39**, 193–195
Curdlan, molecular shapes and interactions **42**, 175–179
Cured meat, antibotulinal activity of fumarate esters **29**, 52
–, – of lactic acid-producing bacteria **29**, 55–56
–, – of nitrate **29**, 13–14
–, – of nitrite **29**, 13–14, 46–48
–, – of research needs **29**, 70–72
–, – of sodium hypophosphite **29**, 52
–, – of sorbic acid **29**, 49–52
–, discolored by light **5**, 36
–, effect of pH **5**, 31
–, flavor, evaluation **29**, 33
–, greening **5**, 21
–, nitrite burn **5**, 20
–, *N*-nitrosamine formation **29**, 57–58
–, –, reduction by blocking agents **29**, 58–61
–, –, – by nitrite–ascorbate combination **29**, 61–62
–, smoking (*see also* Meat smoking) **29**, 21–23
–, –, antioxidant activity **29**, 23
–, –, bacteriostatic action **29**, 23
–, –, color development **29**, 22
–, –, flavor development **29**, 22–23, 33
–, surface fading **5**, 21
–, volatile compounds, nitrite effect **29**, 64–70
Curie **15**, 59
Curing, material states **38**, 214
–, meat (*see also* Dehydration control, IM meat), chemistry of **22**, 4–5
–, –, effects on SH groups **24**, 77–80
Curing smoke, aldehydes in condensate, color formation **29**, 137–139
–, antioxidative, phenolic compounds **29**, 145
–, application **29**, 98–100
–, benzo[*a*]pyrene **29**, 92, 135, 140–141, 147–149
–, chemical composition **29**, 104–135
–, –, analytical methods **29**, 109–112
–, –, electrostatically treated or untreated **29**, 140–141
–, –, for hot smoke processing **29**, 107
–, –, from different wood species **29**, 108
–, –, of condensate **29**, 106–107
–, condensation, laboratory equipment for **29**, 102–103
–, –, technical equipment for **29**, 103
–, formaldehyde formation, toxic effects **29**, 148–149
–, from beech wood, phenol composition **29**, 124–127
–, generation, from smoldering wood **29**, 92–95
–, –, pyrolysis of wood **29**, 93–98
–, –, wood materials for **29**, 90–92
–, identified compounds, alicyclic **29**, 117–118
–, –, aromatic (*see also* Phenols) **29**, 118–135
–, –, –, monocyclic non-phenolic **29**, 132, 134
–, –, heterocyclic **29**, 115–117
–, lysine loss induction in meat **29**, 146–147
–, phenols, *see* Phenols
–, physical properties **29**, 89–90
–, polycyclic aromatic hydrocarbons **29**, 99, 101, 104–106, 110, 112–113, 134–136, 140, 147–148, 150
–, preparations, liquid and solid, application **29**, 100–102
–, –, production, patented methods **29**, 103–104
–, secondary skin formation in fish and meat products **29**, 146
Currant juice, effect of temperature on changes in **1**, 333
–, influence of oxygen on deterioration of **1**, 341
–, measurement of color changes during browning in **1**, 328
Currants, black, pH of **3**, 432
–, brining **5**, 145
–, canned, corrosion by **3**, 353
–, influence of oxygen on deterioration of **1**, 341
–, of red **3**, 432
Curvilinear approach, *see* Nonlinear system
Custard, viscosity of **8**, 33
Cutin, components **31**, 120, 139, 140

–, dietary fiber and **31**, 119
–, in epidermal vegetable cells **2**, 304
–, properties **31**, 161, 163
Cutters in meat processing **16**, 127
Cutting boards, microbial attachment **43**, 332
CVD, *see* Cardiovascular disease
Cyanides, effect on dehydrated potatoes **1**, 272
–, endogenous proteolytic enzymes and **31**, 362
Cyanidin, structure of **19**, 79
Cyanobacteria **41**, 6
Cyanocobalamin, *see* Vitamin B_{12}
Cyclamate, carcinogen risk assessment and **31**, 23
–, chocolate and **31**, 270
Cyclic AMP, effects on cardiolipin content **37**, 300
–, endogenous proteolytic enzymes and **31**, 354, 380
Cycloalliin, biosynthesis of **22**, 88–89
Cyclobenzaprine **44**, 309
Cyclohexanediaminetetraacetate (CDTA), dietary fiber and **31**, 131
Cyclohexanol, DDT solution toxicity to man **2**, 212
–, solubility of DDT in **2**, 203
Cyclohexanone, solubility of DDT in **2**, 203
Cyclone collector in spray dryers **2**, 478–480
Cyclooxygenase, eicosanoids synthesis **35**, 94–97
–, inhibition and inflammation **35**, 140
–, lipid oxidation **33**, 269–270
–, *n*-3 PUFA action **35**, 150–151
Cyclospora cayetanensis **45**, 169
Cylinder geometry, rheology **39**, 31–33
CYP 2C11 **45**, 82
CYP 3A **45**, 82
CYP 3A4 **45**, 82
Cys residues, protein stability **35**, 268
Cystathionine β-synthase deficiency, in homocystinuria **37**, 397
Cysteamine, *N*-nitroso compounds and **31**, 82, 83
Cysteine, artificial meat flavor and **30**, 106, 109
–, chlorine and **7**, 134
–, dough development and **29**, 231, 234
–, effect in dried egg **1**, 172
–, effect on egg albumen **3**, 273, 274
–, – on gel strength of whey protein isolate **34**, 339–340
–, endogenous proteolytic enzymes and **31**, 345
–, –, endopeptidases **31**, 355, 357
–, –, muscle physiology **31**, 381
–, –, proteinase activity **31**, 383
–, in *Allium*, biosynthesis of **22**, 85
–, in bread dough **3**, 82
–, in tallowiness in dry milk **3**, 96
–, irradiation with niacin **3**, 168
–, *N*-nitroso compounds and **31**, 83
Cystine, artificial meat flavor and **30**, 106
–, effect of reducing agents on **1**, 382
–, effect on appetite **1**, 116
–, *N*-nitroso compounds and **31**, 83
Cystine groups, whey proteins, table **33**, 349
Cystine reductase, in wheat germ **23**, 240
Cytidine, reactions with sulfites **30**, 25–26
Cytochrome P450, lipid oxidation **33**, 256–259
–, pyrrolizidine alkaloids metabolism **45**, 81, 82
Cytochrome *b*, deficiency in muscle **37**, 380
Cytochrome *c* **17**, 10–11
–, as oxidative catalyst **17**, 27–28
–, inhibition of oxidation **17**, 30
–, in wheat germ **23**, 240
–, of peroxidase **17**, 29
–, succinylation **35**, 272
Cytochrome *c*-552, reversible unfolding **35**, 244–245
–, thermal stability **35**, 257
Cytochrome oxidase **3**, 9; **17**, 10–11, 20
–, in *Avena* coleoptile **3**, 15
–, in oranges **3**, 16
–, in tea **17**, 258
Cytochrome *c* oxidase, cardiolipin association **37**, 277–279
Cytochromes **17**, 19–20, 59
–, in electron transport **17**, 19–20
Cytokines, characterization **37**, 8
Cytoplasm, endogenous proteolytic enzymes and, endopeptidases **31**, 354, 357
–, muscle physiology **31**, 377, 379, 383
–, proteinase activity **31**, 387, 389
–, proteinase distribution **31**, 369
Cytoplasm vegetable cell, effect of composition on water retention **2**, 309
–, of starch grain **2**, 322
Cytosine, reactions with sulfites **30**, 25–26
Cytoskeletal proteins, endogenous proteolytic enzymes and **31**, 371, 395, 400, 401, 411–413
Cytosol, endogenous proteolytic enzymes and **31**, 411, 412
–, endopeptidases **31**, 354
–, meat technology **31**, 408

Cytosol (*cont'd*)
–, muscle physiology **31**, 378
–, proteinase activity **31**, 383, 386
–, proteinase distribution **31**, 366
–, skeletal muscles **31**, 352
Cytosolic folate **40**, 99, 100–101
Cytotoxicity **40**, 104
–, gut-associated **37**, 19–21

D values (*see also* Decimal reduction time) **44**, 15252
–, *Campylobacter jejuni* **44**, 16262
–, enzymatic time–temperature integrators **44**, 19090
–, *Escherichia coli* O157:H7 **44**, 158–161, 163, 16565
–, *Listeria monocytogenes* **44**, 16060
–, microbiological time–temperature integrators **44**, 17979
–, *Salmonella* **44**, 153–158, 163–16565
Dahlia, inulin **43**, 6, 9, 48
Daidzein **44**, 197, 221
–, anticancer activity **44**, 232
–, antioxidant activity **44**, 225
–, assay methods **44**, 201, 202, 203
–, effects of processing **44**, 213, 214
–, estrogen receptor interactions **44**, 222, 223
–, fungal/bacterial fermentation **44**, 213
–, *in vitro* effects **44**, 223
–, metabolism **44**, 220
–, pharmacokinetics **44**, 218
–, sources **44**, 203, 205
–, toxicity **44**, 226
Daidzin, pharmacokinetics **44**, 218
–, sources **44**, 205
Dairy industry, use of quaternary ammonium compounds in **2**, 175–179
–, waste utilization **38**, 20–22
Dairying, chlorine and **7**, 131
Dairy powders in baking (*see also individual types*) **19**, 147–213
– in –, milk powders, *see* Milk powders
– in –, milk proteins, *see* Milk proteins
Dairy products (*see also* Milkfat), agar in **11**, 123
–, alginates in **11**, 147
–, ascorbic acid inhibition of oxidation in **18**, 287–295
–, bacterial count **6**, 197
–, cholesterol content **37**, 150–152
–, contributions to fat/nutrient intake **37**, 140–143
–, diets meeting current recommendations, available products **37**, 229–232
–, –, by animal husbandry **37**, 233–235
–, –, by food technology **37**, 235–236
–, –, modified products **37**, 232–233
–, effect on CHD risk **37**, 203–206
–, – on serum lipids, animal studies **37**, 200–203
–, – on –, human trials **37**, 194–200
–, fat content **37**, 150–152
–, fermented, immunostimulatory properties **37**, 49–50
–, gum arabic in **11**, 174
–, gum karaya in **11**, 188
–, gums used in **11**, 114
–, insects infesting **4**, 308, 326
–, selenium in **32**, 96, 98
–, ultrasonic composition sensors **45**, 138
–, use of ascorbic acid in **4**, 395–403 *4
–, wastes **17**, 132–133
Dakin's solution **7**, 130
Damol, film formation of **2**, 144
Dandelion (*Taraxacum officinalis*), inulin **43**, 3, 9, 39–40
Danish blue cheese **39**, 201
DAN method **32**, 86–87
Dantrolene sodium **44**, 309
Dapsone **44**, 290
Darcy's law **39**, 185
Dark, firm, and dry pork, *see* Pork
DASSL integrator **40**, 290
Dates, dried, heat sterilization time for **3**, 456
–, polyphenols and enzymic browning in **19**, 119–120
–, souring by osmophilic yeasts **3**, 452
Daucin in carrot leaf **2**, 271
Daucol in carrot seed oil **2**, 271
Daunomycin, cardiolipin association **37**, 288
DDD (1,1-dichloro-2,2-bis(chlorophenyl)-ethane), method of distinguishing from DDT **2**, 205
DDT (dichlorodiphenyltrichloroethane), absorption and distribution **2**, 210
–, antidotes and treatment **2**, 214
–, chemistry of **2**, 202–204
–, effects on cardiac **2**, 207
–, – on nervous system **2**, 206
–, – on skin **2**, 207
–, excretion of **2**, 211
–, infrared spectroscopy of **3**, 147
–, pathology of **2**, 213
–, pharmacology of **2**, 206–211
–, precautions in handling **2**, 213–214
–, properties of **2**, 202

–, stability of **2**, 205
–, tests for **2**, 204–205
–, toxicity of **2**, 208–210
–, toxicity to man **2**, 212
–, trade names for **2**, 202
Deacidification of wine **25**, 1–53
– of –, biological methods for **25**, 25–42
– of –, by amelioration **25**, 13–16
– of –, by carbonic maceration **25**, 38–42
– of –, by ion exchange **25**, 23–25
– of –, by malo-lactic fermentation **25**, 25–32
– of –, by neutralization and precipitation **25**, 16–23
– of –, by *Schizosaccharomyces pombe* **25**, 32–38
– of –, double-salt type **25**, 19–23
– of –, physicochemical methods of **25**, 13–25
Dead-end pipeline **32**, 16
DEAE-cellulose, for monoglutamyl folate separations **33**, 27
Dealkylation, *N*-nitroso compounds and **31**, 59
Deamidation, protein emulsifier modification **34**, 155–156
Deamination, of amino acids **17**, 239
–, oxidative **17**, 246
Death rate, disinfectants and **7**, 137–139
–, nonlogarithmic **7**, 137–139
–, thermal **7**, 137–138
Debaryomyces **12**, 55, 77
Deboned meat, effect on "warmed-over" flavor **23**, 47–48
Deboning, *see* Mechanically deboned fish, Mechanically deboned poultry, Mechanically deboned red meat
Debranching enzymes, degradation **41**, 154–155
–, granule formation **41**, 110–111
Decantation, olive oil and **31**, 475
Decarboxylases **16**, 300; **39**, 331–336
Decarboxylation, cheese **39**, 232
–, fish **39**, 330, 331, 336
–, *N*-nitroso compounds and **31**, 77, 78, 83
–, olive oil and **31**, 458
Decimal reduction time (D value) **17**, 37, 43
–, for oxidase **17**, 43
–, in fruit purées **17**, 43
Decomposition, acid-catalyzed **33**, 278–280
–, acyl hydroperoxides **33**, 270–273
–, chemical indicators of **16**, 161
–, difructoseglycine **12**, 23–24
–, diketosamines **12**, 22–26, 35–56
–, in foods and model systems **12**, 35–59
–, ketosamine **12**, 22–39
–, of carbohydrates **16**, 203ff
–, of cheese **16**, 233
–, –, amino acids in **16**, 245ff
–, –, fatty acids in **16**, 257ff
–, of fats **16**, 198ff
–, of fruits **16**, 203ff
–, of lipids **16**, 425
–, of proteins **16**, 163ff, 237ff
–, of vegetables **16**, 203ff
–, of wheat flour **16**, 425
–, secondary oxidation products **33**, 276–278
–, volatile compounds from **33**, 273–275
Deconjugation, autolytic deconjugation with endogenous conjugases **33**, 17–18
–, efficiency of **33**, 18–19
–, enzymatic, of folates **33**, 17–20
–, pteroylpolyglutarnate hydrolases in **33**, 17
Decyl aldehyde in orange oil **2**, 265
n-Decylic aldehyde in orange peel oil **2**, 264
Defect, flavor **39**, 236, 239–242
Defects in food quality **9**, 192–197
– in –, classification of **9**, 193–195
– in –, instrumental measurement **9**, 195–197
Deflection-modulation display, in scanning electron microscopy **22**, 217
Deflocculation **14**, 358
Deforestation **32**, 187, 191, 195
Deformation (*see also* Rheology, semiliquid foods) **39**, 3–4
Deformation gels **34**, 217–218
Defrosting, of foods **3**, 137; **15**, 289
Degenerative joint disease, alcaptonuria-related **37**, 397
Degerminating mill **38**, 287–288
Degradation, amylase **41**, 153–154
–, chocolate and, alkalization **31**, 247
–, –, cocoa bean chemistry **31**, 233, 234
–, –, emulsifiers **31**, 282
–, –, packaging **31**, 314
–, –, processing **31**, 223, 224
–, –, sweeteners **31**, 270
–, debranching enzymes **41**, 154–155
–, dietary fiber and **31**, 120, 138, 191
–, –, analysis **31**, 142, 143
–, –, components **31**, 139, 140
–, –, dicotyledonous plants **31**, 128–131
–, –, intestinal bacteria **31**, 173–186
–, –, properties **31**, 154–156, 164–166, 169
–, outside chloroplast **41**, 156–157
–, oxidative, folates, energies of activation, table **33**, 50
–, –, free radical mechanism **33**, 45
–, –, resistance to **33**, 45

Degradation, oxidative (*cont'd*)
–, –, tetrahydrofolic acid, mechanism **33**, 42–43
–, pathway **41**, 155–156
–, phosphorylase **41**, 153–154
–, polyglycerolphospholipids **37**, 274–275
–, thermal, 5-methyl-tetrahydrofolate **33**, 49
Dehydrases **16**, 309
–, in wheat germ **23**, 240
Dehydrated mashed potatoes **25**, 55–136
–, antioxidants for **25**, 117–122
–, cell constituent role in **25**, 61–102
–, flavoring constituents in **25**, 102–109
–, –, interaction processes **25**, 108–109
–, lipids in **25**, 61–73
–, –, distribution **25**, 63–68
–, –, processing effects **25**, 68–73
–, –, varietal effects **25**, 61–63
–, microflora in **25**, 111–112
–, pectic substances in **25**, 73–79
–, –, distribution **25**, 73–75
–, –, enzyme effects **25**, 79
–, –, processing effects **25**, 75–78
–, processes for **25**, 56–61
–, –, flakes **25**, 59–61
–, –, granules **25**, 56–59
–, protein in **25**, 79–84
–, –, amino acids **25**, 81–83
–, –, in raw tuber **25**, 79–81
–, –, processing effects **25**, 83–84
–, rancidity in **25**, 112–122
–, –, determination **25**, 117–122
–, –, development **25**, 112–117
–, reconstituted **25**, 122–124
–, –, rehydration rate **25**, 122–123
–, –, texture **25**, 122–123
–, starch in **25**, 85–96
–, –, composition in tuber **25**, 85–87
–, –, processing effects **25**, 87–95
–, –, submicroscopic structure **25**, 85
–, –, texture effects **25**, 95–96
–, sulfite additive role in **25**, 109–111
–, vitamin C in **25**, 96–102
–, –, in aerated slices **25**, 97
–, –, in raw tuber **25**, 96
–, –, processing effects **25**, 97–101
–, –, storage effects **25**, 100–102
Dehydrated products of tropical fruits **17**, 194–195
Dehydraters, classification of **6**, 316
–, compartment **6**, 324
–, criteria for selection **6**, 345
–, development of **6**, 314
–, fruit **6**, 315
–, heating systems **6**, 332
–, instrumentation **6**, 333
–, materials of construction **6**, 335
–, mechanical elements of **6**, 326
–, operating procedures **6**, 363
–, optimum tray loading **6**, 355
–, Oregon tunnel **6**, 314
–, potato granule **6**, 234
–, static pressure drop **6**, 328
–, tunnel, basic theory of **6**, 347
–, typical commercial **6**, 339
Dehydration (*see also* Proteins in foods, future research on) **10**, 64–65; **15**, 240
–, by infrared radiation **3**, 146
–, by microwaves **15**, 288
–, by radio-frequency waves **3**, 142, 143
–, cheese manufacturing **39**, 166
–, economics of **17**, 99
–, foam-mat drying **12**, 323–324
–, of citrus waste **17**, 89–90
–, of fruit **12**, 325
–, undesirable changes in **7**, 172
Dehydration control, IM meat (*see also* names of meats) **39**, 71–161
–, –, absorption **39**, 97–100
–, –, –, bound and unbound water **39**, 97–98
–, –, –, protein denaturation **39**, 100
–, –, –, sorption phenomena **39**, 99–100
–, –, background information **39**, 73–74
–, –, dryer selection **39**, 146–147
–, –, drying equipment **39**, 145–146, 150–151
–, –, energy costs **39**, 143–147
–, –, hazard analysis and critical control point **39**, 151
–, –, mechanisms **39**, 100–114
–, –, –, cooking, raw meat **39**, 107–108
–, –, –, drying rate curves **39**, 102–105
–, –, –, fermentation **39**, 95, 108–110, 118–119, 148–149
–, –, –, moisture removal **39**, 100–102
–, –, –, osmosis **39**, 110–113
–, –, –, physical changes **39**, 105–107
–, –, muscle-meat conversion **39**, 90–97
–, –, –, chopping or grinding **39**, 94
–, –, –, drying rate curves **39**, 102–105
–, –, –, freezing **39**, 93, 148
–, –, –, heating **39**, 95–96
–, –, –, morphological changes **39**, 113–114
–, –, –, myofibers **39**, 92, 94–95, 96
–, –, –, osmotic treatment **39**, 96–97, 101, 149–150
–, –, –, prerigor processing **39**, 93–94, 147–148

–, –, –, rigor mortis **39**, 91–93
–, –, –, storage **39**, 93
–, –, –, tumbling **39**, 103
–, –, pet food production **39**, 83–85, 118, 126
–, –, predrying treatment **39**, 94–97, 102–105
–, –, preservation **39**, 85–88, 93, 118–119
–, –, process optimization **39**, 138–143
–, –, production problems **39**, 88–90
–, –, quality attributes **39**, 114–138
–, –, –, aroma and flavor **39**, 110, 118, 119, 122, 130–136
–, –, –, color **39**, 127–130
–, –, –, microbial control **39**, 119–124
–, –, –, nonheated versus heated meats **39**, 121–124
–, –, –, nonthermodynamic factors **39**, 116–118
–, –, –, nutritive value **39**, 136–138
–, –, –, oxidation control **39**, 133–136
–, –, –, oxygen effects **39**, 121
–, –, –, pH effects **39**, 121, 123, 124, 126, 148
–, –, –, precooking **39**, 126, 130
–, –, –, product acceptability **39**, 118–119
–, –, –, temperature effects **39**, 119–121
–, –, –, texture **39**, 124–126
–, –, –, water activity **39**, 73, 87, 100, 119–127, 139–142
–, –, –, –, definition **39**, 98
–, –, –, –, energy costs **39**, 143
–, –, –, –, equilibrium **39**, 115–116
–, –, –, –, microbial control **39**, 119, 120–124
–, –, –, –, process optimization **39**, 139–142
–, –, research needs **39**, 147–151
–, –, traditional production **39**, 74–83, 145–146
–, –, –, Africa **39**, 79–80, 89
–, –, –, China **39**, 75–77, 90, 119, 123–124
–, –, –, contamination **39**, 75, 77, 78, 80, 82, 89
–, –, –, Europe **39**, 77–79, 118
–, –, –, Indonesia **39**, 75, 89, 119, 136
–, –, –, Latin America **39**, 82–83
–, –, –, Malaysia **39**, 75, 89
–, –, –, North America **39**, 80–82
–, –, –, Turkey **39**, 74–75
–, –, vapor pressure **39**, 98
Dehydration profile **39**, 106
Dehydroascorbic acid **32**, 143
–, in formation of red pigment **32**, 143–144
–, – of yellow pigment **32**, 144–146
–, in kiwifruit juice during vinification **29**, 303–305
–, *N*-nitroso compounds and **31**, 62, 63
–, reaction with alkylamines **32**, 146
–, – with amino acids **32**, 143–146
Dehydroascorbic acid reductase, in wheat germ **23**, 210–211
Dehydrofreezing **9**, 65, 140–141
Dehydrogenase dihydroorotic NAD, in wheat germ **23**, 240
Dehydrogenases **16**, 433
5-Dehydroshikimate reductase, of tea **24**, 234
7-α-Dehydroxylase, fecal, lactic culture effects **37**, 100
Delayed-type hypersensitivity reactions **43**, 197–198
–, contact sensitivity **43**, 200–201
–, gut-associated **37**, 19–21, 29
–, mechanisms **43**, 199–201
Delphinidin, structure of **19**, 79
Denaturation **14**, 63–64
–, by heat, of muscle **20**, 293
–, chocolate and **31**, 257, 258
–, effects on gelation and gel strength **33**, 386
–, – on myofibrillar proteins **19**, 321–322
–, enthalpies, table **33**, 377
–, fast protein liquid chromatography **33**, 372
–, globular proteins **34**, 211
–, heat **34**, 149–150
–, –, effects on emulsifying properties **33**, 407
–, –, factors affecting **33**, 378–379
–, –, 11S globulin emulsification **34**, 148–149
–, kinetics **35**, 344–345
–, myosin, pH dependent **35**, 336
–, of meat, effect on SH groups **24**, 58–63
–, of proteins **10**, 24, 25, 26, 29, 36, 41, 371, 428–433; **39**, 100
–, –, in water and sugar solutions **35**, 291
–, soy proteins **34**, 234–235
–, susceptibility of whey products to **33**, 347
–, temperature **35**, 320
–, –, alkaline pH effect **35**, 323
–, –, effect of sodium salts **35**, 325–326
–, thermally irreversible gels **34**, 240–241
–, utilization and **33**, 371–373
–, whey proteins, assessment methods **33**, 363
–, Wyman-linkage theory **35**, 299
Dending **39**, 75, 89, 119
Dental caries **39**, 283–285
Dental health, inulin carbohydrate replacement **43**, 43
Dental hygiene agents, taste sensation effects **44**, 300–301
Deodorization, chocolate and **31**, 251–253
–, olive oil and **31**, 463

Deoxycortone, licorice and **7**, 356–358
Deoxygalactosone **12**, 24–25
3-Deoxy-D-glucosone, in shoyu during preparation **30**, 249–250
Deoxyosones **32**, 135–142
–, formation **12**, 26
–, isolation **12**, 24
Deoxyosulose **14**, 184
Deoxypentose nucleic acid, halophilic bacteria and **7**, 113
Deoxyribonuclease, in wheat germ **23**, 241
Deoxyribonucleic acid, *see* DNA
3-Deoxy-4-sulfohexosulose, metabolism, mouse, rat **30**, 37–38
Depancreatization, effect on rats **1**, 123
Depletion–repletion bioassay, for folate bioavailability **33**, 59
Depolymerization, endogenous proteolytic enzymes and **31**, 398
Depot fats, age effects on **23**, 32–33
–, composition of **23**, 21–33
–, diet effects on **23**, 25–30
–, environmental effects on **23**, 30–31
–, sex factors affecting **23**, 32
–, species differences in **23**, 21–26
Depsides, in tea **11**, 216–217
Dermatomyositis **37**, 362
Dermatosparaxis **37**, 389–390
Desalination **15**, 305, 343, 355
Desaturase **35**, 26–27, 29–34
–, apparent kinetic parameters **35**, 31–32
–, circadian rhythm **35**, 44
–, *n*-3 PUFA actions **35**, 148–150
–, reaction sequence and components **35**, 30
Δ^4-Desaturase, activity **35**, 50–52, 82–83
Δ^5-Desaturase **35**, 34, 47–50
–, activity **35**, 81–82
–, EFAD effects **35**, 48–50
–, hormonal response **35**, 49–50
–, α-linolenic acid effects **35**, 149–150
–, modified by dietary and hormonal changes **35**, 48
–, relative activities in liver and testes **35**, 47
Δ^6-Desaturase **35**, 31–34
–, activity **35**, 79–81, 148–149
–, –, human **35**, 84
–, competitive inhibition **35**, 107
–, α-linolenic acid effects **35**, 149–150
–, regulation **35**, 34–47
–, –, aging **35**, 46
–, –, dietary unsaturated fatty acids **35**, 35–44
–, –, hormonal effects **35**, 44–46
–, –, relative activity **35**, 27–29
–, –, summary of factors **35**, 35
–, –, temperature **35**, 47
Desaturation, *n*-3 fatty acids **35**, 81–83
–, linoleic acid **35**, 149
–, α-linolenic acid **35**, 24, 27–29
–, PUFA **35**, 35–36
–, rate, dihomo-γ-linolenic acid **35**, 88
–, –, linoleic acid **35**, 88
–, –, α-linolenic acid **35**, 78–81
–, unsaturated fatty acids rates **35**, 31–33
Δ^6-Desaturation, as rate-limiting step **35**, 52, 79
–, depression **35**, 44
Desiccants, freeze-drying and **7**, 189, 202, 214, 224
–, water removal and **7**, 180–181
Desipramine **44**, 311
Desmin, endogenous proteolytic enzymes and **31**, 400, 401, 408
Desmutagen **32**, 165
Desorption, explanation of **3**, 60
–, in packaging dry milk products **3**, 86, 87
Desoxycorticosterone acetate, effect on appetite **1**, 123
Dessert gels, alginates in **11**, 139–144
–, carrageenan in **11**, 125–128
Desserts, gelatin and **7**, 322–323, 325
Desulfiting **5**, 127
Detergency **14**, 326–329
Detergent-extracted residues, dietary fiber and **31**, 151–153, 160
Detergents **14**, 343–345
–, concentration **14**, 409–412
–, disinfectants and **7**, 139–140
–, properties **14**, 343–345, 347–359
–, selection **14**, 345–347
–, solution application **14**, 419–430
–, surface active **14**, 350–358
–, –, agents **14**, 359–368
–, –, anionic **14**, 351–353
–, –, nonionic **14**, 354–355
–, temperature **14**, 412–416
–, testing **14**, 385–394
–, –, direct **14**, 388–394
–, –, indirect **14**, 386–388
–, turbulence **14**, 419
Deterioration (*see also* Decomposition), of frozen food **13**, 311–317, 329–330
–, –, change of state **13**, 313–315, 329–330
–, –, in freezing **13**, 311–315
–, –, in storage **13**, 311–313
–, –, temperature decrease **13**, 311–313
–, –, thawing **13**, 317
Detoxification, histamine **39**, 330–331
Deuterium **40**, 116, 173–174

Deuteromycetes **15**, 167
Development, effect on cardiolipin fatty acyl composition **37**, 297
–, lactose effect, in elderly subjects **33**, 134
–, –, in human infants **33**, 132–134
Dexamethasone **44**, 295, 321
Dextrins **41**, 158, 169
–, binding agent in lozenge paste **6**, 29
–, in diet of rats **1**, 114
–, licorice extract and **7**, 348
Dextroamphetamine **44**, 313
Dextrose, chocolate and **31**, 264, 266, 267, 269, 275, 286
–, in chocolate candies **6**, 44
–, in fruits **17**, 179
–, in ice cream mix **3**, 91
–, in meat curing **29**, 6–7
–, recovery from corn sugar liquor **2**, 30
DFD pork, *see* Pork
DG uptake, *see* Glucose, transport
DHA, *see* Dehydroascorbic acid
Diabetes mellitus **40**, 191–192
–, chocolate and **31**, 268, 269
–, Δ^6-desaturase, regulation effects **35**, 45–46
–, dietary fiber and **31**, 140, 141, 168
–, endogenous proceolytic enzymes and **31**, 375, 389, 390
–, honey use in **24**, 353–354
–, inulin effects **43**, 39–41
–, xylitol use in **25**, 168–169
Diacetates, crystalline **12**, 25
Diacetyl **16**, 206, 212
–, in cocoa **2**, 283
–, in coffee **2**, 280, 281, 282
–, in food deterioration **17**, 20–21
–, in raspberries **2**, 269
–, in strawberries **2**, 270
Diacylglycerol lipids, structure of **23**, 7
Diacylglycerophospholipids, structure of **23**, 6
Dialkoxypolyenes **14**, 313
Dialkylamines, *N*-nitroso compounds and **31**, 61
Dialkyldimethylammonium bromides, solubility of **2**, 130
Diallyl sulfides in *Allium scorodoprasum* L. **2**, 273
Dialysis, micro- **40**, 183–190, 194–195
–, retrograde **40**, 190
Dialysis fiber **40**, 184, 185–186
2,3-Diamino naphthalene, *see* DAN method
Diaporthe citri **15**, 177
Diarrhea, effects of lactic cultures **37**, 84–92
Diarrheal diseases, bacterial **37**, 23–24
–, –, research needs **37**, 118–119
Diathermy **15**, 277
Diazoxide **44**, 304, 307
Dibenzodioxins, carcinogen risk assessment and **31**, 46
Dibucaine **44**, 287
Dibutylamine, *N*-nitroso compounds and **31**, 94
2,6-Di-*tert*-butyl-4-hydroxymethyl phenol **15**, 7
3,5-Di-*tert*-butyl-4-hydroxytoluene **15**, 5, 11, 22, 31, 41
α-Dicarbonyl compounds, shoyu flavor and **30**, 268–270, 271
o-Dichlorobenzene, solubility of DDT in **2**, 203
Dichlorobenzenone, 2,6-indophenol in ascorbic acid test in milk **3**, 75
Dichlorodimethyl hydantoin **7**, 156
–, plant chlorination and **7**, 147
Dichlorophenolindophenol, titration of ascorbic acid with **1**, 293
Di(*p*-chlorophenyl) acetic acid, use in tests for DDT **2**, 211, 213
Diclofenac **44**, 295
Dicotyledons, components **31**, 122, 124
–, dietary fiber and **31**, 136, 137, 159, 165
–, lignified tissues **31**, 132–134
–, parenchymatous tissues **31**, 124–132
–, seeds **31**, 133–135
Dictyostelium, phytase **45**, 12
–, phytate (inositol hexakisphosphate) synthetic pathway **45**, 7
Dicumarin from sweet clover, as stress factor **4**, 116
Dicyclomine **44**, 298
Didanosine **44**, 285
Di(3,5-di-*tert*-butyl-4-hydroxybenzyl) ether **15**, 7
Di-(3,5-di-*tert*-butyl-4-hydroxyphenyl) **15**, 7
Dielectric constant **15**, 280; **43**, 69, 78
–, of emulsifiers **22**, 325
–, water content relationship **43**, 71
Dielectric heating **15**, 278
Dielectric loss factor **15**, 280; **43**, 69, 78
–, water content relationship **43**, 71
Dielectric properties of foods **43**, 69–74
– of –, absorbed microwave power calculation (power equation) **43**, 70–71
– of –, frozen foods **43**, 71, 73–74
– of –, ionic content effects **43**, 74
– of –, measurements **43**, 78–82
– of –, –, foods development **43**, 82

Dielectric properties of foods, measurements (*cont'd*)
– of –, –, frequency domain spectroscopy **43**, 82
– of –, –, resonant cavity method **43**, 79
– of –, –, time domain spectroscopy **43**, 82
– of –, –, waveguide/coaxial lines **43**, 79, 80–82
– of –, microwave foods **43**, 103–104
– of –, microwave penetration depth **43**, 71, 72, 74
– of –, rate of microwave power absorption **43**, 71
– of –, selective heating effects **43**, 76
– of –, water content relationship **43**, 71, 72
Diet, carcinogen risk assessment and **31**, 41
–, effects on animal depot fats **23**, 25–30
–, – on cardiolipin, acyl composition **37**, 291–297
–, – on –, quantity **37**, 300
–, for laboratory animals, irradiation of **24**, 185
–, laboratory data **31**, 25
–, life span relationship **21**, 53–55
–, low-fat, low-cholesterol, effect on vitamin E status **33**, 190
–, modification of gastrointestinal immunity, autoimmunity suppression **37**, 50–51
–, – of –, breast-feeding effects **37**, 45
–, – of –, control of microbial flora **37**, 47–50
–, – of –, food antigens and allergens **37**, 46
–, – of –, hypoallergenic foods **37**, 47
–, – of –, nutritional therapies **37**, 51–52
–, special, irradiation of **24**, 183, 185
–, statistics **31**, 16, 19–22, 24
–, sulfite toxicity assay, pig, rat **30**, 41–44
–, total, effect of weight control **37**, 226–229
–, –, fat deficiency-related diseases **37**, 225–226
–, –, research needs **37**, 237–238
–, –, role of milkfat, CHD and cancer risks **37**, 224–225
–, –, – of –, current fat recommendations, available products **37**, 229–232
–, –, – of –, –, modified products **37**, 232–236
Dietary carbohydrates, effect on plasma cholesterol **36**, 305–306
Dietary fats, lipoprotein, metabolism and **36**, 255–256
–, –, plasma levels, quantity versus quality **36**, 305–315
–, quality, lipoprotein processing and catabolism **36**, 314–315
–, quantity, chylomicron levels **36**, 306
–, –, HDL levels **36**, 311–314
–, –, LDL levels **36**, 309–311
–, –, VLDL levels **36**, 306–309
–, saturation and cardiovascular disease **36**, 261–263
Dietary fatty acids **35**, 2–7; **36**, 253–334, 263
–, cardiovascular disease **36**, 331–333
–, monounsaturated **36**, 264
–, of commonly used dietary fats **36**, 266–267
–, plasma lipids and cholesterol effect **35**, 4
–, plasma lipoprotein levels and genetics **36**, 328–331
–, polyunsaturated **35**, 5–6; **36**, 265
–, saturated **36**, 263–264
–, short and medium chain lengths **35**, 5
–, stereospecific distribution **35**, 4
Dietary fiber (*see also* Fiber) **31**, 118–120, 190–192
–, analysis **31**, 142–146
–, components **31**, 120–124
–, –, dicotyledonous plants **31**, 124–135
–, –, minor constituents **31**, 138–141
–, –, monocotyledonous plants **31**, 135–138
–, degradation **31**, 187–190
–, detergent-extracted residues **31**, 151–153
–, fermentation **31**, 173–186
–, intestinal bacteria **31**, 171–173
–, lignin **31**, 150, 151
–, nonstarch polysaccharide content **31**, 146
–, –, cereal products **31**, 148–150
–, –, fruit **31**, 146–148
–, –, seeds **31**, 148
–, –, vegetables **31**, 146–148
–, properties **31**, 153–156
–, –, bile salt binding **31**, 159–163
–, –, cation exchange capacity **31**, 164–166
–, –, gel formation **31**, 166–169
–, –, intestinal enzymes **31**, 170, 171
–, –, particle size **31**, 156, 157
–, –, starch digestibility **31**, 169, 170
–, –, viscosity **31**, 166–169
–, –, water-holding capacity **31**, 157–159
Dietary folates, *see* Folates, bioavailability
Dietary studies, design **36**, 255–256
Dietary Supplement Health and Education Act (1994) **45**, 74, 91
Dietetic foods, alginates in **11**, 154
–, carrageenan in **11**, 136
–, gums used in **11**, 115
Diethylaminoethyl-cellulose, for monoglutamyl folate separations **33**, 27
Diethyl ketone in coffee **2**, 282
Diethylstilbestrol, residues in food **37**, 42–43

Difference Fourier maps **42**, 143, 146
Difference method, microdialysis **40**, 188–189
Difference tests, value of **7**, 7–8
Differential equation, background information **40**, 283–290
–, commutator **40**, 329–330
–, dynamic system **40**, 328–333
–, graph model **40**, 344–348
–, linear integrators **40**, 283–292
Differential operator **40**, 258–259
Differential scanning calorimetry **35**, 357–358; **41**, 167–168
–, chocolate and **31**, 310, 313, 319
–, egg white **35**, 341
–, endogenous proteolytic enzymes and **31**, 396, 402, 403
–, enzymatic time–temperature integrators **44**, 181, 182
–, fat crystal network fractal dimensions **44**, 115–118
–, heat evolution method **35**, 343
–, low-temperature studies **35**, 346–348
–, meat endpoint temperature monitoring **44**, 175
–, milk proteins **35**, 341
–, muscle **35**, 340
–, peak temperature dynamic method **35**, 343–344
–, proteins **35**, 319–320
–, thermodynamics of whey protein unfolding **33**, 376–377
–, vegetable proteins **35**, 341–342
–, whey protein denaturation **33**, 372
Diffusion, Fickian **39**, 140
–, passive **40**, 248–251
–, rate in ion exchange reactions **2**, 8–9
Diffusion coefficient **39**, 132, 135, 142
–, apparent **34**, 27–29
–, –, abnormalities **34**, 29–30
–, of water and aroma components, in foods **20**, 57–63
–, proteins **34**, 19–20
–, Stokes–Einstein equation **34**, 28–29
Diffusion-limited aggregation **44**, 45, 47
Diffusion pressure in vegetables and fruits, theory of **2**, 308
Difructoseglycine **12**, 23–24, 28
Digestion, enzymic **14**, 124
–, human **41**, 157–158
Digestive enzyme, protein inhibitors of **28**, 128–133
Digital storage oscilloscope **45**, 122–123
Diglutamate, determination in conjugase assay by reversed-phase HPLC **33**, 31
Dihomo-γ-linolenic acid **35**, 47–48
–, desaturation rate **35**, 88
Dihydroconiferyl alcohol, in maple syrup **30**, 111
7,8-Dihydrofolate, folic acid–sodium dithionite reaction **33**, 8
–, preparation, enzymatic reduction **33**, 9
Dihydrofolate reductase, disulfide bond **35**, 289
Dihydroperoxides, from polyunsaturated fatty acid oxidation **33**, 276–277
–, linolenate, breakdown mechanism **33**, 276
Dihydropyridine receptor, in muscular dysgenesis **37**, 371
Dihydroxyacetone, in spoiled table wines **6**, 76
2:3-Dihydroxyacetophenone in coffee **2**, 281
4,7-Dihydroxyflavanone **7**, 342
Dihydroxyphenylalanine, see "Dopa"
Diisobutylcresoxyethoxyltyldimethylbenzyl ammonium chloride, corrosive effect of **2**, 175
–, germicidal action of **2**, 154, 183
–, structure of **2**, 121
–, toxicity of **2**, 130
Diisopropyl fluorophosphate, endogenous proteolytic enzymes and **31**, 353
Diketogulonic acid **3**, 173, 174
Diketosamine **12**, 4–5
–, decomposition **12**, 22–24, 35–36
–, formation **12**, 35–36
–, preparation **12**, 8
Dilatancy, in fluid consistency **11**, 367
Dilatant behavior **39**, 5, 6
Dilauryldimethylammonium bromide, structure of **2**, 123
Dilauryl thiodipropionate, effect on mortality of rats **3**, 205
–, pathologic effects of **3**, 207
–, toxicity of as an antioxidant **3**, 200
Diltiazem **44**, 304, 320
Dilute solution molecular theory **39**, 35–37
Dilution tests, applications of **7**, 9
Dimensional analysis for convection heat transfer **32**, 48–50
Dimensionality **40**, 325–333
–, fractional **40**, 326–328
–, Hausdorff–Besicovic **40**, 328
–, reduction **40**, 328–333
Dimethylamines, fish freshness and **7**, 48–49, 59
–, formation in spoiling fish **2**, 371

Dimethylamines (*cont'd*)
–, fundamentals **31**, 59, 61
–, nitrite/nitrate addition **31**, 78
–, *N*-nitroso compounds and **31**, 55
–, processing **31**, 90
–, test for spoilage of fish **2**, 375–381
Dimethyl phthalate, effects on skin **2**, 207
–, solubility of DDT in **2**, 203
Dimethyl sulfide in coffee **2**, 281
Dimethyl sulfoxide **44**, 295
2,5-Dimethyl-1,3,4-trithiolane, in meaty aroma **18**, 59–60
Diminishing return **40**, 157–166
2,4-Dinitrophenylhydrazone in coffee **2**, 283
Dinucleotides **17**, 19
Dioxane, solubility of DDT in **2**, 203
Dioxin, carcinogen risk assessment and **31**, 26–28, 33
Dipalmitoylphosphatidylcholine liposomes, α-tocopherol transfer to rat liver mitochondria **33**, 195
Dipeptidases, endogenous proteolytic enzymes and **31**, 345, 412
–, in wheat germ **23**, 210
–, meat technology **31**, 411
–, skeletal muscles **31**, 346, 348, 349, 352
Dipeptides, endogenous proteolytic enzymes and **31**, 348–350, 378
–, racemization rates **35**, 207
–, with physiological activity **36**, 180–181
Dipeptidyl aminopeptidases, endogenous proteolytic enzymes and, type I **31**, 350, 411
–, –, type II **31**, 352, 388, 390, 411
–, –, type III **31**, 351, 352, 388
–, –, type IV **31**, 352, 390, 391, 411
Dipeptidylpeptidases, endogenous proteolytic enzymes and **31**, 345, 412
–, meat technology **31**, 410, 411
–, skeletal muscles **31**, 346, 349–352
Diphenylhydantoin, antifolate effects **33**, 71
Diphenyl in fruit wrappings **3**, 465
Diphtheria toxin resistance assay **34**, 392, 395
Diphtheroids in pork **3**, 293
Diplococcus pneumoniae I, germicidal effect of CPCl on **2**, 152
Diplodia natalensis **15**, 177
Dipropylame, *N*-nitroso compounds and **31**, 61
Dips, batter **12**, 327–328
Dipyridamole **44**, 314
Directed graph **40**, 229–230, 340–341
Direct-fired heater, design of burners **2**, 488
–, fuels used for **2**, 487
–, need for complete combustion **2**, 488
–, use in spray-drying **2**, 486–488
Direct-fired indirect heater, use in spray-drying **2**, 486
Direct transformation system **36**, 164–165
Disaccharides, formed by *Kluyveromyces lactis* lactase **38**, 77, 79
Discoloration, chlorine and **7**, 165
–, in meat **10**, 57–58
Diseases, dystrophies **13**, 91, 158–169
–, effect on water-holding capacity of meat **10**, 383–385
–, muscle (*see also* Muscle diseases and disorders) **13**, 156–159
–, postharvest, *see* Postharvest diseases
–, white **13**, 91, 156–158
Disguising potential, medicaments and **7**, 9
Disinfectants, penetration of **7**, 139–140
Disinfection, factories **12**, 410
–, potato starch **12**, 411–412
–, spices and condiments **12**, 412–413
–, water **12**, 413–414
Disjoining pressure, protein-stabilized foams **34**, 64–65
Disodium phosphate in inhibition of corrosion **3**, 342
Disorders, functional **12**, 111–116
–, muscle, *see* Muscle diseases and disorders
Dispersion, effect of travel distance on drying **2**, 465
–, food **13**, 290–291
–, importance of in spray-drying **2**, 465–470
–, terminal velocities of particle **2**, 466–470
Displacements **14**, 295–299
–, on carbon **14**, 295–297
–, steric course **14**, 297
Dissipation factor **15**, 281
Dissociation **41**, 9
Dissociation constants, binding of nonpolar compounds by β-lactoglobulin, table **33**, 410
Distearyl thiodipropionate, effect on mortality of rats **3**, 205
–, pathologic effects of **3**, 207
–, toxicity of as an antioxidant **3**, 201
Distillery wastes **17**, 126–128
Distribution (*see also* Kinetic parameter distribution), posterior **40**, 268
–, prior **40**, 268, 269–271, 273–276
Disulfide bonds, dihydrofolate reductase **35**, 289
–, interchain, amino acid sequences around cysteine residues **36**, 116–118
–, lysozyme **35**, 284–286
–, proteins **34**, 14

–, protein stability **35**, 284–290
–, reduction, protein emulsifier modification **34**, 158
–, subtilisin **35**, 287–289
Disulfide groups, determination of **24**, 28–30
Disulfides, percentage, in garlic oil **2**, 272
–, –, in onion oil **2**, 273
Disulfide–sulfhydryl interchange reactions, wheat proteins **36**, 64
Diterpenes, heat stability **42**, 263
Dithionate, inactivation of disulfide enzymes by **1**, 382
Diuretics, taste sensation effects **44**, 302–307
Diurnal variation, in plasma α-tocopherol concentration **33**, 176
DLVO theory **34**, 95–96
– of colloidal stability **43**, 325
DNA (*see also* Complementary DNA *and* Genetic transfection), ADPGlc **41**, 73–74
–, carcinogen risk assessment and **31**, 25, 45
–, cross-links, formation during pyrrolizidine alkaloid metabolism **45**, 83, 88–90
–, exogenous, characterization **41**, 125–126
–, genomic, cloning **36**, 135, 142–143
–, –, screening of libraries **36**, 143
–, in bacterial destruction **3**, 165
–, lipid oxidation effects **33**, 285–286
–, *N*-nitroso compounds and **31**, 55
–, T_i-plasmid **41**, 126–128
–, reaction with sulfite-produced free radicals **30**, 26
–, repair, inositol phosphate requirement **45**, 31
–, sequencing **36**, 143–144
–, synthetic, insertion in soybean glycinin **36**, 180
DNA damage, cultured mammalian cells **34**, 396–397
DNA polymerase, cardiolipin association **37**, 286
DNA–protein cross-links **45**, 90, 93
DNA/RNA-modifying enzymes **36**, 136–137
Docosahexaenoate, autoxidation, mechanism **33**, 250
Docosahexaenoic acid **35**, 7
–, accumulation in fetus **35**, 122
–, autoxidation **33**, 248–250
–, linseed and fish oil supplementation effects **35**, 55
–, lipid contents **35**, 14–15
–, retina and visual function **35**, 117–118
–, retinal phospholipid content and age **35**, 120
–, vegans and omnivores **35**, 63–64
Docosapentaenoic acid **35**, 14
n-Dodecyldimethylbenzylammonium chloride, germicidal activity of **2**, 137
Dodecyldimethyl-*a*-menaphthylammonium chloride, germicidal activity of **2**, 137, 140
Dogfish, dimethylamine production in **2**, 371, 381
–, rigor mortis in **2**, 364
Dogs, effects of DDT, on brain and liver **2**, 213
–, – of –, on skin **2**, 207
–, secretion of DDT in milk of **2**, 211
–, storage of DDT in **2**, 211
–, toxicity of DDT to **2**, 208
–, use in toxicity tests of CPCl **2**, 153
Doi–Edwards model **39**, 39–41, 52–53
Dole aseptic process **32**, 5–9, 20
Dolphin **39**, 337
Donated foods, for developing countries **22**, 195–196
“Dopa”, as hydrogen carrier in respiration **3**, 13
–, conversion from tyrosine **3**, 23
–, in leaf tissue homogenates **3**, 16
–, occurrence of in fruits **3**, 4
Dopachrome, structure of **19**, 104
“Dopa” oxidase in eggs **1**, 183
Doppler ultrasound, flowmeters **45**, 131–132
–, viscosity determination **45**, 148, 149
Dosage, of pathogens **15**, 151, 155
Dose–response relationship, amino acids **40**, 157–160, 162–166
–, carcinogen risk assessment and **31**, 8, 10
–, laboratory data **31**, 25, 26, 28, 30–34
Dosimetry **15**, 58
Double-blind, placebo-controlled food challenge **42**, 34
Double-effect evaporation, cost of **20**, 89
Doubly labeled water method **40**, 171–180
–, assumptions **40**, 173–174
–, equations **40**, 174–175
–, isotopes **40**, 175–176
–, mass spectrometry **40**, 176–178
–, validations **40**, 178–179
Dough (*see also* Bread *and* Wheat flour) **39**, 53–55, 58–59
–, alginates in **11**, 155
–, analysis of stresses in proofing **11**, 401
–, changes in when stress decreased **11**, 405
–, development, effect of cysteine **29**, 231, 234
–, –, – of loaf score of energy input and intermediate proof time combination **29**, 238–239

Dough, development, effect (*cont'd*)
–, –, – of mixing intensity **29**, 230–234
–, –, – of oxidants **29**, 237–238
–, –, – of passages through sheeting rolls **29**, 238–241
–, –, – of protein in flour **29**, 243–246
–, –, – of sodium metabisulfite **29**, 234, 238
–, –, – of unmixing and remixing **29**, 234–237
–, enzyme effect on **16**, 428
–, evaluating rheological properties of **11**, 402–406
–, extension rate at constant stress **11**, 403
–, flour **8**, 21, 43
–, glutin structure of **8**, 15
–, hard sweet biscuit, sulfite fate **30**, 27
–, lipids **16**, 421
–, membranes in, role in breadmaking **20**, 169–175
–, mixers **8**, 14
–, –, mechanic and mixing efficiencies **29**, 231–234
–, mixing **16**, 371
–, –, increase of wheat proteins solubility by **36**, 14–15
–, oxidation **16**, 367, 418
–, rheology **11**, 401–406; **16**, 357, 417
–, starch **16**, 385
–, sulfur compounds in **16**, 371
–, tensile forces in **11**, 398
–, tests on **8**, 22, 45
Doughnuts, fat absorbed by batter **5**, 177
Dowex 2, for monoglutamyl folate separations **33**, 26
Dowex 50, adsorption of polypeptide fraction by **2**, 12
–, effect of nitric acid on **2**, 6
–, use in finding rate of diffusion **2**, 9
Dowex 30 cation exchanger **2**, 5–6
–, adsorption of polypeptide fraction by **2**, 12
–, effect of nitric acid on **2**, 6
–, flow rate through **2**, 11
Down syndrome **40**, 113
Doxazosin **44**, 304
Doxepin **44**, 311
Doxorubicin **44**, 293
–, cardiolipin association **37**, 287–288
Drawn pouch system, for package air removal **23**, 373–374
–, for retort packaging **23**, 342, 344
Dressings, gums in **11**, 115
Dried foods, preservation of **7**, 117–120
Dried fruits, analyses for SO_2 **5**, 120, 121
–, insects infesting **4**, 306, 309–310, 329
–, sulfured, glucose-bisulfite reaction products in **5**, 59
–, use of SO_2 **5**, 141
Dried pork floss **39**, 76
Dried products, *N*-nitroso compounds and **31**, 91, 92
Dried vegetables, browning pigments in **5**, 88
Drinking water, sulfite toxicity assay, rat **30**, 41, 42
Drosophila assays **34**, 397–398
Drosophila melanogaster **15**, 175
Drugs, as sulfite sources **30**, 31–32
–, immunotoxic, in foods **37**, 43
Drum drying, aroma retention in **20**, 73
Dry distillation, of different woods, products **29**, 93–94
Dryers, chamber designs **13**, 47–63
–, continuous **13**, 57
–, experimental extrusion **13**, 59
–, fixed platen **13**, 47–52
–, –, conventional **13**, 47–50
–, –, cylindrical, integrated **13**, 50–52
–, –, tray, platen spacings **13**, 48–49
–, heating systems **13**, 60–63
–, –, conventional **13**, 60–63
–, –, radio-frequency **13**, 63
–, loading aids **13**, 55–57
–, materials **13**, 59–60
–, movable-platen **13**, 55–57
–, semicontinuous **13**, 57–59
Dry heat **39**, 120
Drying (*see also* Dehydration control, IM meat) **39**, 101–102
–, atmospheric roller **3**, 85
–, convective heating **39**, 113–114
–, energy costs **39**, 146–147
–, of abalone **23**, 172–173
–, process optimization **39**, 140–143
–, rate data **39**, 102–105
–, research needs **39**, 150–151
–, spray **3**, 84
–, temperature and **7**, 198–203
–, theories **39**, 106
–, time and **7**, 198–203
–, vacuum roller **3**, 85
Drying and concentration of foods, aroma retention and recovery in **20**, 1–111
– of –, by evaporation of water **20**, 64–74
– of –, economics of various processes **20**, 85–98
– of –, preconcentration effects on **20**, 96–98
– of –, transport phenomena in **20**, 52–64
– of –, vapor–liquid equilibria in **20**, 10–19
Drying times **13**, 32–34

Dry processing, proteins **35**, 333–334
Dry whole milk (DWM), amino acid composition of **19**, 158
–, lipids in **19**, 187
–, minerals and salts in **19**, 194
–, preparation of **19**, 152–153
–, –, flow diagram **19**, 153
–, use in bakery and confectionery products **19**, 151
–, vitamins in **19**, 192
Duchenne muscular dystrophy **37**, 351–359
Dung, as fuel **32**, 205, 224
–, for biogas generation **32**, 206–209
Duolite A-3, effect of temperature on **2**, 8
–, use in pineapple industry **2**, 19
Duolite C-3, adsorption of polypeptide fraction by **2**, 12
–, use in pineapple industry **2**, 19
Duplications, dystrophin gene **37**, 356–357
Duponol PC, neutralization of cation agents by **2**, 132
Dupré effect **14**, 419
Durum wheat, glutens **36**, 133
Duryea, use in developing South-American countries **22**, 198–199
Dust, *Salmonella* in **3**, 229
Dust collectors, use in spray-drying **2**, 483, 485
Dye-binding capacity, intact proteins **35**, 194
Dyes, azo **15**, 255
Dynamics map **38**, 129, 134, 159–177
–, solute-specific subzero glass transition temperature **38**, 161, 163–166
–, C_g' values **38**, 166–169
–, water and glass dynamics **38**, 160
–, WLF equation **38**, 160, 177–188
Dynamic system **40**, 323–338
–, differential equations **40**, 328–333
–, geometric interpretation **40**, 328–333
–, linear modeling **40**, 324
–, neural networks **40**, 333–337
–, nonlinear modeling **40**, 324–328
Dynamic viscosity **39**, 4–5
Dysgenesis, muscular **37**, 370–371
Dysgeusia (*see also* Taste perception) **44**, 249
–, elderly people **44**, 256
Dysosmia (*see also* Smell perception) **44**, 249
Dysplasia, skeletal **37**, 392–393
–, urinary **37**, 392–393
Dystrophin, function in muscle cells **37**, 355
–, gene **37**, 353–357
–, isoforms **37**, 355
–, structural domains **37**, 354
Eating disorder **40**, 225
Eberthella typhosa, effect of concentration on germicidal power of cationic detergents **2**, 134, 135, 137, 140, 147, 148, 152
–, in milk **2**, 82
Ebonite, expanded **12**, 156
Echimidine **45**, 71, 72, 75
Echinacea angustifolia **43**, 41
Echiumine **45**, 72
Echium plantagineum (Patterson's Curse; Salvation Jane) **45**, 72
Economics, PSE porcine muscle **13**, 165–167
Economics of freeze-drying **13**, 70–73
– of –, equipment **13**, 72
– of –, freezing **13**, 70–73
– of –, loading, unloading **13**, 71–72
– of –, packaging **13**, 72
– of –, processing **13**, 71
– of –, storage, transport **13**, 72
– of of food drying processes **20**, 85–98
Edam cheese **39**, 243, 245
Edema, licorice and **7**, 356–357
Edible coatings/films **44**, 347–389
–, barrier properties **44**, 348, 349–351
–, carrier functions **44**, 348
–, –, antioxidants incorporation **44**, 384
–, coating formation technique **44**, 351
–, definition **44**, 348
–, emulsion formation technique **44**, 351
–, gas permeability **44**, 349, 350
–, polysaccharide–lipid, *see* Polysaccharide–lipid edible films
–, polysaccharide–polysaccharide **44**, 382
–, polysaccharide–protein **44**, 382
–, – with food additives **44**, 382
–, protein–lipid, *see* Protein–lipid edible films
–, protein–protein **44**, 382–384
–, solute permeability **44**, 349
–, volatile permeability **44**, 349
–, water vapor permeability **44**, 349, 350
Edmundson wheels **42**, 99, 101–102
EDTA, treatment of isolated cell walls **34**, 346
Edulan, in passion fruit juice **27**, 277–279
Egg albumen **1**, 150–151, 153–155, 157, 164, 169–172, 176, 178–182, 185–186
–, antitrypsin in **1**, 385
–, compositional analysis **35**, 341
–, effect of alanine on **3**, 274
–, – of amino acids on **3**, 273
–, – of cysteine on **3**, 274
–, – of glycine on **3**, 274
–, – of methylated glubose on **3**, 274
–, – of pH on **3**, 274

Egg albumen, effect (*cont'd*)
–, – of sound waves on **3**, 131
–, infrared dehydration of **3**, 146
–, protective action on thiamine **6**, 261
–, removal of reducing sugars in **3**, 274
–, *Salmonella* infection in **3**, 224–226
–, secondary drying of **2**, 501
–, thermal scanning rheological analysis **35**, 354–357
–, ultraviolet detection of spoilage in **3**, 154
–, use of Hunkel nozzle in drying **2**, 452
Egg industry, use of quaternary ammonium compounds in **2**, 180
Egg proteins, definition and classification **34**, 255
–, egg albumen **34**, 258–259
–, ovalbumin **34**, 255–257
–, –, gelation mechanism **34**, 255–256
–, –, gel properties **34**, 256–257
Eggs **1**, 149–202; **13**, 295–297, 321–322; **14**, 260; **15**, 35, 248; **16**, 166
–, ammonia in **16**, 169
–, chemical changes in **10**, 39–40
–, chemical composition of **1**, 150–162
–, –, influence of hen's diet on **1**, 152–154
–, composition of white **10**, 34–37
–, – of yolk **10**, 37–38
–, cooking for sensory tests **2**, 229–230
–, custards made from **8**, 33
–, dried, application of dilution sensory test to **2**, 224–225
–, –, chemical changes during storage of **1**, 168–187
–, –, cooking properties of **1**, 158, 167–168, 191–194
–, –, criteria of quality and deterioration in **1**, 157–158
–, –, enzymatic changes in **11**, 265–270
–, –, enzyme activity in **1**, 182–187
–, –, factors affecting storage life of **1**, 154–156
–, –, fatty acids in **1**, 174–180, 187
–, –, mineral content of **1**, 151
–, –, palatability of **1**, 150, 158–159, 192–194
–, –, physical properties of **1**, 156–157
–, –, retention of quality in **1**, 187–194
–, –, solubility of **1**, 159–161, 164–167
–, –, vitamin A, loss during storage of **1**, 174–181
–, –, vitamin content of **1**, 153
–, dried state, properties in **10**, 43
–, effect of quality on sensory tests **2**, 230–233
–, – of trained judges on scoring of **2**, 234–235, 239, 242
–, freeze-drying of **7**, 204, 225
–, fresh, cooking for sensory tests **2**, 229
–, frozen state, properties in **10**, 42–43
–, hydrogen sulfide in **16**, 196
–, in consumer preference survey **3**, 403–406, 408, 409
–, in market survey **3**, 415, 416, 419
–, in oriental noodles **43**, 161
–, in shell, characteristics of **10**, 39–41
–, lactic acid in **16**, 191
–, liquid state, properties in **10**, 41–42
–, marine transport **12**, 179
–, nutritional stress factor in **4**, 111–113
–, ozone inactivation of microbial contaminants **45**, 186, 193–194
–, protein in **16**, 24
–, pyrrolizidine alkaloid concentrations **45**, 73, 91
–, quality **8**, 31; **16**, 166
–, role in foods **10**, 33
–, scanning electron microscopy of **22**, 290–291
–, scoring of **2**, 238–239
–, selenium in **32**, 96, 98
–, sensory variations in judging of **2**, 234
–, shell, function of **10**, 34
–, spray, dried whole **6**, 300
–, storage **35**, 338–339
–, use of salt water fluorescense test for **2**, 249
–, – of Swenson dryer for **2**, 420
Eggs and egg products used by the candy industry **6**, 3
Egg white, *see* Egg albumen
Egg yolk **1**, 150–151, 153–155, 157, 164, 168–169, 176, 179–186, 193
–, effect of sample size in judging **2**, 228, 245
–, thawing of frozen **6**, 206
Eh hurdle **39**, 122–123
Ehlers–Danlos syndrome **37**, 391–394
–, classification table **37**, 393
EHT, *see* Extrahepatic tissue
Eicosadienoic acid, desaturase activity, diet effects **35**, 35–36
Eicosanoids **35**, 90–111
–, dietary linoleic acid effects **35**, 91–92
–, dietary PUFA **35**, 105–111
–, effects and functions **35**, 11–12
–, excessive synthesis **35**, 105, 155–156
–, synthesis **35**, 92–97
–, –, cyclooxygenase **35**, 94–97

–, –, macrophages **35**, 140–148
–, –, modification **35**, 105–106
–, –, phospholipases **35**, 93–94
–, synthetic pathway **35**, 90–91
Eicosapentaenoate, autoxidation, mechanism **33**, 249
Eicosapentaenoic acid **35**, 7
–, autoxidation **33**, 248–250
–, α-linolenic acid intake and **35**, 59–60
–, linseed and fish oil supplementation effects **35**, 55
–, lipoxygenase-catalyzed oxidation and generation of oxidative flavor compounds **33**, 301
–, plasma and tissue, heart disease **35**, 135–136
–, rheumatoid arthritis effects **35**, 141–142
–, vegans and omnivores **35**, 63–64
5,8,11,14-Eicosatetraenoic acid, inhibition of lipoxygenases **33**, 306–307
Eicosatrienoic **35**, 10–11
Elaidic acid, olive oil and **31**, 464, 474
Elasmobranchs, oxide content of **2**, 368
Elastase, activity of, in aging meat **20**, 274
Elasticity **39**, 7–8, 9–12
–, protein-stabilized foams **34**, 65–66
Elasticity coefficient **40**, 234–236
Elastic modulus **39**, 7
Elastin **14**, 115–120
–, abnormal calcification **37**, 401
–, and meat quality **26**, 85
–, chemical composition **9**, 9
–, endogenous proteolytic enzymes and **31**, 372–374
–, polysaccharides in **9**, 10
–, preparation **9**, 9
–, properties **9**, 9–10
–, structure and composition of **20**, 266–267
Elastography, carcass grading **45**, 154
Elderberry **15**, 225
–, color detection in grape wine **5**, 446
Elderly people, chemosensory losses **44**, 247–331
–, –, disease-related, *see* Smell perception *and* Taste perception
–, flavor enhancement compensation, *see* Flavor enhancement
–, food preferences **32**, 249–250, 264
–, medication effects, *see* Medication
–, smell perception **44**, 262–264
–, –, suprathreshold perceptual losses **44**, 263–264
–, –, threshold detection elevation **44**, 263
–, –, trigeminal stimulants **44**, 264
–, taste perception **44**, 256–262
–, –, suprathreshold perceptual losses **44**, 260–262
–, –, threshold recognition/detection elevation **44**, 256–260
–, –, trigeminal stimulants **44**, 257–258
Elecampane (*Inula helenium*), inulin **43**, 3, 6, 40
Electrical energy, inactivation of enzymes by **3**, 35
Electrical fields **15**, 277
Electrical stimulation, for muscle function **37**, 347
Electrical stunning **39**, 125
Electric resistance, fish freshness and **7**, 63
Electrochemical techniques, for detection of eluted folates **33**, 30–33
Electrodialysis **15**, 355
Electrolytes, dietary fiber and **31**, 166
–, salting-out effects, bovine casein **34**, 315–316
Electromagnetic radiation, application of in food technology **3**, 120–196
Electromagnetic spectrum **15**, 278
Electromyography, for muscle diseases and disorders **37**, 344
–, myasthenia gravis **37**, 366–367
Electron capture **14**, 18
Electronic imaging system **34**, 170
Electron microscopy **34**, 170–171
–, chocolate and **31**, 222
–, dietary fiber and **31**, 136, 179
–, endogenous proteolytic enzymes and **31**, 369, 387, 399
–, fat crystal network microstructure **44**, 38
–, scanning type, *see* Scanning electron microscopy
Electron probe microanalysis, by scanning electron microscopy **22**, 223–229
Electron spin resonance (ESR), browning reaction between sugars and alkylamines **30**, 81
Electrophoresis, cheese **39**, 210, 226, 230–231, 242–243
–, fish **39**, 357–358
Electrophoretic separation, meat endpoint temperature monitoring **44**, 175
Electrostatic effects, proteins, *see* Protein
Electrostatic interactions, effect on whey protein gelation **33**, 387
Electrostatic potential energy **34**, 32
Electrostatic repulsive theory, emulsion stability **34**, 90–92
Elephant Head (*Pedicularis*) **45**, 77

Elimination **14**, 299–300
β-Elimination **35**, 203–204
Ellagic acid, animal consumption of **27**, 170–172
–, in tea **2**, 284
Elongase **35**, 25–26
Elongation, *n*-3 fatty acids **35**, 81–83
–, α-linolenic acid **35**, 24–27
–, PUFA **35**, 35–36
–, unsaturated fatty acids rates **35**, 31–33
El Salvador, Incaparina use in **22**, 198
Elsberg test **14**, 8–9, 11
Embryonic axis, of wheat germ **23**, 194
Embryos **15**, 35
EMF flavor test **14**, 21
Emmental cheese **39**, 177, 200, 254
Emulsan **43**, 323, 349, 350
Emulsept, germicidal action of **2**, 156, 180
–, structure of **2**, 155
–, use in pickle industry **2**, 183
Emulsification **39**, 265–266
–, modified glycinins **36**, 183
–, seed storage proteins **36**, 131
Emulsification assay **42**, 116–117
Emulsification peptides **42**, 93–122
–, amino acid sequences **42**, 107–109
–, circular dichroism measurements **42**, 116, 118, 120–121
–, design **42**, 104–111
–, future directions **42**, 119, 121–122
–, model peptide 4 **42**, 116, 118
–, model peptide 5 **42**, 116, 119
–, model peptide 6 **42**, 113–115, 116, 119
–, synthesis **42**, 112–115
–, testing of properties **42**, 115–121
Emulsifiers (*see also* Protein emulsifiers *and* Small-molecule emulsifiers) **22**, 318–327; **42**, 115–116
–, calorimetric studies on **22**, 325
–, characterization of **22**, 319–321
–, –, critique of **22**, 327
–, chocolate and **31**, 281–284, 292, 297, 311
–, cloud point of **22**, 324–325
–, composite wheat–sorghum breads **43**, 230
–, concentrations of **22**, 332–336
–, critical micelle concentration of **22**, 322–323
–, dielectric constant of **22**, 325
–, efficiency evaluation **34**, 173–174
–, equilibria of **22**, 334
–, FDA-approved **22**, 444–445
–, FDA regulation of **22**, 442–445
–, hydrocolloids as **22**, 341
–, hydrophile–lipophile balance (HLB) of **22**, 319–321
–, identification of **22**, 446
–, in chocolate candies **6**, 44
–, macromolecular **34**, 128–129
–, mixtures of **22**, 330–331
–, nuclear magnetic resonance spectroscopy of **22**, 323
–, oriental noodles **43**, 162
–, phase inversion temperature (PIT) of **22**, 326
–, polarity index of **22**, 325
–, proteins as (*see also* Proteins) **22**, 339–340
–, role **34**, 181
–, solids as **22**, 340–341
–, solubility partitioning of **22**, 323
–, sorghum cookies **43**, 233
–, structure effects of **22**, 436–438
–, surface and interfacial tension of **22**, 326
–, types **34**, 83
–, types of **22**, 318–319
–, water number of **22**, 323–324
–, wheatless sorghum breads **43**, 231
Emulsifying activity index **34**, 154, 173–174
–, glycosylated β-lactoglobulin **34**, 156–157
Emulsifying agents **16**, 107
Emulsifying capacity **34**, 173
Emulsifying salts **39**, 263, 267–272
Emulsions (*see also* Fish sausage, Meat emulsions, Vegetable oils) **22**, 309–359; **34**, 2, 82
–, aerated **22**, 341–342
–, characterization **33**, 405
–, classification **34**, 83–85
–, composition **34**, 85–86
–, definition **34**, 82–83
–, destabilization of **22**, 312–315
–, droplet size measurement **34**, 170–173
–, emulsifiers for **22**, 318–327
–, formation, equipment and methodology **34**, 168–169
–, free energy of formation **34**, 87
–, gelatin and **7**, 326
–, instability **42**, 94
–, interfacial energy **34**, 87–88
–, internal phase ratio **34**, 84–85
–, microemulsions **34**, 162–165
–, microencapsulation **34**, 165–168
–, multiple **34**, 163–164
–, of fats and oils **22**, 327–330
–, preparation of **22**, 443
–, proteins as stabilizers of **22**, 339–340
–, reduced turbidity **34**, 172
–, research needs **34**, 181–182

–, rheology **39**, 55–58
–, stability **34**, 86, 129–130; **42**, 115–116
–, –, coalescence, *see* Coalescence
–, –, creaming **34**, 130–133
–, –, DLVO theory **34**, 95–96
–, –, electrostatic repulsive theory **34**, 90–92
–, –, flocculation **34**, 133–135
–, –, free polymer effect **34**, 95
–, –, hydration force **34**, 94–95
–, –, London dispersion interaction **34**, 89
–, –, macromolecular films **34**, 181
–, –, measurement **34**, 174
–, –, –, coalescence **34**, 176–181
–, –, –, creaming **34**, 174–175
–, –, –, flocculation **34**, 175–176
–, –, Ostwald ripening **34**, 145–146
–, –, requirements for **34**, 129
–, –, small surface-active agents **34**, 129
–, –, stability rating **34**, 131
–, –, steric interaction **34**, 92–94
–, –, tests **34**, 130
–, –, theory **34**, 129
–, –, thermodynamic theory **34**, 86–88
–, –, total interaction energy **34**, 95–97
–, –, van der Waals interaction **34**, 88–90
–, stability diagram, coalescence measurement **34**, 180
–, stability of **22**, 309–359
–, –, determination **22**, 316
–, –, improvement **22**, 316–317
–, stabilization of **22**, 311–312
–, terminology of **22**, 310
–, types of **22**, 310–311
–, –, emulsifier effects on **22**, 338–339
–, –, tests for **22**, 311
–, ultrasonic characterization **45**, 112, 114–116, 158
–, –, flocculated emulsions **45**, 116, 150
–, –, imaging **45**, 154
–, –, particle sizing **45**, 115–116, 150
–, –, practical applications **45**, 150
–, whey proteins, factors affecting **33**, 408
–, –, properties **33**, 405–406
–, –, protein conformation and **33**, 406–408
–, –, surface hydrophobicity and **33**, 406–408
Emulsitator machine **16**, 128
Emulsitators, *see* Colloid mills
Emulsol 605, film formation of **2**, 144
Emulsol 606, therapeutic action of **2**, 143
Emulsol 607, film formation of **2**, 144
–, therapeutic action of **2**, 143
–, uses on sewage **2**, 183
Enalapril **44**, 305, 320
Enameled cans **3**, 371–374
Encephalomalacia, in chicks, cause of **1**, 125
–, *n*-3 PUFA effects **35**, 127–128
Endocrine disease, smell perception effects **44**, 272
–, taste perception effects **44**, 267
Endocrines, endogenous proteolytic enzymes and **31**, 388, 389
Endocytosis, endogenous proteolytic enzymes and **31**, 378, 388, 390
Endogenous proteolytic enzymes **31**, 344–346, 411–414
–, endopeptidases **31**, 352
–, –, aspartate proteases **31**, 360–362
–, –, metalloproteinases **31**, 362, 363
–, –, serine proteases **31**, 352–355
–, –, thiol proteases **31**, 355–360
–, exopeptidases **31**, 346
–, –, aminopeptidases **31**, 346, 347
–, –, carboxypeptidases **31**, 347, 348
–, –, dipeptidases **31**, 348, 349
–, –, dipeptidylpeptidases **31**, 349–352
–, meat technology **31**, 393
–, –, aging **31**, 394, 395, 403
–, –, connective tissue **31**, 401–403
–, –, contractile proteins **31**, 396–398
–, –, cytoskeletal proteins **31**, 400, 401
–, –, exopeptidases **31**, 410, 411
–, –, glycolysis **31**, 393, 394
–, –, lysosomal proteinases **31**, 403–407
–, –, nonlysosomal proteases **31**, 407–410
–, –, regulatory proteins **31**, 398–400
–, –, sarcoplasmic proteins **31**, 395
–, muscle physiology **31**, 369
–, –, conflicting results **31**, 381, 382
–, –, muscle proteins **31**, 369–373
–, –, protein catabolism **31**, 377–381
–, –, protein turnover **31**, 373–376, 382, 383
–, nonmuscle cathepsins **31**, 364
–, –, serine proteinases **31**, 364, 365
–, –, thiol proteinases **31**, 365, 366
–, –, unclassified proteinases **31**, 366
–, proteinase activity **31**, 383
–, –, animal age **31**, 387
–, –, endocrines **31**, 388, 389
–, –, endogenous inhibitors **31**, 383–385
–, –, muscle type **31**, 385, 386
–, –, muscular dystrophy **31**, 389–391
–, –, nerve system **31**, 387, 388
–, –, nutrition **31**, 386, 387
–, –, physical exercise **31**, 391–393
–, –, weightlessness **31**, 393
–, proteinase distribution **31**, 366–369
Endogenous rhythm (*see also* Bioperiodicity) **40**, 219, 226

Endoglucanase, Albersheim's model and **30**, 162
–, plant cell wall breakdown **30**, 161–162
Endomysial network **39**, 91–92
Endomysium, *see* Connective tissues
Endopeptidases, chocolate and **31**, 223, 224
–, endogenous proteolytic enzymes and **31**, 345, 352, 411–413
–, –, aspartate proteases **31**, 360–362
–, –, meat technology **31**, 403, 404, 410
–, –, metalloproteinases **31**, 362, 363
–, –, muscle physiology **31**, 381
–, –, nonmuscle cathepsins **31**, 364, 366
–, –, proteinase activity **31**, 390
–, –, serine proteases **31**, 352–355
–, –, thiol proteases **31**, 355–360
Endopeptidase system, in dermatosparaxis **37**, 390–391
Endopolygalacturonase, Albersheim's model and **30**, 160–161
–, in ripening fruits, multiple forms **30**, 177
–, –, rhamnogalacturonan hydrolysis **30**, 176
–, –, tissue softening and **30**, 179
–, plant cell wall breakdown **30**, 160–161
Endosperm, components **31**, 120, 122
–, dicotyledonous plants **31**, 133, 135
–, dietary fiber and **31**, 150, 190
–, intestinal bacteria **31**, 181, 183
–, monocotyledonous plants **31**, 136, 137
–, of wheat kernel **23**, 193
Endothelial cells **40**, 245, 246, 248, 250
–, anti-cardiolipin antibody binding **37**, 307–308
End-over-end agitation **32**, 61–62
–, heat transfer in **32**, 65–68
End-point analysis **15**, 163
Endpoint cooking temperature indicators, enzymatic methods **44**, 170–173
–, immunoassays **44**, 173–175
–, meat/poultry products **44**, 169–176
–, physical methods **44**, 175–176
–, USDA tests **44**, 170
Endpoint procedure (quantal response) **44**, 179
Energy, equation of **32**, 42
–, free **14**, 327
–, relationships **14**, 368–370
–, thermal **15**, 281
Energy barrier theory **34**, 20–22
Energy cost, IM meat production **39**, 143–147
Energy dissipation **15**, 71
Energy foods, consumption per capita, worldwide **30**, 334–335
–, interaction with protein foods **30**, 332–334
Energy metabolism (*see also* Nutrient-response curve) **40**, 171–180, 227
–, disorders, glycolysis-related acquired **37**, 379
–, –, glycolytic **37**, 374–379
–, –, lipid metabolism **37**, 381–383
–, –, mitochondrial oxidation **37**, 379–381
–, –, myotonic syndromes **37**, 383–387
–, –, research needs **37**, 408
Energy of activation **38**, 204–205
– of –, degradation of folates in aqueous solution, table **33**, 50
Engineering aspects of food technology **10**, 15–16
Engineering property, rheology **39**, 44–61
Enocianina (grape skin extract) **43**, 212
Enol ester epoxides **14**, 312
Enoxacin **44**, 290
Enrichment ratio method **40**, 45
Ensomysium **14**, 35
Entamoeba histolytica, action of chlorine on cysts of **1**, 377
–, destroyed by quaternary ammonium compounds **2**, 183
Entanglement, rheology **39**, 48–53
Enterobacter cloacae, attachment **43**, 324, 347
Enterobacter faecalis, attachment **43**, 335
Enterococcus faecium, thermal inactivation **44**, 165
Enterocyte **40**, 36–37, 38–39
Enterodiol **44**, 199, 207
–, antioxidant activity **44**, 226
–, metabolism **44**, 221–222
–, toxicity **44**, 226
Enterolactone **44**, 199, 207
–, anticancer activity **44**, 232
–, antioxidant activity **44**, 226
–, cardiovascular health protective effects **44**, 234
–, metabolism **44**, 221–222
–, toxicity **44**, 226
Enteropathies, cow's milk protein intolerance **37**, 30–31
–, food-sensitive, celiac disease **37**, 29–30
–, soy protein **37**, 31
Enthalpy, protein stability **35**, 242
Enthalpy–entropy compensation effect, site-directed mutagenesis **35**, 283
Enthalpy of denaturation **35**, 320
– of –, whey proteins **33**, 377–378
Entrainment separators **15**, 327
Entropy **14**, 318
–, protein stability **35**, 242

Environment, effects on depot fats **23**, 30–32
Environmental Protection Agency, carcinogen risk assessment and **31**, 26, 39
Enzymatic action in food processing **10**, 31
Enzymatically interesterified (EIE) milkfat **44**, 38
Enzymatic browning, reactions in food **19**, 82–123
–, – in –, fundamental aspects **19**, 82
–, – in –, polyphenoloxidases in **19**, 82–97
–, – in –, *o*-quinones in, secondary reactions **19**, 97–104
–, – in –, tea **19**, 109–112
–, theories of **3**, 2–7
Enzymatic changes, in bread **11**, 291–292
–, in cake mixes **11**, 290–291
–, in cereals **11**, 274–278, 280–285
–, in dried apricots **11**, 289–290
–, in dried cabbage **11**, 287
–, in dried carrots **11**, 288
–, in dried egg **11**, 265–270
–, in dried figs **11**, 290
–, in dried fruits **11**, 289
–, in dried meat **11**, 272–273
–, in dried milk **11**, 270–272
–, in dried peaches **11**, 290
–, in dried peas **11**, 288, 289
–, in dried potatoes **11**, 288
–, in dried prunes **11**, 290
–, in dried vegetables **11**, 285–289
–, in flour **11**, 281–285
–, in seed oils **11**, 278–280
–, in walnuts **11**, 309
Enzymatic deconjugation, autolytic deconjugation with endogenous conjugases **33**, 17–18
–, efficiency of **33**, 18–19
–, folates **33**, 17–20
–, pteroylpolyglutamate hydrolases in **33**, 17
Enzymatic digestion-dialysis technique **35**, 218–220
Enzymatic modification, whey proteins **33**, 416–417
Enzymatic time–temperature integrators **44**, 180–182
Enzyme action, catalase in vegetables **8**, 84
–, cause of off-flavors in foods **8**, 84
–, inactivation of **8**, 64
–, in cocoa bean cotyledons **8**, 253
–, in garlic **2**, 272
–, in peppergrass **2**, 275
–, in tea fermentation **2**, 284
–, in vegetables **8**, 78
–, lipase, in vegetables **8**, 86
–, lipoxidase, in vegetables **8**, 86
–, oxidizing, in apples and pears **8**, 354
–, pectinase in fruits **8**, 349
–, polyphenol oxidase, in cocoa beans **8**, 230
–, systems, in wines **8**, 137
Enzyme-catalyzed lipid oxidation, cyclooxygenase **33**, 269–270
–, cytochrome P450 **33**, 256–259
–, fish lipids **33**, 291–297
–, lipoxygenase **33**, 261–269
–, peroxidase **33**, 259–261
Enzyme-catalyzed oxidative browning of fruit products **3**, 1–44
Enzyme inhibitors, naturally occurring, in food preservation **1**, 385
Enzyme-linked immunosorbent assay (ELISA), endpoint cooking temperature indication **44**, 174–175
–, phytoestrogens **44**, 203
Enzymes (*see also individual enzymes and* Proteolysis) **3**, 53–55; **15**, 259, 292
–, absorption of **17**, 50
–, activity, at low temperatures **17**, 47
–, –, –, thermal and environmental factors **17**, 34–53
–, cause of spoilage in fish **2**, 347, 372
–, cell-free, effect of benzoic acid **11**, 347
–, –, – of –, inhibition **11**, 348
–, –, salicylic acid inhibition of **11**, 348
–, cheese curd **39**, 176–177
–, cheese ripening **39**, 211–225, 257–258
–, chlorine and **7**, 134
–, chocolate and, alkalization **31**, 248, 249
–, –, milk **31**, 256
–, –, milk crumb **31**, 291
–, –, processing **31**, 216, 217, 222
–, –, sweeteners **31**, 274
–, content in oats **11**, 293
–, deterioration of foods **17**, 5
–, dietary fiber and **31**, 118, 191
–, –, analysis **31**, 142, 143, 152
–, –, dicotyledonous plants **31**, 126, 129, 132
–, –, intestinal bacteria **31**, 174, 175, 177, 178, 181–183, 186–189
–, –, properties **31**, 154–156, 169–171
–, disulfide, inactivation of by reducing agents **1**, 382–383
–, effect of cathode rays on **3**, 174–176
–, effect on reduction of trimethylamine oxide **2**, 369
–, effects of water **17**, 48
–, endogenous proteolytic, *see* Endogenous proteolytic enzymes
–, future research **39**, 293

Enzymes (*cont'd*)
–, gelatin degradation and **7**, 320–321
–, halophilic **12**, 68
–, heat resistance of **17**, 3–4
–, hydrolysis in barley malt flour and lecithin **11**, 312
–, inactivation of **17**, 3–4, 34–46
–, –, equation **17**, 37
–, –, in fruits **17**, 183–184
–, –, thermodynamics of **17**, 37–39
–, in analyzing pectins **11**, 38–45
–, in breadmaking **16**, 428ff
–, in cheese ripening **16**, 233ff, 255, 281, 287ff
–, in citrus fruits, acetylesterase **9**, 322
–, –, depolymerizing **9**, 321
–, –, glutamic acid decarboxylase **9**, 323
–, –, others **9**, 323–324
–, –, pectinesterase **9**, 320–321
–, –, peroxidase **9**, 323
–, –, phosphatase **9**, 322
–, in extraction of pectins **11**, 38–45
–, in freeze-dried food **13**, 73–74
–, in fruits **17**, 183–186
–, in gene cloning and manipulation **36**, 134, 136–137
–, inhibition of **1**, 380–385; **11**, 348
–, inhibitors **17**, 52–53
–, –, from plants **17**, 59–60
–, in honey **24**, 312–330
–, in liver **15**, 36, 50
–, in low-moisture foods, humidity and reactions **11**, 302–314
–, –, reactions **11**, 263–330
–, –, –, mechanisms **11**, 310–313
–, –, –, models **11**, 303–306
–, –, –, research on **11**, 303–306
–, –, theories on changes **11**, 292–302
–, in milk **10**, 47–48; **19**, 182–183
–, in muscle **19**, 14–16
–, –, and meat quality **26**, 87
–, in peas **9**, 91–93
–, in potatoes **10**, 192–193
–, in tea **17**, 255–259
–, –, effect of thermal treatment **17**, 273
–, in tea leaves **11**, 231
–, involved in food browning, *see* Enzymic browning reactions in food
–, in wheat germ **23**, 209–211
–, irreversible thermal inactivation **35**, 246–249
–, iso, *see* Isoenzymes
–, metabolic control theory (*see also* Substrate) **40**, 233–236
–, microsomal, *see* Microsomal enzymes
–, milk quality **39**, 249
–, molecular forms **17**, 49–50
–, *N*-nitroso compounds and **31**, 64, 73, 97
–, of amino acid metabolism **17**, 22–23
–, of *Byssochlamys* sp. **25**, 264–267
–, of tea **24**, 233–236
–, olive oil and **31**, 461, 463, 478
–, oxidative **17**, 217
–, oxidizing **17**, 4, 7–19
–, –, in plants, classification **17**, 7
–, –, thermal inactivation **17**, 39–47
–, pectic **17**, 21–22
–, pectolytic **17**, 44
–, properties and uses **36**, 136–137
–, proteolytic **14**, 124–125
–, –, as evaluating agents **9**, 44–46
–, –, as tenderizers **9**, 40–46
–, –, in bacon **3**, 303, 304
–, –, in muscle **9**, 35–37
–, *n*-3 PUFA effects **35**, 129
–, reaction of starch with **2**, 321, 322
–, regeneration of **17**, 3, 53–57
–, respiratory **17**, 19–23
–, role in meat tenderness **20**, 273–277
–, salt tolerance of **7**, 112
–, stability **35**, 238–239
–, –, xylitol **35**, 247
–, stabilization, by immobilization **35**, 276–277
–, –, following cross-linking **35**, 274–276
–, –, hydrophilization **35**, 271
–, substrate studies in tea **11**, 234–237
–, systems in pigs **13**, 97, 145–150
–, thermostability **35**, 238–239
Enzymic test **39**, 356–357
Ephedrine **44**, 302
Epiblast, of wheat germ **23**, 195
Epicatechin, structure of **19**, 77
(–)-Epicatechin, chocolate and **31**, 221, 231, 233, 235, 325
l-Epicatechin, in cocoa **2**, 284
–, in green tea **2**, 284, 285
l-Epicatechin gallate in tea **2**, 295
Epichlorohydrin, esterification of carboxyl groups by **1**, 383
Epidemiology, air pollution **31**, 39
–, carcinogen risk assessment and **31**, 5, 41, 47, 48
–, estimates **31**, 39, 40
–, laboratory data **31**, 27, 28
–, statistics **31**, 14, 17
–, testing hypothesis **31**, 38

Epidermal layer of vegetable tissue, parenchyma cells in **2**, 304
Epidermolysis bullosa **37**, 398
–, simplex **37**, 398
Epihydrin aldehyde, Kreis test for **3**, 95
Epi-inositol **45**, 37
Epilepsy **37**, 372; **40**, 333
Epimysium **14**, 37
Epithelial cells, gut, antigen uptake **37**, 12–14
Epithelial tissue, cell membrane **40**, 197–204
–, mammary cells **40**, 207–212
–, vitamin A **40**, 20
Epithelium, carcinogen risk assessment and **31**, 44
–, dietary fiber and **31**, 173, 191
Epitope, cardiolipin **37**, 312–314
Epoxy compounds, wheat germ treatment by **23**, 267
Epoxy-hydroperoxides, from polyunsaturated fatty acid oxidation **33**, 276–277
–, linolenate, breakdown mechanism **33**, 277
Equation of state, proteins at interfaces **34**, 111–113
Equilibration, vitamin B6 metabolism **40**, 126
Equilibrium, chocolate and **31**, 264
–, dietary fiber and **31**, 158
–, *N*-nitroso compounds and **31**, 62, 73
–, water activity **39**, 115–116
Equipment, chlorination of **7**, 161–162
–, control systems **13**, 63–67
–, drying chambers **13**, 47–63
–, economics **13**, 70–73
–, evaluation systems **13**, 67–70
–, freeze-drying **13**, 47–73, 81–82
Equol **44**, 202, 203, 221
–, antioxidant activity **44**, 225
–, metabolism **44**, 220
Eremascus albus, isolation of **7**, 115
Ergosterol, in cocoa bean pulp **8**, 263
Erosion, *see* Soil erosion
Error measurement **40**, 307
Error model **40**, 268
Error sources, rheological instrumentation **39**, 26, 28, 33
Erucic acid, in rapeseeds, antinutritiorial for humans **30**, 371
Erwinia carotovora **15**, 167, 179
Erysipelas insidiosa **37**, 398–399
Erythorbic acid, as substitute for L-ascorbic acid **18**, 297–304
–, inhibition of *N*-nitrosamine formation in cured meat **29**, 59
–, in meat smoking **29**, 32–33
–, *N*-nitroso compounds and **31**, 62
Erythrocyte ghosts, α-tocopherol concentrations **33**, 212
–, α-tocopherol transfer from liposomes to **33**, 195–196
Erythrocyte hemolysis, for vitamin E status **33**, 189
–, α-tocopherol acetate effects **33**, 219
Erythrocyte phospholipids, infants, diet effects **35**, 85–86
Erythrocytes, folate **40**, 87–88
–, membranes, α-tocopherol binding **33**, 198–199
–, –, α-tocopherol turnover **33**, 187
–, tocopherol association with **33**, 177
–, tocopherol-deficient and tocopherol-sufficient, α-tocopherol transfer **33**, 185
–, vitamin B6 **40**, 111
Erythrodiol, olive oil and **31**, 467
Erythromycin treatments, effect of bifidobacteria consumption **37**, 84–86
Escherichia **13**, 358
–, effect of nitrites on **3**, 295
–, enzyme action in **2**, 369
Escherichia coli **40**, 97–101, 105; **41**, 43; **45**, 178, 180, 183, 193
–, attachment **43**, 325, 328, 335, 338
–, –, confocal scanning laser microscopy **43**, 355
–, –, inhibition methods **43**, 353
–, –, plant surfaces **43**, 345
–, carcinogen risk assessment and **31**, 28
–, cloned gene expression **36**, 145–149
–, –, essential units **36**, 145
–, –, expression vector types **36**, 147–149
–, –, factors affecting level of expression **36**, 146–147
–, destruction curve for **3**, 434
–, destruction of **3**, 53, 54
–, –, by sonic vibrations **3**, 130
–, –, by ultraviolet radiation **3**, 148
–, –, by X-rays **3**, 156
–, detachment of daughter cells **43**, 350
–, dietary fiber and **31**, 176
–, effect of radioactive phosphorus on **3**, 155
–, germicidal effect of quaternary ammonium compound on **2**, 137, 140, 142, 147–148, 152–153
–, growth rate of **7**, 101, 105
–, isolated from fish **2**, 349
–, *N*-nitroso compounds and **31**, 96
–, pH in frozen cells of **3**, 449
–, phytase **45**, 9, 10, 11, 21

Escherichia coli (*cont'd*)
–, pulsed electric field (PEF) inactivation **44**, 11, 13
–, soybean glycinin expression **36**, 151, 153–158
–, transgenic expression in *Arabidopsis* **45**, 34
–, wheat HMW glutenin expression **36**, 162
Escherichia coli 8739, pulsed electric field (PEF) inactivation **44**, 13
Escherichia coli O157:H7 **45**, 169, 178, 181, 188, 190, 195, 203
–, foodborne illness **44**, 152
–, pulsed electric field (PEF) inactivation **44**, 13, 14
–, thermal inactivation **44**, 163
–, –, kinetics **44**, 159–159, 160, 161
–, –, mathematical models **44**, 165
–, –, sample variables **44**, 166
–, –, USA meat processor regulations **44**, 150
–, undercooked meat **44**, 148, 149
Esculetin, lipoxygenase inhibition **33**, 317, 318
Esmolol **44**, 305
Esophageal cancer, carcinogen risk assessment and **31**, 14, 16
–, *N*-nitroso compounds and **31**, 56, 65, 72
ESR, *see* Electron spin resonance
Essence recovery **15**, 342, 350
Essential fatty acid deficiency **35**, 6
–, cardiolipin acyl changes **37**, 294–295
–, Δ^5-desaturase effects **35**, 48–50
–, impaired eicosanoids synthesis **35**, 89–90
–, in rats **35**, 66
–, linoleic acid **35**, 10–12
–, α-linolenic acid **35**, 13, 40
–, –, administration **35**, 111–112
–, symptoms **35**, 7–9
Essential fatty acids **35**, 6–14
–, definition **35**, 13
–, desaturation and elongation **35**, 7–8
–, docosahexaenoic acid **35**, 13–15
–, functions **35**, 9–10
–, linoleic acid **35**, 9–13
–, α-linolenic acid **35**, 13–15
–, membrane structure **35**, 9–10
Essential oils, composition in tea **17**, 250–251
–, role in food preservation **42**, 249
–, sampling of **7**, 25
Estazolam **44**, 307
Esterase **39**, 203–205
–, action on galacturonide chain of pectin **1**, 412
Esterification, dietary fiber and **31**, 131, 139, 190
–, –, intestinal bacteria **31**, 186, 187
–, –, properties **31**, 164–166
–, olive oil and **31**, 458
–, protein emulsifier modification **34**, 152–153
–, whey protein modification **33**, 419–420
Esters, aminoethyl **6**, 15
–, carbobenzoxyaminoethyl **6**, 15
–, chlorosulfite **14**, 305
–, contribution to meat flavor **18**, 52
–, hydroxy **14**, 309–310
–, in apple oil **2**, 264
–, in winter and summer pineapple **2**, 267
–, olive oil and **31**, 463, 466, 470
–, shoyu flavor and **30**, 267
Estimation, likelihood **40**, 268–269
–, parameter **40**, 311–312
–, population kinetics **40**, 266–277
–, prior **40**, 273–276
Estrogen receptor binding assay **44**, 196
Estrogen receptor-dependent transcriptional assay **44**, 196–197
Estrogen receptors, phytoestrogen effects **44**, 222–223
Estrogen-related phytoestrogen effects, *in vitro* neoplastic cell growth **44**, 223
–, *in vivo* **44**, 224–225
Estrogens, carcinogen risk assessment and **31**, 15
–, licorice and **7**, 355
Ethacrynic acid **44**, 305
Ethambutol **44**, 291
Ethanol **12**, 123–125
–, chocolate and **31**, 221, 235
–, dietary fiber and **31**, 144, 160, 186
–, effects on cardiolipin content **37**, 301
–, fatty acyl composition **37**, 297
–, in apples **2**, 263
–, in cocoa bean juice **8**, 239
–, ingestion effects on folate bioavailability **33**, 69–71
–, production **32**, 191, 196, 197–204, 211–215, 222
–, –, pollution from **32**, 222, 224
–, soybean protein denaturation **30**, 213
Ethanolamine phosphoglycerides, fatty acid concentrations **35**, 62
Ethers, contribution to meat flavor **18**, 52
–, destruction of yeast cells by **1**, 377
–, mixed cellulose **12**, 332–333
Ethionine **15**, 38
Ethnic origin, and food selection **32**, 260–261

Ethoxyquin, *N*-nitroso compounds and **31**, 81
Ethyl acetate, in apples **2**, 263
–, in bananas **2**, 271
–, in black tea **2**, 286
–, in pineapple **2**, 266–268
–, in raspberries **2**, 269
–, in strawberries **2**, 270
–, solubility of DDT in **2**, 203
Ethyl acrylate in pineapple **2**, 268
Ethyl alcohol **16**, 195, 212
–, effect on rabbits **2**, 207
–, in cherries **2**, 264
–, in coffee **2**, 282
–, in oranges **2**, 264
–, in parsnip seed oil **2**, 274
–, in pineapple **2**, 266, 268
–, in raspberries **2**, 269
–, in Springdale apples **2**, 263
–, in strawberries **2**, 270
–, in table wines **6**, 17
–, solubility of DDT in **2**, 204
Ethylamine, reaction with glycolaldehyde, color formation by smoking **29**, 138–139
Ethyl caproate in apples **2**, 263
Ethyl *n*-caproate in pineapple **2**, 268
Ethylcellulose (EC) **12**, 330–331
Ethylene **15**, 79
–, applied to passion fruit **12**, 223
–, – to –, effect on coloring **12**, 230
–, effect on fruits and vegetables **12**, 127, 186, 189–190
–, – on –, infected with *Penicillium digitatum* **12**, 107
–, – on pectins **1**, 401
–, in storage atmosphere **12**, 100–101
–, production, effect of carbon dioxide **12**, 125–127
–, –, – of oxygen **12**, 126–127
–, –, in passion fruit **12**, 223–229
–, –, on ships **12**, 189–190
–, production by mature kiwifruit **29**, 291
–, – by ripening fruits **30**, 171–172
–, stimulation **12**, 117
–, use in mango ripening **21**, 253–254, 256–258
Ethylenediaminetetraacetic acid (EDTA), chelation **33**, 304–305
–, control of microsomal-enzyme-associated lipid oxidation **33**, 305–306
–, dietary fiber and **31**, 129
Ethylene-induced climacteric **12**, 111
Ethylene oxide, in sterilization **32**, 20, 219 27
–, –, of bacon **3**, 319
–, –, of dried fruits by **3**, 466
–, reaction with amino groups **1**, 383, 386
–, – with carboxyl groups **1**, 386, 389
–, – with phenolic hydroxyls **1**, 383
–, – with sulfhydryl groups **1**, 393
Ethylene vinyl alcohol, chocolate and **31**, 318
Ethyl ester of a C_5 unsaturated acid in pineapple **2**, 268
Ethyl ether, fat extraction by **3**, 52
Ethyl formate in apples **2**, 263
Ethyl gallate added to dry milk **3**, 96
4-Ethylguaiacol, conversion from ferulic acid **30**, 278–280
–, – from –, yeast from shoyu mash and **30**, 278, 280
–, in combination with methionol, flavor evaluation and **30**, 286–287
Ethylhydroxyethylcellulose (EHEC) **12**, 331
Ethyl isovalerate in pineapple **2**, 268
Ethyl linoleate, diet containing **35**, 70
Ethyl linolenate, diet containing **35**, 70
N-Ethylmaleimide, as SH group reagent **24**, 22–24
Ethyl propionate in apples **2**, 263
Etidronate **44**, 315
Etodolac **44**, 295
Etretinate **44**, 315
Eubacterium **43**, 12
–, dietary fiber and **31**, 174, 176
Eukaryote gene, structure and mechanism of expression **36**, 96
Euprocin **44**, 287
Europe, buckwheat products **44**, 414–415
–, cheese production **39**, 166, 167, 193
–, traditional IM meat **39**, 77–79, 118
Europine **45**, 73
Eutectic freezing **27**, 316–320
Eutectics, freeze-drying and **7**, 174
Evacuation systems **13**, 67–70
–, absorbents, adsorbents **13**, 70
–, condensers, refrigerated **13**, 68–69
–, effect on drying **13**, 70
–, ejectors, steam **13**, 69–70
–, pumps, mechanical **13**, 68–69
Evaporation **39**, 101, 107, 117
–, in food industry **15**, 303ff
–, solids and **7**, 191–192
Evaporation-distillation process, in food drying, aroma recovery in **20**, 19–31
–, –, costs of **20**, 89–90
Evaporators, Centri-Therm **15**, 342
–, expanding flow **15**, 342
–, falling film **15**, 331
–, forced circulation **15**, 330

Evaporators (*cont'd*)
–, for cold storage, design of **20**, 130–144
–, –, for fruit precooling **20**, 136–137
–, –, refrigerant-to-air type **20**, 134–136
–, –, refrigerant-to-liquid type **20**, 130–134
–, heat pump **15**, 333
–, plate type **15**, 341
–, thin film **15**, 336
–, tubular **15**, 328
–, vacreators **15**, 340
Examinations, for muscle diseases and disorders **37**, 343
Exchangers, heat **12**, 164–165
Excitation–contraction coupling, in muscular dysgenesis **37**, 371
Excretion, meat mutagens **34**, 410–413
–, α-tocopherol metabolites **33**, 202–204
–, urinary, calcium balance measurements and **33**, 108
–, –, diet effects **33**, 120
Exercise, effects on cardiolipin content **37**, 300–301
–, – on muscle function **37**, 368–369
–, research needs **37**, 407
–, tests for muscle disorders **37**, 348–349
Exocrine glands, xylitol and **25**, 149–152
Exogenous rhythm (*see also* Bioperiodicity) **40**, 219
Exopeptidases, aminopeptidases **31**, 346, 347
–, carboxypeptidases **31**, 347, 348
–, dipeptidases **31**, 348, 349
–, dipeptidylpeptidases **31**, 349–352
–, endogenous proteolytic enzymes and **31**, 345, 346, 411, 412
–, meat technology **31**, 410, 411
–, proteinase activity **31**, 390
Exopolygalacturonase, in ripening fruits, pectin degradation and **30**, 177
–, properties **30**, 177
Experimental methods, rheology **39**, 12–23
Extensibility **14**, 100–106
–, lack of **36**, 74–75
–, Wang method **14**, 101–103
–, wheat proteins **36**, 68–69
Extensional flow **39**, 14–17, 58–59
Extensional viscosity **39**, 16, 17
Extraction, aqueous, effect on losses during cooking **33**, 49
–, folates **33**, 14–17
–, free folate during **33**, 17
–, heat effects during **33**, 16
–, inhibition of oxidative losses **33**, 15
–, nonthermal procedures **33**, 16
–, pH effects during **33**, 15–16
Extractives, fish spoilage and **7**, 50–52
–, for flexible packaging **23**, 313–315
Extractor, passion fruit, centrifugal **12**, 234–235
–, –, mechanical **12**, 235
Extrahepatic tissue (*see also names of specific organs*), β-carotene **40**, 32, 49, 61
–, vitamin A **40**, 9, 11, 17–21
Extrapolation, zero flow **40**, 189
Extrusion cooking, sorghum ready-to-eat products **43**, 237
Eye muscles, ocular myopathies **37**, 361–362
Eyes, vitamin A **40**, 9, 11, 19
Eyring theory, of coefficient of viscosity in liquid structure **11**, 358–362

F_T value **17**, 37, 39
F value, for reducing bacteria at different locations in container **2**, 93–99, 110
–, for thermal death time curve of *Clostridium botulinum* **2**, 76
–, of processes used in industry **2**, 102
Fababean protein **35**, 334–335
Fabaceae (Leguminosae), pyrrolizidine alkaloids **45**, 62
Factor XII, conformation **34**, 59
FAD, *see* Flavin adenine dinucleotide
Fagopyrum cymosum (perennial buckwheat) **44**, 396, 397
Fagopyrum esculentum (common buckwheat) **44**, 396, 397
–, spp. *ancestrale* **44**, 399
Fagopyrum homotropicum **44**, 397
Fagopyrum tartaricum, *see* Tartary buckwheat
Failure properties, gels **34**, 217–218
Familial amyloidotic polyneuropathy **40**, 150–155
Familial periodic paralysis **37**, 384–386
Famotidine **44**, 299
Fans, air movement and temperature control in **20**, 147–150
–, axial flow in dehydraters **6**, 330
–, for cold-storage facilities **20**, 146–150
FAP, *see* Familial amyloidotic polyneuropathy
Farina, enriched with thiamine **6**, 269
FASTA **42**, 50, 52–53, 59–60
–, with transgene proteins **42**, 53–56
Fasting, anti-inflammatory effect **37**, 52
–, tests for muscle disorders **37**, 348–349
Fast protein liquid chromatography, whey protein denaturation **33**, 372
Fat (*see also* Lipids), absorbed by batter of doughnuts **5**, 177

–, acidity of in flour **11**, 282
–, and meat quality **26**, 85–86
–, ascorbic acid as synergist in protection of **18**, 241–248
–, carcinogen risk assessment and **31**, 22, 24
–, chocolate and, alkalization **31**, 248
–, –, cocoa bean chemistry **31**, 229
–, –, cocoa butter **31**, 250–253, 277–281
–, –, conching **31**, 298, 301–303, 307
–, –, emulsifiers **31**, 281, 284
–, –, milk **31**, 253–258, 263, 264
–, –, milk crumb **31**, 284, 286, 291
–, –, packaging **31**, 319
–, –, processing **31**, 244
–, –, sweeteners **31**, 271–274
–, –, tempering **31**, 308, 309, 311–313
–, coefficients of digestibility **35**, 20–21
–, consumption **35**, 2–3
–, content in dairy products **37**, 150–152
–, content of apples and pears **8**, 300
–, – of –, of cocoa **8**, 261
–, cooked at high temperatures **6**, 4
–, copper content **10**, 196, 201
–, decomposition **10**, 195–199, 209; **16**, 198ff
–, deposition **14**, 43–47
–, determination **14**, 120–121
–, dietary fiber and **31**, 168
–, dietary (*see also* Fatty acids), butterfat comparison with other food fats **37**, 168–169
–, –, intake and cancer **35**, 143
–, disappearance data **37**, 133–136
–, dried milk powders and **7**, 230
–, effect of salts on bacon fat **5**, 32
–, effects, on cancer risk, animal studies **37**, 219–223
–, –, –, breast cancer **37**, 211–212
–, –, –, colon cancer **37**, 212–213
–, –, –, fat composition and source **37**, 213–215, 221–222
–, –, –, fat quantity **37**, 210–213, 220–221
–, –, –, milk and dairy products **37**, 215–219
–, –, –, trace lipids **37**, 223
–, –, on coronary heart disease risk **37**, 153–154
–, –, on LDL modification **37**, 171–181
–, –, on serum lipoproteins and apolipoproteins **37**, 154–159
–, –, –, monounsaturated fatty acids **37**, 171–178
–, –, –, *n*-3 polyunsaturated fatty acids **37**, 178–179
–, –, –, saturated and unsaturated fatty acids **37**, 159–170
–, –, on thrombosis tendency **37**, 181–185
–, –, on whey protein foaming properties **33**, 404
–, evaluating oxidative changes **5**, 9, 10, 11
–, filtration **10**, 198
–, freeze-drying and **7**, 217, 219
–, hydrogenated and nonhydrogenated **10**, 194–195
–, in cakes **8**, 36
–, in candies **6**, 29, 32
–, in cheese ripening **16**, 254ff
–, in cocoa beans and nibs **6**, 38
–, in emulsions **16**, 107ff, 116ff, 121ff, 132, 149
–, in fruits **17**, 183
–, ingredients of candy **6**, 12
–, in ice cream mix **3**, 92
–, in meat **5**, 8
–, in pastries **8**, 36
–, in potato chip processing additives in **10**, 196
–, in steers **14**, 44
–, intake data **37**, 136–140
–, mean scores for flavor of pastry made with different **5**, 183
–, measurement **14**, 109–110
–, mutagen formation role **34**, 417–420
–, *N*-nitroso compounds and **31**, 75, 78–81
–, nutrition **39**, 278–280
–, oleic–linolenic in candy production **6**, 32
–, olive oil and **31**, 454
–, optimal balances for CHD protection **37**, 206–208
–, oxidation, chlorophyll as a prooxidant in **4**, 175
–, protection of bacteria during freezing by **6**, 167
–, quasi-properties of **8**, 10
–, rancid, injurious compounds in **1**, 125
–, rancidity **5**, 1
–, –, comparison with fat reversion **4**, 188
–, –, detection by means of chlorophyll fluorescence **4**, 174
–, –, of meat **6**, 138, 142
–, response determinants, genetic factors **37**, 192–194
–, –, quantity and composition **37**, 189–192
–, –, triglyceride structure **37**, 185–188
–, rheology of **8**, 26
–, scores for pastry made with different **5**, 183
–, stability of **6**, 12
–, state of in dry whole milk **3**, 51–53
–, storage **10**, 201

Fat, storage (*cont'd*)
–, – of DDT in **2**, 210–211
–, tocopherols in **33**, 159–164
–, toxicity **10**, 199–200
–, unsaturated **17**, 27
–, –, oxidation of **5**, 22
–, winterized **10**, 195
Fatal familial insomnia **43**, 273, 285
Fat bloom, chocolate and **31**, 312, 313
Fat crystal networks **44**, 33–141
–, atomic force microscopy **44**, 66–75, 88
–, confocal laser scanning microscopy **44**, 63–67, 88
–, formation process, crystallization observations **44**, 80, 81, 82
–, –, microstructural elements **44**, 83
–, –, microstructure clusters **44**, 83
–, –, particle nomenclature **44**, 82–83
–, fractal dimensions, calculation from rheology **44**, 104–106, 108
–, –, crystallization conditions influence **44**, 113–118, 119–120
–, –, density/order of packing relationship **44**, 109–113
–, –, elastic constant influences **44**, 107–109
–, –, physical significance **44**, 107
–, fractal nature **44**, 84–85, 94–100, 123–124
–, –, use of thresholding methodology **44**, 93, 94, 96–100
–, hardness **44**, 36, 37
–, –, macroscopic indicators **44**, 38–41, 57
–, –, processing conditions dependence **44**, 140
–, –, solid fat content dependence **44**, 133
–, mechanical model at low deformations **44**, 121–140
–, mechanical strength modeling **44**, 35
–, microscopic characterization **44**, 61–82
–, –, self-similarity **44**, 71, 72, 73, 74
–, microstructure **44**, 35, 36, 39–42
–, –, structural model **44**, 82–84
–, –, weak link theory **44**, 100–103, 121–122, 124, 132
–, network models **44**, 58–60, 123, 124–129
–, –, forces between microstructures **44**, 125–129
–, particle volume fraction/solid fat content relationship **44**, 103–104, 122
–, polarized light microscopy **44**, 61–63, 65, 75–80, 88
–, –, fractal dimensions calculation **44**, 88–94
–, rheological analysis **44**, 41–42, 55, 56–57, 104–106
–, scaling theory **44**, 55–58
–, scanning electron microscopy **44**, 61, 63, 64, 88
–, sensory impressions of fat-containing foods **44**, 35–36, 37
–, storage modulus **44**, 36, 122–123, 129–131, 133–134
–, –, processing conditions influence **44**, 136–139
–, structural hierarchy **44**, 35, 36, 83, 84
Fat-free diet, α-LNA levels **35**, 71–73
Fatigue, effect on scoring foods **2**, 241, 243
–, muscular **37**, 341–342, 365–368
Fats and oils, emulsion stability of **22**, 327–330
–, –, dielectric constant **22**, 328
–, –, gas chromatography **22**, 328
–, –, HLB value **22**, 327–328
–, –, phase-inversion temperature spreading coefficient **22**, 328–329
–, –, water number **22**, 329
–, reversion problems in **4**, 185–208
–, used by the candy industry **6**, 3
Fats/fatty acids, microwave effects **43**, 92
Fatty acid esters, hydrophilic–lipophilic balance **34**, 99
Fatty acids (*see also* Dietary fatty acids, Essential fatty acids, Fat, Polyunsaturated fatty acids, Unsaturated fatty acids) **39**, 203, 205–209
–, *trans* **36**, 304–305
–, –, incorporation into cardiolipin **37**, 295–297
–, –, in fats and oils **37**, 146–147
–, absorption **35**, 21–22
–, as food preservatives **1**, 386–398
–, cheese flavor and **7**, 27–28
–, chocolate and, alkalization **31**, 247
–, –, cocoa bean chemistry **31**, 234
–, –, cocoa butter **31**, 250–252, 275, 276, 278, 279
–, –, conching **31**, 297
–, –, milk **31**, 254, 264
–, –, milk crumb **31**, 291
–, –, packaging **31**, 324, 325
–, –, sweeteners **31**, 274
–, composition of plant seed oils and products **35**, 18
–, content in animals **5**, 6
–, dietary cardiolipin, positional distribution **37**, 290
–, emulsification of **16**, 119
–, essential fatty acid deficiency **37**, 294–295
–, esters of sorbitan and polyoxyethylene **6**, 15

–, fish spoilage and **7**, 47–48
–, formation in dried raw meat **11**, 303
–, free in wheat flours, breadmaking and **29**, 253, 255–257
–, in abalone **23**, 161
–, in bacon **3**, 301–303, 309–314
–, in cheese ripening **16**, 254ff, 259ff, 270
–, in cocoa fat **6**, 39
–, in cottonseed **3**, 144
–, in depot fats **23**, 22, 23
–, in eggs **1**, 151
–, influence of rations **5**, 6
–, in meats, effects on SH groups **24**, 57–58
–, in milkfat **37**, 144–146
–, –, *n*-3 **37**, 147–148
–, –, *trans* isomers **37**, 146–147
–, –, predominant **37**, 144–146
–, in milk products **16**, 200
–, in protein decomposition **16**, 185
–, in vacuum dehydrated bacon **3**, 320
–, in wheat flour **16**, 426
–, in wheat germ **23**, 225–228
–, liberation of free **6**, 14
–, losses of **17**, 32
–, meat mutagen modulation **34**, 429–430
–, medium-chain, plasma lipid/lipoprotein response **36**, 270–271
–, modification, β-lactoglobutin thermal characteristics effect **35**, 330–331
–, monounsaturated, effects on serum lipoproteins and apolipoproteins **37**, 159–178
–, –, *trans* fatty acids **37**, 175–178
–, –, *cis* monounsaturates **37**, 171–175
–, *N*-nitroso compounds and **31**, 62, 76, 79
–, olive oil and **31**, 458, 463–466, 471, 473, 477
–, oxidation of **5**, 8
–, polyunsaturated, *see* Polyunsaturated fatty acids
–, reactions with sulfites **30**, 27
–, role **36**, 254–255
–, saturated, effects on serum lipoproteins and apolipoproteins **37**, 159–170
–, –, incorporation into cardiolipin **37**, 295–297
–, saturated and monoenoic **35**, 5
–, selectivity for incorporation into cardiolipin **37**, 292–293
Favella ehrenbergii **10**, 141
Favism **16**, 33; **42**, 11
Feces, dietary fiber and **31**, 152, 153, 191
–, intestinal bacteria **31**, 171–176, 178, 179, 181–184, 186, 188
–, properties **31**, 154, 163, 166, 168
Federal Insecticide, Fungicide and Rodenticide Act, carcinogen risk assessment and **31**, 6, 7, 12
Feed, effects on meat flavor **18**, 6–7
Feedback, neural network **40**, 335
Feeds and feedstuffs, effect on milk and meat flavor **23**, 37–38
–, wheat germ use in **23**, 286
Felbarnate **44**, 311
Feline spongiform encephalopathy (FSE) **43**, 278–279
Fenbutrazate **44**, 324
Fenfluramine **44**, 313
Fenoprofen **44**, 295
Fermentation (*see also* Cheese, Salami, Sausage) **16**, 251, 311ff; **17**, 20; **39**, 95
–, chocolate and **31**, 213, 329
–, –, chemical changes **31**, 221–225
–, –, cocoa bean chemistry **31**, 226–229, 231–235
–, –, microbiology **31**, 217–219
–, –, processing **31**, 215–217, 239, 244, 246
–, –, sweeteners **31**, 267
–, continuous **10**, 18–19
–, dehydration mechanisms **39**, 108–110
–, dehydration quality attributes **39**, 118–119
–, dietary fiber and **31**, 172–186
–, in fruit maturation **10**, 294–295, 310, 322
–, in tea manufacture **17**, 264–272
–, milk-based foods **39**, 164–165, 174–175
–, of black tea **24**, 253–260
–, of citrus by-products **17**, 93
–, of honey **24**, 351–352
–, of molasses **17**, 125
–, of sauerkraut, bacterial action in **10**, 240–246, 247–248, 250–253
–, –, lactic acid in **10**, 233, 240–241, 244, 246–250
–, –, salt influence on **10**, 242, 248, 246, 247, 250, 252, 253–259, 260–261
–, –, sugar role in **10**, 240, 247–248
–, –, temperature influence on **10**, 242, 243, 246, 253–259, 261–263
–, –, yeasts in **10**, 241, 242, 243, 249, 252, 275
–, of soy sauce **10**, 85, 87, 111–115
–, of tea **2**, 284
–, –, chemical changes in **11**, 234–241
–, –, composition after **11**, 234
–, –, initiation of **11**, 233
–, of vegetables **10**, 233–235, 278–279
–, olive oil and **31**, 461, 467, 479
–, phytate degradation **45**, 9, 16, 20, 22

Fermentation (*cont'd*)
–, phytic acid destruction and **28**, 55–60
–, products **12**, 76–81
–, –, from tropical fruits **17**, 196–199
–, research needs **39**, 148–149
–, sardines **39**, 346
–, soy products **44**, 213–214
Fermented flat breads **43**, 229
Fermented foods, for developing countries **22**, 201–202
–, wheat germ use in **23**, 285
Ferric iron, chelation **33**, 304
–, fish lipid oxidation **33**, 289–290
Ferricyanide acid, reducing capacity of in dry milk **3**, 75–78
–, reduction of in dry milk, during storage **3**, 101
–, – of –, effect of heat **3**, 84
Ferrous iron, chelation **33**, 304
–, fish lipid oxidation **33**, 289–290
Ferrous sulfate, effects on folate retention **33**, 49–50
Fertilization, in kiwifruit cultivation **29**, 284
–, olive oil and **31**, 455, 458
Ferulic acid, conversion into 4-ethylguaiacol **30**, 278–280
–, –, yeast from shoyu mash and **30**, 278, 280
–, dicotyledonous plants **31**, 124
–, dietary fiber and, components **31**, 139, 140
–, intestinal bacteria **31**, 186, 189
–, in wheat germ **23**, 237
–, monocotyledonous plants **31**, 136, 138
Feta cheese **39**, 177, 193–194
FEV_1, *see* Forced expiratory volume in 1 s
FFA, *see* Free fatty acid
Fiberoptic thermometry, microwave temperature measurements **43**, 84–85, 86
Fibers, area **14**, 47–48
–, carcinogen risk assessment and **31**, 21–23
–, composition **14**, 51
–, crude, in tea **11**, 224
–, differentiation **19**, 29–50
–, effects on calcium bioavailability **33**, 134–135
–, – on –, cereals **33**, 136–139
–, – on –, fruits and vegetables **33**, 139–141
–, – on –, mechanism **33**, 135–136
–, – on –, pH dependence of calcium binding by fiber **33**, 136
–, – on –, purified fibers **33**, 141–142
–, – on folate bioavailability **33**, 76–78
–, – on tocopherol bioavailability **33**, 171–173
–, extensibility **14**, 50–51
–, in cocoa beans and nibs **6**, 38
–, in vegetable tissue, composition and shape of **2**, 302, 304
–, size **14**, 47
–, types of, in muscle **19**, 25–29
Fibrils **9**, 3–4
–, dietary fiber and **31**, 122, 123, 136
–, endogenous proteolytic enzymes and **31**, 372, 403
Fibroblasts, endogenous proteolytic enzymes and, endopeptidases **31**, 362
–, –, meat technology **31**, 407, 411
–, –, muscle physiology **31**, 379
–, –, proteinase distribution **31**, 366, 367, 369
–, uptake of tocopherols **33**, 180–182
Fibrogen, conformation **34**, 59
Fibronectin, deficiency in Ehlers–Danlos syndrome **37**, 392–394
–, role in connective tissue carcinomas **37**, 404–405
Fibrosis, hepatic **37**, 403–404
Fickian diffusion **39**, 140
Figs **15**, 225
–, dried, enzymic changes in **11**, 290
Filaments **9**, 4
–, endogenous proteolytic enzymes and, meat technology **31**, 394, 396, 400, 401
–, –, muscle physiology **31**, 370, 371
Filiform papillae **44**, 251
Fillers in meat emulsions **16**, 138
Fillings, alginates in **11**, 151
Film bag **32**, 20–22, 28, 29, 30
Film model **32**, 57
Films, adsorption **33**, 391–393
–, effects of aging **33**, 394
–, for flexible packaging **23**, 317–322
–, for prepacking passion fruit **12**, 232–233
–, ionic strength effects **33**, 394
–, methylcellulose **12**, 316
–, pH effects **33**, 394
–, protein conformation and **33**, 393–395
–, stability **33**, 394
–, viscoelastic behavior **33**, 394
–, whey proteins **33**, 395–396
Filtration, influence of consistency on **11**, 429–432
–, of fruit juices **9**, 248
–, olive oil and **31**, 462, 470, 471, 475
Fimbriae (pili) **43**, 322
Finfish, amine occurrence **39**, 336–344
Fining, of fruit juices **9**, 247–248

Finnish oils, tocopherols and tocotrienols in **33**, 162
Firing, in tea manufacture **17**, 265–266, 272
Firmness, fish freshness and **7**, 63
Fish (*see also* Mechanically deboned fish) **13**, 13, 300–303, 321; **15**, 238
–, acetylmethylcarbinol in **16**, 196
–, aerobic and anaerobic bacterial flora of **2**, 348–354
–, agar in **11**, 122–123
–, alcohol in **16**, 196
–, alginates in preservation of **11**, 148–150
–, ammonia in **16**, 169
–, ascorbic acid prevention of rancidity of **18**, 256–266
–, – of –, canned fish **18**, 265
–, – of –, fresh, iced, and salted fish **18**, 261–265
–, – of –, frozen fish **18**, 257–261
–, – of –, precautions in **18**, 265–266
–, bacteria in frozen **6**, 190
–, bacterial increase during spoilage **2**, 356
–, bacterial load of gut and skin of **2**, 355
–, bases in **16**, 182
–, biochemical spoilage changes **2**, 367
–, –, changes in pH in **2**, 372–373
–, –, fat spoilage **2**, 373
–, –, formation of dimethylamine in stored **2**, 371
–, –, proteolysis in **2**, 371–372
–, –, trimethylamine oxide reduction in **2**, 367–370
–, biogenic amines, *see* Biogenic amines, fish and shellfish
–, broiled, mutagens **34**, 398
–, canned, corrosion characteristics of **3**, 336
–, carrageenan in **11**, 133–135
–, changes in glycogen, lactic acid and pH in muscle of **2**, 362–364
–, characteristics of fresh **2**, 346
–, – of spoiling **2**, 346–348
–, collectors **12**, 376
–, dehydrated **14**, 79–81
–, effect of heating on nutritive value of protein in **4**, 262–267
–, fatty acids in **16**, 185
–, fatty acids in fat of **23**, 23
–, freeze-drying of **7**, 221–223
–, freshness, estimation of **7**, 58–64, 72–73
–, frozen, and TMAOase activity **26**, 298–304
–, –, interaction between factors **26**, 304–306
–, –, protein denaturation, dehydration **26**, 283–284
–, –, –, divalent cations **26**, 289–290
–, –, –, factors causing **26**, 281–306
–, –, –, ice crystal formation **26**, 281–283
–, –, –, lipid hydrolysis **26**, 294–295
–, –, –, lipid oxidation **26**, 296–297
–, –, –, salt **26**, 286–287
–, –, research needs **26**, 306–307
–, –, tests for **26**, 277–281
–, –, –, degradation products **26**, 280–281
–, –, –, enzymatic activity **26**, 279–290
–, –, –, extracted proteins **26**, 280
–, –, –, microscopic examination **26**, 279
–, –, –, protein extractability **26**, 277–278
–, –, –, protein solubility **26**, 277–278
–, –, –, tissue properties **26**, 278–279
–, –, trimethylamine oxidase, enzymatic activity **26**, 298–304
–, –, –, properties of **26**, 302–304
–, gums in **11**, 116
–, handling and storage of **2**, 384–390
–, histamine in **16**, 193
–, histological analysis **14**, 127–128
–, hot, smoked, sensory indices for color quality of **19**, 242
–, hydrogen sulfide in **16**, 196
–, indole in **16**, 174
–, influence of pH on bacterial growth **2**, 358–367
–, lactic acid in **16**, 190
–, measuring tenderness of **8**, 17, 31
–, mechanism of spoilage of **3**, 184–187
–, methods of preserving in Southeast Asia **4**, 210–212
–, *N*-nitroso compounds and **31**, 86, 92, 93
–, number of organisms reducing trimethylamine oxide in fresh and stale **2**, 355
–, nutritional stress factor in **4**, 111–113
–, objective tests of quality **2**, 375
–, – of –, chemical tests **2**, 375–381
–, – of –, surface pH test **2**, 381
–, – of –, titration test **2**, 382
–, ozone treatment **45**, 197–198
–, preservation **4**, 209–232
–, –, chemical agents and **7**, 64–71, 73–74
–, protein denaturation during storage **26**, 275–30
–, proteins **14**, 222; **16**, 24
–, psychrophilic flora of **6**, 189
–, quality of **7**, 58
–, raw **12**, 376–378
–, –, bleaching **12**, 376
–, –, crushing **12**, 376
–, –, defrosting **12**, 376
–, –, draining **12**, 377

Fish, raw (*cont'd*)
–, –, reddening **12**, 378
–, –, thiamine-destroying enzyme in **1**, 125
–, reactivity with tin **3**, 341
–, red-fleshed **12**, 371–373
–, –, marlin **12**, 372, 397
–, –, salmon **12**, 372
–, –, skipjack and bonito **12**, 372
–, –, tuna **12**, 371–372, 376–377, 397
–, –, whale **12**, 373, 376, 397
–, red-muscled, spoilage of **7**, 50–51
–, reducing substances in **16**, 189
–, rigor mortis in **2**, 364–367
–, salted, not dried **4**, 221–225
–, salted and dried **4**, 225–227
–, sausage **16**, 148
–, sausage and ham industry in Japan **12**, 367–424
–, – in –, quality standards **12**, 420–422
–, – in –, sanitary measures **12**, 415–417
–, selenium in **32**, 96, 97
–, smoking secondary skin induction **29**, 146
–, SO_2 preservation **5**, 98
–, spoilage, changes in **7**, 43–44
–, stews, bacterial count of frozen **6**, 199
–, succinic acid in **16**, 190
–, sulfide discoloration in **3**, 355
–, supercooling of **6**, 164
–, texture **14**, 113–114
–, thermal scanning rheological analysis **35**, 352–354
–, toxins from, *see* Marine toxins
–, trimethylamine in **16**, 178
–, trimethylamine oxidase, distribution in **26**, 298–300
–, ultrasonic composition sensors **45**, 138
–, ultrasonic microscopy for parasite detection **45**, 156
–, use of ascorbic acid in **4**, 390–392
–, verbal ratings **19**, 250
–, "warmed-over" flavor in **23**, 1–74
–, white-fleshed **12**, 373–376
–, –, Alaska pollack **12**, 376
–, –, cod **12**, 375
–, –, eso **12**, 373–374
–, –, flat **12**, 376
–, –, guchi and nibe **12**, 374–375
–, –, kanagashira **12**, 375
–, –, sharks and rays **12**, 373, 377, 397–398
–, –, squid **12**, 376, 397
Fish and fish products, histamine in allowable levels **24**, 146
–, – in –, detection **24**, 130–135
–, – in –, enzymic formation **24**, 121–122
–, – in –, spoilage role **24**, 135–139
–, histamine toxicity from **24**, 113–154
–, histidine decarboxylases in **24**, 122–128
Fishery products, *Clostridium botulinum* in **22**, 135–185
–, consumption of **20**, 192–196
–, preservation of **22**, 160–168
–, production of **20**, 190–191
–, trade in **20**, 191–192
Fish lipids, oxidation, enzyme-catalyzed **33**, 291–297
–, –, factors affecting **33**, 287–289
–, –, metal catalysis of **33**, 289–291
–, –, volatile compound generation **33**, 298–302
–, polyunsaturated fatty acids in **33**, 286
Fishmeal, effect of feeding on palatability of poultry meat **1**, 219–220
–, – of heating on nutritive value of protein in **4**, 250
Fish meat emulsions, development and use of **20**, 207–210
Fish muscle, rigor in **9**, 22
Fishnet gels **34**, 206
Fish oils (*see also* Marine oils), effect on tocopherol bioavailability **33**, 173
–, eicosanoid synthesis suppression **35**, 96
–, feeding studies **35**, 53–55
–, heart disease and **35**, 134–135
–, PUFA **35**, 41–42
–, tocopherol content **33**, 164
Fish pastes **4**, 217–221; **39**, 346
Fish poisons **10**, 137–138
Fish-protein concentrate (FPC) **17**, 135
–, development and use of **20**, 203–204
Fish proteins **10**, 60–61
Fish sauces **4**, 212–217
Fittings and valves, equivalent lengths **11**, 411
Flakes, potato, processes for **25**, 59–61
Flame ionization **14**, 18
Flame sterilization, heat transfer in **32**, 70–73
Flan jelly, furcellaran in **11**, 159
Flat fish, keeping qualities of **2**, 377
–, rigor mortis in **2**, 367
Flat sour bacteria **18**, 163–217
–, biology of **18**, 191–207
–, canning-plant contamination sources **18**, 187–189
–, –, tomato-juice processing **18**, 187–188
–, –, vegetable processing **18**, 188–189
–, classification of **18**, 167–169
–, control of **18**, 190–191
–, distribution of spores of **18**, 169–179

–, – of –, in milk **18**, 173–174
–, – of –, in soil and water **18**, 169–173
–, – of –, in sugar and starch **18**, 174–178
–, – of –, wheat and wheat products **18**, 179
–, enzymes of **18**, 203–206
–, growth of **18**, 192–196
–, metabolism of nitrogen compounds of **18**, 206–207
–, nutrient requirements of **18**, 195
–, research needs for **18**, 208
–, rough and smooth variants of **18**, 169
–, spoilage caused by **18**, 165
–, spore resistance of **18**, 179–187
–, –, antibiotic effect on **18**, 184–186
–, –, chlorine effects on **18**, 186
–, –, measurement **18**, 180
–, –, order of death **18**, 181
–, –, radiation effects on **18**, 186–187
–, –, to heat **18**, 179–180, 181–184
–, spores of, germination and outgrowth of **18**, 197–200
–, –, morphology and chemical composition of **18**, 200–203
–, sporulation of **18**, 196–197
–, thermophily of **18**, 191–192
Flavan molecule **11**, 210
Flavanols (catechins), chromatograms of **11**, 212, 213
–, in tea **11**, 210–214
–, structural formulae **11**, 210–211
Flavanotropilone, structure of **19**, 103
Flavedo, freeze-dried lemon juice and **7**, 226, 228
Flavenoids in citrus fruits **9**, 342
– in –, distribution **9**, 346–347
– in –, identification **9**, 343–346
– in –, properties **9**, 347–348
Flavin adenine dinucleotide (FAD), reactions with sulfites **30**, 25
Flavin-containing monooxygenases **45**, 82
Flavin mononucleotide (FMN), reactions with sulfites **30**, 25
Flavobacter deciduosum, effect of temperature on growth of **2**, 360
Flavobacter in fresh fish **2**, 350
– in –, comparison of fresh and spoiled fish **2**, 353
Flavobacterium, effect of nitrites on **3**, 295
Flavobacterium aquatile **45**, 180
Flavobacterium branchiophilum **45**, 181, 190
Flavones, in discoloration of fruit products **3**, 11, 12
–, in tea, structure **11**, 209
Flavonoid compounds in foods **5**, 261
– in –, action on smooth muscle **5**, 276
– in –, antioxidant action **5**, 271
– in –, color **5**, 271
– in –, fat in the body **5**, 277
– in –, genetic situation in fruits and vegetables **5**, 280
– in –, naturally occurring **5**, 264
– in –, pharmacological action **5**, 275
– in –, properties depending on phenolic character **5**, 268
– in –, properties significant in foods **5**, 268
– in –, reactions with metals **5**, 270
– in –, relation to bloat in ruminants **5**, 276
– in –, systematic distribution **5**, 283
– in –, taste **5**, 273
– in –, tendencies in distribution **5**, 289
– in –, toxicity **5**, 277
Flavonoids **27**, 173–191; **44**, 196, 197
–, antioxidant action **33**, 314–316
–, as drugs **27**, 174–181
–, distribution **33**, 312
–, effects on lipoxygenase **33**, 316–319
–, formation **33**, 312
–, hydroxyl positional isomers, effects on lipoxygenase inhibition **33**, 318–319
–, inhibitory effects on fish gill 12-lipoxygenase, table **33**, 308
–, in higher plants **33**, 313–314
–, metabolism **27**, 184–191
–, mutagenicity of **27**, 181–184
–, nutritional aspects **27**, 173–174
–, optimum antioxidant activity **33**, 316
–, structural alterations, effects on lipoxygenase inhibition **33**, 317–318
–, structural requirements for lipoxygenase inhibition **33**, 319
–, structure **19**, 77; **33**, 311–312
–, toxicity **27**, 173–174, 184–191
Flavonols, as antitumor agents **33**, 319
–, in discoloration of fruit products **3**, 11, 12
–, in food browning **19**, 80–81
–, in tea **11**, 214–215; **17**, 218, 227–231
–, –, chromatogram of **11**, 214
–, in tea plant **11**, 232
–, structural formulae **11**, 214
Flavoprotein enzymes **3**, 9
–, relationship of to respiration in fruits **3**, 17
Flavoproteins **17**, 19
Flavor **14**, 19, 266–267; **15**, 259
–, aftertaste and **7**, 37
–, animal products **14**, 242–244
–, appropriate factors in **7**, 365
–, aroma and **7**, 10

Flavor (*cont'd*)
–, bread and other baked cereal products **30**, 100–102
–, browning reactions **14**, 235–245
–, caramel **6**, 31
–, changes due to peroxidase **17**, 18
–, cheese, *see* Cheese, flavor
–, chlorine and **7**, 162–165
, chocolate and **31**, 329
–, –, alkalization **31**, 247
–, –, cocoa bean chemistry **31**, 225–228, 234–237
–, –, conching **31**, 298, 299, 304, 308
–, –, milk **31**, 255, 260–262, 264
–, –, milk crumb **31**, 285, 290, 291
–, –, packaging **31**, 314, 319, 320
–, –, processing **31**, 215, 237–241, 245
–, –, refining **31**, 292, 295
–, –, tempering **31**, 309
–, –, *Theobroma cacao* L. **31**, 329
–, chocolate and cocoa **30**, 93–100
–, cinnamon and **30**, 78
–, clove and **30**, 78
–, coffee **30**, 109–111
–, definition of **7**, 11
–, detection of **17**, 5
–, deterioration **17**, 31–33
–, detracting factors in **7**, 36–37
–, development of, in onion and garlic **22**, 73–133
–, effect on food intake **21**, 37–48
–, enzyme role **22**, 116–118
–, feeling factors and **7**, 37
–, fish **39**, 349
–, "fishy" **17**, 33
–, fixation with gum arabic **11**, 175
–, food processing **21**, 46–51
–, from Maillard reactions between amino acids and sugars **30**, 91, 92–93
–, history **30**, 77–79
–, IM meat **39**, 110, 122, 130–136
–, in candies **6**, 9, 31
–, in processed milk **10**, 54–55
–, interest and **7**, 37
–, koikuchi shoyu **30**, 257–287
–, maple syrup **30**, 111–112
–, meat **30**, 103–109
–, meat processing **21**, 46, 47
–, milk **39**, 118
–, of abalone **23**, 174, 176–177
–, of cheese **16**, 239, 247, 257, 268ff
–, off-flavor **17**, 21
–, –, caused by oxidation **17**, 33
–, –, in vegetables **17**, 6
–, –, production of **17**, 32–33
–, of foods, advances in research on **19**, 231–240
–, –, flavor conservation **19**, 238–239
–, –, legal requirements **19**, 239–240
–, –, technological impact **19**, 235–237
–, olive oil and **31**, 468–470
–, peanuts **30**, 112–113
–, perception, in meat flavor studies **18**, 66–67
–, philosophy of **7**, 35–37
–, potato products **30**, 113
–, precursors, chocolate and **31**, 221, 226, 231–233
–, reversion, in fats and oils **4**, 188
–, shoyu, components of **30**, 305–313
–, stability, effect of antioxidants **27**, 125–126
–, –, – of carbon dioxide cooling **27**, 126
–, –, – of heme pigments **27**, 123–125
–, –, – of nitrogen cooling **27**, 126
–, –, – of processing variables **27**, 120–122
–, –, – of storage **27**, 122–123
–, thresholds **14**, 244–245
–, vanilla and **30**, 78
Flavor binding, thermodynamic representation **33**, 412
–, whey proteins **33**, 410–413
Flavor chemistry, of muscle **26**, 87–88
Flavor compounds, microwave effects **43**, 94–95
Flavor enhancement, cancer patients **44**, 330
–, effects in elderly people **44**, 325–330
–, lymphocyte count response **44**, 326–328
–, nutritional parameters improvement **44**, 329
–, salivary flow/IgA content improvement **44**, 328–329
–, sodium intake effects **44**, 329–330
Flavor enhancers, intolerances **42**, 30
Flavor formation **32**, 116–117, 118
Flavor impact value, for passion fruit juice **27**, 282–287
Flavoring constituents, in dehydrated mashed potatoes **25**, 102–109
Flavoring oils **34**, 131
Flavoring substances (*see also* Food allergies *and* Food intolerance) **42**, 1–37
–, acting as haptens **42**, 28
–, allergic reactions, published examples **42**, 24–28
–, appropriate diagnostic tests, assessment strategy **42**, 33
–, –, challenge tests **42**, 32, 34–35
–, –, patch tests **42**, 36

–, –, sensitivity to **42**, 31–36
–, –, skin tests **42**, 35
–, classes **42**, 15
–, formation **42**, 15
–, labeling **42**, 20–21, 24
–, manufacturing **42**, 16–18
–, mucosal contact sensitization reactions **42**, 28–29
–, nature and composition **42**, 14–15
–, occupational sensitivities **42**, 31
–, physical classification **42**, 13–14
–, physical or technical functional effects **42**, 21, 24
–, protein content **42**, 17–20
–, sulfur-containing **42**, 17–18
–, usage levels **42**, 20, 22–23
–, volatile components **42**, 14
Flavor profile, after taste and **7**, 13
–, amplitude and **7**, 13–15
–, character notes and **7**, 12
–, detail aids to **7**, 32–33
–, development of **7**, 9–10
–, evolution of **7**, 22–33
–, intensity scale and **7**, 12–13
–, modification of **7**, 33–35
–, order of appearance and **7**, 13
–, panel leader and **7**, 19–20
–, panel selection and **7**, 15–18
–, panel training and **7**, 18–19
–, personality and **7**, 17–18
–, purpose of **7**, 5
–, records of **7**, 30–31
–, reproducibility of **7**, 31–32
–, response sheet and **7**, 28
–, sample numbers and **7**, 26–27
–, smelling techniques and **7**, 26
–, studies on meat flavor **18**, 26–27
–, testing area and **7**, 20–21
–, testing techniques and **7**, 26
–, training and **7**, 10
Flaxseed lignans **44**, 207, 211
–, antiestrogenic effects **44**, 225
–, cancer protective effects **44**, 231
–, effects of processing **44**, 217–218
–, metabolism **44**, 221–222
Flecainide **44**, 305
Flexibacter spp., growth conditions and adhesion **43**, 324
Flexibility indices **35**, 262
Flexible packaging **23**, 305–428
–, air removal from **23**, 369–375
–, bacterial penetration into **23**, 315–317
–, cans compared to **23**, 402
–, current films for **23**, 317–322
–, designs for **23**, 322–324
–, durability of **23**, 399–404
–, early studies on **23**, 309–312
–, equipment development for **23**, 418–419
–, extractives for **23**, 313–315
–, filling of **23**, 364–369
–, flexible film technology in **23**, 418
–, food product development in **23**, 324–335
–, for HT/ST products **23**, 327
–, heat-seal quality, retorting effects on **23**, 352–353
–, interlamina bonds in **23**, 353–354
–, leak detection in **23**, 409–417
–, –, methodology **23**, 415–417
–, materials for **23**, 312–322
–, occluded particles in seals of **23**, 354–355
–, production reliability in **23**, 344–346
–, production systems for **23**, 333–346
–, –, current types **23**, 336–344
–, product research in **23**, 417–418
–, quality and stability of **23**, 328–333
–, quality assurance in **23**, 404–417
–, research and development needs in **23**, 417–418
–, residual gas levels in **23**, 374–375
–, retortability of **23**, 317
–, retorting of **23**, 375–399
–, –, techniques and equipment for **23**, 387–398
–, seal contamination in **23**, 360–363
–, seal defects in, tests for **23**, 407–409
–, sealing in **23**, 346–363
–, –, for retort pouches **23**, 355–359
–, seal wrinkles in **23**, 359–360
–, shipping tests on **23**, 403–404
–, systems approach to **23**, 333–336
–, –, for thermo processed foods **23**, 305–428
–, utility of **23**, 327–328
Flexing, in flexible-package leak studies **23**, 412–413
Flocculation **34**, 130, 133–135
–, measurement **34**, 175–176
Flora, distribution **37**, 71
–, microbial in gastrointestinal tract, control **37**, 47–50
Floridean starch **41**, 5–6
Flory–Huggins expression **34**, 265
Floss, dried pork **39**, 76
Flounder, loss of thiamine in **6**, 280
Flour (*see also* Wheat flour), acidity of fat in **11**, 282
–, ascorbic acid addition to **18**, 272–277
–, bleached, toxic compound in **1**, 124
–, chocolate and **31**, 236

Flour (*cont'd*)
–, color grader, development of **5**, 317
–, correlation of wheat tests for insects to fragment count **5**, 243
–, destruction of beetles in **3**, 135
–, dietary fiber and **31**, 154
–, –, analysis **31**, 148, 150
–, –, monocotyledonous plants **31**, 135–138
–, doughs **8**, 15, 21, 43
–, effect of sonic vibration on **3**, 131
–, enzymatic changes in **11**, 281–285
–, insect fragment counts in **8**, 125
–, milling of, use of infrared radiation in **3**, 146
–, protein content **10**, 62
–, samples, examination of **8**, 113
–, tests for quality **8**, 13
–, thermal characteristics **35**, 341–342
–, thiamine in **6**, 262, 263, 267
–, use of ascorbic acid in **4**, 406–407
–, whiteness in **5**, 311
–, yellowness of **5**, 316
Flour beetles, origin **4**, 283
Flow, frictional loss **14**, 429–430
–, resistance **14**, 423
–, tubing **14**, 424
Flow algorithm **40**, 247–248
Flow behavior index **32**, 47
Flow constants, for ammonium alginate **11**, 387
–, for applesauce **11**, 387
–, for banana purée **11**, 387
–, for blood **11**, 387
–, for honey **11**, 387
–, for various materials **11**, 387
Flow diagram **40**, 340
Flow index **39**, 6, 56
Flowmeters (Doppler) **45**, 131–132
–, transit-time mode **45**, 130–131
–, vortex shedding **45**, 132
Flow models **32**, 44–47
Flow of suspensions **11**, 416
Flow pattern, determination of **32**, 50–56
Flow rate **40**, 342–345, 348–351
–, at various pressure drops **11**, 393
Fluid bed drying, aroma retention in **20**, 73–74
Fluid consistency, dilatancy in **11**, 367
–, in food engineering applications **11**, 355–435
–, in foods **11**, 371–373
–, liquid structure as element in **11**, 358–368
–, rate of shear in **11**, 368–371
–, role of apparent viscosity in **11**, 373
–, – of colloidal suspensions in **11**, 366
–, – of suspensions in **11**, 365
–, shear stress in **11**, 368
–, thixotropy in **11**, 367
Fluid flow, along a curved streamline, a differential element of **11**, 369
–, –, velocity vectors **11**, 369
–, –, –, resolution of **11**, 369
–, ultrasonic sensing **45**, 130–132
Fluid foods, flow models for **32**, 44–47
–, measurement of flow properties of **32**, 47–48
–, transport equations for **32**, 42–43
–, with shear-thinning flow behavior **32**, 45–46
Fluidity **9**, 181
Fluids, center-line temperature in tubes **11**, 420–422
–, non-Newtonian time-dependent **11**, 393–394
–, rheopectic **11**, 394
–, tensile strength **11**, 399
–, thixotropic **11**, 393
–, with yield stress in rotational viscometers **11**, 381–384
Flunisolide **44**, 302, 321
Fluorescence, chocolate and **31**, 322
–, detection of eluted folates with **33**, 28–29
–, dietary fiber and **31**, 136, 148
–, endogenous proteolytic enzymes and **31**, 350
–, freeze-dried beef and **7**, 215–216
–, of dried egg extracts **1**, 159–162, 173
–, of milk fractions **3**, 100
–, use as palatability measure of dried eggs **2**, 249
Fluoride, inhibition of enzymes by **1**, 384
–, in milk **36**, 238
–, in wines **8**, 151
–, microbial inhibition by **1**, 386, 388, 390
Fluorine, effect in diet **1**, 122
–, in diet, adaptation of rats to **1**, 128
Fluoroborates, microbial inhibition by **1**, 386
1-Fluoro-2,4-dinitrobenzene, reactive lysine measurement **35**, 192–193
Fluorometric method for selenium detection **32**, 87–88
Fluorometry assay of histamine **24**, 131–133
Fluorosilicates, microbial inhibition by **1**, 386
Fluorouracil **44**, 294
Fluoxetine **44**, 311
Flurazepam **44**, 307
Flurbiprofen **44**, 295, 321
Flush, core **12**, 114–115

Flushing, chocolate and **31**, 327
Fluvastatin **44**, 288
FMN, *see* Flavin mononucleotide
Foamability, protein-stabilized foams **34**, 70–71
Foaming **15**, 354
Foaming agents, licorice root and **7**, 346
Foam mat drying, aroma retention in **20**, 74
–, cost of **20**, 96
Foams (*see also* Protein-stabilized foams) **34**, 2
–, characterization **33**, 397–399
–, formation **14**, 416–417; **34**, 16
–, stability, protein structure and **33**, 398–400
–, ultrasonic analysis **45**, 150–151
–, whey proteins **33**, 400–402
–, –, foaming properties **33**, 402–404
Foil-free laminations, for thermoprocessed foods **23**, 329–330
Foil laminates, for thermoprocessed foods **23**, 330–333
Foil pouches, ultrasonic leak detection **45**, 154
Folate-binding protein, in jejunal brush border membranes **33**, 54
Folate metabolism **40**, 81–93, 95–106
–, absorption **40**, 82
–, alcoholism **40**, 84–85, 91
–, background information **40**, 81–83, 95–97
–, catabolism **40**, 85–90
–, cytosolic **40**, 99, 100–101
–, dietary factors **40**, 82, 89
–, erythrocytes **40**, 87–88
–, *Escherichia coli* **40**, 97–101, 105
–, folylpolyglutamate chain length **40**, 97–100
–, folylpolyglutamate synthetase **40**, 97–101
–, –, accumulation **40**, 101–104
–, –, chain length **40**, 97–100
–, –, compartmentation **40**, 100–101
–, –, cytotoxicity **40**, 104
–, –, effectiveness **40**, 98–100
–, –, retention **40**, 97–98
–, genetic transfection **40**, 95, 96–101, 105
–, human subject **40**, 86–90
–, intestines **40**, 82, 201
–, membrane vesicles **40**, 201
–, mitochondrial **40**, 99, 100–101
–, pregnancy **40**, 86, 91
–, RDAs **40**, 83
–, stable-isotopic studies **40**, 86–90
–, tracer methods **40**, 86–90
–, turnover **40**, 83–85, 89–90
Folates, antifolates, dietary **33**, 78–80
–, –, ethanol **33**, 69–71
–, –, therapeutic drugs **33**, 70–71
–, bioavailability, absorption **33**, 53–57
–, –, aging effects **33**, 68–69
–, –, assessment methods, bioassays with animals and human **33**, 58–61
–, –, –, isotopic methods **33**, 61–64
–, –, deconjugation **33**, 54–55
–, –, dietary components and **33**, 71–80
–, –, dietary fiber effects **33**, 76–78
–, –, endogenous, in various foods, table **33**, 72
–, –, ethanol effects **33**, 69–71
–, –, folate-binding protein role in jejunal brush border membranes **33**, 54
–, –, gastrointestinal functions and **33**, 67–68
–, –, hepatic uptake and secretion **33**, 54
–, –, inherent **33**, 64–66
–, –, in legumes **33**, 74
–, –, in milk **33**, 75–76
–, –, in orange juice **33**, 74–75
–, –, intestinal conjugases **33**, 55–56
–, –, in vegetables **33**, 75
–, –, *in vivo* turnover kinetics **33**, 57–58
–, –, in yeast **33**, 73–74
–, –, nutrient interactions **33**, 79–90
–, –, pH dependence **33**, 53–54
–, –, K_m transport values **33**, 53
–, C-9–N-10 bond **33**, 34–38
–, chain length, determination with HPLC methods **33**, 34–38
–, chemical properties, concentration-dependent self-association phenomenon **33**, 6
–, –, inherent **33**, 4–6
–, –, ionic **33**, 4–5
–, –, pH effects on behavior **33**, 5–6
–, –, structural **33**, 4
–, chemical structures **33**, 2–3
–, determination, analysis of polyglutamyl forms **33**, 33–38
–, –, HPLC methods **33**, 26–38
–, –, ligand binding methods **33**, 22–26
–, –, microbiological methods **33**, 21–22
–, –, separation and analysis in monoglutamyl form **33**, 26–33
–, deuterated, synthesis, *in vivo* application, and mass spectral analysis **33**, 12
–, distribution in various foods, table **33**, 41
–, enzymatic deconjugation **33**, 17–20
–, extraction **33**, 14–17
–, –, free folate during **33**, 17
–, –, heat effects **33**, 16
–, –, inhibition of oxidative losses **33**, 15
–, –, nonthermal procedures **33**, 16

Folates, extraction (*cont'd*)
–, –, pH effects during **33**, 15–16
–, H_2folate, *see* 7,8-Dihydrofolate
–, H_4folate, *see* 5,6,7,8-Tetrahydrofolate
–, in spinach and Swiss chard, table **33**, 40
–, intrinsic stability **33**, 40–47
–, *in vivo* turnover kinetics **33**, 57–58
–, isotopically labeled and stable, preparation **33**, 12–13
–, one-carbon-substituted, formation **33**, 9–10
–, oxidation potentials, electrochemical detection in reversed-phase HPCL systems **33**, 30–32
–, polyglutamyl, *see* Polyglutamyl folates
–, radioisotopically labeled, preparation **33**, 11–12
–, reactions of nitrite ions with **33**, 44–45
–, Recommended Dietary Allowance **33**, 52
–, Recommended Dietary Intake **33**, 52
–, retention, ascorbate/ferrous sulfate effects **33**, 49–50
–, stability, during cooking or thermal processing **33**, 47–51
–, –, effects of aqueous extraction **33**, 49
–, –, in milk products **33**, 51
–, –, retention after cooking or thermal processing, table **33**, 48
Foliate papillae **44**, 251, 252
Folic acid (*see also* Folate metabolism) **40**, 82, 83, 87–88
–, determination in conjugase assay by reversed-phase HPLC **33**, 31
–, energy of activation for degradation in aqueous solution, table **33**, 50
–, in apples **8**, 369
–, in canned foods **1**, 42, 44, 45, 47
–, in turkey feeding **17**, 31
–, reaction with sodium dithionite reaction for (6-ambo)-5,6,7,8-tetrahydrofolate preparation **33**, 8
–, retention in fortified food **33**, 52
Folylpolyglutamate synthetase **40**, 97–101
Fondant, chemical composition and properties of **6**, 10
–, crystals of **8**, 13
Food, amorphous powder, state diagram, temperature versus water content **38**, 209
–, aqueous glasses, diffusion of water and solute **38**, 169–177
–, ascorbic acid addition to **18**, 219–315
–, concentrated, microbial reduction in **3**, 453–457
–, consumer preference studies on **3**, 386–423
–, dehydrated **14**, 245
–, Drug and Cosmetic Act **42**, 20–21
–, emulsion stability and **22**, 309–359
–, flat sour bacteria spores in **18**, 173–179
–, flour-based products, viscoelasticity **38**, 184–185
–, frozen, *see* Frozen food
–, glass transition temperature measurement **38**, 114–118
–, hypoallergenic **37**, 47
–, labile components, encapsulation **38**, 171
–, liquid type, heat and mass transport in **20**, 52–54
–, losses of thiamine in **6**, 282
–, nitrosamines in **22**, 47–53
–, nonequilibrium nature of products and processes, references **38**, 115–117
–, patents using β-galactosidase activity for galactooligosaccharide production **38**, 87
–, preservation, water and **7**, 117–122
–, processing **14**, 285–324
–, quality, chlorination and **7**, 162–165
–, reactions in **14**, 209–210
–, reactivity with tin **3**, 340–342
–, scanning electron microscopy of **22**, 258–292
–, sensoring stimulus **21**, 35–43
–, structured type, heat and mass transport in **20**, 55–57
–, temperature response characteristics of **23**, 80–82
–, transgalactosylase activity **38**, 84–95
–, types of corrosion by **3**, 337
–, water removal from, processes for **20**, 3
–, world situation of **18**, 85–86
Food additives **15**, 2, 46
Food allergens, characterization and identification **37**, 40–42
–, detection and avoidance **37**, 46
–, research needs **37**, 54
Food allergies (*see also* Food intolerance) **43**, 195–213
–, allergens (*see also* Food allergens) **43**, 197, 198
–, allergic reactions, cell-mediated **42**, 8–9
–, –, delayed-type **42**, 3–4
–, –, IgE-mediated **42**, 4–8, 26–27
–, –, incidence **42**, 63
–, –, likelihood, flavoring substances **42**, 28–29
–, –, oral allergy syndrome **42**, 5, 7
–, avoidance diet **42**, 6
–, characterization and classification **37**, 25–26; **42**, 3
–, common allergenic foods **42**, 5

–, contact sensitivities **42**, 9–10, 24–26
–, definitions **42**, 2; **43**, 197–198
–, delayed hypersensitivity reactions **43**, 197–198
–, –, contact sensitivity **43**, 200–201
–, –, mechanisms **43**, 199–201
–, diagnostic tests, assessment strategy **42**, 33
–, –, challenge tests **42**, 32, 34–35
–, –, patch tests **42**, 36
–, –, sensitivity to flavoring substances **42**, 31–36
–, –, skin tests **42**, 35
–, idiosyncratic reactions **42**, 12–13
–, immediate allergic reactions **42**, 3
–, immediate hypersensitivity reactions **43**, 197, 198–199
–, –, anaphylactic shock **43**, 199
–, –, mechanisms **43**, 198–199, 200
–, –, symptoms **43**, 199
–, intolerances, likelihood, flavoring substances **42**, 30–31
–, metabolic food disorders **42**, 11
–, non-IgE-mediated histamine release **42**, 10–11
–, oral sensitivities **42**, 24–25
–, proteins as **42**, 6–7, 46, 64
–, –, removed or rendered nonallergenic by processing **42**, 6
–, published examples, flavoring substances **42**, 24–28
Food and Drug Administration, carcinogen risk assessment and **31**, 12
–, chocolate and **31**, 225, 264, 320
–, *N*-nitroso compounds and **31**, 86, 87
Food antigens, detection and avoidance **37**, 46
–, research needs **37**, 55
Food applications, seed proteins **36**, 127
Food attitudes, and family setting **32**, 246–247
–, and health as value **32**, 248–250
–, and social setting **32**, 247–248
Foodborne illness, bacterial pathogens **44**, 152
–, –, *Campylobacter* **44**, 162
–, –, *Salmonella* **44**, 153
–, undercooked meat **44**, 148
Food browning **19**, 75–145
–, beer turbidity and **19**, 131
–, enzymic type, *see* Enzymic browning reactions in food
–, in apples **19**, 114–115
–, in asparagus **19**, 127
–, in bananas **19**, 118–119
–, in beets **19**, 121–122
–, in cauliflower **19**, 126–127
–, in cocoa **19**, 112–114
–, in dates **19**, 119–120
–, in grapes and wine **19**, 117–118
–, in peaches **19**, 116–117
–, in pears **19**, 115–116
–, in potatoes **19**, 120–121, 124–125
–, nonenzymic type involving polyphenols **19**, 123–131
–, pink discoloration as **19**, 128–129
–, polyphenoloxidases in **19**, 82–97
–, polyphenols involved in **19**, 76–82
–, –, anthocyanins **19**, 80
–, –, catechin **19**, 77–78
–, –, cinnamic acid derivatives **19**, 81
–, –, flavonols **19**, 80–81
–, –, leucoanthocyanidins **19**, 78–79
–, –, simple phenols **19**, 81–82
–, research needs on **19**, 131–132
Food Chemical Codex, sodium bisulfite purity definition **30**, 6
Food Code, FDA meat products cooking recommendations **44**, 149
Food hypersensitivities, classification **37**, 26
–, delayed-type **37**, 19–21, 29
–, nonreaginic **37**, 28–29
–, reaginic **37**, 27–28
Food intake, adipose tissue, role of **21**, 25–34
–, bioperiodicity **40**, 220–226
–, gastrointestinal role **21**, 17–24
–, obesity impairment of **21**, 51–53
–, regulation of **21**, 1–69
–, sensory stimulus **21**, 35–43
Food intolerance (*see also* Food allergies *and* Intolerance) **37**, 25–26; **43**, 197, 201
–, anaphylactoid reactions **43**, 201
–, definition **43**, 198
–, idiosyncratic reactions **43**, 201
–, metabolic disorders **43**, 201
Food irradiation (*see also* Irradiation) **15**, 105ff; **24**, 155–227
–, combined with other processes **24**, 187–188
–, disinfestation **24**, 198–200
–, economics of **24**, 205–208
–, equipment for **24**, 166
–, future of **24**, 213–216
–, general effects on, proteins **24**, 169–170
–, general effects on carbohydrates **24**, 173
–, – on foods **24**, 168–169
–, – on lipids **24**, 170–173
–, high-dose applications of **24**, 174–188
–, historical aspects **24**, 155–163

Food irradiation (*cont'd*)
–, in various countries **24**, 158–162
–, laboratory plan for **24**, 165
–, low-dose applications of **24**, 188–205
–, radiation sources for **24**, 163–168
–, radicidation **24**, 197–198
–, radurization **24**, 188–197
–, wholesomeness of foods in **24**, 209–213
Food labeling, color additives **43**, 197
–, inulin/oligofructose **43**, 48–50
Food molecule–water systems, characterization **38**, 120, 124–125
Food poisoning (*see also* Contamination) **39**, 290–292, 337, 346–348
Food polymer science (*see also* Dynamics map *and* Glass transition temperature) **38**, 106–143
–, evolution of approach **38**, 109–114
–, glasses and glass transitions **38**, 107–109
–, –, temperature measurement **38**, 114–118
–, ice-melting onset transition **38**, 164–165
–, plasticization, by water **38**, 150–159
–, –, effect on glass transition temperature **38**, 118, 120–125
–, state diagrams **38**, 135–143
–, structure–property relationships, references **38**, 107
–, thermosetting, amorphous polymers **38**, 212–226
–, water and glass dynamics **38**, 127, 129–135
Food–polymer systems, aqueous, viscoelastic behavior **38**, 183–188
Food polysaccharides, *see* Polysaccharides
Food preference, and age of consumer **32**, 242, 253–254
–, and ethnic origin **32**, 260–263
–, and income **32**, 265–266
–, and metabolic function **32**, 245
–, and race of consumer **32**, 258–260
–, and sex of consumer **32**, 255–258
–, and urbanization **32**, 263–265
–, learned **32**, 243–244
–, regional differences in **32**, 259, 263, 264
–, taste and olfaction **32**, 243
Food preservation, essential oils role **42**, 249
Food preservatives, classes of **1**, 389–391
–, toxicity of **1**, 389–391
Food processing, definition **17**, 153
–, equipment for ozone treatment **45**, 192
–, flavors **21**, 46–51
–, importance of **17**, 154–155
–, pork, normal, PSE, and DFD **21**, 124–128
Food products, for improved world nutrition **22**, 187–203
–, small-molecule emulsifiers in **34**, 108–109
Food protein engineering **36**, 172–187
–, field bean legumin **36**, 184–185
–, french bean phaseolin **36**, 185
–, objectives **36**, 172–173
–, procedures **36**, 173–176
–, rice proteins **36**, 187
–, soybean glycinin **36**, 176–184
–, –, ability to form correct conformation **36**, 181–183
–, –, domain exchange **36**, 179
–, –, functional properties **36**, 183–184
–, –, insertion of synthetic DNA or foreign gene fragments **36**, 180
–, –, methods **36**, 178–181
–, –, modifications and glycinin quality **36**, 178
–, –, oligonucleotide-mediated mutagenesis **36**, 180–181
–, –, region deletion **36**, 179–180
–, –, susceptible regions **36**, 176–177
–, wheat proteins **36**, 186
–, zein **36**, 185–186
Food proteins (*see also* Seed storage proteins), physiological activities **36**, 91
Food quality, *see* Decomposition
Food record **40**, 171
Food science, and World War II **10**, 16
–, as a research field **10**, 2–4
–, definition **17**, 154
–, enzyme chemistry in **10**, 6–8
–, future of **10**, 63, 67
–, history of **10**, 2–16
–, industrial advances since 1948 **10**, 16–19
–, literature of **10**, 1, 4, 5
–, methodology, developments in **10**, 4–5
–, quality, measurement of **10**, 11–12
Food shortage **32**, 187
Food storage **15**, 288
Food systems **13**, 289–311
–, dispersions **13**, 290–291
–, freezing changes **13**, 292–311
–, gross intact tissue **13**, 291–292
Food technology, definition **17**, 153–154
–, intermediate, for developing countries **22**, 199–201
–, modification of milkfat composition **37**, 235–236
Food texture, definition **29**, 162
–, dimensions **29**, 176–179
–, effect on mastication **29**, 171–173
–, – on salivation **29**, 173–175

–, fracturability **29**, 190–194
–, –, auditory cues, not essential for perception **29**, 193–194
–, –, crushing sounds **29**, 192–194
–, –, instrumental measures **29**, 191
–, –, vibratory sensations **29**, 191–192
–, hardness **29**, 185–189
–, –, force–compression functions **29**, 186–188
–, –, instrumental and sensory measures **29**, 187–189
–, oral cavity responses to **29**, 170–175
–, perception (*see also* Oral cavity), complexity of sensations **29**, 159–162
–, –, future research needs **29**, 194–195
–, roughness **29**, 189–190
–, –, non-oral perception **29**, 189–190
–, –, oral perception **29**, 190
–, viscosity **29**, 179–185
–, –, instrumental and sensory values **29**, 184–185
–, –, shear stress–shear rate for samples **29**, 180–185
Food toxicant, *see* Phenol
Forced expiratory volume in 1 second (FEV_1), sulfite-induced asthma and **30**, 48–49, 53, 55–57, 60
Forces, net **14**, 371–375
Forcing function method **40**, 19–21
Foreign bodies, ultrasonic detection **45**, 151
Forestry (*see also* Social forestry) **32**, 186, 194
–, and erosion **32**, 220–221
Formaldehyde, gelatin and **7**, 271
–, inactivation of disulfide enzymes by **1**, 382
–, – of enzymes by **1**, 386, 388–389
–, in curing smoke, toxic effects **29**, 148–149
–, in onion oil **2**, 273
–, *N*-nitroso compounds and **31**, 82–84
–, reaction with amino and amide groups **1**, 383, 386
Formalin, estimation of fish freshness and **7**, 62
Formamide, gelatin manufacture and **7**, 240
Formate, acceleration of trimethylamine oxide reduction in fish by **2**, 369
Formic acid **16**, 185, 216
–, esters of, in carrot seed oil **2**, 271
–, –, in peaches **2**, 265
–, fish spoilage and **7**, 48
–, found in decomposing salmon **2**, 371
–, in apples **2**, 262, 263
–, in coffee **2**, 280
Formononetin **44**, 197, 203, 221
–, sources **44**, 203, 207
Formulations development, rheology **39**, 59–61
Formylation, formyl-tetrahydrofolates **33**, 10
Formyl nitrogen, shoyu color intensity and **30**, 248
5-Formyl-tetrahydrofolate, 6-ambo form, availability **33**, 9
–, –, preparation **33**, 10
–, oxidation **33**, 78
10-Formyl-tetrahydrofolate, oxidation **33**, 46, 78
Formyl-tetrahydrofolates, formylation before/after pteridine reduction **33**, 10
Fortification of foods, folic acid retention **33**, 52
Foscarnet sodium **44**, 300
Fosinopril **44**, 305
Fourier heat conduction equation **20**, 219
–, solutions for **20**, 239–246
Fourier transform infrared (FT-IR) spectroscopy, gluten proteins **45**, 239, 278
Fractal **40**, 327–328
Fractal dimensions **44**, 45
–, box-counting dimension calculation **44**, 86–88
–, determination methods **44**, 85–88
–, fat crystal networks **44**, 84–85, 94–100
–, –, calculation from rheology **44**, 104–106, 108
–, –, crystallization conditions influence **44**, 113–118, 119–120
–, –, density/order of packing relationship **44**, 109–113
–, –, elastic constant influences **44**, 107–109
–, –, physical significance **44**, 107
Fractal geometry **44**, 42–45
–, colloidal aggregates **44**, 45–46
Fractional catabolic rate, β-carotene **40**, 61
–, folate **40**, 88–89, 90
–, population kinetics **40**, 273
–, transthyretin **40**, 152
–, vitamin A **40**, 7, 13
Fractional dimensions **40**, 326–328; **44**, 43–44
Fractional standard deviation **40**, 29, 41
Fractional transfer coefficient **40**, 31, 40–43, 267–268, 312
Fractionation, analysis **31**, 142, 143, 146, 152, 153
–, dietary fiber and **31**, 119, 124, 138
–, of amino acids **2**, 34
–, of bread **2**, 276
–, of cucumbers **2**, 275

Fractionation (*cont'd*)
–, of rare earths by ion exchangers **2**, 33
Fragaria ananssa (strawberry) **44**, 207
Fragility plot **38**, 193
Frameshift mutations **34**, 390
Framingham Study **36**, 263
Frankfurters **39**, 108
–, flavor, nitrite effect **29**, 29–30, 32–33
–, gray color **5**, 18
–, *N*-nitroso compounds and **31**, 80
–, radar cooking of **3**, 139
–, sterilization of casings **3**, 163
–, thermal scanning rheological analysis **35**, 354–355
–, use of polyphosphates to preserve color **5**, 39
FranRica Drum Filler **32**, 13
Free available chlorine, definition of **7**, 143
Free energy of adsorption, air–water interface **34**, 10
– of formation, emulsions **34**, 87
Free fatty acid **39**, 203, 205–206, 208
Free polymer effect, emulsion stability **34**, 95
Free radicals, carcinogen risk assessment and **31**, 24
–, in biological systems **10**, 8–9
–, in browning reaction **32**, 123–127
–, *N*-nitroso compounds and **31**, 78
–, olive oil and **31**, 471, 472
Free water in muscle protein **10**, 360–362, 363, 364
Freeze concentration, aroma recovery in **20**, 39–45
–, cost of **20**, 91
Freeze-drying **13**, 1–88; **15**, 290; **39**, 144, 146
–, advantages of **7**, 173, 207
–, applications **13**, 73–80
–, –, biological aspects **13**, 73–75
–, –, organoleptic aspects **13**, 76–80
–, aroma retention in **20**, 75–85
–, contact **13**, 19–20
–, cost of **20**, 96
–, effects on meat flavor **18**, 19–20
–, equipment **13**, 47–73, 81–82
–, –, commercial **7**, 186–187
–, –, laboratory **7**, 185–186
–, for scanning electron microscopy **22**, 233–237
–, fundamentals **13**, 3–46
–, –, end-point determination **13**, 43–46
–, –, heat-transfer **13**, 11–32
–, –, mass-transfer **13**, 32–43
–, –, mechanism **13**, 9–11
–, –, theories **13**, 3–9
–, heat-transfer and **7**, 198
–, *N*-nitroso compounds and **31**, 78
–, research needs **7**, 231–232; **13**, 80–82
–, stages of **7**, 189
–, temperature working zone for **27**, 331
–, vacuum **13**, 67–70
Freeze-etching, for scanning electron microscopy **22**, 233–237
Freezing (*see also* Proteins in foods), abalone **23**, 168–170
–, beefsteak **13**, 267
–, changes caused **13**, 292–311
–, chick embryo **13**, 266–267
–, commercial processes **13**, 317–329
–, –, air blast **13**, 318
–, –, food selection **13**, 319
–, –, immersion **13**, 318–319
–, –, indirect contact **13**, 318
–, –, prefreezing treatments **13**, 320–322
–, –, rate, quality **13**, 322
–, –, storage **13**, 323–327
–, –, thawing **13**, 327–329
–, concentration, nonaqueous constituents **13**, 270–271
–, effects on meat emulsions **16**, 135
–, – on meat flavor **18**, 14–16
–, – on protein extraction **16**, 122
–, enhanced coalescence **34**, 143, 145
–, evaporative **7**, 175–176
–, foods **15**, 240, 343
–, –, heat transfer of **20**, 217–256
–, –, time estimation of **20**, 235–251
–, fruits **17**, 185–188
–, future research on **10**, 64
–, gels, artifacts and **34**, 282
–, IM meat **39**, 93
–, meat **35**, 339
–, –, hydration of, effects on **10**, 372, 403–408
–, –, SH groups in **24**, 73–76
–, methods **7**, 175–176
–, phenomena **13**, 3–9
–, –, eutectic temperature **13**, 7–9
–, –, rate **13**, 4–7
–, proteins **35**, 336
–, rates **7**, 175; **13**, 274–287
–, –, determining **13**, 275–278
–, –, factors affecting **13**, 278–283
–, –, normally rigid aqueous materials **13**, 283–287
–, simple solutions **13**, 259–261
–, slow **13**, 263, 265
–, volume changes **13**, 272–274

–, water **13**, 259–261
Freezing point, depression, oligosaccharide formation and **38**, 30
French bean phaseolin, expression in micro-organisms **36**, 161–162
–, food protein engineering **36**, 185
French buckwheat products **44**, 415
Freon, solubility of DDT in **2**, 204
–, toxicity to man of DDT solution **2**, 212
Frequency, of microwaves **15**, 287, 292
Frequency domain spectroscopy, dielectric properties measurement **43**, 82
Fresh acid-curd cheese **39**, 178–193
Fresh food, preservation of **7**, 117
Freshness indicator, seafood **39**, 348–351
Fresh water fish farming **20**, 205
Freundlich's isotherm **20**, 36
Frictional coefficient **34**, 29
Friction factor, in determining pumping requirements **11**, 409
–, vs. generalized Reynolds number **11**, 410, 414
Friction-factor factor, as a function of porosity and sphericity **11**, 430
Friction smoke, steam-volatile and -nonvolatile fractions **29**, 107–108
Fried bacon, *N*-nitroso compounds and, *see* Bacon
Fried instant noodles (*see also* Oriental noodles) **43**, 148, 155, 160, 162, 170
–, quality evaluation **43**, 178, 179
Fringed micelle model, crystalline–amorphous structure of partially crystalline polymers **38**, 129, 133
Frisse conche, chocolate and **31**, 301–303
Fromage frais **39**, 178, 179
Frost, effects on fruit composition **9**, 301–302
–, – on plant **25**, 208–209
–, kiwifruit damage **29**, 283
Frost damage, prevention of by infrared radiation **3**, 146
Frozen fish, ascorbic acid in prevention of rancidity of **18**, 257–261
Frozen foods **15**, 289
–, cold storage of **20**, 116–117
–, cooking of **6**, 210
–, defrosting of **6**, 204
–, firmness of **2**, 335–336
–, firmness of thawed **2**, 338
–, hygienic aspects of **6**, 210
–, ice crystal formation in **2**, 337
–, microbiological methods of analysis **6**, 173
–, occurrence of bacteria in **6**, 172
–, packaging problems **6**, 209
–, pathogenic bacteria in **6**, 201
–, precooked, bacteria in **6**, 169, 198
–, preservation of **7**, 120
Frozen foods industry, use of quaternary ammonium compounds in **2**, 181
Frozen fruit, browning protection by ascorbic acid **18**, 250–252
Frozen fruits and vegetables, processing of **25**, 181–235
Frozen storage, effect on folate in human milk **33**, 51
Fructan–fructan fructosyl transferase **43**, 3, 5
Fructans **41**, 5; **43**, 3
β-Fructofuranisidase **43**, 6
Fructoglycine **14**, 189
Fructooligosaccharides (*see also* Oligofructose) **43**, 2, 6
–, dental health effects **43**, 43
–, intestinal microflora response **43**, 16, 18
–, lipid metabolism effects **43**, 29
–, mineral absorption effects **43**, 32
Fructosamines **12**, 5, 7, 11–13
–, absence of carbonyl absorption **12**, 11–13
–, crystalline **12**, 7
Fructose **14**, 221–222
–, acceleration of trimethylamine oxide reduction by **2**, 369
–, anhydrides **6**, 17
–, chocolate and **31**, 265, 266, 269
–, –, cocoa bean chemistry **31**, 232
–, –, milk crumb **31**, 286
–, –, refining **31**, 295
–, content of apples and pears **8**, 300, 313
–, crystallization by ion exchange **2**, 30
–, effect in dried egg **1**, 172
–, – in potato powder during storage **1**, 289–270
–, effect on calcium absorption **33**, 127
–, in cocoa beans, fermentation and **30**, 94
–, increase, in apples during storage **8**, 318
–, in fresh cocoa bean juice **8**, 239
–, in raw cocoa bean **8**, 262
–, in spoiled table wines **6**, 76
–, in table wines **6**, 72
–, loss in dehydrated potatoes **1**, 274
–, Maillard reaction of **32**, 168
–, olive oil and **31**, 459
–, reaction with amino acids **3**, 249
–, roasting and **30**, 97
–, structure and simpler reactions of **6**, 4
–, utilization by spoilage bacteria in wine **6**, 91
Fructoseglycine **12**, 28

Fructosylamine, Heyns rearrangement **30**, 87–88
–, product of fructose reaction with amine **30**, 87
Fruit beverages, alginates in **11**, 152
–, preparation of **17**, 172–173
–, –, juice **17**, 190–194
–, –, pulp **17**, 191–194
Fruit fiber, effect on calcium bioavailability **33**, 139–141
Fruit-fly control **12**, 210
Fruitiness, cheese **39**, 241
Fruit juices **5**, 127
–, ascorbic-acid addition to **18**, 223–226, 253–254
–, ascorbic-acid content **4**, 373
–, for candies **6**, 28
–, freeze-drying of **7**, 204, 225–228
–, in American dietary **4**, 371–372
–, Love wave-based component analysis **45**, 153
–, microbial inactivation **44**, 12–15
–, ozone treatment of ingredients **45**, 196–197
–, phase transition temperature of **27**, 339
–, preservation with carbon dioxide **3**, 444
–, puff-drying of **7**, 204
–, pulsed electric field (PEF) processing **44**, 26
–, quality impact **44**, 16–21
–, –, color changes **44**, 17
–, –, flavor **44**, 16–17
–, –, nutritional aspects **44**, 17
–, –, shelf-life **44**, 15–16
–, sulfiting **5**, 134
–, use of ascorbic acid in **4**, 371–381
–, viscosity **39**, 45–46
Fruit products, carrageenan in **11**, 137
–, frozen, use of ascorbic acid in prevention of discoloration in **3**, 31
–, used by the candy industry **6**, 3
Fruit pulps, brined **5**, 98
–, desulfiting **5**, 127
–, sulfiting **5**, 136
Fruit ripening, physiology of mango **21**, 249–270
Fruit ripening retardation, polysaccharide–lipid edible films **44**, 370
Fruits (*see also individual names*), acid content of **17**, 177
–, acidity of **10**, 301–304
–, analysis **31**, 146–148, 150, 152
–, aroma of **17**, 174–179
–, ascorbic acid prevention of browning **18**, 249–255
–, – of –, canned fruit **18**, 254–255
–, – of –, frozen fruit **18**, 250–253
–, – of –, fruit juices **18**, 253–254
–, astringency **13**, 195–209
–, atmospheric conditions in storage of **3**, 467–470
–, boundary temperatures for freeze-drying **27**, 335
–, brined **5**, 98
–, *Byssochlamys* spp. in **25**, 237–288
–, canned, use of ascorbic acid in **4**, 368
–, carbohydrates in **17**, 182–183
–, carbon dioxide in transport and storage **12**, 95–146
–, chemical preservation of **3**, 458–463
–, chemical properties of **17**, 174–185
–, chlorine treatment **45**, 188
–, classification of **17**, 158
–, climacteric **15**, 107
–, color of **17**, 174–179
–, culture of **15**, 122
–, definition **17**, 157
–, dehydrated products of **17**, 194–195
–, development, degradative and synthetic changes **30**, 170
–, –, enlargement, cell expansion **30**, 168–169
–, –, maturation **30**, 169
–, –, ripening, climacteric **30**, 169
–, –, –, nonclimacteric **30**, 169
–, –, senescence **30**, 170
–, –, set, cell multiplication **30**, 168
–, dicotyledonous plants **31**, 127, 130
–, dietary fiber and **31**, 119, 120, 139, 191
–, differential thermograms for **27**, 334
–, dried, enzymic changes in **11**, 289
–, –, protection of by packing **3**, 457
–, –, sterilization of **3**, 466
–, effect of climate **15**, 122
–, – of injury on discoloration of **3**, 3, 4
–, – of ozone **15**, 135
–, ethylene production in **15**, 109
–, exocarp, composition of **10**, 304–307
–, flavor, classification of **17**, 174–179, 180
–, flexible packaging for **23**, 326
–, freeze-drying of **7**, 204, 223–224
–, frozen **25**, 181–235
–, –, freezing effects on **25**, 214–218
–, –, ice formation in **25**, 183–193
–, –, problems in **25**, 229–230
–, –, steps prior to freezing **25**, 219–221
–, –, storage changes in **25**, 227–228
–, –, treatment for micro-organisms in **3**, 449–450

–, fungicidal wrappings for **3**, 463–466
–, high-protein **10**, 301–302
–, in candies **6**, 29, 45, 48
–, –, dehydration of **6**, 367
–, –, dried, used by confectionery industry **6**, 48
–, –, frozen **6**, 169, 174, 177
–, –, micro-organisms on **6**, 179
–, –, thawing of frozen **6**, 206
–, –, thiamine loss in **6**, 296
–, injury of **15**, 110, 116
–, inositol phosphates **45**, 22–23
–, intestinal bacteria **31**, 176, 180, 182, 187, 189
–, irradiated **15**, 57ff, 105ff, 147ff, 173; **24**, 183
–, jellies **8**, 33
–, juices, *see* Fruit juices
–, measuring tenderness of **8**, 17
–, metabolism during ripening, ethylene production **30**, 171–172
–, –, glycolysis **30**, 172–173
–, –, mitochondrial activity **30**, 173–174
–, –, phosphorylation **30**, 173
–, –, protein synthesis **30**, 176
–, –, starch hydrolysis **30**, 172
–, morphology of **17**, 163–165
–, nonclimacteric **15**, 114
–, nutrients **17**, 159
–, oxidative systems **17**, 1–76
–, ozone treatment **45**, 190, 191, 192, 194–195
–, particulate, processing of **32**, 30–32
–, passion fruit **12**, 203–282
–, –, agri-horticultural aspects **12**, 207–209
–, –, mycological and entomological aspects **12**, 209–210
–, –, physiology and storage **12**, 211–233
–, –, pulp, juice, and related products **12**, 234–258
–, –, research needs **12**, 271–273
–, –, taxonomic aspects **12**, 205
–, pathogens **15**, 135
–, pectin degradation with, α-L-arabinosidase **30**, 178
–, –, endopolygalacturonase **30**, 176–177
–, –, exopolygalacturonase **30**, 177
–, –, β-galactosidase **30**, 177–178
–, –, hemicellulase **30**, 178
–, –, pectinmethylesterase **30**, 175
–, peeling of **17**, 188–190
–, pesticide residues reduction **45**, 199
–, pH **3**, 432; **17**, 178
–, physical properties of **17**, 165–172
–, post-harvest chemical changes **10**, 308–315
–, precooling of, evaporators in **20**, 136–137
–, –, facilities for **20**, 118–119
–, –, specialized designs for **20**, 125–128
–, prefreezing **13**, 320–321
–, preservation of **17**, 185–188
–, –, at low temperatures **3**, 446–450
–, processing wastes **17**, 88–96
–, properties **31**, 155, 165, 170
–, quality of **16**, 203ff
–, radurization of **24**, 194–196
–, respiration **15**, 107; **17**, 186–187
–, ripeness **15**, 108, 131
–, sanitary handling of **3**, 470–471
–, selenium in **32**, 95
–, significance of **17**, 157–163
–, sterilization of by heat **3**, 433–443
–, sulfur dioxide absorption **5**, 89
–, supercooling **27**, 307–315
–, –, cryoscopic temperature of **27**, 310–315
–, survival of *Salmonella* in **3**, 219, 220
–, technology, tropical **17**, 155–156
–, texture (rheological properties), ultrasonic sensing **45**, 142
–, transport by ship **12**, 179–184
–, tropical, classification **17**, 162–163
–, washing water-related disease outbreaks **45**, 169, 194
–, wastes **17**, 104–106
–, xylitol, occurrence in **28**, 376–377
Fruit spread cookers **15**, 342
FSD, *see* Fractional standard deviation
FTC, *see* Fractional transfer coefficient
Fudge, chemical composition and properties of **6**, 10
–, drying **6**, 7
–, improved by sorbitol **6**, 11
–, ingredients in **6**, 29
–, stability of fats in **6**, 13
Fuel alcohol, from corn wet milling **38**, 295
Fuel oil, solubility of DDT in **2**, 203, 204
Fuelwood **32**, 186, 189, 191, 194, 195, 196, 204–206
–, toxic products of **32**, 223–224
Fulvine **45**, 71, 74
Fumarate esters, antibotulinal activity in cured meat **29**, 52
Functional groups, modification, protein stability **35**, 269–274
Functionality **34**, 300
Function-linked binding analysis **34**, 347
Function-linked multivalent cation binding **34**, 354–357

Fungi (*see also* Micro-organisms) **15**, 149, 289
–, as sources of protein **18**, 116
–, chocolate and **31**, 218, 219, 328
–, endogenous proteolytic enzymes and **31**, 362
–, from fermenting cocoa beans **8**, 231, 288
–, germination **15**, 150
–, irradiation **15**, 153
–, mutations **15**, 158
Fungicidal gases for treatment of stored fruit **3**, 465–466
Fungicidal wrappings for fruits and vegetables **3**, 463–466
Fungiform papillae **44**, 251
Furanone **32**, 137–138
Furan ring compounds, contribution to meat flavor **18**, 55–56
Furcellaran, general properties **11**, 157
–, in flan jelly **11**, 159
–, in icing **11**, 159
–, in jam **11**, 160
–, in marmalade **11**, 160
–, in milk products **11**, 159
–, in miscellaneous foods **11**, 160
–, in piping jelly **11**, 160
–, in Tortenguss **11**, 160
–, in water-based foods **11**, 159–161
–, viscosity **11**, 118
Furfural **12**, 36, 42, 407; **14**, 184, 186, 227; **32**, 135–138, 141, 142, 143, 164
–, formation **12**, 36
–, in brown pigment **12**, 42
Furfural alcohol, in coffee **2**, 281
–, in peaches **2**, 265
Furfuraldehyde, formation during browning **1**, 357–359
–, in bread **2**, 276
–, in coffee **2**, 280, 282
–, in crab apples **2**, 263
Furfuraldehyde in nonenzymic browning **3**, 180–184
Furfuryl acetate in coffee **2**, 282
Furfuryl alcohol in coffee **2**, 280, 282
Furfuryl esters, preparation of **2**, 36
l-Furfurylpyrrole in coffee **2**, 281
Furyl ketone in coffee **2**, 281
Furyl mercaptans in coffee **2**, 281
Fusarium **12**, 110; **15**, 180
Fusarium mycotoxins **44**, 196
Fusicladium dendriticum, resistance of to cold **3**, 468
Fusion, in flexible-packaging sealing **23**, 348–349
G-actin, endogenous proteolytic enzymes and **31**, 398
G-protein, involvement in mediation of cellular cAMP formation **42**, 220
G_α-subunit, GTPase activity **42**, 230–231
"G"-value **15**, 59
Gabo near isogenic line **45**, 252
–, dough properties **45**, 260, 261
–, transgenic HMW glutenin subunit studies **45**, 263–264
Gadodiamide **44**, 316
Galactans, dietary fiber and **31**, 130, 131, 146
Galactobiose, in yogurts **38**, 84
Galactoglycerides, unsaturated acids of **17**, 33
Galactolipids, in wheat germ **23**, 223
Galactomannans, dietary fiber and **31**, 135, 155, 181
–, molecular shapes and interactions **42**, 155–156
Galactose, chocolate and **31**, 263, 272
–, concentration changes and allolactose production **38**, 83
–, dietary fiber and **31**, 123, 148, 176
–, –, dicotyledonous plants **31**, 126, 132, 135
–, effect on lactase activity during milk processing **38**, 12
–, endogenous proteolytic enzymes and **31**, 403
–, enzymatic modification **38**, 10
–, gelatin and **7**, 271
–, in pears **8**, 313
–, in pectins **1**, 397–399; **11**, 75
–, in raw cocoa **8**, 262
–, olive oil and **31**, 459
β-Galactosidase (*see also* Lactase), catalysis of lactose hydrolysis **38**, 24–25
–, from *Bifidobacterium bifidium* **38**, 85
–, hydrolysis **38**, 23–24
–, in ripening fruits, multiple forms **30**, 177–178
–, patents using, for production of galactooligosaccharides **38**, 87
–, purified **38**, 23
–, specificity for lactose portions **38**, 63
β-Galactosidase-deficient subjects, calcium absorption **36**, 216–217
Galactosyl, enzymatic transfer reactions **38**, 60
Galactosyl isomaltol **14**, 182–183
Galacturonic acid **16**, 216
–, dietary fiber and **31**, 126, 130, 137
–, effect on browning in fruit products **1**, 367

–, in pectins **11**, 74
–, –, presence proved **1**, 397
–, intestinal bacteria **31**, 175, 186, 187
–, properties **31**, 164, 166
Galahad near isogenic line **45**, 252
–, γ-gliadins **45**, 222
Gallate, alkyl **5**, 271
–, esters **5**, 271
Gallic acid, animal consumption of **27**, 170–172
–, in tea **2**, 285
l-Gallocatechin gallate, quantity in tea **2**, 284, 285
Gallocatechins, in tea **2**, 285
–, –, oxidation of **11**, 235–236
Galloryl ester in tea **2**, 285
Gallstones, prevalence in men on low-cholesterol diets **37**, 225
Gamma radiation (*see also* X-rays) **14**, 111–112; **15**, 71, 110, 241
–, sterilization by **32**, 21
Gantrez AN **12**, 346–449
–, applications **12**, 348–349
–, –, cosmetics **12**, 349
–, –, pharmaceuticals **12**, 349
–, background **12**, 347–348
–, properties **12**, 347–348
–, –, compatibility **12**, 348
–, –, films **12**, 348
–, –, solubility **12**, 347
–, –, toxicology **12**, 348
–, –, viscosity **12**, 347–348
Garbanzo beans, *see* Chickpeas
Garden cress, *see* Peppergrass
Garlic (*see also Allium*), constituents of oil of **2**, 272
–, dehydrated **6**, 315
–, flavor and odor development in **22**, 73–133
–, inulin **43**, 9
–, ozone treatment **45**, 198
–, volatile organic sulfur compounds **5**, 120
Garnet, volume per oxygen atom in **2**, 3
Gas, equilibria in milk powder **3**, 60–63
–, techniques for measurement of in dry milk **3**, 60–61
Gas chromatography, chocolate and **31**, 319, 320
–, dietary fiber and **31**, 119
–, in studies of meat flavor **18**, 26
–, IRMS **40**, 66–70, 71, 73–74, 177
–, *N*-nitroso compounds and **31**, 66–68
–, olive oil and **31**, 469, 470, 474
–, use in flavor chemistry **9**, 2, 211
Gas chromatography–mass spectrometry, folate bioavailability measurement **33**, 61–62
–, phytoestrogens **44**, 201
Gases, flow through dried meat **7**, 194–195
–, residual, in flexibly packaged foods **23**, 376–380
Gas–liquid chromatography, of histamine **24**, 133
Gas stripping process, of food drying, aroma recovery in **20**, 31–32
Gastric cancer **40**, 57
Gastrointestinal delay **40**, 36–37
Gastrointestinal health, inulin effects **43**, 42–43
Gastrointestinal tract, anatomy **37**, 2–4
–, immune response, modification, by breast-feeding **37**, 45
–, –, –, food antigens/allergens **37**, 46
–, –, –, hypoallergenic foods **37**, 47
–, –, –, microbial flora control **37**, 50
–, –, –, nutritional therapies **37**, 51–52
–, –, –, oral tolerance induction **37**, 50–51
–, –, nutrition effects **37**, 44–45
–, –, research needs **37**, 53–56
–, immune system diseases, autoimmunity **37**, 32–33
–, –, food hypersensitivity **37**, 25–26
–, –, food intolerance **37**, 25–26
–, –, food-sensitive enteropathies **37**, 29–31
–, –, immune complex-related **37**, 32–33
–, –, inflammatory bowel disease **37**, 31–32
–, –, intestinal cancer **37**, 24–25
–, –, microbial infections **37**, 23–24
–, –, nonreaginic hypersensitivities **37**, 28–29
–, –, reaginic hypersensitivities **37**, 27–28
–, immunosuppression **37**, 33–34
–, microbial ecology **37**, 71–72
–, nonspecific immune mechanisms **37**, 4–6
–, role of bacterial agents **37**, 35–37
–, – of foodborne chemicals **37**, 41–43
–, – of parasitic agents **37**, 39
–, – of viral agents **37**, 38
–, specific immune response **37**, 6–8
–, –, antigen uptake **37**, 12–15
–, –, cell-mediated responses **37**, 19–21
–, –, common mucosal immune system **37**, 21
–, –, gut-associated lymphoid tissue **37**, 10–12
–, –, humoral responses **37**, 15–19
–, –, immunocompetent cells **37**, 8–10
–, –, nonspecific mechanisms **37**, 4–6
–, –, oral tolerance **37**, 22
–, –, phases **37**, 7

Gastrointestinal tract, specific immune response (*cont'd*)
–, –, stimulation of specific immunity **37**, 21–22
GBSS, *see* Granule-bound starch synthase
GC, *see* Chromatography
GC-C-IRMS, *see* Gas chromatography, IRMS
Gear pump, for thermoprocessed food filling **23**, 366–367
Gelatin **10**, 59; **43**, 298–299, 303, 305
–, acid–base behavior of **7**, 272–279
–, amino acid composition of **7**, 261–265
–, amino acid sequence of **7**, 265–270
–, applications, food **7**, 322–326
–, –, pharmaceutical **7**, 326–327
–, –, photographic **7**, 327–328
–, –, specialized **7**, 328
–, as cryostabilizer **35**, 347
–, binding agent in lozenge paste **6**, 29
–, color and clarity of **7**, 246–249
–, degradation of **7**, 309–322
–, denaturation of **7**, 321–322
–, effect of drying on bulk density of **2**, 423, 473, 476
–, elasticity, swelling and **7**, 298
–, freeze-dried orange juice and **7**, 228
–, gels, properties of **8**, 33
–, gel–sol transition, functionality and **7**, 306–307
–, –, gelation mechanism **7**, 306–309
–, –, light scattering **7**, 304–306
–, –, melting point **7**, 300–304
–, –, optical rotation **7**, 306
–, gel state, films **7**, 299–300
–, –, light scattering **7**, 297–298
–, –, rigidity of **7**, 290–297
–, –, stress relaxation **7**, 297
–, –, swelling and **7**, 298–299
–, homogeneity of **7**, 279–280
–, in abalone **23**, 175, 179
–, in production of marshmallows **6**, 24
–, ionic groups of **7**, 263, 272–273
–, isoelectric point of **7**, 273–274
–, isoionic point of **7**, 274
–, manufacture, acid processing and **7**, 242
–, –, extraction process and **7**, 242–244
–, –, filtration and drying **7**, 244–246
–, –, liming and **7**, 238–242
–, –, ossein and **7**, 242
–, –, raw materials of **7**, 238
–, –, testing and **7**, 249–250
–, modification of sugar properties produced by **6**, 53
–, molecular weight **7**, 265
–, –, chemical methods for **7**, 282–285
–, –, gel and **7**, 295
–, –, miscellaneous methods for **7**, 285–287
–, –, physical methods for **7**, 280–282
–, properties of **7**, 236–237
–, protective action on thiamine **6**, 261
–, sol state **7**, 279–290
–, –, rheology of **7**, 289–290
–, –, shape and configuration in **7**, 287–289
–, source of **7**, 236
–, sugars in **7**, 270–272
–, *N*-terminal residues of **7**, 264–265, 314–315, 320
–, titration curves of **7**, 274–279
–, types of **7**, 246
–, X-ray diagrams of **7**, 299–300
Gelatin components, of, from collagen **20**, 288
Gelatin–egg white gels **34**, 274–281
–, network inversion **34**, 278–279
–, network structure **34**, 275–277
–, phase inversion **34**, 274, 276
–, polymer–solvent interaction parameters **34**, 280
–, shear modulus **34**, 278, 280
Gelatin gels, critical concentration **34**, 224, 226
–, heat of formation, junction zones **34**, 227–228
–, pH and shear modulus **34**, 230–231
–, preaging **34**, 227
–, rheology **34**, 224, 226–231
–, rigidity development kinetics **34**, 226–227
–, rubber elasticity **34**, 228–229
–, shear modulus, dependence on gelation concentration **34**, 229–230
–, temperature and mechanical properties **34**, 227
Gelatinization **41**, 165–168
–, dietary fiber and analysis **31**, 142–144
–, in breadmaking **16**, 386
–, properties **31**, 154, 155, 159, 169, 170
–, sugar role **38**, 158
Gelatin–lipid films **44**, 372–373
Gelation, cheese **39**, 173–174, 182–188, 191–193
–, collagen triple helix **34**, 219
–, cooling **34**, 224
–, curing reaction and **38**, 214
–, definition **34**, 204–205, 218–219
–, factors affecting gel composition and properties **33**, 385–389
–, fiber network **34**, 221–222

–, forces in gel formation and stabilization, table **33**, 384
–, forces involved **34**, 207–212
–, gel formation **34**, 220–222
–, gel structure **33**, 383–384
–, IM meat **39**, 108, 150
–, in proteins **10**, 28, 42–43, 53
–, junction zones **34**, 221, 224–225
–, β-lactoglobulin **34**, 244
–, load as function of concentration **34**, 117–118
–, mechanism, actomyosin **34**, 253–254
–, –, egg albumen **34**, 258
–, –, myosin **34**, 250–251
–, –, ovalbumin **34**, 255–256
–, –, plasma proteins **34**, 260
–, –, salt-soluble proteins **34**, 254
–, –, serum albumin **34**, 259–260
–, milk **39**, 165
–, origin **34**, 219–220
–, quarter-staggered fibers **34**, 220
–, renaturation **34**, 223–225
–, rheology **39**, 41–43, 60–61
–, rigidity factor **34**, 222
–, seed storage proteins **36**, 126, 128–131
–, sorption **39**, 99
–, temperature effects on gel **34**, 223–224
–, thermally irreversible gels **34**, 241–242
–, ultrasonic analysis **45**, 152
–, versus precipitation **39**, 183–184
–, whey proteins **33**, 381–385
Gel electrophoresis **39**, 242–243
Gel filtration chromatography, β-lactoglobulin binding of *p*-nitrophenyl phosphate **33**, 409
–, separation of polyglutamyl folates **33**, 33
–, whey protein preparation **33**, 361
Gelling applications, whey proteins in **33**, 389–391
Gel point **38**, 214
Gels, additional research needs **34**, 285–286
–, classification **34**, 205–207
–, complex **34**, 263
–, composite or multicomponent **34**, 262–263
–, critical opalescence **34**, 209
–, definition **34**, 204–205
–, equilibrium elastic shear modulus **34**, 217
–, extent of hydration **34**, 208–209
–, filled **34**, 263
–, final pH **6**, 26
–, formation, denaturation and **34**, 211
–, –, gelation **34**, 220–222
–, –, soy proteins **34**, 232–236
–, ion pressure **34**, 208
–, isoelectric **34**, 222
–, measurement of **7**, 249
–, microstructure **34**, 209, 211
–, –, artifact potential **34**, 281–284
–, –, critical point drying **34**, 282–284
–, –, environmental SEM **34**, 284
–, –, innovative approaches and future **34**, 284–285
–, –, modified oil-emulsion freezing **34**, 282–283
–, –, preparation technique effects **34**, 281–282
–, –, ultrasound imaging **34**, 284
–, nucleated filament model **34**, 206
–, physical integrity **34**, 207
–, pore size distribution **34**, 211–212, 283
–, properties of **6**, 35
–, protein–protein interactions **34**, 208
–, protein–solvent interactions **34**, 208
–, random aggregation model **34**, 206
–, rheology, classes of methods **34**, 213
–, –, equation **34**, 212–216
–, –, gel point **34**, 214–215
–, –, large deformation and failure properties **34**, 217–218
–, –, ratio of stress to strain **34**, 214
–, –, rubber elasticity **34**, 217
–, –, strength **34**, 215–216
–, –, stress wave **34**, 214
–, –, viscoelasticity **34**, 212–214
–, rubber elasticity **34**, 217
–, rubberlike elasticity **34**, 207–208
–, strength **34**, 213, 215–216
–, –, liming and **7**, 239
–, –, whey proteins (*see also* Whey protein concentrates and isolates) **34**, 247
–, temperature effects **34**, 223–224
–, thermally irreversible, *see* Thermally irreversible gels
–, transitions between transparency and opacity **34**, 209
Gemfibrozil **44**, 288
Gempylid poisoning **18**, 155
Gene disruption **41**, 10
Gene interference, microbial inhibition by **1**, 375–376
Gene mapping, for muscle diseases and disorders **37**, 409
Gene mutation, dystrophin gene **37**, 355–356
Generalized Reynolds number, in determining pumping requirements **11**, 409
Generally Regarded as Safe requirement, carcinogen risk assessment and **31**, 12
Generators, microwave **13**, 63
Genes, cloning, *see* Seed storage proteins

Genes (*cont'd*)
–, dystrophin **37**, 353–357
–, foreign fragments, insertion in soybean glycinin **36**, 180
–, manipulation, properties and uses of enzymes used in **36**, 136–137
–, Steinert's disease **37**, 361
Genetic diseases, in connective tissue **37**, 389–401
Genetic engineering **41**, 125–126
–, wheat proteins **36**, 75–76
Genetic factors, in response to dietary fat **37**, 192–194
Genetic factors in fruit composition **9**, 292
Genetics, effect of radiation on **15**, 152
–, plasma lipoprotein levels and **36**, 328–331
Genetic transfection **40**, 95, 96–101, 105
Gene transfer, pAMβ1 from *Lactobacillus reuteri* to *Enterococcus faecalis in vivo* **37**, 114–115
Genistein **44**, 197
–, anticancer activity **44**, 232
–, antioxidant activity **44**, 225
–, assay methods **44**, 201, 202
–, cancer treatment **44**, 230
–, effects of processing **44**, 214
–, estrogen receptor interactions **44**, 222, 223
–, *in vitro* effects **44**, 223
–, pharmacokinetics **44**, 218, 219, 220
–, sources **44**, 203, 205
–, toxicity **44**, 226
Genistin **44**, 218
Genotoxicity, pyrolysis products **34**, 393, 399
GenPept database **42**, 66
Gentiobioside, in wheat germ **23**, 241
Geometry, rheological instrumentation **39**, 23–33
Geotrichum candidum **15**, 177
Geraniol, in apples **2**, 263
–, in cherries **2**, 264
–, in oranges **2**, 264
–, in tea **2**, 286, 287, 288
Geranyl-geranyl-pyrophosphate **15**, 205
Germanium oxide, meat mutagen modulation **34**, 433
Germ breads, preparation and nutritive value of **23**, 282–284
Germicidals, cationic and anionic agents as **2**, 132
–, factors affecting activity of **2**, 133–137
–, requirements for **2**, 129
–, structure of quaternary ammonium compounds **2**, 127–128
Germicidal tests for quaternary ammonium compounds **2**, 157–158
Germine monoacetate **44**, 316
Gerstmann–Straussler–Scheinker syndrome **43**, 284–285, 287
Gherkins, pH value of **3**, 432
Gibberellic acid, chocolate and **31**, 327
Gibbs adsorption equation **34**, 102
Gibbs free energy, protein stability **35**, 242
–, unfolding, wild-type and mutants of tryptophan synthase α-subunit **35**, 262–264
GI delay, *see* Gastrointestinal delay
Gidley endotherm **38**, 172
Glaced products, desulfiting **5**, 127
Glandless cottonseed flour, defatted, meat mutagen modulation **34**, 432
Glass dynamics **38**, 133–135, 160
Glass-forming liquids, behavior classification **38**, 192–195
–, super-structuring effects **38**, 197–198
Glass-slide method of testing germicidal action of quaternary ammonium compounds **2**, 162
Glass thermometers, microwave temperature measurements **43**, 83–84
Glass transition **38**, 107–109; **39**, 117–118, 134–135, 150
–, definition **38**, 108
–, ice-melting onset transition **38**, 164–165
–, recent publication **38**, 111–113
–, research needs **38**, 226–233
–, studies using methods other than DSC or DMA **38**, 115, 119–120
–, texture of cereal and **38**, 185
Glass transition temperature, as function of, log degree of polymerization **38**, 138, 144
–, –, moisture, hand-washed and lyophilized wheat gluten **38**, 153–154
–, diluent–monomer blend **38**, 175–176
–, effects of water as plasticizer **38**, 151–159
–, gluten, moisture effect **38**, 219
–, low-molecular-weight carbohydrates **38**, 148–149
–, measurement, in foods **38**, 114–118
–, –, methods **38**, 227–228
–, molecular weight effect **38**, 138, 144–150
–, –, maltooligosaccharides **38**, 144, 147
–, plasticization effect **38**, 118, 120–125
–, polymer–polymer and polymer–plasticizer blends **38**, 145–150
–, relaxation phenomena **38**, 195–196
–, solute-specific subzero **38**, 136–137, 139–143, 161, 163–166

–, –, as function of dextrose equivalent **38**, 144–145
–, –, – of molecular weight, maltooligosaccharides **38**, 144, 146
–, –, low-molecular-weight carbohydrates **38**, 139–143
–, temperature–composition domain above **38**, 207–208
–, temperature location, determined by free volume **38**, 198
–, temperature–time conditions of measurement **38**, 227
Glassy state, recent publication **38**, 111–113
Glauconite, volume per oxygen atom in **2**, 3
Glengarry spray dryer, operation of **2**, 435–437
Glenodinine, structure and pharmacology of **18**, 158
glg C gene **41**, 132–13434
α-Gliadin, expression in micro-organisms **36**, 162
γ-Gliadin **36**, 133
–, expression in micro-organisms **36**, 162–163
ω-Gliadin **36**, 132–133
Gliadins **16**, 347, 353, 376; **38**, 216; **45**, 221
–, amino acid composition **36**, 17–19
–, dough viscoelasticity gluten fractionation/reconstitution experiments **45**, 242, 243, 245
–, electrophoretic separation **45**, 222, 223
–, in wheat flours, breadmaking and **29**, 248, 251
–, –, composition, effect on baking quality **29**, 268
–, –, dough properties and **29**, 242–246
–, local intermolecular disulfide crosslinking **38**, 217, 222
–, protein fraction incorporation studies **45**, 245–246
–, structural studies **45**, 278
–, structure **36**, 38
–, thermolabile disulfide bonds **38**, 225
–, wheat proteins **36**, 27–29
–, –, genetic control **36**, 36
Glipizide **44**, 307
Global identifiability **40**, 313
Globe artichoke, inulin **43**, 9
Globoid, composition from cottonseed **28**, 9
Globular proteins, denaturation **34**, 211
–, viscous films **34**, 125
7S Globulin genes, CACA box sequences and positions **36**, 10909
–, compared to 11S globulins **36**, 122–12323
–, construction **36**, 10606
–, structure **36**, 104–10909
11S Globulin genes, CACA box sequences and positions **36**, 10909
–, compared to 7S globulins **36**, 122–12323
Globulins **16**, 353
–, HMW, wheat proteins **36**, 24, 26
–, legume seeds **36**, 103–104
–, wheat proteins **36**, 28
–, –, genetic control **36**, 36–37
–, with sequenced cDNA and genes **36**, 105
7S Globulins, domain structure **36**, 11616
–, nucleotide sequences around exon and intron junctions **36**, 10707
–, sequences and positions of vicilin box **36**, 10808
–, structure and conformation **36**, 113–114, 11616
–, transgenic plants **36**, 166, 16868
11S Globulins, construction **36**, 109, 11111
–, domain structure **36**, 12222
–, gene structure **36**, 109–11313
–, interchain disulfide bonds **36**, 116–11919
–, intradisulfide bonds **36**, 119–12020
–, nucleotide sequences around junctions of exons and introns **36**, 109, 11212
–, primary structure **36**, 119–12020
–, quaternary structural model **36**, 120–12121
–, sequences and positions of legumin boxes **36**, 109, 11313
–, structure and conformation **36**, 114–12222
–, subunits **36**, 116–11818
–, –, biosynthesis **36**, 124–12525
–, thermodynamic characteristics **35**, 321–32222
–, transgenic plants **36**, 168–16969
–, with sequenced cDNAs and genes **36**, 11010
Gloeosporium **15**, 177
Gloeosporium album, resistance of to cold **3**, 468
Gloeosporium fructigenum, resistance of to cold **3**, 468
Glu-A1 **45**, 224, 226, 256–257, 258, 260, 263
–, near isogenic lines **45**, 251, 252
Glu-A3 **45**, 258
Glu-B1 **45**, 224, 226, 257, 258, 262, 263
–, near isogenic lines **45**, 251, 252
Glu-B3 **45**, 258
Glu-D1 **45**, 224, 226, 256, 257, 258, 260, 262
–, near isogenic lines **45**, 251, 252
Glu-D3 **45**, 258

Glu-P1, distribution and excretion **34**, 411–412
Glucagon, Δ^6-desaturase, regulation effects **35**, 44–45
–, endogenous proteolytic enzymes and **31**, 357
β-Glucan, dietary fiber and **31**, 136, 137, 148, 150, 155
–, molecular shapes and interactions **42**, 175–179
Glucans, dietary fiber and **31**, 128, 176
–, reserve **41**, 5
–, starch degradation **41**, 153
β-D-Glucans, dietary fiber and **31**, 122, 126, 128
Glucocorticoids, Δ^6-desaturase, regulation effects **35**, 45
Glucomannans, dietary fiber and **31**, 122, 128, 135, 136
Gluconeogenesis, endogenous proteolytic enzymes and **31**, 375, 386, 391
Glucosamine, amides of **3**, 260–261
Glucosan, from glucose **6**, 16
Glucose **14**, 221
–, acceleration of trimethylamine oxide reduction by **2**, 369
–, addition to dough, aroma and **30**, 100–101
–, amino acid esters of **3**, 258–259
–, browning reaction with casein **30**, 89–90
–, chocolate and, cocoa bean chemistry **31**, 231–233
–, –, conching **31**, 297
–, –, milk **31**, 255, 263
–, –, processing **31**, 218
–, –, refining **31**, 295
–, –, sweeteners **31**, 267, 272
–, –, *Theobroma cacao* L. **31**, 326, 327
–, concentration changes and allolactose production **38**, 83
–, content of apples and pears **8**, 300, 313
–, dietary fiber and **31**, 137, 141, 148
–, –, dicotyledonous plants **31**, 127, 128, 135
–, –, intestinal bacteria **31**, 174, 179, 182, 188
–, –, properties **31**, 167–169
–, effect in dried egg **1**, 172–173
–, effect on calcium absorption **33**, 127
–, – on dried egg albumen **3**, 274
–, – on thiamine destruction **6**, 261
–, endogenous proteolytic enzymes and **31**, 394
–, fermentation by *Saccharomyces rouxii* **12**, 75–76
–, formed from sucrose **6**, 16
–, freeze-dried beef and **7**, 213
–, gelatin and **7**, 271
–, in browning reaction **32**, 151–152
–, in cocoa beans, fermentation and **30**, 94
–, –, roasting and **30**, 97
–, increase of, in apples during storage **8**, 318
–, in fresh cocoa bean juice **8**, 239
–, in raw cocoa **8**, 262
–, in spoiled table wines **6**, 76
–, in table wines **6**, 72
–, loss, activation energies **35**, 196, 198
–, loss to amino groups **12**, 35–36
–, metabolism of **1**, 131
–, need by central nervous system **1**, 131
–, *N*-nitroso compounds and **31**, 80
–, olive oil and **31**, 459
–, reaction with alanine **3**, 253
–, – with amino acids **3**, 249, 255
–, – with bovine serum albumin **3**, 275
–, – with casein **3**, 274–275, 276–277
–, – with dipeptides **3**, 254
–, – with glycerol **3**, 252
–, – with glycine **3**, 250–251, 265
–, relation to browning in dehydrated potatoes **1**, 269–270, 273–274
–, separation of reaction products of glycine and by anion exchanger **2**, 35
–, structure and simple reactions of **6**, 4
–, sweetness of **2**, 261
–, transport **40**, 207–213
–, ultrafiltration **40**, 191–192
–, utilization by spoilage bacteria in wine **6**, 91
Glucose–casein reaction **14**, 212–213
Glucose-6-P dihydroxyacetone-P **41**, 120
Glucose oxidase, enzymatic acidification of milk by **38**, 16
–, in honey **24**, 325–329
Glucose 6-phosphate **15**, 39; **41**, 30–31
Glucose *l*-phosphate, method of preparation **2**, 35
Glucose 6-phosphate dehydrogenase, deficiency of, xylitol effects on **25**, 169–170
–, in wheat germ **23**, 240
Glucose transport **41**, 159
α-1,4-Glucosidic linkages **41**, 33–34
Glucosinolates, in rapeseeds, antinutritional for nonruminants **30**, 371
Glucuronic acid, glycyrrhizin and **7**, 359–360
β-Glucuronidase, fecal, lactic culture effects **37**, 99–101
Glucuronides **15**, 11
Glutamate dehydrogenase, cardiolipin association **37**, 285–286

Glutamate salts, age-related taste thresholds **44**, 257, 261
Glutamic acid **10**, 80–81, 112–113, 117
–, chocolate and **31**, 224
–, dietary fiber and **31**, 129
–, in fruit products, leaking from cells treated with detergents **1**, 379
–, –, relation to browning **1**, 352
–, –, – to microbial inhibition **1**, 387
–, *N*-nitroso compounds and **31**, 76
–, reaction with sugars **3**, 266
–, separation from sugar beet molasses **2**, 35
Glutamic acid decarboxylase **16**, 301
–, in wheat germ **23**, 240
Glutamic dehydrogenase, in wheat germ **23**, 240
Glutamic oxalacetic transaminase as endpoint cooking temperature indicator **44**, 171
Glutamic pyruvic transaminase as endpoint cooking temperature indicator **44**, 171
Glutamine, *N*-nitroso compounds and **31**, 76
Glutamine synthetase, thermal stability **35**, 257
γ-Glutamyl peptidase, in onion and garlic flavor development **22**, 122–124
γ-Glutamyl peptides, biosynthesis **22**, 90
–, in *Allium* **22**, 79–83
γ-Glutamyl transpeptidase, in onion and garlic flavor development **22**, 122–124
Glutathione **16**, 366
–, chlorine and **7**, 134
–, in bread dough **3**, 82
–, in wheat germ **23**, 270
–, –, effect on baking quality **23**, 274–275
–, –, inactivation **23**, 277
–, metabolism **45**, 79
–, reduction of α-tocopherol intermediate oxidation products **33**, 212
Glutathione peroxidase, removal of hydrogen peroxide with **33**, 303
Glutathione *S*-transferase **45**, 83
Glutelin **36**, 93, 95, 115–116
Gluten **16**, 347, 353, 356, 361, 376; **36**, 131–132
–, amorphous, thermosetting behavior **38**, 218–223
–, aqueous systems, thermoplastic and thermoset behavior **38**, 223–226
–, as microemulsion system **34**, 164
–, classification of proteins **38**, 216
–, corn **38**, 288, 296
–, disulfide crosslinks, no change in free–SH groups **38**, 224
–, dough performance relationship **45**, 259
–, durum wheat **36**, 133
–, glassy state **38**, 123, 126–127
–, hand-washed and lyophilized, glass transition temperature as function of moisture **38**, 153–154
–, infrared dehydration of **3**, 146
–, insolubility, thermodynamic aspects **45**, 274–275, 276
–, interaction with lipids, effect on baking quality **29**, 263–264
–, interchange experiments **36**, 49
–, in wheat flours, acid-soluble and -insoluble fractions **29**, 249–251
–, –, amide content, effect on baking quality **29**, 265–267
–, –, breadmaking and **29**, 246–251
–, –, dough properties and **29**, 242–251
–, –, fractionation and reconstitution **29**, 224–226
–, –, gliadin, *see* Gliadin
–, –, glutenin, *see* Glutenin
–, –, interchanging between two samples **29**, 228–230
–, macropolymer **45**, 258–259
–, membranes in, role in breadmaking **20**, 169–175
–, molecular weight distribution, effect on baking quality **29**, 265
–, partially deamidated, surface and emulsifying properties **34**, 155
–, pathways leading to ultimate thermosets **38**, 225–226
–, plasticization, bread-baking **38**, 218–219
–, protein fractions, quality and composition data **36**, 45, 47–48
–, separation **29**, 222–224
–, solubility and pH relations **36**, 4–5
–, sulfur-containing amino acids, effect on baking quality **29**, 267–269
–, viscoelasticity **45**, 279–280
–, viscosity **36**, 41–43
–, water-plasticized, thermosetting **38**, 222–223
–, wheat, as viscoelastic polymer system **38**, 215–218
Glutenin **38**, 216–217; **45**, 221
–, amino acid composition **36**, 17–19
–, content, extensibility and resistance as function of **36**, 52–53
–, dough viscoelasticity, gluten fractionation/reconstitution experiments **45**, 242–245
–, –, protein fraction incorporation studies **45**, 245–246

Glutenin (*cont'd*)
–, electrophoretic subunit separation **45**, 222, 223
–, food protein engineering **36**, 186
–, –, genetic control **36**, 33–34
–, –, structure **36**, 38–39
–, high-molecular-weight subunits **36**, 100, 132; **45**, 222, 223
–, –, amino acid sequences **45**, 228–233
–, –, atomic force microscopy **45**, 233, 235
–, –, composition manipulation **45**, 249, 251–256
–, –, cross-link formation, disulfide bonds **45**, 240–242, 278, 284
–, –, –, low-molecular-weight subunit branches **45**, 240, 242, 278
–, –, –, mechanical behaviour of dough **45**, 280
–, –, –, transgenic lines **45**, 265
–, –, –, tyrosine bonds **45**, 242
–, –, dough viscoelasticity influence **45**, 242–249
–, –, –, dough mixing process **45**, 284–288
–, –, –, gluten fractionation/reconstitution experiments **45**, 242–245
–, –, –, incorporation into dough, purified subunits **45**, 247–249
–, –, –, –, subunit peptides **45**, 249, 250
–, –, –, *in vitro* polymerization **45**, 246
–, –, –, 'loop and train' hypothesis **45**, 281–283, 284, 285, 286, 288–289
–, –, –, macropolymer interactions **45**, 280–281
–, –, –, protein fraction incorporation studies **45**, 245–247
–, –, –, theoretical models **45**, 279–284
–, –, expression in micro-organisms **36**, 162
–, –, genetic control **36**, 32–33
–, –, genetics **45**, 224–226
–, –, grain breadmaking quality relationship **45**, 226–228, 259–265, 266
–, –, –, biophysical models **45**, 273–289
–, –, –, gluten macropolymer composition **45**, 259
–, –, –, molecular basis **45**, 265, 267–273
–, –, –, quality scoring system **45**, 227
–, –, –, ranking of subunit loci **45**, 258
–, –, –, relation to dough rheology **45**, 279
–, –, –, variation between cultivars **45**, 256–259
–, –, hydration-related molecular rearrangements **45**, 278–279, 284
–, –, insolubility, thermodynamic aspects **45**, 274–278
–, –, mixing/rheological properties influence **45**, 256–265
–, –, molecular basis of processing properties, amino acid sequences **45**, 267–269, 271
–, –, – of –, subunit interactions **45**, 271–273
–, –, – of –, subunit stability **45**, 270, 271
–, –, – of –, total amount of protein **45**, 267
–, –, molecular dimensions **45**, 233, 234
–, –, near isogenic lines **45**, 251–253
–, –, –, dough quality differences **45**, 259–262
–, –, –, Gabo **45**, 252, 260, 261
–, –, –, Galahad **45**, 252
–, –, –, Pegaso **45**, 252–253
–, –, –, Sicco **45**, 251–252, 259–261
–, –, –, single subunit **45**, 253
–, –, null lines **36**, 56–57
–, –, polymorphisms **45**, 224–226
–, –, SDS-polyacrylamide gel electrophoresis **45**, 224, 225
–, –, solubilization **36**, 14–17
–, –, structure **36**, 37–38
–, –, –, repetitive domains **45**, 237–239
–, –, –, terminal domains **45**, 234, 236–237
–, –, transgenic lines **45**, 253–256
–, –, –, dough quality differences **45**, 262–265, 266
–, –, transgenic plants **36**, 170–171
–, in wheat flours, breadmaking and **29**, 248, 251
–, –, dough properties and **29**, 243–246
–, –, subunits, effect on baking quality **29**, 268–269
–, long-range intermolecular disulfide network formation **38**, 217, 222
–, low-molecular-weight subunits **36**, 133–134; **45**, 222, 223
–, –, cross-links **45**, 240, 242, 278
–, –, –, mechanical behaviour of dough **45**, 280, 281
–, –, dough viscoelasticity, incorporation studies **45**, 247
–, –, genetic variation, influence on technological properties **45**, 257, 258
–, –, gluten macropolymer composition **45**, 259
–, –, *in vitro* polymerization **45**, 246
–, –, B-type **45**, 222
–, –, C-type **45**, 222
–, –, D-type **45**, 222
–, structure, future directions **36**, 77–78
–, subunits **36**, 132

–, –, arrangement in native molecules **36**, 42, 44
–, –, comparison of high- and low-molecular-weight subunits **36**, 57–60
–, –, effects on dough properties **36**, 58–59
–, –, physical studies **36**, 39
–, –, *see entries for Glutenin, high- and low-molecular-weight subunits*
–, thermolabile disulfide bonds **38**, 225
–, viscosity **36**, 41–43
–, wheat proteins **36**, 22–25
Gluten intolerance **37**, 29–30
Gluten–keratin multicomponent films **44**, 382
Gluten-sensitive enteropathy **42**, 9
Glyceraldehyde-3-phosphate dehydrogenase, from thermophilic and mesophilic bacteria **35**, 261
–, stability **35**, 251
Glyceral production, from *Saccharomyces rouxii* **12**, 76–81
–, from *Zygosaccharomyces* **12**, 76–77
Glycerides **16**, 255
–, in cocoa fat **6**, 39
–, olive oil and **31**, 463–466, 471, 473, 475, 477
Glycerin, in fruit juices **9**, 261–262
–, in solution of CPCl **2**, 153
–, in soy sauce **10**, 82–83
Glycerol **13**, 288–289
–, anhydrous **6**, 20
–, effect on phenolases in fruit products **3**, 35
–, gel rigidity and **7**, 297
–, in candies **6**, 13
–, in cocoa beans **8**, 262
–, in laboratory rations **6**, 301
–, in table wines **6**, 72
–, olive oil and **31**, 458, 463, 466
–, osmophilic yeasts and **7**, 114–115
–, preferential hydration **35**, 291
–, reaction with glucose **3**, 252
–, solute-specific subzero glass transition temperature **38**, 228–229
–, use of **6**, 11
–, –, in frozen food **6**, 169
Glycerol monostearate **43**, 230, 231
Glycerol phosphate, olive oil and **31**, 458
α-Glycerol-phosphate dehydrogenase, cardiolipin association **37**, 283
Glycerophosphatase, in wheat germ **23**, 241
Glycine **40**, 98–99
–, acceleration of trimethylamine oxide reduction by **2**, 369
–, activity with sugars **3**, 265–266
–, chocolate and **31**, 269
–, effect on browning in potato chips **1**, 277
–, – on dried egg albumen **3**, 274
–, gelatin structure and **7**, 262–263, 314
–, in browning reaction **32**, 138–141
–, in dried egg **1**, 172–173
–, reaction with glucose **3**, 250–251, 255
Glycinin (*see also* Soybean glycinin) **36**, 119, 125
–, amino acid sequences around free cysteine residues **36**, 129–130
–, gelation **36**, 126, 128–130
–, –, heat-induced **36**, 126, 128
–, subunits **36**, 116–119
–, –, gelation **36**, 128–129
Glycitein **44**, 197, 202
–, fungal/bacterial fermentation **44**, 213
–, sources **44**, 203, 205, 207
Glycoalkaloid, control of formation in potato **21**, 331–342
–, formation in *Solanun tuberosum* **21**, 312–331
–, pharmacology and toxicology **21**, 342–348
Glycocyamine, separation from arginine by silicate exchanger **2**, 38
Glycogen, breakdown in muscle **1**, 3
–, characterization **41**, 6
–, endogenous proteolytic enzymes and **31**, 394
–, in abalone **23**, 162, 176, 179
–, –, in can liquor **23**, 178
–, in muscle **1**, 11; **6**, 122; **19**, 4–5
–, –, effect of exercise on **1**, 11
–, –, – of fatigue on **1**, 14
–, –, – of feeding on **1**, 13
–, –, poultry meat, effect of feeding on **1**, 218
–, synthesis **41**, 125
Glycogen content of fish muscle **2**, 361–362
Glycogenesis, type 1, Von Gierke's disease **37**, 374–377
–, type 2, Pompe's disease **37**, 377
–, type 3, Cori–Forbes disease **37**, 377
–, type 4, Andersen's disease **37**, 377
–, type 5, McArdle's disease **37**, 377–378
–, type 6, Hers' disease **37**, 378
–, type 7, Tauri's disease **37**, 378–379
Glycogenolysis **40**, 136
Glycogen phosphorylase β, reductive alkylation **35**, 271
Glycogen phosphorylase metabolism (*see also* Vitamin B6 metabolism) **40**, 135–147
–, cofactor, labeling **40**, 137–140
–, –, role **40**, 135–136
–, growth, muscle **40**, 142
–, labeling methods **40**, 137–140

Glycogen phosphorylase metabolism, labeling methods (*cont'd*)
–, –, radiolabeling **40**, 137–138
–, –, stable isotope **40**, 138–140
–, McArdle's disease **40**, 142–145
–, messenger RNA **40**, 141, 144, 145
–, model systems **40**, 140–142
–, pyridoxal phosphate **40**, 135–136
–, turnover **40**, 124, 137–140, 142
–, vitamin B6 **40**, 115–116, 118, 121
–, wasting, muscle **40**, 140–141
Glycogen synthase **41**, 100
–, characterization **41**, 107–108
–, sequences **41**, 85
Glycogen-synthesizing enzymes **41**, 110
Glycolaldehyde, reaction with ethylamine in color formation by smoking **29**, 138–139
Glycolipids, interaction with wheat flour in baking **20**, 153–188
–, – with – in –, description of **20**, 161–164
–, – with – in –, evidence for **20**, 154–159
–, – with – in –, mechanism **20**, 166–167
–, in wheat flours, breadmaking and **29**, 253, 257
–, –, cookie quality and **29**, 259
–, structural formulas of **20**, 163
–, structure and biosynthesis of **23**, 15–17
Glycollate oxidase **17**, 13–14, 26
Glycollic acid, oxidation of **17**, 14
Glycolysis (*see also* Fermentation) **13**, 89–178; **17**, 225; **39**, 196, 198–201, 255
–, acquired diseases **37**, 379
–, anaerobic **17**, 120
–, endogenous proteolytic enzymes and **31**, 370, 385, 393, 394
–, enzyme deficiencies, table **37**, 375
–, fruit ripening and **30**, 172–173
–, in porcine stress syndrome **28**, 185–186
–, olive oil and **31**, 458
–, relationship to meat quality **37**, 379
Glycolytic enzymes, in wheat germ **23**, 240
Glycoproteins, content **30**, 147
–, dietary fiber and, components **31**, 120, 122, 123
–, –, properties **31**, 126, 128, 129, 132, 135
–, endogenous proteolytic enzymes and **31**, 355
–, plant cell wall, composition, binding to other fractions **30**, 151–152
–, –, –, hydroxyproline-rich **30**, 147–149
–, –, hydroxyprolinyl *O*-arabinosides **30**, 149
–, –, serinyl *O*-galactosides **30**, 149
Glycopyrrolate **44**, 299
Glycoside appin in celery roots **2**, 271
Glycoside hydrolases **38**, 23–25
–, in plant primary cell wall **30**, 157, 159
N-Glycosides, formation in browning reactions **30**, 81
Glycosides (flavonol), in tea **17**, 228–230
–, preparation of **3**, 256–258, 259–260
Glycosidol, hydrolysis of in mushroom **2**, 277
Glycosyl, enzymatic transfer reactions **38**, 60
Glycosylamines, Amadori rearrangement **30**, 82, 87–88
–, products of aldose reaction with amines **30**, 87
–, reaction of during storage **3**, 247
Glycosyl amino acids, reactions of **3**, 262
Glycosylation, endogenous proteolytic enzymes and **31**, 355, 363, 374
–, protein emulsifier modification **34**, 156–157
–, whey proteins **33**, 421–422
Glycyl-glycine dipeptidase, endogenous proteolytic enzymes and **31**, 349, 389
Glycyrrhetic acid, absorption spectrum of **7**, 362
–, assay of **7**, 370–371
Glycyrrhiza glabra, varieties of **7**, 340–341
Glycyrrhizic acid, excretion of **7**, 354
Glycyrrhizin, aglycon of **7**, 360–362
–, assay **7**, 366–371
–, –, colorimetric **7**, 370
–, –, copper precipitation **7**, 368
–, –, gravimetric **7**, 367–368
–, –, oxidimetric **7**, 369–370
–, –, physiological **7**, 369
–, –, titrimetric **7**, 368–369
–, chemical structure of **7**, 358–366
–, chocolate and **31**, 271
–, commercial preparation of **7**, 346
–, composition of **7**, 342
–, functional groups of **7**, 362–366
–, licorice extract and **7**, 347
–, plants containing **7**, 343
–, salt balance and **7**, 357
–, spasmolytic effect of **7**, 355–356
–, sugar moiety of **7**, 359–360
Glyoxalcyclohexylamine, formation in browning reactions **30**, 91
Goat, secretion of DDT in milk of **2**, 211
–, toxicity of DDT to **2**, 208
Goat meat in diet **1**, 109
Goiter **16**, 33
Goiter-producing food factors **10**, 14
Gold **44**, 296

Golgi, endogenous proteolytic enzymes and **31**, 369, 375, 387
Gonyaulax catenella **10**, 138–142, 156, 173, 174, 175
–, shellfish toxicity from **18**, 155–157
Gonyaulax tamarensis **10**, 141, 174
Goodpasture's syndrome **37**, 33
Gooseberries, canned, corrosion by **3**, 338
–, pH of **3**, 432
–, with added copper **3**, 355
–, with added sulfur **3**, 352
Gordon–Taylor equation **38**, 150
Gossypol, in cottonseed **17**, 109
–, in diet **1**, 124–125
–, toxic, in cotton seeds **30**, 371
Gouda cheese, contamination **39**, 289
–, flavor **39**, 243, 245
–, lipolysis **39**, 201, 205
–, proteinases **39**, 231
–, salting **39**, 177
–, texture **39**, 176, 254
–, ultrafiltration **39**, 194
Graded levels, nutrient **40**, 157–166
Grading scheme, cheese **39**, 252, 295–296
Grains (*see also* Caryopsis *and* Cereal grains) **15**, 289
–, as feeds **17**, 114–115
–, insect-infested **8**, 111
–, radiography **8**, 121
–, utilization of **17**, 106–115
Gramine, *N*-nitroso compounds and **31**, 90, 91
Granisetron **44**, 316
Granule-bound starch synthases, antisense **41**, 129
–, characterization **41**, 78–81, 111–113
Granules, amylopectin **41**, 13, 16, 20–23
–, amylose **41**, 13, 16, 20–23
–, dried **41**, 165
–, formation **41**, 110–111
–, lipids in **41**, 30
–, minor constituents **41**, 30
–, orientation **41**, 27–29
–, phosphorusin **41**, 30
–, potato, processes for **25**, 56–59
–, proteins in **41**, 31–32
–, starch synthases bound **41**, 78–81
–, structure **41**, 13
Grape anthocyanins **43**, 212
–, adverse reactions **43**, 212–213
Grape concentrate, browning in **1**, 341, 354, 362
Grapefruit **10**, 314–315, 317; **15**, 223
–, bitterness **5**, 273
–, canned, corrosion characteristics of **3**, 336, 846
–, –, nutrients in **1**, 43, 46–49
–, extraction of pectin from peel **2**, 21
–, juice, ascorbic acid content, effect of nitrogen on **1**, 308
–, –, canned, ascorbic acid content **1**, 54–55; **4**, 373, 380
–, –, –, nutrients in **1**, 43, 46–50
–, –, concentrate, yeast infections **5**, 79
–, –, in tin plate porosity test **3**, 362
–, –, B vitamins in **1**, 42, 44, 45
–, peels, brining **5**, 144
–, –, pectin in **1**, 400
–, phosphorus content of, effect of fertilizers on **1**, 313
Grape gels, changes in during aging **1**, 420
Grape industry, use of ion exchangers in **2**, 15–18
Grapes **15**, 225
–, acidic components of **25**, 3–10
–, –, factors affecting **25**, 5–10
–, anthocyanin pigment in skins **5**, 282
–, calcium in **8**, 174
–, Concord, inactivation of polyphenol oxidase in **3**, 29
–, effect of ozone on **3**, 466
–, flavonoids **5**, 282
–, fungicides and insecticides on **8**, 138
–, importance in wine making **25**, 2
–, iodine in wrapping for **3**, 465
–, juice, browning **1**, 328, 333–334; **5**, 54
–, –, –, chemical changes during **1**, 349–350
–, –, color of **5**, 311
–, –, combination of sulfur dioxide **5**, 79
–, –, copper content of **8**, 118
–, –, destruction of antineuritic activity by SO_2 **5**, 103
–, –, – of wine yeast in **3**, 436
–, –, free SO_2 **5**, 139
–, –, peroxidase activity in **3**, 28
–, –, use of ascorbic acid in **4**, 375–376, 381
–, leuco-anthocyanins **5**, 288
–, Muscat, peroxidase activity of **3**, 10
–, nitrogenous compounds **5**, 448
–, polyphenols and enzymic browning in **19**, 117–118
–, recommended amount of sulfur dioxide added to musts **6**, 89
–, sodium in **8**, 196
–, solubility of carbon dioxide in **8**, 148
–, sulfiting for transportation **5**, 146
–, Thompson Seedless, peroxidase activity of **3**, 10

Grapes (*cont'd*)
–, treatment of, by ammonia **3**, 465
–, –, by sulfur dioxide **3**, 466
–, volatile constituents of **2**, 270
Grape skin extract **43**, 196
Graph, definition **40**, 339
Graph theory **40**, 339–352
–, computer implementation **40**, 348
–, model analysis **40**, 348–351
–, model building **40**, 340–348
Grashof number **32**, 58, 64, 76, 79
Grasses **41**, 2
–, dietary fiber and **31**, 139, 152, 187, 188
Grave's disease **37**, 33
Gravity, specific **14**, 110–112
Gravity-induced separation, emulsions **34**, 174–175
Grayling, aerobic bacteria in **2**, 350
Green algae **41**, 4
Green mold, *see Penicillium digitatum*
Green tea, organoleptic properties of **24**, 265–266
–, production changes in **24**, 261–262
–, storage of **24**, 267
Grey feather (*Liatris punctata*) **45**, 77
Grinders, food **14**, 95–97
–, in meat processing **16**, 126
Grinding, chocolate and **31**, 241–243, 304
–, effects on water-holding capacity of meat **10**, 433–436
Grindrod, George **32**, 4
Griseofulvin **44**, 291
Gross national product **32**, 189
Ground meat **39**, 94
Groundnuts, *see* Peanuts
Ground substance, structure and composition of **20**, 267
Group-specific proteinase, endogenous proteolytic enzymes and **31**, 353, 354
Growth hormone, and meat quality **21**, 88–89
Growth inhibitors, structurally non-specific **11**, 333
Growth promoters, residues in food **37**, 42–43
Growth regulators, fruit **10**, 336
Gruyère cheese **39**, 243, 254
Guacamole spread, alginates in **11**, 156
Guaiacol in coffee **2**, 281, 282
Guanfacine **44**, 305
Guanidination, protein stability **35**, 273–274
Guanidine hydrochloride, lysozyme denaturation **35**, 299–300
Guanidyl groups, gel formation and **7**, 255
Guano, in animal protein food chain **20**, 201
Guar gum **39**, 34–35
–, dietary fiber and **31**, 140, 141, 191
–, general properties **11**, 166–168
–, in bakery products **11**, 168
–, in beverages **11**, 169
–, in cheese products **11**, 168
–, in ice cream stabilization **11**, 168
–, in meat products **11**, 169
–, in miscellaneous foods **11**, 168–170
–, in salad dressing **11**, 169
–, in sauces **11**, 169
–, intestinal bacteria **31**, 172, 174, 175, 182
–, properties **31**, 166–171
–, viscosity **11**, 118
Guar solution **39**, 49–51
Guatemala, Incaparina use in **22**, 197
Guavas, composition **17**, 160
–, distribution of oxidase in **3**, 10
–, extract, catalytic effect of **3**, 7
–, peroxidase activity in **3**, 27
Guided wave sensors **45**, 128
Guinea pig, effects of DDT on skin of **2**, 207
–, toxicity of DDT to **2**, 208
–, use in tests for toxicity for quaternary ammonium compounds **2**, 130, 153
Guinea pig ileum contraction assay, for histamine **24**, 130–131
Gum arabic, candy applications of **6**, 29
–, drops **6**, 29
–, –, produced with tapioca **6**, 34
–, general properties **11**, 171
–, in bakery products **11**, 173
–, in beverages **11**, 175
–, in confectionery **11**, 172
–, in dairy products **11**, 174
–, in flavor fixation **11**, 175
–, in miscellaneous foods **11**, 180
–, tragacanth, candy applications of **6**, 29
–, viscosity **11**, 118
Gum guaiac, as antioxidant **3**, 28, 201, 203
–, –, effect on mortality of rats **3**, 205
–, –, – on tallowiness in dry milk **3**, 95
–, –, in dried egg **1**, 181
–, –, pathologic effects of **3**, 207
Gum karaya, general properties **11**, 186
–, in bakery products **11**, 188
–, in dairy products **11**, 188
–, in ice cream, ices, and sherbets **11**, 187
–, in meat products **11**, 187
–, in miscellaneous foods **11**, 187–189
–, viscosity **11**, 118
Gums (*see also specific gums*), dietary fiber and **31**, 140, 141, 158
–, economics in foods **11**, 111–112

–, history of use in foods **11**, 110
–, in bakery products **11**, 114–115
–, in beverages **11**, 114
–, in cocoa beans and nibs **6**, 38; **8**, 263
–, in confectionery **11**, 116
–, in dairy products **11**, 114
–, in dietetic foods **11**, 115
–, in dressings and sauces **11**, 115
–, in meat and fish **11**, 116
–, in miscellaneous foods **11**, 116
–, natural **6**, 29; **12**, 284–285
–, natural vs. synthetic in foods **11**, 112
–, needed research on **11**, 189
–, properties and uses **11**, 112–117
–, protective action on thiamine **6**, 261
–, synthetic **12**, 283–366
–, –, advantages **12**, 286
–, –, completely **12**, 289–290
–, –, economics **12**, 284–287
–, –, research needs **12**, 357–358
–, traditional classification **11**, 116–117
–, typical functions in foods **11**, 113
–, use in the food industry **11**, 109–200
–, viscosities **11**, 118
Gum tragacanth, general properties **11**, 181
–, in bakery products **11**, 185
–, in confectionery **11**, 185
–, in ice cream and ices **11**, 184
–, in meringues **11**, 185
–, in miscellaneous food applications **11**, 185
–, in pie fillings **11**, 185
–, in salad dressings and sauces **11**, 182–184
–, in sherbets **11**, 184
–, viscosity **11**, 118
Gustducin, involvement in sweetener-induced taste **42**, 227–229, 234–235
Gut-associated lymphoid tissue **37**, 10–12
Gut microbial metabolism, isoflavones **44**, 218–220
–, lignans **44**, 199, 207, 221
Gymnodinium **10**, 174
Gymnothorax, *see* Moray eel poisoning

Haber–Weiss reaction **33**, 237–238
HACCP, *see* Hazard analysis and critical control point
Haddock **39**, 341–342, 349
–, bacterial increase on skin after storage of **2**, 356
–, Canadian, aerobic bacteria in **2**, 350
–, –, anaerobic bacteria in **2**, 351
–, effect of cathode rays on **3**, 172, 174
–, formation of dimethylamine in **2**, 371
–, North sea, aerobic bacteria in **2**, 350
–, –, anaerobic bacteria isolated from **2**, 353
–, –, comparison of fresh and spoiling **2**, 353, 354
–, organoleptic spoilage of **2**, 377
–, percentage glycogen in **2**, 362
–, percentage lactic acid in **2**, 362
–, pH value of **2**, 363, 381
–, radar cooking of **3**, 139
–, reduction of trimethylamine oxide in **2**, 355
–, rigor mortis in **2**, 364–366
–, route of bacterial attack in **2**, 375
–, spoilage of **3**, 186
–, tests for quality of **2**, 380, 381
Halibut, changes in pH **2**, 372
–, loss of thiamine in **6**, 280
–, relation of pH value to keeping qualities of **2**, 363
–, spoilage of **7**, 50
–, tests for quality of **2**, 380
Haliotis sp., *see* Abalone
Hall spray dryer, operation of **2**, 414
Halogens, oxidation of sulfhydryl enzymes by **1**, 381
Halothane, effect on muscle metabolism **21**, 84–87; **28**, 207–209
Ham **39**, 79, 81, 110, 123
–, curing brines **5**, 31
–, fish **12**, 367–424
–, nitrite effects on flavor **29**, 26–29
–, – on volatile compounds **29**, 65–70
–, *N*-nitroso compounds and **31**, 57
–, patties, home frozen **6**, 207
–, salt-cured **6**, 123
–, smoked, phenol composition **29**, 133
–, souring **6**, 138, 141
–, thiamine loss in **6**, 275, 276
Hamaker constant **22**, 313
Hamburger, radar cooking of **3**, 139
–, sterilization of by cathode rays **3**, 167, 174
Handling, chilling **13**, 159–160
–, exsanguination **13**, 164–165
–, liquid nitrogen treatment **13**, 160–164
–, post-mortem **13**, 159–165
–, poultry **13**, 164
–, stunning **13**, 165
Hansenula, destruction of by heat **3**, 435
Haptens, contact sensitivity **43**, 200–201
Hardness meter **9**, 106
Hardwood, lignin pyrolysis **29**, 121–122
–, phenol composition **29**, 127
Hartman apparatus **14**, 20

Harvest, research on factors surrounding **10**, 65–66
Hash, F value for industrial processing of **2**, 102
Hausdorff–Besicovic dimension **40**, 328
Havarti cheese **39**, 194
Hazard analysis and critical control point (HACCP) **39**, 151
–, program of meat processors **44**, 148
HCA, *see* Hydrophobic cluster analysis
HCF process **32**, 2–4
HDL (*see also* Lipoproteins) **36**, 259–260
–, levels, fat quantity and **36**, 311–314
–, metabolism, animal studies **36**, 286–287
–, –, HDL receptor **36**, 290–291
–, –, human studies **36**, 287–290
–, –, *n*-3 PUFA **36**, 324
–, –, *n*-6 PUFA **36**, 285–291
–, receptor, *n*-6 PUFA effects **36**, 290–291, 327
HDL cholesterol, effects of lactic acid cultures **37**, 93
Headspace **32**, 64, 68, 74
Heart, glycyrrhizin in **7**, 354–355
–, α-LNA conversion **35**, 72–74
–, membrane transport **40**, 259
–, microsomes, peroxidation, α-tocopherol effects **33**, 213
–, of meat animals **6**, 133
Heart disease, inulin effects **43**, 41
–, olive oil and **31**, 477
–, *n*-3 PUFA effects **35**, 134–138
Heat, cycle **12**, 160–161
–, dielectric, freeze-drying and **7**, 183–185, 203, 209
–, effects on milk proteins **19**, 163–165
–, – on "warmed-over" flavor **23**, 48–53
–, – on water-holding capacity of meat **10**, 428–433
–, exchangers, *see* Heat exchangers
–, forced air circulation **12**, 161–164
–, grid-cooled space **12**, 160–161
–, leakage into ships **12**, 157–160
–, –, control of outside conditions **12**, 159
–, –, convection **12**, 160
–, –, estimation by relaxation **12**, 158
–, –, measurements **12**, 158–159
–, –, Niemann's test **12**, 159–160
–, –, theory **12**, 158
–, protein emulsifier modification **34**, 147–150
–, radiant, freeze-drying and **7**, 182–183
–, specific, of foods **13**, 278–281
–, –, of ice **13**, 240
–, –, of water **13**, 240
–, sublimation and **7**, 181–185
–, transfer, *see* Heat transfer
Heat effects (*see also* Temperature effects *and* Thermal processing), folates during extraction **33**, 16
–, ligand binding by β-lactoglobulin **33**, 415
–, α-tocopherol content of vegetable oils **33**, 164–165
–, whey proteins, concentrate foaming properties, table **33**, 402
–, –, conformation **33**, 376–378
–, –, foams **33**, 401
–, –, partial unfolding **33**, 404
–, –, solubility **33**, 375
Heat evolution method **35**, 343
Heat exchangers **32**, 15–16
–, on ships **12**, 164–165
Heating (*see also* Temperature) **39**, 101–102, 106–107, 187, 262
–, convective **39**, 113–114
–, effects **39**, 95–96
–, flavor **39**, 131–132
–, microbial control **39**, 120–121
–, osmosis **39**, 110–113
–, preservation **39**, 85–88
–, process optimization **39**, 138–143
–, research needs **39**, 149
–, ripening **39**, 196–197
Heating curve, curvilinear portion of **23**, 81
Heat of formation, junction zones **34**, 227–228
Heat penetration, effect on bacterial survival **2**, 93–96
–, – on quality of canned food **2**, 104
–, factors in plotting curves **2**, 53, 58, 83
Heat processes, *see* Thermal processes
Heat sterilization, effect on ascorbic acid **1**, 89
–, – on carotene **1**, 89
–, – on niacin **1**, 87–89
–, – on riboflavin **1**, 87–89
–, – on thiamine **1**, 84, 89
Heat transfer, by forced convection **32**, 60–74
–, by natural convection **32**, 50–59
–, characteristics of non-Newtonian fluids **11**, 416–423
–, coefficients for pseudoplastic fluids in tubes **11**, 417–420
–, conduction-heating products **2**, 90–91
–, convection-heating products **2**, 95, 99
–, convective, dimensional analysis for **32**, 48–50
–, dimensionless groups for **32**, 49–50

–, during freezing and thawing of foods **20**, 217–256
–, freeze-drying and **7**, 188–189, 198
–, heat conduction with phase change in **20**, 223–235
–, – with –, at single temperature **20**, 224–226
–, – with –, in a range of temperatures **20**, 226–235
–, high-temperature short-time processes **2**, 104
–, in ammonium alginate **11**, 419
–, in applesauce **11**, 419
–, in banana purée **11**, 419
–, in food processing **2**, 90–91, 96–99
–, in motor oil **11**, 419
–, in non-Newtonian fluids with turbulent flow **11**, 422
–, in refrigerated ships **12**, 160–164
–, in thermal processing of foods **23**, 376–380
–, mechanism in food processing **2**, 89
–, methodologies for studying **32**, 43–44
–, principles of **20**, 218–220
–, –, boundary conditions **20**, 219–220
–, –, initial conditions **20**, 220
–, product agitation during **2**, 103
–, rates, with natural convection **32**, 56–59
–, theory of **32**, 42–43
–, to suspensions **11**, 422
–, transfer coefficients **32**, 43, 44, 57–58, 67–69, 72–73, 75–76
–, –, calculated vs. experimental values **11**, 419
–, F values of industrial processes by **2**, 102
–, with particulate matter **32**, 74–76
Heat transfer treatments, proteins **35**, 336–337
Heat treatment, of fruit juices **9**, 249–250
–, use in storage of mango fruits **21**, 281–282
Hegsted equation **36**, 272
Heleurine **45**, 73
Helianthus tuberosus, *see* Jerusalem artichoke
Heliosupine **45**, 66, 67
Heliotrine **45**, 70, 71, 73, 78
Heliotrine *N*-oxide **45**, 78
Heliotropium contamination of staple foods **45**, 68, 70
– of –, prevention **45**, 91
Heliotropium europaeum **45**, 73
Heliotropium popvoii **45**, 70
Helix capping **42**, 96
Hematin, catalytic activities **17**, 27–29
Hematin pigments in fatty fishes **2**, 373
Hematopoiesis, characterization **37**, 8
Heme, fish lipid oxidation **33**, 290
Heme compounds, as catalysts of lipid oxidation **23**, 40–43, 59–60
–, – of –, in meat **29**, 37–38
–, as prooxidants **23**, 45
HEMF, *see* 4-Hydroxy-2(or 5)-ethyl-5(or 2)-methyl-3(2H)-furanone
Hemicellulase, absence in fruits **30**, 178
Hemicelluloses (*see also* Pentosans), analysis **31**, 150, 153
–, components **31**, 120, 122–124
–, dicotyledonous plants **31**, 124, 126, 128, 129, 132, 133, 135
–, dietary fiber and **31**, 191
–, ester formation between pectins and **11**, 70–80
–, glucuronoarabinoxylan **30**, 147
–, intestinal bacteria **31**, 176–182, 185, 188
–, monocotyledonous plants **31**, 136, 138
–, plant, biosynthesis from nucleotide sugars **30**, 164
–, properties **31**, 165
–, xyloglucans **30**, 145–146
Hemocyanin, in abalone **23**, 162
Hemoglobin, effect on color in bacon **3**, 314
–, endogenous proteolytic enzymes and **31**, 362, 366
–, freeze-dried beef and **7**, 211–212
–, green discoloration and **7**, 57
–, muscle **14**, 51–52, 122
Hemolysis, erythrocyte, α-tocopherol acetate effects **33**, 219
–, glycyrrhizin and **7**, 355
–, vitamin E status with **33**, 189
Hemolytic anemia, xylitol therapy of **25**, 169–170
Hemoproteins, *N*-nitroso compounds and **31**, 73
Hemp seed, effect of heat on nutritive value of protein in **4**, 249
Hencky strain rate **39**, 15
Hepatic fibrosis **37**, 403–404
Hepatic triglyceride lipase, dietary fat quality and **36**, 314
–, *n*-3 PUFA effects **36**, 325
–, *n*-6 PUFA effects **36**, 292–293
Hepatic veno-occlusive disease, herbal teas **45**, 74
–, pyrrolizidine alkaloid toxicity **45**, 69–70, 72, 75–76, 77, 79–80, 91
–, synergism with copper **45**, 79
Hepatitis A **45**, 178
Hepatoxins **15**, 38
n-Heptacosone in coffee **2**, 282

Heptoic acid, in manufactured tea **2**, 286
–, in parsnip seed oil **2**, 274
Herbal medicines, pyrrolizidine alkaloids, adverse health effects awareness **45**, 91, 93
–, –, sources **45**, 66, 68, 73–78
Herbicides, carcinogen risk assessment and **31**, 28
Heredity **14**, 53
–, carcinogen risk assessment and **31**, 3
HERP, carcinogen risk assessment and **31**, 35
Herring **39**, 339, 341–343, 348–349
–, amine production in spoiling **2**, 368
–, anaerobic bacteria isolated from **2**, 351
–, bacterial increase in stored **2**, 356
–, fat spoilage in **2**, 373
–, formation of dimethylamine in **2**, 371
–, handling and stowage of **2**, 387–388
–, North sea, anaerobic bacteria isolated from **2**, 351
–, Norwegian winter, aerobic bacteria in **2**, 350
–, –, anaerobic bacteria isolated in **2**, 351
–, –, comparison in fresh and spoiling **2**, 353
–, rigor mortis in **2**, 365
–, Shetland, aerobic bacteria in **2**, 350
–, tests for quality of **2**, 380
–, tyrosine test for spoilage of **2**, 371–372
Herschel–Bulkley model **39**, 6, 34, 46
Hers' disease **37**, 378
Hertzian waves, *see* Radio waves
Hesperidin in oranges **2**, 260
Hevea rubber, local viscosity **38**, 192
Hexadecenoic acid in poultry fat **1**, 212
n-Hexadecyldimethylallylammonium bromide, germicidal activity of **2**, 137
n-Hexadecyldimethylethylammonium bromide, germicidal activity of **2**, 137
n-Hexadecyltrimethylammonium bromide, germicidal activity of **2**, 137
n-Hexaldehyde in apples **2**, 263
Hexamethylenetetramine **2**, 126
Hexamine, *N*-nitroso compounds and **31**, 54, 66
Hexanal, in frozen vegetables **17**, 6
n-Hexanal, in rancidity **23**, 2, 38
Hexane, extraction method, coalescence measurement **34**, 179–180
–, olive oil and **31**, 463
Hexanol, in black tea oil **2**, 287
–, in Formosan black tea oil **2**, 287
n-Hexanol alcohol, in apples **2**, 263
–, in strawberries **2**, 270
2-Hexeneal in apples **2**, 263
Hexenoic acid in Formosan black tea oil **2**, 287
a,B-Hexenol alcohol in black tea oil **2**, 33
B,y-Hexenol in black tea oil **2**, 28787
2-Hexen-1-ol in tea **2**, 288
3-Hexen-1-ol in tea **2**, 285
Hex II form, cardiolipin **37**, 271–273
Hexitidine **44**, 298
Hexobarbitone oxidase **15**, 37
Hexoic acid, in black tea oil **2**, 286
–, in cocoa **2**, 283
Hexokinase, in wheat germ **23**, 240
–, relationship to carbohydrate metabolism **1**, 131
Hexosamines, gelatin and **7**, 271–272
Hexose-P **41**, 122
Hexose diphosphate, formation during rigor mortis **1**, 5
Hexose monophosphate, acceleration of trimethylamine oxide reduction by **2**, 369
–, formation during breakdown of glycogen **1**, 4–6
Hexose-phosphate isomerase in wheat germ **23**, 240
Hexoses, reactivity **35**, 200
Hexose sugars, effect on browning in dehydrated potatoes **1**, 273–274
n-Hexyl alcohol in manufactured tea **2**, 286
Hexyl alcohol in tea **2**, 288
Hexylresorcinol, virucidal action of **2**, 138
Heyns rearrangement **14**, 207–208
HGPRT test system **34**, 395
High-calcium activated factor, endogenous proteolytic enzymes and **31**, 359
High-density lipoprotein, *see* HDL
High-performance liquid chromatography (HPLC) (*see also* Chromatography) **40**, 29, 60, 66, 72, 74
–, C-9–N-10 bond **33**, 34–38
–, chocolate and **31**, 221, 229
–, detection of eluted folates, electrochemical techniques **33**, 30–33
–, – of –, fluorescence **33**, 28–29
–, – of –, microbiological assays **33**, 29–30
–, – of –, UV absorbance **33**, 28
–, folates, chain length determination **33**, 34–38
–, inositol phosphates analysis **45**, 2, 5–6, 13, 41
–, ion-exchange, monoglutamyl folates **33**, 27–28
–, *N*-nitroso compounds and **31**, 67, 68, 89
–, reverse-phase, monoglutamyl folates **33**, 27–28

–, –, polyglutamyl folates as azo dye derivatives of *p*-aminobenzoyl(poly)glutamates **33**, 35
–, –, pteroyltriglutamate, diglutamate, and folic acid in conjugase assay **33**, 31
–, –, reduced folates **33**, 30
–, –, urinary folates, with UV absorbance **33**, 29
High-pressure multipiston homogenizers **34**, 169
High-protein foods **36**, 91
High-temperature/short-time products, packaging for **23**, 327
Hippocampus, modeling **40**, 333
Hippuricase in eggs **1**, 183
Hira-men **43**, 146
His⁻ mutation, Ames test **34**, 391–392
Hispanic immigrant, food selection by **32**, 262–263
Histaminase, role in histamine toxicity **24**, 144–145
Histamine **16**, 193
–, bacterial destruction of **24**, 128
–, bacteria responsible for formation of **24**, 122–124
–, cheese **39**, 234, 346
–, colorimetric assay of **24**, 133–134
–, defect action level **39**, 351–352
–, early reviews **24**, 120–121
–, –, symptomatology **24**, 114–115
–, –, synergists or potentiators of **24**, 142–146
–, enzymatic isotopic assay of **24**, 134
–, fish **39**, 337, 341–344, 346, 350–357
–, –, detection **24**, 130–135
–, –, spoilage **7**, 46–47, 50–51, 52
–, fluorometric assay of **24**, 130–131
–, gas–liquid chromatography of **24**, 133
–, guinea pig ileum contraction assay of **24**, 130–131
–, histidine as precursor of **24**, 124–125
–, in putrid abalone **23**, 166
–, occurrence of precursors, of **24**, 124
–, release reactions, non-IgE-mediated **42**, 10–11
–, scombroid toxicity and **24**, 139–140
–, thin-layer chromatography of **24**, 134–135
–, toxicity from, cases of **24**, 115–120
–, –, in fish **24**, 113–154
Histamine detoxification **39**, 330–331
Histamine-forming bacteria **39**, 331–336
Histamine phosphate **44**, 316
Histamine poisoning **39**, 290, 291, 337, 346–348; **42**, 10
Histidine, action of formaldehyde on **1**, 389
–, as histamine precursor **24**, 124–125
–, carcinogen risk assessment and **31**, 28
–, endogenous proteolytic enzymes and **31**, 352, 353, 355
–, separation from other amino acids **2**, 34
Histidine decarboxylases, carbohydrate effects on **24**, 127
–, fish **24**, 122
–, –, spoilage **7**, 47
–, oxygen tension effects on **24**, 127–128
–, pH effects on **24**, 126–127
–, temperature effects on **24**, 125–126
–, vitamin effects on **24**, 127
Histological changes in cellular adhesions **2**, 310–316
– in –, changes in chromoplasts of vegetable tissue by blanching **2**, 328–330
– in –, – in starch grain **2**, 316–328
– in –, – in –, effects of blanching **2**, 322, 328
– in –, – in –, – of milling **2**, 321–322
– in –, changes of vegetable tissue induced by processing technique **2**, 310–339
– in –, effect of chemicals **2**, 314–316
– in –, – of heat **2**, 310–314
– in –, low temperatures and food processing **2**, 333–338
– in –, structure of **2**, 316–318
– in –, texture **2**, 310
Histology, irregular bands **13**, 114–120
–, –, association **13**, 115–120
–, –, contracture band similarity **13**, 114–115
–, of normal vegetable tissue, cell types **2**, 298–306
–, –, contents of normal cells **2**, 306–307
–, PSE porcine musculature **13**, 107–120
–, structure **13**, 107–114
–, –, micro- **13**, 107–108
–, –, ultra- **13**, 108–114
Histones, endogenous proteolytic enzymes and **31**, 366
Histozyme in eggs **1**, 183
HIV infection, *see* Human immunodeficiency virus infection
HIV-therapeutic drugs, smell sensation effects **44**, 320
–, taste sensation effects **44**, 285–286
Hiya-mugi **43**, 146
Hock cleavage **33**, 279–380
Hodgkin–Huxley equations **40**, 331–332
Hofmeister effect, neutral salts **35**, 294–295
Hofmeister series **35**, 294–297
Hogs, butchered on the farm **6**, 123
–, carcasses of **6**, 149

Hogs (*cont'd*)
–, slaughter of **6**, 125
Hollow fiber **40**, 184
Hollow-fiber enzymatic reactor **38**, 52–53
–, loaded on lumen side of membrane **38**, 52–54
Holothurins, as marine toxins **18**, 157
Homocystinuria **37**, 397
Homogenization, of cheese **39**, 192
–, of milk **3**, 83
–, –, effect of sound waves on **3**, 131
–, –, iron supplementation **36**, 222
Homogenizers, *see* Colloid mills
Homogentisic acid oxidase deficiency **37**, 397
Homolinolenic acid, desaturation **35**, 39
Homolytic cleavage, hydroperoxides of polyunsaturated fatty acids **33**, 272–275
Homopolymer tailing method **36**, 141
Honey **14**, 237–238; **24**, 287–374
–, acids in **24**, 304–305
–, analysis and composition of **24**, 297–333
–, aroma of **24**, 331–332
–, carbohydrates in **24**, 299–304
–, color **24**, 332
–, –, specifications **5**, 315
–, consistency of **8**, 38
–, crystallization of **24**, 339–344
–, diabetic use of **24**, 353–354
–, enzymes in **24**, 312–330
–, fermentation in **24**, 351–352
–, flavor of **24**, 331
–, flow constants for **11**, 387
–, folklore of **24**, 354
–, harvesting in **24**, 293
–, hygroscopicity of **24**, 338–339
–, market forms of **24**, 295–297
–, melezitose crystallization from **24**, 343–344
–, minerals in **24**, 305, 354
–, moisture content of **24**, 298–299
–, nutritive value of **24**, 352–354
–, physical characteristics of **24**, 333–344
–, plant layout **24**, 295
–, pollination in **24**, 293
–, processing of **24**, 293–295
–, production and processing of **24**, 289–292
–, production methods for **24**, 292–293
–, proteins and amino acids in **24**, 305–312
–, pyrrolizidine alkaloids contamination **45**, 72, 91
–, quasi-properties of **8**, 10
–, research needs on **24**, 363–364
–, rheology of **24**, 333–335
–, standards and quality control of **24**, 358–363
–, storage changes in **24**, 344–352
–, thermal properties of **24**, 335–338
–, toxic constituents of **24**, 333
–, ultrasonic viscosity measurement **45**, 147
–, uses of **24**, 354–358
–, –, as food **24**, 354–357
–, –, as nonfood **24**, 357–358
–, vitamins in **24**, 332, 354
Hoof and mouth disease virus, destruction of by radio-frequency waves **3**, 133
Hookean body **39**, 7–8
Hooke's law **39**, 7
Hop residue **17**, 131
Hops, beer flavor and extracts of **19**, 235
C-Hordein **36**, 10000
Hordenine, *N*-nitroso compounds and **31**, 90
Hordeum chilense **45**, 256
Hormodendrum in bacon **3**, 298
Hormones **13**, 150–152
–, carcinogen risk assessment and **31**, 13, 18
–, chocolate and **31**, 321, 322, 327
–, Δ^6-desaturase, regulation effects **35**, 44–46
–, Δ^5-desaturase response **35**, 49–50
–, effects on cardiolipin content **37**, 300
–, endogenous proteolytic enzymes and **31**, 379, 383, 388, 389
–, in porcine stress syndrome **28**, 190–192
–, interaction with enzymes **10**, 7
Horse chestnut starch, gelatinization temperature of **2**, 319
Horse mackerel **39**, 344
Horse muscle, rigor in **9**, 20
Horseradish, volatile organic sulfur compounds **5**, 120
Horseradish peroxidase, acylated **35**, 270
Host specificity, adherence of probiotic cultures **37**, 75
Hot-bar scaling, of retort pouches **23**, 355–359
Housefly, toxicity of DDT to **2**, 208
Household composition **32**, 241–242
HPLC, *see* High-performance liquid chromatography
HPLC-mass spectrometry, phytoestrogens **44**, 201, 202
Human immunodeficiency virus infection **37**, 34
–, effects of hydrogen peroxide-producing *Lactobacillus acidophilis* **37**, 114
–, enteric pathogens in **37**, 34
Human milk, calcium content **36**, 214–215
–, chromium content **36**, 237

–, copper concentration **36**, 228–229
–, fluoride content **36**, 238
–, iodine content **36**, 234
–, iron content **36**, 221–224
–, magnesium content **36**, 219
–, manganese in **36**, 230–231
–, mineral and trace element content **36**, 211–212
–, minerals and trace elements **36**, 239
–, molybdenum content **36**, 236
–, phosphorus content **36**, 220
–, selenium content **36**, 232–233
–, zinc concentration **36**, 226–227
Humans, essentiality of *n*-3 PUFA **35**, 113–115, 151–153
Human spongiform encephalopathies **43**, 280–285
–, transmission **43**, 280
Human subject, bioperiodicity **40**, 225
–, β-carotene metabolism **40**, 29–32, 62–67
–, energy metabolism **40**, 176, 178
–, folate metabolism **40**, 86–90
–, total energy expenditure **40**, 171–180
–, transthyretin metabolism **40**, 150–154
–, vitamin B6 metabolism **40**, 115, 121, 145
Humectant **39**, 84, 85, 126–127
Humidity, chocolate and, milk **31**, 260
–, –, packaging **31**, 317, 318
–, –, processing **31**, 239, 240, 244
–, –, refining **31**, 295
–, –, sweeteners **31**, 264–269, 272
–, control **7**, 88–92
–, –, equilibrium rate and **7**, 90–91
–, –, temperature and **7**, 91
–, effects on disease spread **15**, 169
–, – on enzyme inactivation temperatures in low-moisture foods **11**, 314–316
–, – on enzymic reactions in low-moisture foods **11**, 314–316
–, – on meat emulsions **16**, 143
–, – on spray-drying **2**, 496–591
–, olive oil and **31**, 470
–, solutions and **7**, 86
Humin formation of during acid hydrolysis of zein **3**, 272
Humin nitrogen in fruit products, relation to browning **1**, 352
Humoral immunity, effects of lactic cultures **37**, 107–110
–, gut **37**, 15–19
Hunter color meter **9**, 168–169
Hurdle, microbial control **39**, 122–123
HVP, *see* Hydrolyzed vegetable proteins
Hyaluronate synthesis, in Marfan syndrome **37**, 396
Hyamine 1622, germicidal effect of **2**, 183
Hybridization, carcinogen risk assessment and **31**, 26
Hydrates, gas **13**, 229–234
–, host water cages **13**, 231
–, properties **13**, 233
Hydration, of proteins in muscle **9**, 32–35
–, of whey proteins **33**, 373–374
Hydration force, emulsion stability **34**, 94–95
Hydrazine, *N*-nitroso compounds and **31**, 56
Hydrobromide **44**, 298
Hydrocarbons, contribution to meat flavor **18**, 52
–, in celery seed oil **2**, 271
–, in coffee **2**, 281
–, measurement for vitamin E status **33**, 191
–, olive oil and **31**, 466, 467, 470
Hydrocarbon/water interface, protein adsorption **34**, 121
Hydrochloric acid, addition to milk **2**, 21
–, chocolate and **31**, 229
–, dietary fiber and **31**, 164
–, effect on adhesive properties of pea coats **2**, 315
–, – on saltiness sensation **2**, 260
–, rate of diffusion of **2**, 9
–, separation of acids from exchanger by **2**, 34
–, use in treating anion exchange **2**, 17
Hydrochloride of parsley oil **2**, 273
Hydrochlorothiazide **44**, 305, 307
Hydrocolloids, as emulsifiers **22**, 341
–, chocolate and **31**, 273
–, creaming and **34**, 132–133
Hydrocortisone **44**, 296
Hydrocyanic acid, inactivation of disulfide enzymes by **1**, 382–383
–, inhibition of oxidation by **3**, 30
–, interference with prosthetic groups of the enzymes by **1**, 384
Hydrogen **12**, 123
–, dietary fiber and **31**, 161, 162
–, in exchange reactions **2**, 8, 9, 11
–, inhibition of enzymes by **1**, 384
–, olive oil and **31**, 471, 472
Hydrogenation, chocolate and **31**, 278, 284
–, effect on tocopherol content of vegetable oils **33**, 163
Hydrogen bonding, dicotyledonous plants **31**, 126–128
–, dietary fiber and **31**, 122, 187
–, gelation and **7**, 308

Hydrogen bonding (*cont'd*)
–, properties **31**, 158, 163
Hydrogen bonds, protein stability **35**, 252–253
Hydrogen evolution test for corrosion in tin plate **3**, 367–370
Hydrogen ion, association with sour taste **2**, 260
Hydrogen peroxide, as substrate **17**, 16
–, control **33**, 303
–, enzymic production of **17**, 13–14, 17, 26
–, formation **33**, 237
–, in enzyme temperature experiment **3**, 28
–, in enzymic browning **3**, 8, 9
–, inhibition of soybean lipoxygenase **33**, 307
–, in oxidation of pyrogallol **3**, 22
–, – of –, of substrate **3**, 18, 19
–, oxidation of sulfhydryl enzymes by **1**, 381
Hydrogen peroxide sanitization **45**, 189
–, ozone combined procedures **45**, 200–201
Hydrogen peroxide sterilization **32**, 18–19, 24–25, 27–30
Hydrogen sulfide **16**, 195, 276, 367
–, adsorption by anion exchanger **2**, 38
–, chlorine demand and **7**, 142
–, contribution to meat flavor **18**, 56–58
–, green discoloration and **7**, 57
–, inactivation of disulfide enzymes by **1**, 382
–, in coffee **2**, 281, 283
–, in "putrid" fish **2**, 372
–, interference with prosthetic groups of the enzymes by **1**, 384
–, release of, during meat heating **24**, 64–69
Hydrolases, in wheat germ **23**, 241
Hydrolok continuous retort system **23**, 395–397
Hydrolysis **39**, 271
–, chocolate and, alkalization **31**, 247
–, –, cocoa butter **31**, 252, 279
–, –, milk **31**, 263
–, –, processing **31**, 220
–, –, sweeteners **31**, 269, 270
–, dietary fiber and **31**, 118, 138, 141
–, –, analysis **31**, 142, 143, 145, 146, 150, 151, 153
–, –, dicotyledonous plants **31**, 126, 127, 130–132
–, –, properties **31**, 155, 169, 170
–, endogenous proteolytic enzymes and **31**, 344, 414
–, –, endopeptidases **31**, 352, 354, 361, 363
–, –, exopeptidases **31**, 346–349
–, –, meat technology **31**, 404, 408, 410
–, –, muscle physiology **31**, 374, 375, 378
–, –, proteinase activity **31**, 386
–, in softening pickles **2**, 315
–, in starch grains on killing plant **2**, 309
–, lactose, chemical reactor **38**, 45–46
–, –, in milk **38**, 10–12
–, olive oil and **31**, 467, 471
–, partial, protein emulsifier modification **34**, 159–160
–, peptide bond, measurement **35**, 223
–, reverse, versus transgalactosylation **38**, 61–64
–, starch grains resistance to **2**, 321
–, thermal inactivation **35**, 247
–, whey, immobilized lactase reactors **38**, 46–47
Hydrolytic rancidity in dry milk **3**, 93
Hydrolyzed proteins, idiosyncratic reactions **42**, 31
Hydrolyzed vegetable proteins (HVP), artificial meat flavor and **30**, 106–109
–, –, cystine and cysteine role **30**, 106, 109
–, heating with reducing sugars **30**, 106–109
Hydromorphone **44**, 296, 323
Hydropac system, for retort packaging **23**, 342
–, –, diagram **23**, 343
Hydroperoxides, decomposition of **17**, 28–30
–, formation of **17**, 31
–, of linolenate **17**, 29–30
–, olive oil and **31**, 471, 472
Hydroperoxy bis-epidioxide, from polyunsaturated fatty acid oxidation **33**, 276–277
Hydroperoxy cyclic peroxides, from polyunsaturated fatty acid oxidation **33**, 276–277
–, linolenate, breakdown mechanism **33**, 277
Hydroperoxyeicosatetraenoic acids **35**, 101, 104
Hydrophile–lipophile balance (HLB), applications of **22**, 331–332
–, limitations of **22**, 332
–, of emulsifiers **22**, 319–321
–, small-molecule emulsifiers **34**, 99–100
Hydrophobic amino acids, thermal stability **35**, 261–262
Hydrophobic cluster analysis **41**, 68–72
Hydrophobic groups, covalent attachment, protein emulsifier modification **34**, 156
Hydrophobic index **35**, 258–260
Hydrophobic interactions, proteins **35**, 239–240
–, –, stability **35**, 257–266
–, salt effects **35**, 296

Hydrophobicity, average **36**, 8–10
–, effects on whey proteins, emulsifying properties **33**, 406–408
–, – on –, functional properties **33**, 369
–, surface **34**, 33–34; **36**, 11–12
–, wheat proteins **36**, 7
Hydrophobic ligands, protein emulsifier modification **34**, 160–162
Hydrophobic moment **42**, 101–102
Hydroquinone, as antioxidant **3**, 201
–, –, effect on growth **3**, 203
–, –, – on mortality of rats **3**, 206
–, –, – on tallowiness in dried milk **3**, 95
–, –, pathologic effects of **3**, 207
–, in coffee **2**, 279
Hydrostatic pressure in plants, effect on diffusion pressure **2**, 308
Hydrosulfites, gelatin manufacture and **7**, 248
Hydroxy amino acids, gelatin and **7**, 263
Hydroxybenzoate, microbial inhibition by **1**, 386
Hydroxy α-carotene **15**, 218
Hydroxycinnamate, as food toxicant **27**, 167–170
Hydroxycobalamin, reaction with sulfites **30**, 24
Hydroxyeicosatetraenoic acids **35**, 101, 104
Hydroxyethylcellulose (HEC) **12**, 328–329
4-Hydroxy-3-furanones, shoyu flavor and **30**, 272–277
Hydroxyfurfuraldehyde in rye bread **2**, 276
Hydroxylamine, effect on browning in dehydrated potatoes **1**, 272
–, fish preservation and **7**, 69
–, inhibition of enzymes by **1**, 384
Hydroxylation, meat mutagens **34**, 408–409
–, *N*-nitroso compounds and **31**, 65
Hydroxyl groups, chocolate and **31**, 290
Hydroxyl radical, formation **33**, 236
–, scavengers, control of lipid oxidation with **33**, 303
o-Hydroxymethylbenzoate in manufactured tea **2**, 286
Hydroxymethylfurfural, end products of **6**, 17
–, in honey **24**, 345–349
5-Hydroxymethylfurfural **32**, 163
4α-Hydroxy-5-methyl-tetrahydrofolate, structure **33**, 46
4-Hydroxy-2(or 5)-ethyl-5(or 2)-methyl-3(2H)-furanone (HEMF), shoyu flavor and **30**, 273, 275, 276, 287
Hydroxyproline **14**, 117–119
–, dietary fiber and **31**, 123, 126, 129, 132
–, endogenous proteolytic enzymes and **31**, 349
–, gelatin structure and **7**, 268–270
–, *N*-nitroso compounds and **31**, 76
β-Hydroxypropanthial, structure of **22**, 97
Hydroxypropyl methylcellulose **12**, 314–328
–, composite edible films based on **44**, 351, 352–356, 358
–, –, applications **44**, 370
–, –, gas permeability **44**, 365
–, –, relative humidity effects **44**, 363
–, –, solute barrier properties **44**, 368, 369
–, –, temperature effects **44**, 364, 369
Hydroxyquinone, formation of in fruit products **3**, 20–22
Hyoscamine **44**, 298, 299
Hypercholesterolemia, dietary fiber and **31**, 160, 167, 168, 190
Hyperexia, malignant **37**, 386–387, 408
Hyperglycemia, dietary fiber and **31**, 167
Hyperglycemic agents, taste sensation effects **44**, 307
Hyperkalemic periodic paralysis **37**, 385–386
Hyperlipidemia **35**, 4–5
Hypersensitivities, delayed-type **37**, 19–21, 29
–, food-related, classification **37**, 26
–, nonreaginic **37**, 28–29
–, reaginic **37**, 27–28
Hyperthermia, malignant **37**, 386–387
Hyperthyroidism, cardiolipin content **37**, 301
–, cardiolipin fatty acyl composition **37**, 297–298
Hypertrophy, muscle **37**, 363–364
Hyperuricemia, after xylitol infusion **25**, 172–173
Hypnotics, taste sensation effects **44**, 307–308
Hypobaric storage **21**, 340
Hypochlorites, plant chlorination and **7**, 147
–, production of **7**, 146
–, sanitization **45**, 169–170
–, stabilization **7**, 146
Hypochlorous acid, germicidal activity and **7**, 135, 136
Hypogeusia (*see also* Taste perception) **44**, 249
–, elderly people **44**, 256
Hypoglycemia, dietary fiber and **31**, 168
–, relation to appetite **1**, 131
Hypoglycemic agents, taste sensation effects **44**, 307
Hypokalemic periodic paralysis **37**, 384–385
Hypophosphites, effect on appetite **1**, 133

Hypophysectomy, effect on rats **1**, 122
Hyposmia (*see also* Smell perception) **44**, 249
Hypotension, reaction to sulfites **30**, 47, 58
Hypothalamus, relation to appetite **1**, 137
Hypoxanthine **14**, 122
–, formation from adenosine triphosphate **1**, 10
Hysteresis loop **39**, 9, 57

Ibogaine, glenodinine and **18**, 158
Ibuprofen **44**, 296
Ice, and deterioration **13**, 311–313
–, and water **13**, 221–235, 238–244
–, antibiotic, carrageenan in **11**, 133
–, crystal(s), effect on fruit **13**, 330
–, –, growth **13**, 247–252, 260
–, –, size **13**, 252–253
–, evaporation from **7**, 190–191
–, formation of, in frozen fruits and vegetables **25**, 183–193
–, phase diagram **27**, 302–307
–, physical characteristics **27**, 302
–, structure **13**, 221–235; **27**, 301–302
–, –, half-hydrogen **13**, 224–225
–, –, hydrogen bonded **13**, 224–226
–, tetrahedral coordination of water molecules in **11**, 363, 364
Ice cream, alginates in stabilization **11**, 145
–, carrageenan in stabilization **11**, 131–132
–, gelatin and **7**, 325
–, guar gum in stabilization **11**, 168
–, gum karaya in **11**, 187
–, gum tragacanth in **11**, 184
–, lactase in **38**, 13–15
–, locust bean gum in stabilization **11**, 162
–, sterile cocoa for use in **8**, 278
–, use of ascorbic acid in **4**, 402–403
Ice cream bar, flow diagram for manufacturing **4**, 65
–, flow process chart for making **4**, 52
Ice cream mix, composition requirements for **3**, 91
–, deteriorative changes in **3**, 92
–, effect of sound waves on **3**, 131
–, – of ultraviolet radiation on **3**, 151
–, military specifications for **3**, 91, 92
–, moisture content of **3**, 92
–, problems in manufacture of **3**, 91, 92
–, spray-dried **3**, 85
Ice cream powder, use of Bishop spray dryer for **2**, 410
–, – of Swenson dryer for **2**, 420
Ice–liquid separators, for aroma recovery in freeze concentration **20**, 43
Ices, alginates in **11**, 147
–, gum karaya in **11**, 187
–, gum tragacanth in **11**, 184
Ichthyocol, "parent gelatin" and **7**, 260
Icing, alginates in **11**, 151
–, –, furcellaran in **11**, 159
–, gelatin and **7**, 324
IDEA digestibility, compared with rate bioassays **35**, 223–224
Identifiability, conditional **40**, 314
–, global **40**, 313
–, interval **40**, 314
–, local **40**, 313, 318–320
–, quasi **40**, 314
–, structural **40**, 313
Identifiability problem **40**, 305–321
–, background information **40**, 305–310
–, checking methods **40**, 314–317
–, –, linear systems **40**, 315–317
–, –, nonlinear systems **40**, 317
–, classification of identifiability **40**, 313–314
–, – of parameters **40**, 310–311
–, correlations **40**, 320
–, estimation problem, compared to **40**, 311–312
–, nutrient-response analysis **40**, 235, 240
–, population kinetics **40**, 276–277
–, single point **40**, 318–320
Identifiable parameter **40**, 311
IDENT software **40**, 318
Idiosyncratic food/food additive reactions **43**, 201
Idiosyncratic reactions **42**, 12–13
–, MSG **42**, 30–31
IDL, *see* Lipoprotein
Idoxuridine **44**, 300
IgE antibodies, carmine **43**, 203, 204, 205–206
–, immediate hypersensitivity reactions **43**, 198, 199
–, saffron **43**, 212
IgE-mediated allergic reactions **42**, 4–8, 26–27
Ileostomy, dietary fiber and **31**, 169, 170, 173, 178
5-Iminodaunomycin, cardiolipin association **37**, 288
Imipenem-cilastatin **44**, 291
Imipramine **44**, 311
IM meat, *see* Dehydration control, IM meat
Immediate hypersensitivity reactions **43**, 197, 198–199

–, anaphylactic shock **43**, 199
–, mechanisms **43**, 198–199, 200
–, symptoms **43**, 199
Immobilization, protein stability **35**, 276–277
Immobilized digestive enzyme assay, protein digestibility **35**, 222–225
Immune cells, *n*-3 PUFA effects **35**, 109–111
Immune function **40**, 58
–, *n*-3 PUFA **35**, 146–148
Immune response, cell-mediated **37**, 19–21
–, common mucosal immune system **37**, 21
–, effect of foodborne chemicals **37**, 41–43
–, – of microbes and microbial products **37**, 35–40
–, gastrointestinal tract antigen uptake **37**, 12–15
–, gut-associated lymphoid tissue **37**, 10–12
–, humoral responses **37**, 15–19
–, immunocompetent cells **37**, 8–10
–, modification, food antigens/allergens **37**, 46
–, –, hypoallergenic foods **37**, 47
–, –, microbial flora control **37**, 50
–, –, nutritional therapies **37**, 51–52
–, –, oral tolerance induction **37**, 50–51
–, –, role of breast-feeding **37**, 45
–, nonspecific **37**, 4–6
–, nutritional effects **37**, 44–45
–, oral tolerance **37**, 22
–, research needs **37**, 53–56
–, specific **37**, 6–8
–, stimulation of specific immunity **37**, 21–22
Immune surveillance, in intestinal cancer **37**, 24–25
Immune system, carcinogen risk assessment and **31**, 24, 44, 45, 48
–, common mucosal **37**, 21
–, inulin effects **43**, 41–42
–, leukotriene effects **35**, 104
–, stimulation with lactic cultures **37**, 107–110, 120
Immunoassays, meat/poultry endpoint cooking temperature indicators **44**, 173–175
Immunoelectrophoresis **16**, 362
Immunoglobulins, chocolate and **31**, 255, 261
–, IgA, adjuvants for gut responses **37**, 22
–, –, deficiency, selective **37**, 33–34
–, –, induction by oral immunization **37**, 21–22
–, –, related hephropathy **37**, 33, 35, 40
–, –, secretory, malnutrition effects **37**, 44
–, –, –, structure and functions **37**, 17–18
–, –, structure and functions **37**, 16–17
–, IgE, functions **37**, 18–19
–, IgG, functions **37**, 19
–, IgM, functions **37**, 19
–, isotypes **37**, 16–17
–, properties, table **37**, 17
–, F_c region **37**, 16
–, structure **33**, 357–358; **37**, 15–16
Immunology, endogenous proteolytic enzymes and **31**, 360
Immunostimulation, ingested bacteria **37**, 49–50
Immunosuppression, gastrointestinal immune system **37**, 33–34
–, nutritional therapies **37**, 51–52
Immunosuppressive agents, taste sensation effects **44**, 293–294
Immunotoxicity, ingested chemicals **37**, 41–43
Impedance testing **32**, 15
Impulse process, isolation of lipid–protein complexes **17**, 104
Incaparina **16**, 63; **17**, 110
–, use in developing South-American countries **22**, 197–198
Incap mixtures **16**, 40, 48, 64
Incidence matrix, graph theory **40**, 342–347
Income, effect on food selection **32**, 265–266
Indalone, solubility of DDT in **2**, 203
Indanyl sodium **44**, 289
India, annual agricultural and forestry harvest **32**, 193
–, annual biomass production **32**, 192
–, biomass energy used **32**, 191
–, biomass resources **32**, 194–195
–, consumption of commercial energy **32**, 190
–, forest utilization **32**, 194
–, gross national product **32**, 189
–, land distribution by use **32**, 190
–, soil erosion in **32**, 216–221
Indian childhood cirrhosis **45**, 79
Indian paint brush (*Castellija*) **45**, 77
Indian Warrior (*Pedicularis*) **45**, 77
Indicators, fecal **13**, 349–350, 358–360, 382
–, low growth temperature **13**, 359–360
Indicine *N*-oxide **45**, 66, 67, 88
Indinavir **44**, 285
Indirect calorimetry **40**, 171, 172, 178–179
Indole **16**, 173ff
Indoleacetic acid **15**, 85, 128
Indole in "putrid" fish **2**, 348, 372
Indomethacin, cancer and **35**, 145
Indonesia, IM meat **39**, 75, 89, 119, 136

Induced-current mode, in scanning electron microscopy **22**, 216–217
Industrial chemicals, from corn wet milling **38**, 295
Industrial engineering in food industry **4**, 38–43
Industrial exposure, carcinogen risk assessment and **31**, 19, 20
Industrial processes, high temperature **35**, 238
Infant formula, artificial, calcium/phosphorus ratio **36**, 220
–, iodine in **36**, 234
–, iron fortification **36**, 224–225
–, manganese in **36**, 231
–, selenium content **36**, 233
–, whey proteins and **33**, 422–423
–, zinc supplementation **36**, 228
Infection-prevention tests for quaternary ammonium compounds **2**, 164
Inflammation, *n*-3 PUFA effects **35**, 139–143
Inflammatory bowel disease **37**, 31–32
Inflammatory myopathies **37**, 362
Influenza virus, effect of quaternary ammonium compounds on **2**, 138
Infradian rhythm (*see also* Bioperiodicity) **40**, 219, 225, 226
Infrared, freeze-drying and **7**, 182, 209, 217
Infrared imaging, microwave temperature measurements **43**, 84
Infrared radiation **3**, 126, 146–147
Infrared scanning, for flexible-package seal defects **23**, 407–409
Infusion **39**, 112
Inherited myoclonus **37**, 373
Inhibition, lactase **38**, 42–43
–, *N*-nitroso compounds and **31**, 60–64
–, transgalactosylase activity of lactases **38**, 82–83
Inhibitors, endogenous proteolytic enzymes and **31**, 383–385
–, enzyme **17**, 51–53
–, water requirements and **7**, 110
Initial value problem (*see also* Differential equation) **40**, 284, 325
Initiation, olive oil and **31**, 471, 472
Initiators, carcinogen risk assessment and **31**, 28
Injury, carbon dioxide **12**, 113–114
–, –, external **12**, 113
–, –, low-temperature **12**, 114
Inorganic constituents in citrus fruits **9**, 313–315
Inositol, content of apples **8**, 314
–, in cocoa beans **8**, 262
–, in tea **17**, 225
Inositol hexakisphosphate (InsPU6u; phytate) **45**, 1–2
–, analytical methods **45**, 4–5
–, anticancer activity **45**, 37, 38–39
–, antioxidant activity **45**, 23, 39
–, –, food preservative effects **45**, 39–40
–, blood glucose-lowering effects **45**, 40
–, cholesterol/triglyceride-lowering effects **45**, 40
–, degradation **45**, 8–12
–, –, digestive processes **45**, 9, 24
–, –, food processing/preparation **45**, 9, 16
–, –, thermal **45**, 12
–, extraction during seed processing **45**, 13
–, functions in animal tissues **45**, 30–31
–, – in –, calcium flux regulation **45**, 30–31
–, – in –, DNA repair **45**, 31
–, – in –, nuclear mRNA export **45**, 31
–, high-performance liquid chromatography (HPLC) **45**, 5, 6
–, mineral absorption impairment **45**, 2, 32–33
–, –, iron **45**, 32, 33–34, 40–41
–, optimal dietary levels **45**, 42
–, seed content, processed foods **45**, 16–22
–, –, reduction strategies **45**, 34–35
–, –, whole raw seeds **45**, 12–15
–, synthetic pathway **45**, 7–8
Inositol kinases **45**, 7, 8, 31–32
Inositol phosphate phosphatases **45**, 11, 12
Inositol phosphates **45**, 1–43
–, analytical methods **45**, 4–6
–, animals **45**, 23–32
–, –, absorption **45**, 23–25
–, –, biological functions **45**, 27–32
–, –, tissue content **45**, 26–27
–, anticancer activity **45**, 37, 38–39
–, antioxidant activity **45**, 23, 28, 29, 30, 39
–, calcium mobilisation **45**, 27–28, 29, 30–31
–, chemistry **45**, 2–6
–, chloride channel regulation **45**, 29
–, degradation **45**, 8–12
–, –, breadmaking processes **45**, 16, 20
–, –, digestive processes **45**, 9, 24
–, hemoglobin oxygen affinity regulation **45**, 30
–, iron binding **45**, 28–29, 30
–, malting **45**, 22
–, –, fruit/vegetable content **45**, 22–23
–, metabolism **45**, 7–12
–, nomenclature **45**, 2–3
–, nutritional importance **45**, 32–41, 42

–, –, health disorders prevention **45**, 36–41
–, –, mineral bioavailability influence **45**, 32–36, 42
–, –, receptors **45**, 27, 28
–, seed contents **45**, 12–23
–, –, processed foods **45**, 16–22
–, –, whole raw seeds **45**, 12–15
–, signaling activities **45**, 7, 27, 28, 29
–, synthesis **45**, 7–8
–, –, animal cells **45**, 7–8
–, –, micro-organisms **45**, 7
–, –, plants **45**, 8
Inositol pyrophosphates **45**, 31
Inositol(1,4,5)trisphosphate (Ins(1,4,5)PU3u) **45**, 5, 7
–, animal cells **45**, 26
–, receptors (calcium channels) **45**, 27–28
–, signaling function **45**, 27–28
–, –, plant cells **45**, 23
Inositol(1,2,6)trisphosphate (α-trinositol) **45**, 28, 40
Insecticides, vegetables and **7**, 24
Insects **15**, 289
–, attacking stored food products, life history and development **4**, 299–305
–, attacking stored foods, classification **4**, 284–298
–, –, definition **4**, 283–284
–, –, effect of temperature **4**, 333–339
–, –, food requirements **4**, 328–333
–, attacking stored products **4**, 281–358
–, destruction of, in grain **3**, 134–136
–, –, in packaged foods **3**, 145
–, effect of DDT on **2**, 206
–, infesting foods, as cause of heating **4**, 339–342
–, infesting stored foods, moisture content as factor **4**, 317–325
–, radiation disinfestation of **24**, 199–200
Insensible parameter **40**, 311, 319
"Instant" spray dryer, operation of **2**, 410–412, 474
Instrumentation, rheology **39**, 23–33
Instruments, odor **14**, 5–24, 26
Insulation, inefficiency **12**, 152–153
–, leakage **12**, 157–160
–, materials **12**, 153–157
–, –, cork **12**, 153
–, –, expanded **12**, 155–157
–, –, foamed plastics **12**, 156–157
–, –, mineral wool **12**, 155
–, –, rigid foams **12**, 157
–, ship fibrous **12**, 160
–, technique **12**, 153–154
Insulin, biological activity of **1**, 383
–, chocolate and **31**, 267
–, desaturase activity effects **35**, 44
–, Δ^5-desaturase effect **35**, 50
–, dietary fiber and **31**, 166, 169
–, effect on appetite **1**, 123
–, endogenous proteolytic enzymes and, endopeptidases **31**, 357, 360, 361
–, –, muscle physiology **31**, 375
–, –, proteinase activity **31**, 389
–, receptor, *n*-3 PUFA effects **35**, 132
Intakes, calcium, long term **33**, 112
–, –, table of **33**, 106
–, –, within groups **33**, 105–106
–, folates, recommended **33**, 52
–, tocopherols **33**, 166–168
–, vitamin D, calcium absorption and **33**, 115–116
Integrator, linear, *see* Linear integrator
Intercellular air in plant matter, effect of blanching on **2**, 330–333
Intercellular spaces in plant tissue **2**, 309
– in –, formation of ice crystals in during freezing **2**, 336
Intercellular substances in plants, effect of cooking potato on **2**, 311, 315
Interfacial properties, pressure, proteins **34**, 123
–, proteins **34**, 110–111
–, surfactants **34**, 104–106
Interfacial rheology, protein films **34**, 124–126
Interfacial tension **34**, 4–6
–, oil/water, microemulsions **34**, 163
–, water–hydrocarbon **34**, 5–6
Interferons **44**, 294, 300
Intermediate-moisture meat, *see* Dehydration control, IM meat
Intermedine **45**, 71, 72, 75, 77
Internal burst test, for seal integrity in flexible packaging **23**, 349–350
Internal phase ratio **34**, 84–85
International Agency for Research on Cancer, carcinogen risk assessment and **31**, 10–12, 25, 34, 35
– on –, *N*-nitroso compounds and **31**, 56
International Olive Oil Council **31**, 474–476
Interpenetrating polymer network, mixed protein gels **34**, 263
Interstitial lung disease **37**, 402–403
Interstitial retinol-binding protein, role in tocopherol binding and transport **33**, 194
Intestinal diseases, nutritional therapies **37**, 51

Intestinal microflora, beneficial health effects **43**, 10–11, 12
–, breastfed infants **43**, 12
–, exogenous/endogenous modifiers **43**, 13
–, impact of antibiotics **43**, 13
–, modification, prebiotics **43**, 16, 17
–, –, probiotics **43**, 15–16, 17
–, –, synbiotics **43**, 16, 17
–, pathogenic bacteria **43**, 12, 13–14
–, toxic metabolites/carcinogens **43**, 13, 35, 36
Intestinal tract cancer **37**, 24–25
Intestines, adherence of probiotic cultures **37**, 74–77
–, calcium absorption, dietary requirements and **33**, 118–119
–, –, during development **33**, 117–118
–, –, effects of, fiber and phytate **33**, 134–142
–, –, –, oxalic acid **33**, 142
–, –, lactose effect, *see* Lactose effect
–, –, regulation **33**, 114–117
–, β-carotene **40**, 49
–, folate **40**, 82, 201
–, folate absorption **33**, 53–57
–, –, age effects **33**, 68–69
–, –, altered gastrointestinal function and **33**, 67–68
–, –, conjugases and **33**, 55–56
–, –, deconjugation of dietary polyglutamyl folate **33**, 54–55
–, –, dietary components and **33**, 71–72
–, –, ethanol ingestion effects **33**, 69–70
–, –, folate-binding protein in jejunal brush border membrane **33**, 54
–, –, pH dependence **33**, 53–54
–, –, pH effects **33**, 67
–, –, K_m transport values **33**, 53
–, membrane transport **40**, 245–251, 255–257, 259
–, membrane vesicle **40**, 198–199
–, pteroylpolyglutamate hydrolases **33**, 55–56
–, tocopherol absorption, destruction effects **33**, 169–170
–, –, efficiency **33**, 168–171
–, –, mechanism **33**, 168–171
–, –, via lymphatic system **33**, 168–169
–, vitamin A **40**, 9, 11, 19
–, vitamin B6 **40**, 109–110, 115, 121
Intolerance (*see also* Food allergies and intolerance), cow's milk protein **37**, 30–31
–, food **37**, 25–26
–, gluten **37**, 29–30
–, lactose **37**, 79–84
–, research needs **37**, 118
Intradisulfide bonds, amino acid sequences around cysteine residues **36**, 119–120
Intrinsic viscosity **39**, 116
Inula helenium (elecampane), inulin **43**, 3, 6, 40
Inulin **43**, 1–51
–, anticancer activity **43**, 34, 37
–, bifidogenic properties **43**, 10–26
–, biosynthesis **43**, 3, 5
–, calorific value **43**, 28
–, characteristics **43**, 3–6
–, –, functional **43**, 45–46
–, dental health **43**, 43
–, diabetes mellitus **43**, 39–41
–, dietary supplementation, applications **43**, 18
–, –, intestinal microflora response **43**, 16, 19
–, estrogen recyling enhacement **43**, 44
–, fermentation products **43**, 23–26
–, –, carbon dioxide/hydrogen gas **43**, 23, 25, 26
–, –, short-chain fatty acids **43**, 24–26, 32
–, food applications **43**, 45–46
–, food sources **43**, 6, 7, 8, 9
–, functions in plants **43**, 6
–, gastrointestinal health benefit **43**, 42–43
–, gastrointestinal side effects **43**, 42–43, 46–47
–, glucose absorption influence **43**, 26
–, heart disease **43**, 41
–, historical background **43**, 6–8
–, immune system effects **43**, 41–42
–, intake **43**, 8
–, intestinal/hepatic enzyme responses **43**, 22–23
–, legal/regulatory status **43**, 48
–, lipid metabolism effects **43**, 28–32, 41
–, mineral metabolism effects **43**, 32–34
–, nutritional labeling **43**, 48–50
–, origin **43**, 6
–, osteoporosis prevention **43**, 43–44
–, prebiotic substrate **43**, 18, 20, 21, 22
–, production **43**, 8–10, 11
–, safety/tolerance **43**, 46–47
–, soluble dietary fiber properties **43**, 26–27
–, structural aspects **43**, 3, 4, 5
Invertase **17**, 198
–, in fruits **17**, 184
–, in honey **24**, 313–321
–, of yeast cells **1**, 389
–, used to develop fluidity in candies **6**, 36
Invertebrates, aquatic, consumption of **20**, 194

In vitro mutagenicity tests, Ames test **34**, 390–392
–, diphtheria toxin resistance assay **34**, 392, 395
–, DNA damage, cultured mammalian cells **34**, 396–397
–, HGPRT test system **34**, 395
–, mammalian cell culture mutagenicity tests **34**, 392–396
–, ouabain resistance assay **34**, 395–396
In vivo mutagenicity tests **34**, 397–399
Iodide, in musts and wines **8**, 152
Iodination **40**, 8
Iodine, as impregnant for wrapping of fruit **3**, 464–465
–, deficiency **36**, 233–234
–, estimation of fish freshness and **7**, 63
–, radioactive **3**, 156
–, RDAs **36**, 234
–, therapeutic action of **2**, 144
Iodine content of plants, deficiency **1**, 121
– of –, effect of fertilizers on **1**, 314
– of –, inhibition of enzymes by **1**, 383
Iodine–iodide titration method, for estimating high-molecular quaternary ammonium compounds **2**, 170
–, for testing for starch conversion **2**, 323
Iodine sanitizers **14**, 439–440
Iodoacetate, inhibition of enzymes by **1**, 382
Iodoform test, on apples **2**, 263
–, on raspberries **2**, 269
–, on strawberries **2**, 270
Iodosobenzoate in heat treatment of milk serum protein **3**, 82
Iohexol **44**, 316
Ion, in muscle, and meat quality **26**, 87
Ionac A-300, stability of **2**, 8
Ion exchange, controlling factors in reactions **2**, 8–13
–, effects of concentration on cations **2**, 10
–, electrical charge and radius of ions **2**, 9–10
–, equilibrium concentrations **2**, 11
–, flow rate in **2**, 11
–, pilot plant, operation of **2**, 13–14
–, rate of diffusion in **2**, 8–9
–, temperature effects **2**, 11
–, wine deacidification by **25**, 23–25
Ion-exchange chromatography, monoglutamyl folates **33**, 26
–, polyglutamyl folates **33**, 33–34
–, whey protein preparation **33**, 361
Ion-exchange resins, gelatin degradation and **7**, 318–320
–, gelatin manufacture and **7**, 248–249
Ion exchangers, analytical type **2**, 38
–, catalysts for **2**, 36
–, concentration and separation with **2**, 35–36
–, fractionation with **2**, 33–35
–, laboratory uses of **2**, 33
–, purification of **2**, 37
–, size of organic cations for **2**, 11
Ionic strength, effects on enzymes **17**, 47–48
–, – on foaming properties of whey proteins **33**, 403
–, heat treatment of whey proteins **33**, 376–378
Ionic yield **15**, 59
Ionization, freeze-drying and **7**, 184
Ionizing radiation (*see also* γ-Radiation) **15**, 119, 147ff
–, effect on flat sour bacteria spores **18**, 186–187
β-Ionone, role in off-flavors **17**, 6
B-Ionone in raspberries **2**, 209
Ionophores, cardiolipin **37**, 273–274
Ionox antioxidants **15**, 6, 9, 17, 21, 28, 30, 39
Ion permeability, membranes, α-tocopherol effects **33**, 218
Ions, decreasing adsorbability for **2**, 9
–, effect of concentration on **2**, 10
–, electrical charge and radius of hydrated **2**, 9
–, exchange reactions **2**, 8, 10
Ipriflavone **44**, 228
IQ, *see* 2-Amino-3-methylimidazo[4,5-*f*]-quinoline
IQ-like compounds, antioxidants and formation during frying **34**, 435
–, formation, Fe^{2+} and Fe^{3+} effects during frying **34**, 436
–, –, modulators **34**, 428
–, –, pyrolysis role **34**, 434–435
–, formation mechanisms, creatine and creatinine role **34**, 414–417
–, –, fat role **34**, 417–420
–, –, Maillard reaction **34**, 413–414
–, –, pyrolysis role **34**, 420
–, –, relationship with pH **34**, 435
–, relation to moisture retention and internal temperature **34**, 435
Irish moss, effect of drying on bulk density of **2**, 473–474
IRMS, *see* Isotope ratio mass spectrometry
Iron **36**, 221–225
–, absorption, fructooligosaccharide effects **43**, 33, 34
–, –, impairment **45**, 32, 33–34, 40–41

Iron, absorption, impairment (*cont'd*)
–, –, –, low-phytic acid grains **45**, 34–35
–, anticancer activity **45**, 38–39
–, as catalyst of lipid oxidation **23**, 43–44, 59
–, bioavailability **36**, 223–224
–, content, of canned foods **1**, 44, 49
–, –, of peas **9**, 78
–, –, of plants, effect of fertilizers on **1**, 313–314
–, content of apples and pears **8**, 371
–, corrosion of **3**, 341
–, effect on low-ester pectins **1**, 415
–, – on tallowiness in dried milk **3**, 95
–, Fe^{2+}, oxidative browning acceleration, in shoyu during storage **30**, 257
–, –, –, in sugar-amino acid model systems **30**, 254
–, –, –, of Amadori compounds from shoyu **30**, 255–256
–, –, soy protein effects on absorption and metabolism, human **30**, 364–368
–, gelatin color and **7**, 247
–, importance of, in apples and pears **8**, 378
–, in browning reaction **32**, 133, 135
–, in mechanically deboned red meat **27**, 86–88
–, inositol phosphates binding **45**, 28–29
–, in tea **17**, 248
–, in wines **8**, 136, 137, 138, 139, 181
–, lactoferrin **36**, 222–224
–, nonheme, warmed-over flavor development in cooked meat and **29**, 39–40
–, olive oil and **31**, 473
–, overall dietary absorption impact **45**, 40–41, 42
–, phytic acid and bioavailability **28**, 33–36
–, polyphenol complexes with, in food browning **19**, 123–127
–, RDAs **36**, 221
–, supplementation **36**, 224
–, with tin in acid solutions **3**, 334, 335
Iron ions, effects on IQ-like compound formation during frying **34**, 436
Iron salts, effect on pectin viscosity **1**, 406
Iron sorbitex **44**, 316
Irradiated beef, flavor of **18**, 21–23
Irradiation (*see also* Radiation), effect on auxins **15**, 128
–, – on chemical compounds **15**, 123
–, – on genetics **15**, 152
–, – on metabolism **15**, 82
–, – on pigments **15**, 126, 132
–, – on taste **15**, 129
–, – on texture **15**, 116
–, – on vitamins **15**, 124
–, fish preservation and **7**, 71
–, gamma **12**, 86
–, in fruit preservation **17**, 204
–, of foods **15**, 105ff; **24**, 155–227
–, of fruit **15**, 116
–, of fungi **15**, 149ff
–, –, *in vitro* **15**, 159
–, –, *in vivo* **15**, 166
–, side-effects, *Lactobacillus acidophilus* effects **37**, 90–91
Irreversible thermal inactivation, enzymes **35**, 246–249
Irreversible utilization **40**, 12
Irrigation, in kiwifruit cultivation **29**, 283
–, olive oil and **31**, 454
Irritable bowel syndrome **43**, 203
–, inulin effects **43**, 43
–, unfermented acidophilus milk effects **37**, 86
Ischemia **40**, 194–195
–, effects on cardiolipin content **37**, 301–302
Isethionate **44**, 292
Isoamyl alcohol, in black tea **2**, 288
–, in lemons **2**, 271
–, in raspberries **2**, 269
–, in strawberries **2**, 270
–, solubility of DDT in **2**, 204
Isoamylamine, fish spoilage and **7**, 46
Isoamyl *n*-caproate, in strawberries **2**, 270
Isoascorbic acid, effect on mortality of rats **3**, 205
–, in meat curing, color stabilization **29**, 14
–, –, *N*-nitrosamine formation blocking **29**, 14
–, pathologic effects of **3**, 207
D-Isoascorbic acid, *see* Erythorbic acid
Isoascorbyl palmitate, as antioxidant in dried egg **1**, 181
–, effect on mortality of rats **3**, 205
–, pathologic effects of **3**, 207
–, toxicity of as an antioxidant **3**, 201
Isobutanol in apples **2**, 263
Isobutyl aldehyde in black tea oil **2**, 287
Isobutyric acid in decomposing salmon **2**, 371
Isocitrate dehydrogenase, *see* Bovine isocitrate dehydrogenase
Isocitric dehydrogenase, in wheat germ **23**, 240
Isocitric dehydrogenase as endpoint cooking temperature indicator **44**, 171
Isocoumarin and related compounds, from *Aspergillus oniki* 1784 **30**, 295

Isodityrosine, dietary fiber and **31**, 132
Isoelectric pH, of whey proteins, table **33**, 349
Isoelectric point, gelatin and **7**, 273–274
Isoenzymes **17**, 49–50
–, of lactic dehydrogenase **17**, 49
–, of peroxidase **17**, 49
–, of phenol oxidase **17**, 49–50
dl-Isofenchyl alcohol in strawberries **2**, 270
Isoflavones **44**, 196, 197
–, analytical methods **44**, 201, 202
–, antioxidant activity **44**, 225–226
–, bioavailability/metabolism **44**, 218–220
–, chemistry **44**, 197
–, effects of processing **44**, 212–217
–, fungal/bacterial fermentation **44**, 213
–, gut microbial metabolism **44**, 218–220
–, health protective effects, bone **44**, 227–228, 229
–, –, cancer **44**, 229–230
–, –, cardiovascular **44**, 232–234
–, role in plants **44**, 200
–, sources **44**, 203–207
–, –, database **44**, 205–207
Isoionic point, gelatin and **7**, 274
Isomaltose, from lactose via Maillard reaction **19**, 186
Isomerization of carotenoids **15**, 197, 239
Isoprene **15**, 205
Isopropanol in apples **2**, 263
Isopropyl alcohol, solubility of DDT in **2**, 204
Isopropylaldehyde in black tea **2**, 287
Isoquinoline in cyclic type of quaternary ammonium **2**, 125
Isosaccharosan, anhydride of sugar **6**, 16
Isosorbide mononitrate **44**, 314
Isotherms, adsorption, for measuring water-binding in proteins **10**, 357–358
–, sorption, for predicting storage stability **11**, 313–314
Isothiocyanate glycosides **14**, 312
Isotope ratio mass spectrometry, GC **40**, 66–70, 71, 73–74, 177
Isotopes, in tea research **11**, 250
Isotope tracer, stable, *see* Stable isotope tracer
Isotopic labeling, calcium bioavailability, foods **33**, 123–124
–, –, tracer techniques **33**, 122–124
–, folate bioavailability **33**, 61–64
–, folates with deuterium and other stable isotopes **33**, 12–13
Isotropic pressure **39**, 13
Isovalderaldehyde in black tea oil **2**, 287
Isovaleric acid **16**, 185
–, fish spoilage and **7**, 48, 55
–, in coffee **2**, 281
–, in Formosan black tea oil **2**, 287
–, in lemons **2**, 270
Italian buckwheat products **44**, 414–415
Italy, retort packaging (STAR) system for **23**, 341–342

Jack mackerel, ozone treatment **45**, 197
Jacobine **45**, 72
Jacoline **45**, 70, 72
Jaconine **45**, 72
Jacozine **45**, 72
Jaffe color test, for shellfish poison **10**, 170–172
Jams **15**, 342
–, from kiwifruit **29**, 307
–, furcellaran in **11**, 160
–, in candies **6**, 45
–, mold growth on **3**, 455
–, propagation of *Bacillus saccharolyticus* in **3**, 450
Japan, retort packaging for processed foods in **23**, 341
Japanese buckwheat noodles **44**, 412–413, 416, 417
Japanese cup noodles, microwave drying **43**, 123
Japanese flounder, ozone treatment **45**, 197
Japanese udon noodles (*see also* Oriental noodles) **43**, 146, 148, 155, 168, 181
–, quality evaluation **43**, 171, 174
Jejunal brush border membranes, folate-binding protein in **33**, 54
Jejunum (*see also* Intestines) **40**, 82, 115
Jellies **15**, 342
–, alginates in **11**, 152
–, chemical composition and properties of **6**, 10
–, fruit **6**, 26
–, furcellaran in **11**, 160
–, rheology of **8**, 33
–, toughening of **6**, 7
Jelly units of pectin solutions **1**, 401–404
Jerky **39**, 81
Jerusalem artichoke (*Helianthus tuberosus*), inulin **43**, 3, 6, 8, 9, 40, 46, 48
Jet ejectors **15**, 316
JM105, production of $A_{1a}B_{1b}$ protein **36**, 154–156
Joints, temperomandibular, oral cavity sensitivity to position of **29**, 169–170

Judges, attitude of **2**, 239–241
–, checking performance of **2**, 237–239
–, effect of fatigue on **2**, 241–244
–, selecting of **2**, 235–236
–, training of **2**, 235
–, variation in sensory ability of **2**, 234–244
Juice, chemical constituents **12**, 236–245
–, –, carbohydrates **12**, 236–237
–, –, cartenoids **12**, 238–239
–, –, ester-distillation **12**, 238
–, –, nitrogeneous substances **12**, 240
–, –, organic acids **12**, 238
–, –, pectic substances **12**, 240–241
–, –, polypbenols **12**, 240
–, –, vitamins **12**, 242–245
–, –, volatile flavoring **12**, 241–242
–, frozen fruit **6**, 169
–, –, sources of infection of **6**, 182
–, fruit, micro-organisms on **6**, 179
–, –, preparation of **17**, 172–173, 190–194
–, kiwifruit, chemical changes during vinification **29**, 303–305
–, –, production **29**, 301–302
–, passion fruit **12**, 234–258
–, recovery **12**, 234–236
–, –, small-scale **12**, 234
–, technological aspects **12**, 245–258
–, –, blends **12**, 251–252
–, –, concentrates **12**, 254–256
–, –, cordials **12**, 252–254
–, –, nectar **12**, 252–254
–, –, powder **12**, 255–257
–, –, preservation **12**, 245–249
–, –, spoilage **12**, 250–251
–, –, squash **12**, 252–254
–, –, storage **12**, 249–250
–, –, syrup **12**, 252–254
Juiciness measurements **14**, 95
–, centrifugal **14**, 109
–, mechanical **14**, 107
Jumping genes **41**, 7
Junction zone, polymer **39**, 42

Kaempferol **44**, 197
–, inhibition of soybean lipoxygenase **33**, 317
–, oxidation, mechanism **33**, 315
–, percentage in green tea **2**, 284
–, structure **19**, 80; **33**, 311
Kaffeol in coffee **2**, 279
Kafirins **43**, 235, 242
Kahawai **39**, 339
Kahweal, properties of **2**, 281–282
Kale, ascorbic acid content of, effect of sunlight on **1**, 300
–, calcium content of, effect of limestone on **1**, 310
–, effect of blanching on **1**, 77
–, iron content of, effect of fertilizers on **1**, 314
–, loss of thiamine on processing **6**, 288
Kamaboko, manufacture of **20**, 207–209
Kanamycin nucleotidyltransferase, site-directed mutagenesis **35**, 281–282
–, thermal stability **35**, 262–263
Karlsruhe device **14**, 104–106
Kelvin model **39**, 9–10
Kenya, annual agricultural and forestry harvest **32**, 193
–, annual biomass production **32**, 192
–, biomass energy used **32**, 191
–, biomass resources **32**, 195–196
–, consumption of commercial energy **32**, 190
–, forest utilization **32**, 194
–, gross national product **32**, 189
–, land distribution by uses **32**, 190
Kernels, *see* Caryopsis *and* Palm kernels
Kerosene, solubility of DDT in **2**, 203, 204
–, toxicity to man **2**, 212
Kestner atomizer, operation of **2**, 454–455
Kestner spray dryer, operation of **2**, 413–414, 439
–, production of specified bulk density by **2**, 472, 474
–, use in manufacture of toilet soap **2**, 432
Ketene, acetylation of amino and phenolic groups by **1**, 383
Keto-gluconic acids, in spoiled table wines **6**, 76
Ketones, chocolate and **31**, 234, 251, 297
–, hydroxy **14**, 309–310
–, in black tea oil **2**, 287–288
–, in coffee **2**, 283
–, in parsley oil **2**, 274
–, in strawberries **2**, 270
Ketoprofen **44**, 296
Ketorolac **44**, 296
Ketosamines **12**, 4–39
–, and aldosylamines **14**, 169–177
–, decomposition **12**, 22–39; **14**, 169, 177–185
–, –, oxidation **12**, 27–28
–, determination **14**, 174
–, formation **12**, 14–20; **14**, 174–175
–, –, acid–base catalysts **12**, 15–16

–, –, mechanism **12**, 16–20; **14**, 175–176, 207–208
–, –, rate **14**, 174–175
–, –, substituents **12**, 15
–, in foods **14**, 176–177, 183–185
–, preparation **14**, 171–172
–, properties **12**, 8–13; **14**, 172–173
–, –, infrared spectra **12**, 9
–, –, reaction with oxidation–reduction indicators **12**, 9
–, –, solubility **12**, 8
–, –, structure **12**, 10–13
–, quantitative determination **12**, 14
–, simplest **12**, 7
–, structure **14**, 173–174
Ketoses **14**, 199–210, 264
–, browning reactions with amines, fructosylamine formation **30**, 87
–, chocolate and **31**, 232
–, Heyns rearrangement **30**, 87–88
Ketosylamines **14**, 200–201
Keys equation **36**, 272
Khandi, Arabic candies **6**, 6
Kidney cancer, carcinogen risk assessment and **31**, 14
Kidneys, calcium handling, protein and phosphate effects **33**, 143–144
–, β-carotene **40**, 33, 49
–, distribution of DDT in **2**, 210, 211
–, loss of thiamine on processing **6**, 278
–, membrane vesicle **40**, 197, 200, 201, 202
–, microdialysis **40**, 194–195
–, of meat animals **6**, 133
–, urinary excretion, α-tocopherol **33**, 202–204
–, –, γ-tocopherol **33**, 205–206
–, –, δ-tocopherol **33**, 205–206
–, vitamin A **40**, 4, 9, 11, 20–21
–, vitamin B6 **40**, 201
Kilishi **39**, 80
Killer cells, mononuclear **37**, 10
–, natural **37**, 10
Kimchi preparation **45**, 192
Kinetic modeling, process optimization **39**, 141–143
Kinetic parameter distribution **40**, 265–279
–, adaptive control **40**, 270
–, applications **40**, 271–273
–, Bayesian estimation **40**, 269–270
–, covariates **40**, 272–273
–, identifiability **40**, 276–277
–, missing values **40**, 271–272
–, Monte Carlo simulations **40**, 270–271
–, prior, estimation **40**, 273–276
–, –, naive data pooling **40**, 273
–, –, nonparametric **40**, 276
–, –, parametric **40**, 275
–, –, semiparametric **40**, 275–276
–, –, two-stage methods **40**, 273–274
–, –, uses **40**, 268, 269–271
–, sparse data **40**, 265–266, 272
–, theory **40**, 266–269
–, –, error model **40**, 268
–, –, likelihood **40**, 268–269
–, –, parameter estimation **40**, 269
–, –, system model **40**, 267–268
Kinetics, chemical, in food science **10**, 8–10
Kinetin, chocolate and **31**, 327
Kingfish **39**, 339
Kiwifruit (*Actinidia chinesis*), biology and vineyards **29**, 279–280
–, canning of peeled fruits **29**, 299–300
–, chemical composition of fruits **29**, 294–298
–, – of –, actinidin, proteolytic activity **29**, 297–299
–, – of –, chlorophyll after storage and canning **29**, 295
–, – of –, fresh, frozen, and canned **29**, 294
–, – of –, organic acids **29**, 294–297
–, – of –, sugars **29**, 294–295
–, cultivation, diseases **29**, 294, 297
–, –, fertilization **29**, 284
–, –, frost damage **29**, 293
–, –, irrigation **29**, 283
–, –, pruning **29**, 284–285
–, –, training **29**, 284–285
–, –, wind sensitivity **29**, 283
–, growth and ripening **29**, 288–294
–, –, cell growth during **29**, 288–289
–, –, chemical changes during **29**, 291–294
–, –, ethylene production during **29**, 291
–, –, fruit weight-seed numbers in cultivars **29**, 293
–, –, physiological changes during **29**, 290–292
–, –, respiration during **29**, 288, 290–291
–, harvesting **29**, 295–286
–, low-salt water requirement **29**, 282
–, packing **29**, 286–287
–, processing **29**, 298–307
–, –, drying, effect of slice thickness **29**, 300–301
–, –, freezing preservation of slices **29**, 300
–, –, peeling **29**, 298–299
–, –, production of candy from peeled slices **29**, 306–307
–, –, – of jam **29**, 307

Kiwifruit (*Actinidia chinesis*), processing, production (*cont'd*)
–, –, – of juice, procedure and vinification **29**, 301–305
–, –, – of leather from fruit pulp **29**, 306
–, –, – of wine, procedure and composition **29**, 302–306
–, production areas **29**, 282
–, propagation, container plants **29**, 281–282
–, –, grafting seedlings **29**, 281
–, –, rooting cuttings **29**, 281–282
–, soil needs **29**, 282
–, standards, grades **29**, 297–288
Kjeldahl nitrogen analyses **10**, 78
–, whey protein denaturation **33**, 372
Klason lignin, dietary fiber and **31**, 151, 160
Klebsiella pneumoniae, fructooligosaccharide substrate **43**, 20
–, germicidal action of CPCl on **2**, 152
Klucel **12**, 332–333
Kluyveromyces fragilis, β-galactosidase **38**, 25, 78–79
Kluyveromyces lactis, β-galactosidase, hydrolysis catalyzed by **38**, 72–73
–, –, specificity **38**, 81
–, –, transgalactosylase activity and substrate components **38**, 77–78
–, –, velocity for production of allolactose **38**, 65, 70
–, lactase, concentration effect on lactase-catalyzed hydrolysis **38**, 54–55
–, –, disaccharides and oligosaccharides formed by **38**, 77, 79
–, –, temperature requirements **38**, 34
–, lactase stability, enzyme concentration effect **38**, 37–38
–, –, function of protease contamination **38**, 40
–, product inhibition **38**, 9–10
KOH-amylose complex, molecular shapes and interactions **42**, 165
Kohlrabi, pH value of **3**, 455
Koikuchi shoyu, chemical composition **30**, 238–241
–, fermentation, scheme **30**, 203
–, flavor evaluation **30**, 257–261
–, –, chemical components and **30**, 257–258, 260
–, –, odorous components and **30**, 258–259
–, –, taste components and **30**, 261
–, koji making **30**, 204
–, mash making and aging **30**, 204–205
–, mash pressing **30**, 205
–, refining **30**, 205
–, soybean treatment **30**, 204
–, volatile flavor compounds, acetals **30**, 277–278
–, –, alcohols **30**, 265–266
–, –, alkylcyclopentadiones **30**, 277
–, –, carbonyls, aldehydes, from Strecker degradation **30**, 267–268
–, –, α-dicarbonyl compounds **30**, 268–270, 271
–, –, esters **30**, 267
–, –, 4-hydroxy-3-furanones **30**, 272–277
–, –, identification method **30**, 262
–, –, lactones **30**, 280–281
–, –, of topnote aroma concentrate **30**, 283–285
–, –, –, concentration and odor units **30**, 284
–, –, organic acids **30**, 264–265
–, –, phenols **30**, 278–280
–, –, –, alkylphenol formation **30**, 278–279
–, –, –, ferulic acid conversion into 4-ethylguaiacol by yeasts **30**, 278–280
–, –, pyrazines **30**, 281–282
–, –, –, pasteurization and **30**, 282
–, –, γ-pyrones **30**, 272
–, –, quantitative analysis, methods **30**, 285–286
–, –, sensory evaluation **30**, 262–263
–, –, –, 4-ethylguaiacol-methionol combination and **30**, 286–287
–, –, sulfur-containing **30**, 282–283
–, –, –, comparison with soybean protein hydrolysate **30**, 283
–, –, terpenes **30**, 283
–, –, weak acidic fraction and **30**, 263–264
Koji, as soy sauce material **10**, 108–111
–, for shoyu preparation, bacterial contamination **30**, 224–225
–, –, cultivation, air supply **30**, 226–227
–, –, mechanical equipment **30**, 225–226
–, –, soybean/wheat ratio **30**, 224
–, –, temperature **30**, 222–224
–, molds (*see also specific molds*), enzymatic activities **30**, 196–197, 220–221
–, –, strain selection **30**, 220
–, wheat germ use in **23**, 285
Konjak **44**, 407, 408
Konti conche, chocolate and **31**, 303
Korean buckwheat products **44**, 414
Korean fried instant noodles (*see also* Oriental noodles) **43**, 155
–, quality evaluation **43**, 179
Kosmotropes **35**, 296
Kosmotropic salts **34**, 47–48

Krause spray dryer, operation of **2**, 428–429, 432–433
Krebs cycle **17**, 19–20, 25
Kreith and Romie's solution, of heat conduction problems **20**, 226
Krill, as food source **20**, 201, 202
Kudzu root isoflavones **44**, 205
Kuru **43**, 280, 281, 293
Kwashiorkor **16**, 1, 43, 54, 58, 64

LAB, *see* Lactic acid bacteria
Labeling, flavoring substances **42**, 20–21, 24
Labetolol **44**, 306
Labiatae (*see also* Rosemary) **42**, 245–267
–, compound activities **42**, 256–261
–, essential oils as antioxidants **42**, 249–252
–, evolution as antioxidant sources **42**, 247
–, health implications **42**, 263–267
–, plant tissue studies **42**, 247–249
–, species, active compounds **42**, 246–247
Labneh cheese **39**, 190
Laboratory animals, diets for, irradiation of **24**, 185
Laboratory spray dryers, operation of **2**, 433–439
Lachrymatory factor, in onion **22**, 96–97
Lactacin B **43**, 14
Lactacin F **43**, 14
α-Lactalbumin, amino acid composition of **19**, 157
–, residues **35**, 207
–, structure **33**, 354–357
–, structure and composition of **19**, 163
–, thermal stability **35**, 254
β-Lactam antibiotics, in foods **37**, 43
Lactase (*see also* β-Galactosidase), commercial, future potential **38**, 56–59
–, –, properties **38**, 30–39
–, –, purity **38**, 39–41
–, –, sources **38**, 5–6
–, –, technical data **38**, 32
–, –, transgalactosylase assay conditions **38**, 64, 66–68
–, deficiency **38**, 3
–, effect on sensory properties of nonfat ice milk **38**, 14–15
–, enzyme modification **38**, 57–58
–, fungus-derived, optimum temperatures **38**, 33–34
–, hydrolase, assay methods and enzyme activity, chemically modified substrates **38**, 27–29
–, –, colorimetric analysis **38**, 26–27
–, –, hydrolysis rates **38**, 30–31
–, hydrolase activity **38**, 22–59
–, –, activation and inhibition **38**, 41–43
–, –, assay methods and **38**, 25–31
–, –, enzyme mechanism **38**, 23–26
–, –, future potential for commercial sources **38**, 56–59
–, –, immobilization mechanisms and reactor systems **38**, 43–51
–, –, ultrafiltration bioprocess reactors **38**, 47, 50, 52–56
–, immobilization **38**, 18–20
–, –, commercially available technologies **38**, 47–48
–, immobilized systems **38**, 16, 18–20, 44
–, impact of microbial source **38**, 80
–, in fermented milk **38**, 14–17
–, in ice cream **38**, 13–15
–, level decrease with age **38**, 3–4
–, linked to modified corn grits **38**, 45
–, low-lactose milk **38**, 6–7
–, –, processing by consumers **38**, 7–9
–, powders, lactase units **38**, 28–29
–, pressure-induced immobilization **38**, 19
–, product inhibition **38**, 9–13
–, protease activity **38**, 40–41
–, research needs **38**, 89–90
–, selection, pH **38**, 33
–, –, stability **38**, 35–39
–, –, temperature **38**, 33–35
–, stability, pH change effects **38**, 39
–, –, skim milk, enzyme concentration effect **38**, 37–38
–, –, –, media and temperature effect **38**, 37
–, transgalactosylase activity **38**, 59–89
–, –, activation and inhibition **38**, 82–83
–, –, assay methods **38**, 64–69
–, –, commercial source effect **38**, 77–80
–, –, compounds formed **38**, 86, 88
–, –, donor plus acceptor molecules **38**, 76–79
–, –, future sources **38**, 86, 89
–, –, future utilization **38**, 85–89
–, –, in food **38**, 84–85
–, –, lactase concentration **38**, 76
–, –, pH **38**, 65, 69–70
–, –, potential uses **38**, 89–90
–, –, specificity **38**, 80–82
–, –, substrate concentration **38**, 76–70
–, –, temperature and reaction time **38**, 70–76
–, –, transgalactosylation versus reverse hydrolysis **38**, 61–64
–, waste lactose utilization **38**, 20–21
–, yeast, immobilization of whole cells **38**, 45

Lactase, yeast (*cont'd*)
–, –, stability **38**, 35
Lactate, acceleration of trimethylamine oxide reduction by **2**, 369
–, production in porcine stress syndrome **28**, 214
Lactate dehydrogenase, acetamidation **35**, 272–273
–, amino acid residues **35**, 269
–, endpoint cooking temperature indicator **44**, 171, 172
–, guanidination **35**, 273
–, immunoassay (ELISA) **44**, 174–175
–, thermal stability **35**, 267
Lactate levels, blood **37**, 349
Lactate metabolism **39**, 198–200
Lactation **40**, 112–113
Lactic acid **16**, 190, 216, 251
–, addition to milk **2**, 21
–, changes in content in fish muscle **2**, 362
–, chocolate and **31**, 217, 218, 221
–, dehydrogenase, inhibition of **1**, 388
–, effect of degree of acidity in milk **2**, 22
–, – of temperature on taste intensity **2**, 246
–, effect on pH of beef muscle **1**, 6
–, – on – of –, post-mortem formation in beef **1**, 3, 6–8
–, – on saltiness **2**, 260
–, fish preservation and **7**, 46, 68
–, in laboratory steeping **38**, 289–290
–, in rye bread **2**, 276
–, intestinal antibacterial activity **43**, 14, 15, 34
–, *N*-nitroso compounds and **31**, 81, 82, 84
–, oxidation as cause of fish spoilage **2**, 369–370
–, pH of fish and **7**, 48
–, role, in corn wet milling **38**, 281–282
–, sorghum foods fermentation **43**, 252–254
Lactic acid bacteria (*see also* Nonstarter lactic acid bacteria) **39**, 164–165, 174–175
–, bacteriocin production **37**, 77–78
–, cultures, constipation **37**, 110–111
–, –, diarrhea **37**, 84–92
–, –, health targets, cancer suppression **37**, 99–107
–, –, immune system stimulation **37**, 107–110
–, –, lactose digestion **37**, 79–84
–, –, vaginitis **37**, 111–114
–, effect of pH on growth of **3**, 431
–, fecal recovery **37**, 72–74
–, fermentation, preservation of vegetables by **3**, 457–458
–, health effects **37**, 70
–, history **37**, 69–70
–, peptidases **39**, 215, 216–218
–, proteolysis **39**, 211
–, research needs **37**, 116–120
–, reviews **37**, 70
–, safety issues **37**, 114–115
–, strain selection **37**, 115–116
Lactic acidosis, in xylitol metabolism **25**, 171–172
Lactic dehydrogenase **17**, 20, 49
–, isoenzymes of **17**, 49
Lactobacilli **43**, 12
–, adhesion to gut **43**, 322
–, bacteriocin production **37**, 77–78
–, cancer protective effects **43**, 36, 37
–, chocolate and **31**, 218
–, effects on cancer-related fecal enzyme levels **37**, 99–101
–, – on cancer suppression **37**, 99–103
–, – on cholesterol reduction **37**, 92–97
–, intestinal microflora **43**, 10, 12, 14
–, –, health benefit **43**, 14
–, inulin fermentation products **43**, 23
–, prebiotics **43**, 16
–, prevention of enterotoxigenic *Escherichia coli*-induced diarrhea **37**, 86
–, probiotics **43**, 15
Lactobacillus **32**, 15
–, in bacon **3**, 308
Lactobacillus acidophilus **43**, 36, 44
–, bacteriocidal substances production **43**, 14
–, effects on, candidal vaginitis **37**, 112–114
–, –, immune response **37**, 108–109
–, –, irradiation side-effects **37**, 90–91
–, fecal recovery **37**, 72–74
–, germicidal action of CPCl on **2**, 152
–, hydrogen peroxide-producing, effects on HIV **37**, 114
Lactobacillus brevis, pulsed electric field (PEF) inactivation **44**, 11
Lactobacillus bulgaricus **43**, 14
–, potential lactase sources **38**, 86
Lactobacillus casei **43**, 36, 37
–, assay for folate in foods **33**, 21–22
–, biological synthesis of long-chain folates **33**, 11–12
Lactobacillus casei reductase, reduction of oxidized folates **33**, 9
Lactobacillus delbrueckii **43**, 253
Lactobacillus leichmannii **45**, 203
Lactobacillus lindneri, destruction of by heat **3**, 436
Lactobacillus pasteurianus, destruction of by heat **3**, 436

–, survival of at low temperatures **3**, 446
Lactobacillus plantarum **16**, 211; **45**, 22
Lactocidin **43**, 14
Lactocin 27 **43**, 14
Lactoferrin **36**, 222–224
–, bovine milk, structure **33**, 358–359
β-Lactoglobulin, alkyl chain length effect **34**, 153
–, amino acid composition of **19**, 157
–, binding of nonpolar compounds, dissociation constants, table **33**, 410
–, creaming stability, phosphorylated and native **34**, 154–155
–, denaturation kinetics **35**, 344
–, desorption and surface pressures **34**, 53
–, film-forming properties **33**, 396–397
–, flavor binding **33**, 412–413
–, genetic variants **33**, 353–354
–, glycosylated, emulsifying activity indices **34**, 156–157
–, –, film-forming properties **33**, 396–397
–, heat effects on **19**, 165–168
–, ionic strength and rate of change of surface pressure **34**, 42–44
–, ligand binding **33**, 413–415
–, $\ln(d\pi/dt)$ versus π plots **34**, 43, 45
–, neutral salt effect **35**, 300–301
–, PEG effects **35**, 293
–, reducing agent effect on thermal characteristics **35**, 329
–, residues **35**, 207
–, secondary structure **33**, 352–353
–, steady-state surface pressure, ionic strength and **34**, 43, 45
–, –, net charge and **34**, 42–43
–, structure **33**, 350–354
–, structure and composition of **19**, 161–163
–, succinylation **35**, 272
–, surface area cleared during surface penetration and molecular rearrangement **34**, 45–46
–, surface pressure versus concentration **34**, 41
–, thermal characteristics, fatty acid modification effects **35**, 330–331
–, –, pH effects **35**, 324
–, –, succinylation effects **35**, 330
–, thermodynamic and binding constants, table **33**, 414
–, vapor-pressure–moisture-content curve for **3**, 57
β-Lactoglobulin-stabilized emulsions, coalescence rate constants **34**, 140, 142
Lactones, contribution to **18**, 54–55
–, formation of **19**, 190, 191
–, in butterfat **19**, 191
–, shoyu flavor and **30**, 280–281
Lactone sedanolid, in celery seed oil **2**, 271
Lactose **12**, 8; **14**, 182–183; **38**, 37
–, α and β forms of in dried milk products **3**, 49–51, 59
–, calcium absorption effect **36**, 217
–, carmellization of **3**, 99
–, chocolate and, milk **31**, 253, 255, 256, 260, 261, 263
–, concentration effect on allolactose production **38**, 65, 69–70
–, – on production of oligosaccharides by transgalactosidation **38**, 74–76
–, content of in whey **3**, 89
–, crystallization of **3**, 50, 51, 56, 59
–, –, in drying of whey **3**, 90, 91
–, decomposition of during storage **3**, 101
–, digestion, effects of lactic cultures **37**, 79–84
–, effect of temperature on taste intensity of **2**, 246
–, effect on dehydration process **3**, 59, 60
–, – on thiamine destruction **6**, 261
–, half-life in column reaction **38**, 47, 50
–, hydrolysis, catalyzed by β-galactosidase **38**, 24–25
–, –, chemical reactor **38**, 45–46
–, –, maximum product synthesis **38**, 72
–, in candies **6**, 30, 44
–, in milk crumb **31**, 286
–, in milk powders **19**, 183–184
–, in test for "remade" milk **3**, 70
–, intolerance, research needs **37**, 118
–, isomaltose from, via Maillard reaction **19**, 186
–, melanoidin in **3**, 267–268
–, precipitation in milk **2**, 24
–, reaction on sulfhydryls **3**, 75
–, spray-dried **3**, 58
–, sweeteners **31**, 266
–, syrup production **38**, 21–22
–, uptake of water by in dry milk **3**, 97
Lactose effect **33**, 124–125
–, in animals **33**, 125–126
–, in dried egg **1**, 173
–, in elderly subjects **33**, 134
–, in humans **33**, 128–132
–, –, infants **33**, 132–134
–, of carbohydrates **33**, 130–131
–, of other sugars **33**, 127
Lactose glass **3**, 50–51, 56, 97
Lactose intolerance **42**, 11; **43**, 201

Lactose metabolism **39**, 174–177, 198–200
Lactose-reduced foods **38**, 5
Lactulose, formation **38**, 69
LaGrangian flow **40**, 247
Lamb **14**, 41
–, fat **14**, 44, 46
–, fatty acids in fat of **23**, 23
–, freeze-drying of **7**, 220
–, organisms in frozen **6**, 188
–, processing **21**, 178–186, 193–194, 196, 203, 204
–, retention of thiamine in **6**, 283
λ repressor, disulfide bonds **35**, 289
–, site-directed mutagenesis **35**, 279–280
Lamellae, components **31**, 120, 139, 140
–, dietary fiber and **31**, 129, 131
–, in frozen plant products **2**, 336
–, in peas **2**, 315
–, in starch grain **2**, 318
–, properties **31**, 155, 164, 165
Lamina propria, components **37**, 10
Laminarin **41**, 5
Laminin, role in connective tissue carcinomas **37**, 404–405
Lamivudine **44**, 285
Lanolin, viscosity reducer in chocolate **6**, 40
Lanosterol, structure of **23**, 18, 19
Laplace equation, spherical foam particle **34**, 68
Laplace transform, identifiability **40**, 316–317
Larchwood, dietary fiber and **31**, 177, 187
Lard, ascorbic acid as antioxidant synergist in **4**, 388
–, effect of ascorbic acid **5**, 29
–, oxidation of **5**, 29
Lard in diet of rats **1**, 114
Lasiocarpine **45**, 71, 73
Lathyrism **16**, 33; **37**, 388
Latin America, IM meat **39**, 82–83
Lattice gels **34**, 206
Lauric acid, plasma lipid/lipoprotein response **36**, 268
Lauric fats, chocolate and **31**, 278
Lauryldimethylbenzylammonium chloride, germicidal action of **2**, 155
–, structure of **2**, 120, 155
–, trade names for **2**, 155
Lauryldimethylchlorethoxyethylammonium chloride, structure of **2**, 123
Laurylisoquinolinium bromide, structure of **2**, 123, 124
Laurylpyridinium bromide, structure of **2**, 123
Laxative, chocolate and **31**, 269, 275
La Zang **39**, 76–77
LDL (low-density lipoproteins) (*see also* Lipoproteins) **36**, 259
–, cholesterol, effects of lactic acid cultures **37**, 93–96
–, –, modification, dietary fat effects **37**, 171–181
–, levels, fat quantity and **36**, 309–311
–, lowering mechanism and MUFAs **36**, 301–302
–, metabolism, animal studies **36**, 278–280
–, –, composition and size **36**, 283–285
–, –, human studies **36**, 280–281
–, –, *n*-3 PUFA **36**, 322–324
–, –, *n*-6 PUFA **36**, 278–285
–, –, receptor mass and gene expression regulation **36**, 281–283
–, receptor, expression and dietary fat quality **36**, 314–315
–, –, *n*-3 PUFAs and **36**, 326–327
Lead, in wines **8**, 135, 139, 189
–, removal from maple syrup **2**, 37
–, use of ion exchangers for removal of in apple industry **2**, 15
Lead-phytate (inositol hexakisphosphate) interactions **45**, 32
Lead salts, effect on pectin viscosity **1**, 406
Leaks, detection of, in flexible packages **23**, 409–417
Leak test apparatus **23**, 410
Learning ability, *n*-3 PUFA **35**, 120–127
Learning problem **40**, 333–335
Least squares, bioperiodicity **40**, 221–224
–, identifiability **40**, 318
Leather, from kiwifruit pulp **29**, 306
Leaves **41**, 3–4, 148
–, proteins of **16**, 16, 72
Lebanon bologna **39**, 81–82
Lecithin, added to chocolate **6**, 40
–, as factor in fat reversion **4**, 195
–, chocolate and, alkalization **31**, 247
–, –, conching **31**, 300, 303, 306
–, –, emulsifiers **31**, 281–284
–, –, refining **31**, 292
–, –, tempering **31**, 311
–, enzymatic hydrolysis in **11**, 312
–, in non-enzymic browning **17**, 33
–, *N*-nitroso compounds and **31**, 78
–, reversion in pastes **11**, 298–301
–, sorption isotherms for **11**, 305, 307, 312
–, use with quaternary ammonium compounds **2**, 160
Lecithinase in eggs **1**, 183

Lecithin:cholesterol acyltransferase, activity and PUFAs **36**, 293, 325–326
Lecithin content of egg yolk **1**, 151
Lectin, dietary fiber and **31**, 132
–, distribution in plants **28**, 114–115
–, from bean seeds **28**, 122
–, importance **28**, 114–115
–, in beans, composition **28**, 115–123
–, –, physicochemical properties **28**, 115–123
–, medical and nutritional importance **28**, 123–128
–, nomenclature **28**, 112–113
–, occurrence **28**, 112–113
L.E.E.–Kramer shear press **14**, 74–79, 132
Leeks, inulin **43**, 9
Left ventricular function, effects of age **37**, 369
Legg cutter **11**, 206
Legislation, on poisonous shellfish **10**, 162–164
Legumes **41**, 2
–, composition **36**, 93
–, dietary fiber and **31**, 155, 170, 181, 187, 191
–, folate bioavailability **33**, 74
–, phytase enzyme of **28**, 21–23
–, phytate degradation during processing **45**, 16
–, phytic acid phosphorus content **28**, 10–13
–, storage proteins **36**, 103–123
–, –, biosynthesis **36**, 124–125
–, –, classification **36**, 103–104
–, –, comparison of structure and conformation of 7S and 11S globulins **36**, 122–123
–, –, 7S globulin, gene structure **36**, 104–109
–, –, –, structure and conformation **36**, 113–114, 116
–, –, 11S globulin, gene structure **36**, 109–113
–, –, –, structure and conformation **36**, 114–122
Legume seeds **16**, 9ff
–, digestibility **16**, 75
–, proteins **16**, 9ff, 24
Legumin (*see also Vicia faba* legumin pea) **36**, 160–161
Leguminosae (Fabaceae), chymotrypsin and trypsin inhibitors **28**, 138
–, pyrrolizidine alkaloids **45**, 62
Leino-α-protease, endogenous proteolytic enzymes and **31**, 353
Leino-β-protease, endogenous proteolytic enzymes and **31**, 361
Lemon albedo, pectin from **1**, 398–399
Lemon concentrate, minimizing browning in **1**, 364, 366
Lemon juice, effect on corrosion **3**, 338
–, freeze-drying of **7**, 226
–, measurement of color changes during browning in **1**, 328
–, photomicrographs of spray-dried **2**, 517
–, spray-drying of **2**, 486
Lemon pectinate, changes in gels made from **1**, 420
Lemon peel, brining **5**, 144
–, disappearance of chlorophyll **5**, 326
–, pectin in **1**, 400
Lemon pulp, pectin in **1**, 400
Lemons **10**, 297, 298, 805, 308, 315, 317, 326–327; **15**, 225
–, pH value of **3**, 432
–, sodium orthophenylphenate treatment of **3**, 464
–, use of juice for capillary resistance **5**, 276
–, volatile constituents of **2**, 270–271
Lemon sole, rigor mortis in **2**, 366
Lentil lignans **44**, 207
Lentils **16**, 9
–, inositol phosphates degradation **45**, 20, 22
Leonov model **39**, 59
"Lethal mutations", microbial inhibition by **1**, 375–376
Lethal radiation doses **15**, 153
Lettuce, ascorbic acid content, effect of fertilizers **1**, 310
–, chlorination **45**, 188
–, dietary fiber and **31**, 158, 183
–, in children's diet **1**, 109
–, inulin **43**, 9
–, ozone treatment **45**, 192, 195–196, 206
Leucine aminopeptidase, as endpoint cooking temperature indicator **44**, 170
–, endogenous proteolytic enzymes and **31**, 346, 347
–, endopeptidases **31**, 356
–, proteinase activity **31**, 386, 388–390
Leucine α-ketoglutarate transaminase, in tea **24**, 235
Leucoanthocyanidins, in food browning **19**, 78–79, 128–130
–, in grapes **8**, 263
–, structures of **19**, 79
Leucoanthocyanins, in tea **11**, 215
–, structural formulae **11**, 215
Leuconostoc mesenteroides **45**, 188
Leucoplasts, in parenchyma vegetable cells **2**, 306
–, in starch grains **2**, 322

Leukemia, carcinogen risk assessment and 31, 14, 17
Leukocytes, characterization 37, 8
–, distribution 37, 10
–, endogenous proteolytic enzymes and 31, 364, 365, 367
–, functions in specific immunity 37, 9
–, inflammation 35, 139
–, tocopherol association with 33, 177
Leukoplakia, oral 40, 57
Leukotrienes, inflammation and 35, 140–141
–, synthesis 35, 92–93, 101–105
Leuprolide acetate 44, 316
Levamisole 44, 294, 324
Level sensors, ultrasonic 45, 129–130
Levodopa 44, 309
Levulinic acid, ultraviolet absorption of 3, 182, 183
Levulinic acid in apples 2, 263
Levulosan, formed from sucrose 6, 16
Levulose, production plants of 2, 29, 30
Liatris punctata (cachana; grey feather; blazing star) 45, 77
Licorice, confectionery and 7, 348–350
–, detection of 7, 342
–, hormonal activity of 7, 356–358
–, pharmaceutical preparations of 7, 353–354
–, pharmacology, history of 7, 351–353
–, physiological properties of 7, 354–355
–, uses of 7, 350–351
Licorice extract, constituents of 7, 347
–, impurities in 7, 347–348
–, manufacture 7, 344–346
–, –, by-products of 7, 346–347
Licorice root, constituents of 7, 341–343
–, sources of 7, 340–341
Lidocaine 44, 287
Ligand binding 40, 122–127
–, by whey proteins, by β-lactoglobulin 33, 413–415
–, –, flavor binding 33, 410–413
–, –, lipid binding 33, 408–409
–, –, thermodynamic and binding constants, table 33, 414
–, folate determination methods 33, 22–26
–, –, alternative approach to 33, 25–26
–, –, differences between procedures 33, 23
–, –, plasma and red cell folate measurement 33, 24
–, –, problems and limitation 33, 24–25
–, –, selectivity of assay 33, 23
–, protein stability 35, 253–257
Ligases, in wheat germ 23, 241
Light 14, 190, 222
–, glycoalkaloid formation in potato 21, 324–330
–, influence on tea constituents 11, 233
–, water requirements and 7, 110
Light microscopy 41, 167
–, fat crystal network microstructure 44, 38
Lignans 44, 196, 197
–, analytical methods 44, 201
–, antioxidant activity 44, 226
–, bioavailability/metabolism 44, 221–222
–, cancer protective effects 44, 230–231
–, chemistry 44, 199
–, effects of processing 44, 217–218
–, gut microbial metabolism 44, 199, 207, 221
–, *in vivo* antiestrogenic effects 44, 225
–, role in plants 44, 200
–, sources 44, 207–211
–, structure 44, 208
Lignins 44, 200
–, analysis 31, 142, 146, 150, 151, 153
–, chemical characteristics 27, 208
–, combination with pectins 11, 82
–, components 31, 120, 122, 123
–, dicotyledonous plants 31, 127, 132–134
–, dietary fiber and 27, 209–210; 31, 118, 190, 191
–, digestibility of 2, 304
–, in annular vessels 2, 301
–, in fiber cells of veins 2, 302
–, intestinal bacteria 31, 172, 178, 180–184, 186, 188, 189
–, monocotyledonous plants 31, 136–138
–, properties 31, 159–163, 165
–, pyrolysis, phenol production 29, 121–123
–, secondary cell walls 31, 138, 139
Likelihood estimation 40, 268–269
Lily pollen phytase 45, 11
Lima beans, canned, nutrients in 1, 43, 46–49
–, nutritional stress factor in 4, 111–113
–, thiamine content of 1, 66
Lima beans starch, gelatinization of 2, 327
Limb girdle muscular dystrophy 37, 359
Limbic system 44, 255
Lime, gelatin manufacture and 7, 238–242
–, use in pineapple industry 2, 18
Liming, chemistry of 7, 241–242
d-Limonene, effect on storage of oranges 2, 265
–, in canned orange juice 2, 265
–, in carrot seed oil 2, 271
–, in celery seed oil 2, 271
–, in orange peel 2, 264
l-Limonene, in carrot seed oil 2, 273

Limonoids in citrus fruits **9**, 348–349
– in –, chemistry **9**, 352–353
– in –, delayed bitterness **9**, 351–352
– in –, distribution **9**, 349
– in –, effect of maturity on **9**, 349
– in –, – of rootstock on **9**, 349
Linalool **42**, 251
–, in cocoa **2**, 283
–, in Formosan black tea oil **2**, 286, 287
–, in oranges **2**, 264
–, in peaches **2**, 265
d-Linalool in orange peel oil **2**, 265
Linalyl acetate **42**, 251
Lincomycin **44**, 291
Lindemann–Hinshelwood theory **14**, 315–316
Linear energy transfer **15**, 60, 70
Linear integrator **40**, 281–303
–, background information **40**, 281–283
–, Bulirsch Stoer **40**, 290, 297, 299–303
–, CBCCDS **40**, 297, 299–303
–, Chu Berman **40**, 290–292
–, DASSL **40**, 290
–, differential equations **40**, 283–292
–, evaluation **40**, 293–300
–, Petzold **40**, 297, 299–303
–, Runge Kutta **40**, 290, 291, 297, 299–303
Linear system (*see also* Rectilinear approach), graph model **40**, 349–351
–, identifiability **40**, 315–317
–, limitations **40**, 324, 335, 337
–, membrane transport model **40**, 246
Linear viscoelasticity **39**, 10, 18–23
Liners, apples **12**, 132–134
–, consumer prepacks **12**, 135–136
–, film **12**, 132–136
–, pears **12**, 134
–, plastic tents **12**, 136
–, polyethylene **12**, 133–136
–, temperature control **12**, 135–136
Ling, comparison of aerobic bacteria of fresh and spoiling **2**, 353
Lingonberry (*Vaccinium vitusidea*) **44**, 207, 211
Linked-atom least squares analysis **42**, 145
Linked-function analysis, bovine isocitrate dehydrogenase inhibition by citrate **34**, 360–361
trans,trans-Linoelaidic acid **35**, 41–42
Linoleate, by singlet oxygen **33**, 253
–, carbonyl compounds generated from, table **33**, 265
–, oxidation, autoxidation mechanism **33**, 242
–, –, free radical and photosensitized, distributions of isomeric hydroperoxides, table **33**, 254
–, PUFA effects **35**, 38–39
Linoleic acid **35**, 9–13
–, autoxidation **33**, 242–243
–, benefits **35**, 6
–, blood cholesterol **10**, 200
–, conversion to PUFA **35**, 29
–, desaturase activity, diet effects **35**, 35–36
–, Δ^6-desaturase conversion **35**, 31
–, desaturation **35**, 39, 149
–, –, human skin cells **35**, 53–54
–, –, rate **35**, 88
–, –, unsaturated fatty acids effects **35**, 31, 33
–, dietary **35**, 6–7
–, dietary α-LNA effects, animals **35**, 86–88
–, –, humans **35**, 83–84
–, EFA activity **35**, 9
–, elongation, human skin cells **35**, 53–54
–, essential fatty acid deficiency **35**, 10–12
–, feeding studies **35**, 67–68
–, in natural fats **23**, 8
–, in poultry fat **1**, 212
–, metabolism **35**, 90–91, 150
–, olive oil and **31**, 463, 464
–, plant content **35**, 16–17
–, platelet aggregability **35**, 89–90
–, α-tocopherol sources and **33**, 167–168
Linoleic acid deficiency, dietary PUFA and **35**, 106
–, signs **35**, 111
Linolenate, autoxidation and formation of hydroperoxy cyclic peroxide **33**, 244
–, bicycloendoperoxide formation from 13-hydroperoxide precursor **33**, 245
–, bis-epidioxide, breakdown mechanism **33**, 278
–, carbonyl compounds generated from, table **33**, 265
–, dihydroperoxide, breakdown mechanism **33**, 276
–, –, formation from hydroperoxide precursors **33**, 246
–, epoxy-hydroperoxide, breakdown mechanism **33**, 277
–, feeding studies **35**, 67–68
–, free radical and photosensitized oxidations, distributions of isomeric hydroperoxides, table **33**, 254
–, hydroperoxy cyclic peroxide, breakdown mechanism **33**, 277
–, PUFA effects **35**, 38–39

Linolenic acid, autoxidation **33**, 243–246
–, in natural fats **23**, 9
–, oxidation by tea leaf **24**, 235
α-Linolenic acid (*see also* Desaturase system *and* Dietary fatty acids) **35**, 1–160
–, acylation patterns **35**, 23–24
–, appropriate dose **35**, 158–159
–, availability from edible oils **35**, 19–20
–, average dietary intakes **35**, 159–160
–, biosynthesis **35**, 16–17
–, cerebral injection **35**, 75–76
–, concentration in lipids **35**, 17
–, consumption **35**, 19–20
–, conversion, *see* α-Linolenic acid, metabolism and conversion
–, deficiency **35**, 13–14
–, Δ^6-desaturase, conversion of linoleic acid **35**, 31
–, –, inhibition **35**, 39–40
–, desaturation **35**, 24, 27–29
–, –, human skin cells **35**, 53–54
–, –, *n*-3 in other tissue **35**, 81–83
–, –, limitation **35**, 85
–, –, rates **35**, 78–81
–, –, unsaturated fatty acids effects **35**, 31, 33
–, dietary, as *n*-3 PUFA source **35**, 107–109, 122–123
–, –, requirements **35**, 151–155
–, –, sources and supply **35**, 14, 16–19
–, elongation **35**, 24–27
–, –, human skin cells **35**, 53–54
–, –, *n*-3 in other tissue **35**, 81–83
–, –, limitation **35**, 85
–, essential fatty acid deficiency **35**, 13
–, interactions with *n*-6 PUFA **35**, 83–90
–, – with –, animals **35**, 86–89
–, – with –, human studies **35**, 83–86
–, – with –, tissue arachidonic acid effects **35**, 89–90
–, metabolism and conversion **35**, 20–24, 52–83
–, –, adipose tissue **35**, 74–75
–, –, animal studies **35**, 65–78
–, –, brain **35**, 74–78
–, –, breast milk lipids **35**, 62–64
–, –, deficient diet **35**, 69
–, –, *n*-3 desaturation and elongation **35**, 81–83
–, –, desaturation rates of *n*-6 and *n*-3 fatty acids **35**, 78–81
–, –, fat-free diet **35**, 71–73
–, –, feeding studies **35**, 53–61
–, –, heart **35**, 72–74
–, –, human studies **35**, 52–65
–, –, isolated human cells **35**, 53–54
–, –, linseed and fish oil effects **35**, 53–57, 66–67
–, –, liver and plasma lipids in animals **35**, 66–72
–, –, maternal and infant levels **35**, 61–65
–, –, rapeseed and peanut oil effects **35**, 60–61
–, –, to PUFA **35**, 29
–, –, vegan and omnivores **35**, 63–64
–, nutritional effects and functions **35**, 111–132
–, –, EFAD symptoms **35**, 111–112
–, –, essentiality **35**, 112–116
–, –, nerve tissue and learning ability **35**, 120–127
–, –, *n*-3 PUFA and membranes **35**, 116–127
–, –, retina and visual function **35**, 117–120
–, β-oxidation **35**, 34
–, plant content **35**, 16–17
Linolenic fats, use in candy **6**, 32
Linseed, nutritional stress factor in **4**, 111–113
Linseed meal **17**, 107
–, effect on chicks **1**, 124
–, – on pigs **1**, 124
Linseed oil, feeding studies **35**, 53–55
–, fishy flavors in **4**, 191
–, platelet aggregability **35**, 136
–, reversion problems in **4**, 187, 190, 193–195, 199, 202–203
Lintnerized starch **41**, 168
Lipases **16**, 254; **17**, 24–25; **39**, 201–205
–, chocolate and **31**, 263, 264, 291
–, deterioration of peas **17**, 32
–, dietary fiber and **31**, 170, 171
–, inactivation of by heat **3**, 93
–, inactivation temperature in oats **11**, 294
–, inactivation time–temperature relationships **3**, 53, 54
–, in eggs **1**, 183
–, in wheat germ **23**, 210, 237–239
–, olive oil and **31**, 471
–, presence of in milk **3**, 78, 79
Lipid binding, in breadmaking **20**, 156–161
Lipid content, in mechanically deboned red meat **27**, 78–84
Lipid metabolism, disorders **37**, 381–383
–, inulin effects **43**, 28–32, 41
Lipid oxidation **14**, 225–226; **39**, 134
–, in food **17**, 31–33
–, in meat **29**, 35–46
–, –, catalysis by, heme compounds **29**, 37–38

–, –, –, metal ions **29**, 38–39
–, –, mechanism **29**, 36–37
–, mechanisms **23**, 39–48
–, –, catalysts of **23**, 40–45
–, oxidative changes **17**, 23–34
"Lipid oxidation potential" **17**, 33
Lipid-protein isolates **17**, 104
Lipids **14**, 242; **16**, 397ff; **41**, 30
–, amino group in fluorescence of **3**, 100
–, autoxidation of **17**, 27–28; **23**, 39–40
–, binding by whey proteins **33**, 408–409
–, biological oxidation of **17**, 25–26
–, breast milk **35**, 62–64
–, carbonyl compounds in country-style cured ham **29**, 67
–, carcinogen risk assessment and **31**, 24
–, changes in storage **16**, 425
–, chocolate and, emulsifiers **31**, 281
–, –, milk **31**, 253
–, –, milk crumb **31**, 291
–, –, *Theobroma cacao* L. **31**, 320, 322–325
–, classification and significance of **23**, 3–5
–, contribution to meat flavor **18**, 39–40
–, degradation of **17**, 24–26
–, depot fats, *see* Depot fats
–, deterioration of in dried milk during storage **3**, 93–97
–, dietary fiber and **31**, 139, 143, 163, 168, 169
–, docosahexaenoic acid content **35**, 14–15
–, effect on dough **16**, 421
–, – on whey protein foaming properties **33**, 404
–, fish, *see* Fish lipids
–, in abalone **23**, 160–162
–, in blood, plant and animal protein effects **30**, 372–375, 376
–, in breadmaking **16**, 399, 410ff
–, in citrus fruits **9**, 329–332
–, in dehydrated mashed potatoes **25**, 61–73
–, in egg yolk **10**, 37
–, in meat **29**, 33–39
–, –, composition **29**, 33–35
–, –, oxidation, *see* Lipid oxidation, in meat
–, in milk proteins **19**, 187–191
–, in muscle **19**, 5–6
–, in peas **9**, 73–74
–, in plants, winter hardiness and **25**, 206–208
–, in tea **11**, 226–227
–, in tissues, composition of **23**, 33–37
–, in wheat **16**, 397ff
–, in wheat flours **29**, 217–222
–, –, analysis **29**, 221–223
–, –, effect on baking quality **29**, 251–260
–, –, – on bread **29**, 251–258
–, –, – on cakes **29**, 260–261
–, –, – on cookies **29**, 259–260
–, –, extraction **29**, 217–218
–, –, fractionation **29**, 221
–, –, functionality **29**, 218–220
–, –, nonpolar fraction, breadmaking and **29**, 253–256, 258
–, –, –, cookie quality and **29**, 259
–, –, polar fraction, breadmaking and **29**, 253–256
–, –, –, cookie quality and **29**, 259
–, –, polar fraction–protein interaction, effect on baking quality **29**, 263–264
–, α-linolenic acid concentration **35**, 17
–, material extracted from vegetables **8**, 99
–, meat flavor and **23**, 37–39
–, *N*-nitroso compounds and, fundamentals **31**, 62–64, 66
–, –, nitrite/nitrate addition **31**, 73, 78–81
–, of wheat germ **23**, 220–230
–, olive oil and **31**, 461, 467, 472
–, oxidation, *see* Lipid oxidation *and* Oxidation
–, peroxidation during Maillard reaction **30**, 121
–, plant-oxidation mechanisms **17**, 59
–, polar, effect on wheat germ **23**, 279–280
–, radiation effects on **24**, 170–173
–, reactions **14**, 223–226, 265
–, reducing capacity of in dried milk **3**, 101
–, resistance of to oxidation **3**, 74
–, structure of **23**, 5–20
–, –, in membrane's **23**, 20, 35–37
–, –, nonsaponifiable lipids **23**, 18–20
–, –, phospholipids **23**, 9–15
–, –, sphingolipids and glycolipids **23**, 15–17
–, –, triglycerides **23**, 5–9
–, unsaturated, in oxidation **17**, 6
Lipid transfer protein, tocopherol transfer between lipoproteins and **33**, 175
Lipid uptake **40**, 197, 198, 202–203
Lipoids, effect on quaternary ammonium compounds **2**, 132
Lipolysis **16**, 255; **39**, 201–209, 255
–, chocolate and **31**, 253, 264, 291
–, effect of temperature of fish on **2**, 361
–, endogenous proteolytic enzymes and **31**, 389
–, in spoiling fish **2**, 373
–, olive oil and **31**, 461, 463, 471, 473
Lipomannan **43**, 322
Lipopolysaccharide **43**, 322
–, effects on gastrointestinal immunity **37**, 35

Lipopolysaccharide (*cont'd*)
–, inhibition of CL binding to IgG aCL **37**, 310
Lipoprotein in egg yolk **1**, 150–151
Lipoprotein lipase **39**, 201–202
–, activity and *n*-6 PUFAs **36**, 291–292
–, dietary fat quality and **36**, 314
–, *n*-3 PUFA effects **36**, 325
–, role in α-tocopherol transfer **33**, 183–184
Lipoproteins (*see also* Plasma lipoproteins), bacterial cell envelope **43**, 322
–, classes **36**, 256
–, dietary fat type and source effects **37**, 154–159
–, halophilic bacteria and **7**, 113
–, high-density **40**, 38–39, 57
–, –, mediation of tissue α-tocopherol uptake **33**, 183
–, in egg yolk **10**, 37–38
–, in MUFA-rich vs. lowfat diets **37**, 174, 189
–, intermediate-density **40**, 69
–, lactic acid cultures effects **37**, 93–96
–, low-density **40**, 38–39, 58, 62, 69
–, –, mediation of tissue α-tocopherol uptake **33**, 180–182
–, metabolism and dietary fats **36**, 255–256
–, plasma, diurnal/seasonal variations **33**, 176
–, –, exchange between classes **33**, 174–175
–, –, incorporation, tracing with *d*-α-tocopherol acetate **33**, 176–177
–, –, lipid transfer protein role **33**, 175
–, –, postprandial changes **33**, 176
–, –, tocopherol in, distribution **33**, 174
–, *n*-3 PUFA effects **35**, 133–134; **37**, 178–179
–, serum, butter effects **37**, 166–169
–, very-low-density **36**, 259; **40**, 38–39, 69
–, –, inulin response **43**, 29
–, –, levels, fat quantity and **36**, 306–309
–, –, mediation of tissue α-tocopherol uptake **33**, 183
–, –, metabolism, animal studies **36**, 275–277
–, –, –, human studies **36**, 277–278
–, –, –, *n*-3 PUFA **36**, 319–322
–, –, –, *n*-6 PUFA **36**, 275–278
Liposomes, chocolate and **31**, 220
–, dipalmitoylphosphatidylcholine, α-tocopherol transfer to rat liver mitochondria **33**, 195
–, phosphatidylcholine, α-tocopherol transfer to rat liver microsomes **33**, 194
Lipoteichoic acid **43**, 322, 324
Lipovitellenin in egg yolk **1**, 150–151, 182
Lipoxidase (*see also* Lipoxygenases) **16**, 431
–, in wheat germ **23**, 210–211, 239
Lipoxygenases **17**, 52, 59
–, activity in beans **17**, 31
–, – in fish gill and skin tissues, table **33**, 294
–, control of oxidative activities **33**, 306–309
–, effects of flavonoids **33**, 316–319
–, fish lipid oxidation **33**, 294–297
–, free radical formation **17**, 28–29
–, from plant and animal tissues, positional specificity, table **33**, 262
–, gill, effect of thiol groups **33**, 296–297
–, heat inactivation of **17**, 42
–, in carotene destruction **17**, 30
–, inhibition and inflammation **35**, 140
–, inhibition by sulfiting agents **30**, 11
–, in off-flavor production **17**, 32
–, lipid oxidation **33**, 261–269
–, metabolites **33**, 297
–, oxygen insertion, positional specificity **33**, 266–267
–, *n*-3 PUFA action **35**, 151
–, specificity of **17**, 26–27
–, synthesis **35**, 101–105
Liquid, cross section of **11**, 359
Liquid crystalline phases, formation, small-molecule emulsifiers **34**, 106–108
Liquid drainage method, measuring foam stability **34**, 67–68
Liquid extraction process of food drying, aroma recovery in **20**, 32–34
Liquid food, heat processing of **23**, 106
Liquid formula diet, selenium in **32**, 98–99
Liquid-phase methods, for polyglutamyl folate synthesis **33**, 7
Liquid smoke, meat mutagen modulation **34**, 433–434
Liquid structure, as element in fluid consistency **11**, 358–368
–, Eyring theory of coefficient of viscosity **11**, 358–362
Liquiretin **7**, 355
–, structure of **7**, 342
Liquor, chocolate and, alkalization **31**, 247–249
–, –, cocoa butter **31**, 249, 250, 275
–, –, conching **31**, 304, 307
–, –, milk **31**, 258, 262
–, –, milk crumb **31**, 284, 286–290
–, –, processing **31**, 237, 238, 241–243
–, –, refining **31**, 292
–, –, roasting **31**, 243–246
Lissant method, small-molecule emulsifiers **34**, 100–101

Listeria, pulsed electric field (PEF) inactivation **44**, 11, 13
–, thermal inactivation kinetics **44**, 159–160, 162
Listeria monocytogenes **45**, 169, 188, 193, 203
–, attachment **43**, 327, 328
–, –, glass surfaces **43**, 330
–, –, growth condition effects **43**, 324
–, –, inhibition methods **43**, 353
–, –, meat tissue **43**, 335, 339
–, –, properties of attached cells **43**, 347, 348
–, –, stainless steel surfaces **43**, 330, 331, 333
–, –, starvation stress **43**, 325
–, thermal inactivation, kinetics **44**, 159–160, 162
–, –, USA meat processor regulations **44**, 150
Lithium, in wines **8**, 137
Lithium carbonate **44**, 311
Litton device **15**, 284
Liver, calf's **12**, 21–22
–, carcinogen risk assessment and **31**, 26, 28
–, β-carotene **40**, 38–40, 46–48, 60, 69, 71
–, chocolate and **31**, 267
–, desaturase and elongate activity **35**, 81–82
–, distribution of DDT in **2**, 210–211
–, effect of DDT on **2**, 213
–, – of sonic vibration on **3**, 131
–, essential fatty acids desaturation **35**, 29
–, folate uptake and secretion **33**, 54
–, hog's **12**, 21
–, in meat animals **6**, 113, 133
–, lipids, α-linolenic acid conversion **35**, 66–72
–, loss of thiamine on processing **6**, 277
–, microsomal enzyme-catalyzed lipid oxidation **33**, 256–259
–, microsomes, α-tocopherol concentrations **33**, 212
–, –, α-tocopherol transfer factors **33**, 194–195
–, mitochondria, α-tocopherol concentrations **33**, 212
–, *N*-nitroso compounds and **31**, 54, 55
–, –, fundamentals **31**, 64, 65
–, –, nitrite/nitrate addition **31**, 86
–, role in α-tocopherol clearance from blood **33**, 184
–, tissue, tocopherol content **33**, 178–179
–, –, α-tocopherol turnover **33**, 187
–, α-tocopherol metabolism **33**, 199–201
–, γ-tocopherol metabolism **33**, 205–206
–, δ-tocopherol metabolism **33**, 205–206
–, unknown nutrient in **1**, 114, 130
–, vitamin A **40**, 4, 21
–, –, compartmental modeling **40**, 14–18
–, –, empirical compartmental analysis **40**, 12–14
–, –, whole-body models **40**, 9–11
–, vitamin B6 **40**, 108, 110–112, 115, 121
–, xylitol effects on **25**, 173
Liver-cell microsomal enzymes **15**, 36ff, 50
Liver powder intake by depancreatinized rats **1**, 123
Livetin fraction in egg yolk **1**, 150–169; **10**, 38
Living cells, factors affecting inhibition of processes in **11**, 332
Loading pattern **39**, 18
Loaf volume in breadmaking **10**, 51
Lobatto formula **23**, 94
Lobster **39**, 355
Local identifiability **40**, 313
Locust bean gum, general properties **11**, 161–162
–, in bakery products **11**, 165
–, in cheese products **11**, 163
–, in ice cream stabilization **11**, 162
–, in meat products **11**, 164
–, in miscellaneous food products **11**, 165
–, viscosity **11**, 118
Loganberries, canned, effect of copper on **3**, 364
–, processing of **3**, 349
–, with added sulfur **3**, 353
Logistic equation, nutrient response **40**, 159–160
Lomefloxacin **44**, 291
Long life (LL) noodles (*see also* Oriental noodles) **43**, 159, 167
Looper worms, kiwifruit damage **29**, 284
Loquats, leuco-anthocyanins **5**, 288
Loratadine **44**, 289
"Lossiness" **15**, 280
Loss modulus **39**, 23
Lousewort (*Pedicularis*) **45**, 77
Lovastatin **44**, 288
Love waves **45**, 104
–, sensors **45**, 128–129, 147
–, –, arrays **45**, 129
–, –, smart tongue and nose **45**, 153
Low acid IM meat **39**, 79
Low-calcium activated factor, endogenous protelytic enzymes and **31**, 359
Low-cost nutritious foods (LCNF), for improved world nutrition **22**, 187–203
Low-density lipoproteins, *see* LDL

Low-moisture foods, bitterness in oats **11**, 292–298
–, earlier studies on **11**, 265–292
–, enzymic reactions **11**, 263–330
–, –, effects of humidity and temperature **11**, 314–316
–, humidity and enzymic reactions **11**, 302–314
–, humidity-dependence of temperature standards **11**, 314–316
–, inactivation temperatures as affected by humidity **11**, 314–316
–, lecithin reversion in pastes **11**, 298–301
–, mechanism of enzymic reactions **11**, 310–313
–, model enzymic reactions **11**, 303–306
–, of animal origin **11**, 265–274
–, of plant origin **11**, 274–292
–, predicting storage stability **11**, 313–314
–, reactions leading to spoilage **11**, 264
–, research on enzymic reactions **11**, 303–306
–, – on –, research needs **11**, 316
–, sorption isotherms for predicting storage stability **11**, 313–314
–, souring of cereals **11**, 301–302
–, temperature optima as affected by humidity **11**, 314–316
–, theories on enzymic changes in **11**, 292–302
Low-phytic acid grains **45**, 34–35
Low temperatures, chemical reactions at **25**, 188–192
–, plant survival at **25**, 193–211
–, storage of mango fruits at **21**, 255, 275–278
Lozenge paste, binding agent in **6**, 29
LPL, *see* Lipoprotein lipase
LTB_4 **35**, 102–104, 139
LTC_4 **35**, 101, 103
Lucerne, dietary fiber and **31**, 160, 163, 175
Lucuma glycyphylla, glycyrrhizin and **7**, 343
Luikov's solutions, of heat conduction problems **20**, 225–226
Lung cancer **40**, 57
–, carcinogen risk assessment and **31**, 47
–, epidemiology **31**, 39, 40
–, laboratory data **31**, 29
–, statistics **31**, 13–17, 22
Lung disease, interstitial **37**, 402–403
Lungs, β-carotene **40**, 49
–, microsomes, α-tocopherol effects on peroxidation **33**, 213
–, tissue, α-tocopherol turnover **33**, 187
–, vitamin A **40**, 9, 11
Lup Cheong **39**, 76–77
Lupin, inositol phosphates degradation **45**, 22
Lupus anticoagulant, anti-cardiolipin antibody binding **37**, 308–309
Lutein **15**, 218, 239
Lutidine in cyclic type of quarternary ammonium **2**, 125
Lycopene **15**, 126, 132, 218, 223, 241
Lycopersene **15**, 205
Lycopsamine **45**, 71, 72, 75, 77, 78
Lymphatic system, tocopherol absorption via **33**, 168–169
Lymphocytes (*see also* B lymphocytes, T lymphocytes), in lamina propria **37**, 10–12
–, intraepithelial **37**, 10–12
Lymphoma, carcinogen risk assessment and **31**, 17
Lyotropic effect, neutral salts **35**, 294–295
Lysine **14**, 214–215; **41**, 53–55
–, action of formaldehyde on **1**, 389
–, additive to pig feed **30**, 344–345
–, deficiency in seed **17**, 107, 112, 117
–, effect on calcium absorption **33**, 127
–, endogenous proteolytic enzymes and **31**, 350, 371
–, fish spoilage and **7**, 45
–, loss, activation energies **35**, 196, 198
–, –, during Maillard reaction **30**, 120–121
–, –, from detergent-treated cells **1**, 379
–, –, in milk powder during storage **3**, 64
–, –, protein digestibility **35**, 224–225
–, reactive, measurement methods **35**, 192–195
–, separation from other amino acids **2**, 34
–, smoking-induced losses in meat **29**, 146–147
Lysine decarboxylase **16**, 301
Lysinoalanine, biological effects **35**, 210–211
–, cytotoxicity **35**, 210–211
–, in commercial foods **35**, 205–206
–, metabolism **35**, 208–209
Lysol, concentration to destroy staphylococci **2**, 135
Lysosomes, endogenous proteolytic enzymes and **31**, 411–413
–, endopeptidases **31**, 355, 356
–, exopeptidases **31**, 347
–, –, carboxypeptidases **31**, 347, 348
–, –, dipeptidylpeptidases **31**, 350, 351
–, meat technology **31**, 403–407, 411
–, muscle physiology **31**, 374, 377–380, 382
–, nonmuscle cathepsins **31**, 366
–, proteinase activity **31**, 385–392
–, proteinase distribution **31**, 366–369

Lysozyme **10**, 36, 39–41, 42
–, bovine milk, structure **33**, 359
–, configurations **34**, 58
–, destruction of cell membrane by **1**, 377–378
–, disulfide mutants, melting temperature **35**, 286–287
–, engineered disulfide bonds **35**, 284–286
–, first-order kinetic plot of adsorption **34**, 24–25
–, foam volume increase rate **34**, 61
–, guanidine hydrochloride **35**, 299–300
–, in egg albumen **1**, 150, 183
–, irreversible thermal inactivation **35**, 248–249
–, molecular properties **34**, 23–24
–, π–a plots **34**, 57–58
–, polyols and stability **35**, 292
–, rate of collapse of foams **34**, 61–62
–, site-directed mutagenesis **35**, 278–279
–, stability **35**, 253
–, –, thermal, mutants **35**, 263–264
–, thermal transition curve **35**, 187
Lysozyme–dextran conjugate, emulsifying activity **34**, 157

M cells, function **37**, 15
Maasdam cheese **39**, 243
Macaroni, alginates in **11**, 157
Mackerel **39**, 337, 341, 344, 352
–, aerobic bacteria in **2**, 350
–, anaerobic bacteria isolated from **2**, 351
–, bacterial attack on **2**, 357
–, effect of ascorbic acid on storage life **4**, 391
–, fat spoilage in **2**, 373
–, rigor mortis in **2**, 364
–, spoilage of **3**, 185, 186; **7**, 50, 51–52
–, sterilization of by cathode rays **3**, 176
Macroemulsions **34**, 83–84
Macrominerals **36**, 210
Macromolecular emulsifying agents, flocculation induction **34**, 134–135
Macromolecular films, stability **34**, 181
Macromolecular food emulsifiers **34**, 128–129
Macrophages, endogenous proteolytic enzymes and, endopeptidases **31**, 362
–, muscle physiology **31**, 378
–, proteinase activity **31**, 385
–, proteinase distribution **31**, 367, 369
–, n-3 PUFA **35**, 146–148
Magnesium, chocolate and **31**, 246
–, content of apples and pears **8**, 371, 386
–, dietary fiber and **31**, 140
–, effect on low-ester pectins **1**, 415
–, – on meat quality **21**, 102, 110, 136
–, endogenous proteolytic enzymes and, exopeptidases **31**, 347
–, –, meat technology **31**, 396–398, 408
–, inhibition of enzymes by **1**, 384
–, in milk **36**, 218–219
–, in muscle chemistry **9**, 26–28
–, in wines **8**, 138, 139, 191
–, –, determination of **8**, 137
–, morphology and **7**, 112
Magnesium absorption, inulin/fructooligosaccharide effects **43**, 32, 33
–, phytate (inositol hexakisphosphate) impairment **45**, 32, 35
Magnesium deficiency **1**, 120
Magnesium ions, effects on β-galactosidase **38**, 82
Magnesium salts, effect on potato tissue **2**, 315
Mahi-mahi **39**, 337
Maillard compounds, mechanisms for formation **35**, 190–191
Maillard reactions (*see also* Browning, nonenzymatic *and* Food browning) **15**, 293; **34**, 413–414; **35**, 190–191; **39**, 128–129, 132, 135
–, activation energies **35**, 196–199
–, aldoses heated with amines **30**, 87–88
–, artificial meat flavor and **30**, 106–109
–, bread crust color and **30**, 100
–, broiled meat aroma and **30**, 104
–, browning in dehydrated potatoes due to **1**, 278
–, causing nutritional stress **4**, 120–121
–, chocolate and, alkalization **31**, 247
–, cocoa bean chemistry **31**, 233, 236
–, cocoa flavor and **30**, 98
–, coffee bean roasting and **30**, 110–111
–, discovery and early study **30**, 79–80
–, factors affecting degree of **35**, 195–199
–, future research **30**, 123–124
–, glucose heated with casein **30**, 89–90
–, in breadmaking **19**, 198–199, 202
–, in foods **3**, 97
–, –, carbon dioxide production resulting from **3**, 100
–, –, water production resulting from **3**, 100
–, in shoyu preparation **30**, 245, 264
–, –, aldehyde production, Strecker degradation **30**, 268

Maillard reactions (*cont'd*)
–, isomaltol from lactose by **19**, 186–187
–, ketoses heated with amines **30**, 87–88
–, maple syrup patents and **30**, 112
–, meat flavor and **18**, 61–64
–, milk **31**, 255, 257, 260, 262
–, milk crumb **31**, 286–288, 290
–, moisture and temperature requirements **30**, 85–86
–, *N*-nitroso compounds and **31**, 55, 56
–, nutritional problem **30**, 119–122
–, peanut roasting and **30**, 112
–, pH effect **35**, 199
–, possible mutagenicity **30**, 122–123
–, processing **31**, 244
–, products as antioxidants inhibiting warmed-over flavor in cooked meat **29**, 45–46
–, protein digestibility **35**, 200–201
–, reducing sugars heated with, alkylamines **30**, 81
–, –, amino acids, browning and products **30**, 89
–, –, –, volatiles and aromas **30**, 91, 92–93
–, –, nitrogen compounds **30**, 81–84
–, sweeteners **31**, 266
–, volatiles, characteristics **30**, 113, 114–119, 120
–, water activity and **35**, 195–196
–, whey proteins **33**, 373
Maize (*see also* Corn) **16**, 7, 27
–, as starch model **41**, 7–9
–, biosynthesis rate **41**, 38–39, 135
–, branching enzymes in **41**, 92–93
–, degradation during processing **45**, 22
–, dietary fiber and **31**, 159
–, enzymes **41**, 47–48
–, phytases **45**, 9
–, phytate (inositol hexakisphosphate) **45**, 9
–, reduced content gene mutations **45**, 34
–, SSS in **41**, 76–77
–, starch synthases **41**, 80–81
–, waxy gene **41**, 82
Malate dehydrogenase, as endpoint cooking temperature indicator **44**, 171
–, of tea **24**, 236
Malate synthase, thermal stability **35**, 251
Malaxation, olive oil and **31**, 462
Malaysia, IM meat **39**, 75, 89
Maldigestion, lactose **37**, 79–84
Maleic acid in corrosion **3**, 338
Male sterility **41**, 131
Malic acid, effect on browning in fruit products **1**, 358, 367
–, – on saltiness **2**, 260
–, fermentation of, by *Saccharomyces pombe* **25**, 32–38, 40
–, –, during vinification **25**, 12
–, in fruit juices **9**, 264–269
–, in grape waste **2**, 16
–, precipitation in pineapple juice **2**, 20
–, removal in apple juice **2**, 15
Malic acid in corrosion **3**, 338, 339
Malic dehydrogenase, in wheat germ **23**, 240
Malignancy, acyl differences in cardiolipin **37**, 298–299
–, effects on cardiolipin content **37**, 302
Malignant hyperexia **37**, 386–387, 408
Malignant hyperthermia **21**, 82–87
–, in porcine stress syndrome **28**, 173–175
Malnutrition, effects on gastrointestinal immunity **37**, 44–45
–, research needs **37**, 55
Malo-lactic fermentation, wine deacidification by **25**, 25–32
Malonaldehyde **17**, 33
Malondialdehyde, mutagenicity **33**, 285–286
Malonic acid, fish preservation and **7**, 68–69
–, inhibition of enzymes by **1**, 384
Malonic acid in corrosion **3**, 339, 340
Malonyl coenzyme A, in wheat germ **23**, 240
Malt, melanoidins in **3**, 267
–, *N*-nitroso compounds and **31**, 86–91, 93, 986
Malt diastase, effect of spray dryer on **2**, 400
Malting, applications **43**, 238–239
–, inositol phosphates degradation **45**, 22
–, scanning electron microscopy of **22**, 278–281
–, sorghum **43**, 238–243
–, technologies **43**, 239–243
Maltodextrins **38**, 295
Maltol **12**, 33–34
Maltooligosaccharides, glass transition temperature as function of molecular weight **38**, 144, 146–147
–, C'_g values **38**, 168–169
Maltose **12**, 75–76; **14**, 182–183
–, hydrate **6**, 19
–, reaction with amino acids **3**, 249
–, sweetness of **2**, 261
Mammalian cell culture mutagenicity tests **34**, 392–396
Mammals, DHA concentration in brain phosphatidylethanolamine **35**, 121
–, effects of DDT on **2**, 206–207, 209, 212
–, essentiality of *n*-3 PUFA **35**, 113–116
–, excretion of DDT by **2**, 211

Mammary tissue culture **40**, 207–213
Mandarins, pH value of **3**, 432
Manganese **14**, 190
–, absorption, inositol phosphate effects **45**, 36
–, bioavailability **36**, 231
–, content, of apples and pears **8**, 371
–, –, of plants, effect of fertilizers on **1**, 314
–, –, –, effect on ascorbic acid content of plants **1**, 307–310
–, –, –, – on – of –, calcium absorption by plants **1**, 312
–, deficiency, of apples **8**, 378
–, –, of plants **1**, 121
–, endogenous proteolytic enzymes and **31**, 347, 349
–, in milk **36**, 230–231
–, in wine **8**, 191
–, phytic acid and bioavailability **28**, 41–42
Mango **10**, 311, 317, 324
–, composition of **17**, 160
–, flour **17**, 194
–, physical properties **17**, 173
–, physicochemical changes **17**, 164–165
–, physiology and biochemistry **21**, 223–306
–, starch micrograins from **17**, 168
–, storage and transport of **21**, 271–288
Mangold stems, corrosiveness of **3**, 341
Manipulation facilities, modeling **40**, 282, 283
Mannans **41**, 5
–, molecular shapes and interactions **42**, 152–155
Mannitol, chocolate and **31**, 268, 269, 274
–, effect on calcium absorption **33**, 127
–, from *Byssochlamys* spp. **25**, 277
–, in spoiled table wines **6**, 77, 91
Mannose, dietary fiber and **31**, 135
–, effect on dried egg **1**, 172
–, gelatin and **7**, 271
–, olive oil and **31**, 459
–, presence in candies **6**, 17
Mannuronic acid, glycyrrhizin and **7**, 359
Manufacture, ham, fish **12**, 390–392
–, sanitary measures **12**, 417
–, sausage, casings **12**, 384–389
–, –, final processing **12**, 389–390
–, –, fish **12**, 376–390
–, –, raw materials **12**, 376–384
–, tea **17**, 260
–, –, black tea **17**, 261
Manufacturing technology, cheese **39**, 166, 168, 193–195
MAPLE software **40**, 330
Maple syrup **14**, 237–238; **15**, 306
–, color specifications **5**, 315
–, extraction of dihydroconiferyl alcohol **30**, 111
–, – of syringaldehyde **30**, 111
–, – of vanillin **30**, 111
–, flavor constituents of **2**, 277
–, patents, Maillard technology **30**, 112
–, removal of lead from **2**, 37
–, volatiles, identification **30**, 111
Maprotiline **44**, 312
Marasmus **16**, 2
Marbling **14**, 44–47
–, determination **14**, 109–111
Marbling fat, composition of **23**, 33–34
Marfan syndrome **37**, 396
Margarine **15**, 248
–, blending and mixing of **8**, 13
–, reversion problems in **4**, 202
–, tocopherol content **33**, 163
Marginal chlorination, definition of **7**, 143
Margules equations **39**, 32
Marine ecosystem (*see also* Biogenic amines, fish and shellfish) **39**, 336
Marine oils, reversion problems in **4**, 192
Marine products, nutrients in **1**, 41, 45–49
Marine species, essentiality of *n*-3 unsaturated fatty acids **35**, 112–113
Marine toxins **18**, 141–161
–, in ciguatera **18**, 143–147
–, miscellaneous types **18**, 157–158
–, nereistoxin **18**, 157
–, pahutoxin **18**, 151–154
–, prymnesin **18**, 157
–, saxitoxin **18**, 155–157
–, tetrodotoxin **18**, 147–151
Marine waste products **17**, 132–135
Marjoram, antioxidant activity **42**, 248
Market surveys **3**, 412–423
Marmalade, furcellaran in **11**, 160
Marshmallows, chemical composition and properties of **6**, 10
–, gelatin and **7**, 323–324
–, gelatin in production of **6**, 24
–, setting of **6**, 36
–, toughening of **6**, 7
Martin, William McKinley **32**, 5–9, 10
Marzipan, in candies **6**, 45
Mash, fermentation **30**, 228–230
–, –, composition during **30**, 233–234
–, –, enzyme activities during **30**, 232–233
–, –, lactic and alcoholic **30**, 231
–, –, lactobacilli, metabolic pattern during **30**, 231

Mash, fermentation (*cont'd*)
–, –, microbial contamination prevention **30**, 229–230
–, filtrate pasteurization **30**, 237–238
–, for shoyu preparation, agitation during fermentation **30**, 234–235
–, pressing, degradation **30**, 235–237
–, –, enzyme activities **30**, 235–237
–, temperature **30**, 227–228
–, –, composition and **30**, 228
Mass fractal dimension **44**, 45
Mass spectrometry **39**, 227, 231, 238
–, β-carotene **40**, 66–70, 71, 73–74
–, deuterated folates **33**, 12
–, dietary fiber and **31**, 119
–, folate bioavailability measurement **33**, 61–62
–, *N*-nitroso compounds and **31**, 56, 57, 67, 91
–, of nitrosamines **22**, 16–17
–, olive oil and **31**, 469
–, total energy expenditure **40**, 176–178
Mass transfer **39**, 140–141, 151
–, dehydration mechanisms **39**, 101–102, 107, 110, 112
Mast cells, characterization **37**, 10
–, endogenous proteolytic enzymes and **31**, 366, 367, 407, 409, 411
Mastication, crushing sounds during **29**, 192–194
–, effect of food texture **29**, 171–173
Masticogna, licorice extract and **7**, 347–348
Material function, rheology **39**, 23
Mathematical modeling **39**, 139–143, 150
–, importance **40**, 26, 244, 261
MATHEMATICA software **40**, 330
Matrices, graph theory **40**, 342–347
–, identifiability **40**, 315–316
Maturation, passion fruit **12**, 211–214
Maturity, effects on fruit composition **9**, 294–296
Maturometer **9**, 63, 74, 105, 115, 119–121, 122; **14**, 83–85
Maximum oxygen uptake capacity, effects of age **37**, 368–369
Maximum tolerated dose, carcinogen risk assessment and **31**, 26
Maxwell–Boltzmann, distribution law **17**, 36
Maxwell model **39**, 9–10, 43, 58
Mayonnaise (*see also* Salad dressing), freeze-dried egg yolk and **7**, 225
Mazindol **44**, 313
McArdle's disease **37**, 377–378; **40**, 142–145
McKenna spray dryer, operation of **2**, 410
Meal patterns, and age **32**, 248, 250–253
Meander system **15**, 285
Mean residence time, *see* Residence time
Meat (*see also* Beef, Pork, Lamb, Muscle, Muscle proteins, Myofibrillar proteins, Poultry) **14**, 242–244
–, aging of **10**, 56, 59, 371, 385–493
–, alginates in preservation **11**, 148–150
–, animals, microbiology of **6**, 109, 111
–, ascorbic acid as color stabilizer of **18**, 266
–, bacterial count during freezing **6**, 188
–, by-products **17**, 133
–, canned, corrosion characteristics of **3**, 336
–, carrageenan in **11**, 133–135
–, chilling of **6**, 135
–, color **9**, 2, 3
–, –, changes **5**, 21
–, components of **10**, 396–398
–, contamination of in self-service stores **6**, 189
–, cooked, flavor development, chemistry **29**, 62–64
–, –, mutagens in **32**, 157–161
–, –, selenium in **32**, 92–98
–, –, warmed-over flavor development **29**, 35–36, 39–41
–, –, –, inhibition by curing and natural antioxidants **29**, 41–46
–, cooking method effects on **20**, 300–303
–, criteria for evaluating **9**, 2
–, curing **5**, 16; **10**, 58, 423–428; **29**, 1–86
–, –, by ascorbic acid, color stabilization **29**, 14
–, –, –, flavor development **29**, 15, 32
–, –, –, *N*-nitrosamine formation blocking **29**, 14–15, 59–60
–, –, by isoascorbic acid, color stabilization **29**, 14
–, –, –, *N*-nitrosamine formation blocking **29**, 14
–, –, by nitrate **29**, 7–17
–, –, –, bacteriostatic action **29**, 13–14
–, –, –, color stabilization **29**, 7–8, 10–12
–, –, –, flavor production **29**, 11–13
–, –, by nitrite, bacteriostatic action **29**, 13–14, 46–48
–, –, –, color stabilization **29**, 7–8, 10–12
–, –, –, flavor production **29**, 11–13
–, –, by nitrite alternatives, evaluation **29**, 56
–, –, by phosphates, color improvement **29**, 16
–, –, –, flavor development **29**, 32
–, –, –, water binding increase **29**, 15–16

–, –, by radiation as nitrite alternative **29**, 52–55
–, –, by sodium chloride, antioxidation–prooxidation **29**, 3–5
–, –, –, flavor development, comparison with nitrite **29**, 30–32
–, –, by sodium erythorbate **29**, 32–33
–, –, by sugars **29**, 6–7
–, –, by sweetening agents **29**, 6–7
–, –, chemistry **22**, 4–5
–, –, history **29**, 2
–, –, methods **29**, 16–21
–, –, –, artery pumping **29**, 18–19
–, –, –, conventional dry **29**, 17
–, –, –, dry salt **29**, 17
–, –, –, pickle **29**, 18
–, –, –, stitch pumping **29**, 19–20
–, –, –, thermal **29**, 20
–, –, –, Wiltshire **29**, 20–21
–, cysteine in **24**, 50–52
–, –, heat effects on nutritive value of **24**, 63–64
–, dehydrated, disadvantages of **7**, 206
–, –, rehydration of **7**, 206
–, dehydration, effects on **10**, 409–413
–, –, *see* Dehydration control, IM meat
–, determination **10**, 364–368
–, discolorations **5**, 2, 12, 14, 30, 31
–, drying, temperature and **7**, 198–203
–, –, time of **7**, 198–203
–, effect of cathode rays on **3**, 167
–, – of heating on nutritive value of protein in **4**, 262–267
–, elastographic carcass grading **45**, 154
–, enzymatic changes in **11**, 272–273
–, evaluating oxidative changes in fats **5**, 9
–, factors affecting **10**, 368–398
–, fatty acid formation in **11**, 303
–, flavor **9**, 2; **18**, 1–84
–, –, acids, esters, and ethers, contribution to **18**, 52
–, –, age effects on **18**, 4–6
–, –, alcohol contribution to **18**, 52–53
–, –, amino acid contribution to **18**, 40–42, 56–58
–, –, H_2S and sulfur compound contribution to **18**, 56–58
–, –, ante- and post-mortem effects on **18**, 4–16
–, –, aroma GC fractions and **18**, 58–60
–, –, artificial **18**, 46–48; **30**, 106–109
–, –, –, patents **30**, 106–107, 109
–, –, beef flavor isolates **18**, 48–51
–, –, benzene-ring compound contribution to **18**, 54
–, –, breed effects on **18**, 4–6
–, –, carbohydrate contribution to **18**, 38–39
–, –, carbonyl contribution to **18**, 39–40
–, –, carcass condition and **18**, 7–9
–, –, compounds important for **18**, 54–58
–, –, development, boiling and **30**, 103
–, –, –, broiling and **30**, 104
–, –, –, roasting and **30**, 104
–, –, due to processing **21**, 46, 47
–, –, feeding effects on **18**, 6–7
–, –, flavor perception and compounds in **18**, 64–67
–, –, flavor profile studies **18**, 26–27
–, –, freezing and storage effects on **18**, 14–16
–, –, furan-ring compound contribution to **18**, 55–56
–, –, gas chromatography studies on **18**, 26, 58–60
–, –, hydrocarbon contribution to **18**, 52
–, –, in canned, dried, and freeze-dried beef **18**, 19–20
–, –, in cured and smoked meat **18**, 21
–, –, in raw and cooked beef **18**, 16–17
–, –, lactone contribution to **18**, 54–55
–, –, lipid contribution to **18**, 39–40
–, –, lipid effects on **23**, 37–39
–, –, Maillard browning and **18**, 61–64
–, –, mineral contribution to **18**, 38–39
–, –, model systems for study of **18**, 32–33
–, –, newer findings on **18**, 45–51
–, –, nitrogen-compound contribution to **18**, 40–43, 60–61
–, –, nonmeaty compounds in **18**, 51–54
–, –, nonvolatile compounds in **18**, 36–38
–, –, nucleotide contribution to **18**, 43–45
–, –, of frozen **9**, 23–26
–, –, of heated meat **18**, 27–45
–, –, of irradiated beef **18**, 21–23
–, –, of precursors **18**, 28–32
–, –, origin of compounds in **18**, 38–45, 51–64
–, –, precursors of **30**, 103–104
–, –, problems in research of **18**, 23–27
–, –, – in –, formed flavor studies **18**, 24–27
–, –, – in –, precursor studies **18**, 23
–, –, sex effects on **18**, 4–6
–, –, slaughtering effects on **18**, 9–14
–, –, uses for knowledge of **18**, 2–3
–, –, volatile compounds in **18**, 33–36
–, –, volatiles of cooked meat **30**, 104–106
–, flavor studies on **19**, 234

Meat (*cont'd*)
–, flexible packaging for **23**, 325
–, fluid flow through **7**, 192–196
–, foodborne disease outbreaks **45**, 169
–, freeze-dried **7**, 175, 203–204
–, –, advantages of **7**, 207
–, –, production of **7**, 205
–, –, uses of **7**, 205–206
–, freezing **13**, 267, 297–306, 321
–, freezing and thawing, effects on **10**, 403–408
–, frozen **6**, 164, 188
–, gelatin and **7**, 325
–, greening **5**, 16
–, ground, deterioration of **5**, 23
–, gums in **11**, 116
–, hydration of, definition **10**, 356–364
–, hydrogen sulfide release from, during heating **24**, 64–69
–, importance for special products **10**, 438–443
–, importance of muscle biochemistry in **19**, 57–61
–, in diet **1**, 110
–, irradiation of **24**, 174–182
–, juiciness of **9**, 2
–, –, water-holding capacity and **20**, 280
–, keeping quality **5**, 9
–, lipids, composition **29**, 33–35
–, –, mechanisms **29**, 36–37
–, –, oxidation **29**, 35–46
–, –, –, catalysis **29**, 37–39
–, low-heating methods for **20**, 303–312
–, mammals **13**, 303–305
–, measurement of tenderness **9**, 40–41
–, molds and yeasts on **6**, 139
–, myoglobin derivatives **5**, 20
–, normal pigments **5**, 12, 13
–, off-flavors **5**, 2
–, organoleptic testing **14**, 129–136
–, oxidative rancidity **5**, 3
–, ozone treatment **45**, 186, 190, 191, 192, 193–194
–, pigments, changes during curing **29**, 8–12
–, –, nitrate effect **29**, 10–12
–, –, nitrite effect **29**, 10–12
–, pressure required to chew **8**, 42
–, processing, effects on **10**, 413–438
–, products, agar in **11**, 122–123
–, –, alginates in **11**, 150
–, –, guar gum in **11**, 169
–, –, gum karaya in **11**, 187
–, –, insects infesting **4**, 308, 326, 330
–, –, locust bean gum in **11**, 164
–, –, thermal processing, *see* Thermal processing
–, protein ultrasonic analysis **45**, 152–153
–, pyrrolizidine alkaloid residues **45**, 73
–, quality (*see also* Pork) **6**, 121
–, –, and muscle biophysics **26**, 90–94
–, –, animal physiology and **21**, 71–155
–, –, ante-mortem factors affecting **26**, 94–95
–, –, beef **21**, 187–193, 195, 203–206
–, –, carcass tissues **26**, 104–106
–, –, –, chemical composition **26**, 106–108
–, –, –, enzymes **26**, 112–113
–, –, –, labile proteins in tissues **26**, 108–112
–, –, –, macro- and microstructure **26**, 113–116
–, –, –, specific nutrients **26**, 119–120
–, –, carnitine relationship **37**, 382–383
–, –, color chemistry **26**, 88–90
–, –, conditioning **21**, 173–178, 185–186, 190–191, 197–198
–, –, control methods to maintain **21**, 134–138
–, –, cooling and quality relationship **21**, 137–138
–, –, detection methods **21**, 131–134
–, –, effect of ammonia **16**, 169
–, –, – of hydrogen sulfide **16**, 196
–, –, – of reducing substances **16**, 189
–, –, effects on **10**, 398–402
–, –, electrical stimulation of rigor **21**, 198–199
–, –, flavor chemistry **26**, 87–88
–, –, high-temperature conditioning **21**, 197–198
–, –, hormonal affects **21**, 87–98
–, –, hot cutting and boning **21**, 194–197
–, –, influence of, age **26**, 98–100
–, –, –, blood characteristics **26**, 95–96
–, –, –, carcass morphology **26**, 104
–, –, –, climatological stressors **26**, 127–128
–, –, –, exercise **26**, 128
–, –, –, genetics **26**, 95
–, –, –, hormones **26**, 120–125
–, –, –, –, adrenal **26**, 122
–, –, –, pancreatic **26**, 123
–, –, –, periodic electrical stimulation **26**, 128–129
–, –, –, pituitary hormones **26**, 120–121
–, –, –, –, ions **26**, 127
–, –, –, –, lathyrogens **26**, 126–127
–, –, –, –, nutrition **26**, 100–120
–, –, –, –, –, high levels **26**, 100–102
–, –, –, –, sex **26**, 123–125
–, –, –, –, thyroid hormone **26**, 121–122

–, –, –, post-mortem changes **26**, 132–151
–, –, –, –, aging **26**, 140–142
–, –, –, –, biochemical **26**, 132–135
–, –, –, –, cold shortening **26**, 138–140
–, –, –, –, –, phenomenon **26**, 137–138
–, –, –, –, cooking **26**, 146–151
–, –, –, –, glycolysis **26**, 136–137
–, –, –, –, tenderization **26**, 142–146
–, –, –, –, ultrastructural **26**, 135–140
–, –, –, proteolytic enzymes **26**, 125–126
–, –, –, sex **26**, 96–98
–, –, –, slaughtering methods **26**, 129–132
–, –, –, undernutrition **26**, 102–103
–, –, –, –, body organs **26**, 104
–, –, lamb **21**, 178–186, 193–194, 196, 203, 204
–, –, mutton **21**, 186–187, 193–194
–, –, new concepts **21**, 157–222
–, –, of muscle, evaluation **26**, 76–82
–, –, preslaughter environment **21**, 74–79
–, –, research needs **26**, 152–157; **37**, 406–407
–, –, rigor mortis relationship **21**, 80–81
–, –, role in mitochondrial metabolism disorders **37**, 380–381
–, radurization of **24**, 189–192
–, reactivity with tin **3**, 341
–, resistance of anaerobic bacteria in **2**, 67
–, retention of nutrients during electronic cooking of **3**, 142
–, ripening of **8**, 12
–, *Salmonella* in **3**, 220–222
–, sanitizing agents **45**, 189
–, sensory tests for **2**, 227, 232, 240
–, smoking (*see also* Cured meat, smoking *and* Meat smoking) **29**, 87–158
–, –, carcinogenic polycyclic aromatic compound increase **29**, 147–149
–, –, color formation **29**, 137–139
–, –, effects, *see* Meat smoking
–, –, flavoring **29**, 139–144
–, –, formaldehyde formation in smoke **29**, 148–149
–, –, history **29**, 87–89
–, –, lysine loss **29**, 146–147
–, –, mutagenic phenol formation **29**, 150
–, –, preservation **29**, 144–146
–, –, secondary skin formation **29**, 146
–, –, technology **29**, 90–102
–, –, –, wood materials **29**, 90–92
–, spoilage of **6**, 110, 115
–, storage **35**, 338–339
–, –, effects on **10**, 402–403
–, –, oxidation during **23**, 51–53
–, structure **14**, 35–38
–, sulfhydryl and disulfide groups in **24**, 1–111
–, –, curing effects **24**, 77–80
–, –, factors affecting **24**, 55–58
–, –, freezing effects on **24**, 73–76
–, –, irradiation effects on **24**, 81–83
–, –, muscles **24**, 45–50
–, –, organs **24**, 52–55
–, –, processing effects on **24**, 58–83
–, –, shelf-life effects **24**, 84
–, –, toxicological aspects **24**, 84–85
–, sulfide discoloration in **3**, 355
–, temperature rise in **20**, 297–300
–, tenderness (*see also* Meat tenderness), cold shortening effect **21**, 137, 159–170, 187–190
–, –, enzyme role in **20**, 273–277
–, –, factors affecting **20**, 257–323
–, –, heating effects on **20**, 281–297
–, –, low-temperature cooking effects on **20**, 308–312
–, –, muscle aging and **20**, 268–277
–, –, muscle components and **20**, 258–267
–, –, temperature rise effects on **20**, 297–300
–, –, thaw shortening **21**, 170–173, 182–185
–, –, water-holding capacity role in **20**, 277–281
–, texture **14**, 33–165
–, –, disulfide group effects on **24**, 71–73
–, thermal conductivity of **7**, 198
–, thermal losses of thiamine in **6**, 275
–, ultrasonic composition sensors **45**, 138
–, ultrasonic imaging of carcasses **45**, 154
–, ultraviolet treatment of **3**, 152
–, use of ascorbic acid in **4**, 392
–, "warmed-over" flavor in **23**, 1–74
–, Warner–Bratzler test for **2**, 250
–, water-binding capacity **9**, 2
–, X-ray sterilization of **3**, 157
Meat balls, *see* Spaghetti and meat balls
Meat chilling, cooling phase **21**, 206–211
–, storage phase **21**, 211–213
Meat emulsions **16**, 105ff
–, binders **16**, 138
–, casings for **16**, 144, 152ff
–, color **16**, 150
–, effect of rigor on **16**, 135
–, equipment for **16**, 126ff
–, factors affecting **16**, 111ff, 143
–, fillers **16**, 138
–, formulation **16**, 131ff, 146ff
–, freezing **16**, 135
–, preblending **16**, 136

Meat emulsions (*cont'd*)
–, production **16**, 130ff
–, stability **16**, 119ff, 124ff, 141ff
–, texture **16**, 148
Meat industry, in United States **18**, 3
Meat mutagens (*see also* IQ-like compounds) **34**, 388–389
–, absorption and excretion **34**, 410–413
–, canning effects **34**, 422–423
–, classification **34**, 389
–, cooking conditions **34**, 416–417
–, cooking effect **34**, 420–422
–, cooking methods **34**, 424–425
–, differentiation of high- and moderate-temperature-induced **34**, 404–405
–, fat role in formation **34**, 417–420
–, formed at high temperatures **34**, 398, 400–401
–, formed at moderate temperatures **34**, 400, 402–403
–, from cooking and processing **34**, 389, 423–424
–, hydroxylation **34**, 408–409
–, metabolic activation **34**, 408
–, modulators **34**, 426–434
–, –, antioxidants **34**, 427
–, –, biogenic amines **34**, 433
–, –, defatted glandless cottonseed flour **34**, 432
–, –, fatty acids **34**, 429–430
–, –, germanium oxide and cobaltous chloride **34**, 433
–, –, human saliva **34**, 432
–, –, liquid smoke **34**, 433–434
–, –, peroxidases with H_2O_2 **34**, 429
–, –, plant extracts **34**, 429
–, –, pyrrole pigments **34**, 431–432
–, –, soy protein concentrate **34**, 432
–, –, β-thiols **34**, 431
–, –, vitamins **34**, 430–431
–, –, xanthine derivatives **34**, 433
–, *N*-oxidation **34**, 409–410
–, pyrolysis role **34**, 420, 434–435
–, structures **34**, 403–404
–, temperature effects **34**, 425–426
–, toxicology **34**, 405–408
Meat processors, USA time/temperature procotol regulations **44**, 149–152
Meat technology, aging **31**, 394, 395, 403
–, connective tissue **31**, 401–403
–, contractile proteins **31**, 396–398
–, cytoskeletal proteins **31**, 400, 401
–, endogenous proteolytic enzymes and **31**, 393, 412–414
–, exopeptidases **31**, 410, 411
–, glycolysis **31**, 393, 394
–, lysosomal proteinases **31**, 403–407
–, nonlysosomal proteases **31**, 407–410
–, regulatory proteins **31**, 398–400
–, sarcoplasmic proteins **31**, 395
Meat thermometers, cooking adequacy verification **44**, 166–167
Meat tissue, attachment sites **43**, 336
–, bacterial motility **43**, 336
–, confocal scanning laser microscopy **43**, 355
–, contamination of food processing environment **43**, 339
–, cultural condition effects **43**, 338
–, extracellular polymer secretion **43**, 338
–, hydrophobic/electrostatic interactions **43**, 337
–, lean versus adipose tissue **43**, 335
–, microbial attachment **43**, 334–339
–, penetration of muscle tissue **43**, 337–338
–, physical entrapment **43**, 335–336, 347
–, physicochemical detachment **43**, 351
Meat wrapping, development of methods for **4**, 49
–, operator chart for **4**, 69
Mechanical deboning (*see also* Mechanically deboned . . .) **27**, 110–111
Mechanical dough development (Chorleywood) process **43**, 229–230
Mechanical energy balance, in determining pumping requirements **11**, 408
Mechanically deboned fish, bone particle content **27**, 119–120, 141
–, bone residue, utilization **27**, 137–138
–, calcium content **27**, 141
–, cholesterol content **27**, 141–142
–, color stability **27**, 127–129
–, –, myoglobin and **27**, 128–129
–, –, processing variables, influence of **27**, 127–128
–, fatty acid content **27**, 117–119
–, flavor stability **27**, 120–129
–, –, effect of antioxidants **27**, 125–126
–, –, – of carbon dioxide cooling **27**, 126
–, –, – of heme pigments **27**, 123–125
–, –, – of nitrogen cooling **27**, 126
–, –, – of processing variables **27**, 120–122
–, –, – of storage **27**, 122–123
–, fluorine content **27**, 141
–, functional characteristics **27**, 129–136
–, –, effect of composition **27**, 129–132
–, –, – of food additives **27**, 134–136
–, –, – of processing variables **27**, 132–134

–, heme pigments **27**, 120
–, lipid content **27**, 141–142
–, microbial quality **27**, 138–140
–, mineral composition **27**, 115–117
–, nutritive properties **27**, 111–120
–, –, proximate composition **27**, 113–115
–, –, structural characteristics **27**, 111–113
–, protein content **27**, 141
–, protein quality **27**, 117
–, regulations for **27**, 140
–, research needed **27**, 142–143
Mechanically deboned poultry, bone particle content **27**, 119–120, 141
–, bone residue, utilization **27**, 137–138
–, calcium content **27**, 141
–, cholesterol content **27**, 117–119, 141–142
–, color stability **27**, 127–129
–, –, myoglobin and **27**, 129–129
–, –, processing variables, influence of **27**, 127–128
–, fatty acid content **27**, 117–119
–, flavor stability **27**, 120–129
–, –, effect of antioxidants **27**, 125–126
–, –, – of carbon dioxide cooling **27**, 126
–, –, – of heme pigments **27**, 123–125
–, –, – of nitrogen cooling **27**, 126
–, –, – of processing variables **27**, 120–122
–, –, – of storage **27**, 122–123
–, fluorine content **27**, 141
–, functional characteristics **27**, 129–136
–, –, effect of composition **27**, 129–132
–, –, – of food additives **27**, 134–136
–, –, – of processing variables **27**, 132–134
–, heme pigments **27**, 120
–, lipid content **27**, 141–142
–, microbial quality **27**, 138–140
–, mineral composition **27**, 115–117
–, nutritive properties **27**, 111–120
–, –, proximate composition **27**, 113–115
–, –, structural characteristics **27**, 111–113
–, protein content **27**, 141
–, protein quality **27**, 117
–, regulations for **27**, 140
–, research needed **27**, 142–143
Mechanically deboned red meat **27**, 23–95
–, bone fragments in **27**, 56–62
–, calcium content **27**, 84–86
–, composition of **27**, 39–53
–, –, fat **27**, 39–42
–, –, mineral content **27**, 42–56
–, –, –, antimony **27**, 50
–, –, –, arsenic **27**, 51
–, –, –, ash **27**, 42–43
–, –, –, cadmium **27**, 50–51
–, –, –, calcium **27**, 42–43
–, –, –, cobalt **27**, 49–50
–, –, –, copper **27**, 49–50
–, –, –, fluoride **27**, 51–53
–, –, –, iron **27**, 49
–, –, –, lead **27**, 50
–, –, –, magnesium **27**, 48
–, –, –, mercury **27**, 51
–, –, –, nickel **27**, 49–50
–, –, –, phosphorus **27**, 43, 48
–, –, –, potassium **27**, 48–49
–, –, –, selenium **27**, 50–51
–, –, –, sodium **27**, 48
–, –, –, tin **27**, 50
–, –, –, zinc **27**, 49
–, –, moisture content **27**, 39–42
–, –, protein **27**, 39–42
–, cost impact **27**, 37
–, definition **27**, 23–24
–, development of **27**, 26
–, economic implications **27**, 35–39
–, –, employment **27**, 37
–, –, social effects **27**, 38–39
–, functional properties of **27**, 68–74
–, –, color **27**, 68–70
–, –, emulsion characteristics **27**, 70–72
–, –, pH and water-holding capacity **27**, 72–74
–, iron content **27**, 86–88
–, lipid make-up **27**, 78–84
–, mineral toxicity of **27**, 53–56
–, –, fluoride **27**, 54–55
–, –, lead **27**, 54
–, –, strontium-90 **27**, 55–56
–, palatability **27**, 88–93
–, –, and oxidative stability **27**, 88–90
–, –, –, sensory characteristics **27**, 90–93
–, potential yield **27**, 26–31
–, –, from different meat sources **27**, 28
–, process of **27**, 24–25
–, protein quality **27**, 74–78
–, regulations governing **27**, 31–35
–, –, in Australia **27**, 32
–, –, in Denmark **27**, 32
–, –, in the United States **27**, 33–35
–, –, U.S. Department of Agriculture and **27**, 33–35
–, research needs **27**, 93–95
–, safety **27**, 53–68
–, –, and bone particle size **27**, 56–62
–, –, –, microbiological properties **27**, 62–65
–, –, –, mineral toxicity **27**, 53–56
–, –, –, nucleic acids **27**, 65–68
Medicaments, flavor and **7**, 9

Medication, hyposalivary side effects **44**, 319, 325
–, smell perception effects **44**, 283–284, 319, 320–324
–, taste perception effects **44**, 283–284, 285–318, 319
Megalocytosis, pyrrolizidine alkaloid-induced **45**, 88, 89
Megastigmatriene, in passion fruit juice **27**, 279–281
Megrim, rigor mortis in **2**, 366
MeIQ, *see* 2-Amino-3,4-dimethylimidazo-[4,5-*f*]quinoline
Melanins, in abalone **23**, 163–164
–, in enzymic food browning **19**, 103–104
–, production of **3**, 23
–, structure of **19**, 104
Melanoidins **32**, 121, 132
–, chemistry of **32**, 146–150
–, formation of **32**, 132–142
–, –, in acid solution **3**, 271–273
–, –, in neutral and alkaline solution **3**, 264–268
–, in dried apricots **3**, 263
–, in lactose **3**, 267–268
–, in malt **3**, 267
–, in molasses **3**, 243–244
–, in shoyu browning during storage **30**, 255–256
–, laboratory preparation of **3**, 244–245
–, mutagenicity **32**, 161–163
–, properties of **3**, 268–271
–, reactions **3**, 262–273
–, –, inhibition of **3**, 272–273
Melezitose, from honey **24**, 343–344
Melibiose, in cocoa beans **8**, 262
Melittin, amino acid sequences **42**, 107–109
–, amphipathic structures **42**, 102
–, emulsion stability **42**, 116, 118
Melons, iodine wrappings for **3**, 465
Melting, chocolate and **31**, 250, 278, 308
Melting points, proteins **35**, 258, 260, 295
Melt theory, rheology **39**, 37–41
Membrane-bound lipids, composition of **23**, 20, 35–37
Membrane conductance, *see* Membrane transport, conductance
Membrane disordering, ethanol-induced, cardiolipin-related resistance **37**, 302–304
Membrane fluidity, ethanol-induced, cardiolipin-related resistance **37**, 302–304
–, phospholipid acyl changes **37**, 299
Membrane pore formation, microbial inactivation by pulsed electric field (PEF) **44**, 10
Membrane probe **40**, 183–184, 185–186
Membranes, in theory of glycolipid–protein interaction in breadmaking **20**, 167–169
–, lipid oxidation effects **33**, 283–285
–, lipids in **23**, 20
–, permeability to ions/small molecules, α-tocopherol effects **33**, 218
–, *n*-3 PUFA effects **35**, 129
Membrane transport **40**, 243–262
–, aroma recovery by **20**, 45–50
–, background information **40**, 243–245
–, carrier-mediated **40**, 251–257, 261–262
–, –, saturability **40**, 251, 261
–, –, single-site **40**, 252–255
–, –, tracer studies **40**, 255–257
–, conductance **40**, 248–249, 252–257, 331–332
–, differential operators **40**, 258–259
–, multiregion model **40**, 245–248
–, –, assumptions **40**, 246
–, –, solution methods **40**, 247–248
–, organ models **40**, 259
–, passive diffusion **40**, 248–251
–, potential **40**, 331–332
–, tracer washout rate **40**, 249–250
–, whole-body models **40**, 259–260
Membrane vesicle **40**, 197–206
–, brush border **40**, 197–199, 200–204
–, intestinal basolateral **40**, 198–200
–, intestinal luminal **40**, 198–199
–, lipid uptake **40**, 197, 198, 202–203
–, preparation **40**, 199–200
–, structure **40**, 202–203
–, transport **40**, 200–202, 203, 204
Memory, immune system **37**, 6, 8
Men, food preferences and attitudes **32**, 255–258
Menthol in raspberries **2**, 269
Menthone in raspberries **2**, 269
Mercaptans **16**, 278
–, ethyl, in young wines **8**, 159
Mercaptans in coffee **2**, 278, 281
Mercaptide-forming agents, inhibition of enzymes by **1**, 382
Mercaptides, formation of, from sulfhydryl groups **24**, 13–22
2-Mercaptoethanol, inhibition of oxidative losses to reduced folates **33**, 15
Mercaptols in coffee **2**, 281
3-Mercaptopyruvate, reaction with sulfites **30**, 35

3-Mercaptopyruvate sulfurtransferase, sulfite conversion to thiosulfate **30**, 35
Mercuric chloride, estimation of fish freshness and **7**, 62
Mercury, accumulation in edible fish **18**, 155
–, in wines **8**, 193
Mercury compounds, as SH reagents **24**, 19–22
Mercury–inositol phosphate interactions **45**, 32, 36
Mercury ions, inhibition of enzymes by **1**, 382
Meringues, gum tragacanth in **11**, 185
Merrell–Soule spray dryer, operation of **2**, 402–403, 405–406
Merthiolate, therapeutic action of **2**, 144
Mesalamine **44**, 299
Mesna **44**, 317
Mesophilic enzymes **35**, 239
Mesophyll **41**, 150
MESOSAUR software **40**, 221, 223
Messenger RNA **40**, 141, 144, 145
Metabisulfite capsules, asthmatic symptoms and **30**, 50–53, 56–57
Metabolic activation, meat mutagens **34**, 408
Metabolic control theory **40**, 233–236
Metabolic disease, smell perception effects **44**, 271
Metabolic disorders, food intolerance **43**, 201
Metabolic food disorders **42**, 11
Metabolic pathways **40**, 107–110, 227, 233–234, 240
–, altering **41**, 125–126
–, in fruit maturation **10**, 294–296, 301, 306–307, 310, 321, 329, 335, 336–343, 344–346
–, vectors **41**, 126–127
Metabolism, abnormal **12**, 111
–, acid **12**, 122
–, *Arabidopsis thaliana* model **41**, 10
–, carbohydrate **41**, 144–145
–, *Chlamydomonas reinhardtii* model **41**, 11
–, maize model **41**, 7–9
–, model comparisons **41**, 6–7
–, of micro-organisms, as affected by acids **11**, 336–339
–, –, – by benzoic and salicylic acids **11**, 331–353
–, –, pH influence on **11**, 333–336
–, of senescent fruit **12**, 119
–, potato model **41**, 9–10
–, snapdragon model **41**, 10–11
–, volatile products of **12**, 125–127
–, wheat model **41**, 6–7
Metabolite antagonists, competitive inhibition of enzymes by **1**, 384
Metairesinol **44**, 199, 207, 218
–, metabolism **44**, 221
Metal ions, as catalysts of lipid oxidation **23**, 43–45
–, – of –, in meat **29**, 38–39
–, effects on bound acid phosphatase activity **34**, 353–354
–, influence on peroxidase **17**, 16
–, variation of acid phosphatase with, *see* Acid phosphatase
Metalloenzyme, endogenous proteolytic enzymes and **31**, 381
Metallopeptidases, endogenous proteolytic enzymes and **31**, 345
Metalloproteinases, endogenous proteolytic enzymes and **31**, 345, 352, 362, 363
Metal–oxygen complexes, initiation of polyunsaturated fatty acid oxidation **33**, 237–238
Metals, complexes with polyphenols in nonenzymic food browning **19**, 123–127
–, effects on water-holding capacity of meat **10**, 373–376
–, in wines **8**, 135
Metaphen, therapeutic action of **2**, 144
Metaphosphates, effect on appetite **1**, 133
Metaphosphoric acid, use to inhibit oxidation of ascorbic acid **1**, 293–294
Metaproterenol **44**, 302
Methamphetamine **44**, 313
Methanol, in apples **2**, 263
–, soybean protein denaturation **30**, 213
Methanol extract, rosemary **42**, 253
Methazolamide **44**, 317
Methimazole **44**, 298, 322
Methional **16**, 278
–, in potato products **25**, 105
Methionine, additive to poultry feed **30**, 344–345
–, deficiency in leaf proteins **17**, 102
–, effect on appetite **1**, 133, 135–136
–, – on chicks **1**, 128
–, FAP disease **40**, 150–155
–, in diet of rats **1**, 116
–, supplementation **40**, 161–162
–, volatile thermal decomposition products of **19**, 201
Methocarbamol **44**, 309
Methocel **12**, 315, 317–319
Methotrexate **44**, 293
–, effects on folate absorption and metabolism **33**, 70

Methoxyhydroquinone glycosides, in wheat germ **23**, 237
Methoxyl groups in pectin **1**, 397, 399, 405, 407–410, 413–418
– in –, pectinic acids, relation of combining weight to **1**, 408
Methyl acetylcarbinol in bread **2**, 276
Methyl alcohol, in apples **2**, 263
–, in cherries **2**, 264
–, in coffee **2**, 281
–, in parsnip seed oil **2**, 274
–, in peaches **2**, 265
–, in raspberries **2**, 269
–, solubility of DDT in **2**, 204
Methylamine, gelatin manufacture and **7**, 240
Methylamine in coffee **2**, 279
Methyl anthranilate in grapes **2**, 270
Methylation, dietary fiber and **31**, 119, 138, 177
–, whey proteins **33**, 421
d-2-Methylbutanol in apples **2**, 263
B-Methylbutan-*a*-ol in tea **2**, 286
a-Methyl-*n*-butyraldehyde in coffee **2**, 281
Methyl butyrate in apples **2**, 263
Methylcellulose **43**, 231
–, and hydroxypropylmethylcellulose **12**, 314–328
–, –, properties **12**, 316–317
–, bakery products **12**, 317–320
–, –, chemically leavened systems **12**, 318–319
–, –, functional properties **12**, 317–318
–, –, yeast-leavened systems **12**, 319–320
–, dehydrated foods **12**, 322–324
–, –, chocolate milk **12**, 324
–, –, juices **12**, 322–324
–, dietetic foods **12**, 320–322
–, –, gluten-free flours **12**, 321–322
–, –, jams and jellies **12**, 321
–, –, salad dressings **12**, 322
–, –, soft drinks **12**, 322
–, –, syrup **12**, 320–321
–, –, wafers and crackers **12**, 321
–, frozen foods **12**, 324–327
–, –, confections **12**, 326
–, –, fruit **12**, 325
–, –, potatoes **12**, 325–326
–, preparation **12**, 314–315
Methylcellulose-based composite edible films **44**, 351, 352–355
–, applications **44**, 370
–, gas permeability **44**, 365
–, relative humidity effects **44**, 363, 369
–, solute barrier properties **44**, 368–369
–, temperature effects **44**, 364, 369
Methylcyclohexanone, DDT emulsion of, fatal to man **2**, 212
Methylene blue, effect of size on adsorption **2**, 11–12
–, test for oxide reducers **2**, 389
Methylene chloride, *N*-nitroso compounds and **31**, 66
–, solubility of DDT in **2**, 203
Methylene dihydroxycoumarin, interference with prothrombin formation **1**, 125
Methylene sulfonic acid types of ion exchangers **2**, 5
Methylergonovine **44**, 317
Methyl ester of C_5 hydroxy acid in pineapple **2**, 268
– of a C_5 keto acid in pineapple **2**, 268
– of a C_5 unsaturated acid in pineapple **2**, 268
Methyl esters, in pectin **1**, 397, 399, 406–407, 409–411, 413–414, 416, 420
–, *N*-nitroso compounds and **31**, 79
Methyl ether of saligenin in coffee **2**, 279
Methyl ethylacetaldehyde in black tea **2**, 287
Methylethyl (furyl)-*a*-oxysulfide in coffee **2**, 281
Methylglyoxal **32**, 163–164
3-Methylhistidine, research needs **37**, 406–407
Methyl iscaproate in pineapple **2**, 268
Methyl isovalerate in pineapple **2**, 268
Methyl ketones **16**, 257, 273; **39**, 206–208
–, binding to unprocessed whey proteins **33**, 411
–, in butterfat **19**, 191
–, α-lactalbumin binding **33**, 415
Methyl linolenate, brain phosphoglyceride effects **35**, 77–78
Methylmercaptan in Formosan black tea **2**, 288
Methyl *B*-methylsulfonylproprionate in pineapple **2**, 269
Methyl *B*-methylthiolproprionate in pineapple **2**, 269
Methyl-*a*-oxysulfide in coffee **2**, 281
Methyl *n*-propyl ketone in pineapple **2**, 268
Methylpyrazine in coffee **2**, 281
N-Methylpyrrole in coffee **2**, 281
Methyl salicylate phenylethyl alcohol, in black tea oil **2**, 287
Methyl sulfide in Formosan black tea **2**, 287
5-Methyl-tetrahydrofolate, 6-ambo form, availability **33**, 9

–, chemical synthesis of 6-ambo or 6S form **33**, 10
–, energy of activation for degradation in aqueous solution, table **33**, 50
–, oxidative degradation **33**, 45–47
–, thermal degradation **33**, 49
Methylthiouracil **13**, 143–144; **44**, 299, 322
Methyl transferase *S*-adenosyl methionine, in wheat germ **23**, 240
Methyl *n*-valerate in pineapple **2**, 268
Methylxanthines, chocolate and **31**, 325, 326
Metmyoglobin, derivatives important for meat **18**, 267
–, fish lipid oxidation **33**, 291
–, reduction and meat mutagens formation **34**, 436
–, thermal behavior **35**, 331–332
Metolazone **44**, 306
Metronidazole **44**, 286
Met3O transthyretin **40**, 150–155
Mevalonic acid **15**, 205
–, structure of **23**, 19
Mexico, IM meat **39**, 82–83
Mexiletine **44**, 306
Mezocillin **44**, 291
MG uptake, *see* Glucose, transport
Mice, protection against influenza **2**, 138
–, toxicity of DDT to **2**, 208
–, use in toxicity tests of CPCl **2**, 153
Micelles, chocolate and **31**, 255
–, effect on alimentary adsorption **15**, 32
Michaelis constant **40**, 234
Michaelis–Menten equation, analogy with WLF equation **38**, 200–204
Michaelis–Menten kinetics, enzyme substrate **40**, 158
–, initial velocity **40**, 307–309
–, population kinetics **40**, 268
–, vitamin B6 **40**, 117
Microbacterium arborescens **44**, 213
Microbial activity, *N*-nitroso compounds and **31**, 96, 97
Microbial attachment **43**, 319–357
–, attached cells **43**, 347–349
–, –, heat resistance **43**, 348
–, –, microbial activity **43**, 348–349
–, –, sanitizer resistance **43**, 347
–, bacterial cell envelope **43**, 321–323
–, conditioning films **43**, 326–327
–, confocal scanning laser microscopy **43**, 354–357
–, cutting boards **43**, 332
–, detection methods **43**, 351–352
–, excreted polymers **43**, 323, 327, 328–329, 330, 331, 338, 347, 348
–, food contact surfaces **43**, 329–334
–, –, arrival at surface **43**, 329–330
–, food matrix effects **43**, 333
–, food processing equipment **43**, 333–334
–, growth media influences **43**, 324–325, 338
–, inhibition methods **43**, 353–354
–, initial reversible stage **43**, 325–326
–, –, DLVO theory of colloidal stability **43**, 325
–, –, electrostatic interactions **43**, 328, 337
–, –, hydrophobic effects **43**, 327–328, 337
–, irreversible stage **43**, 326, 328–329
–, meat tissue **43**, 334–339
–, mechanisms **43**, 325–329
–, microbial footprints **43**, 327
–, microbial motility **43**, 330, 336
–, microbial survival function **43**, 320
–, physical entrapment **43**, 341, 343, 347, 355
–, plant tissues **43**, 344–347
–, poultry skin **43**, 339–343
–, response to environmental change **43**, 324–325
–, selective **43**, 332
–, stainless steel **43**, 330–331, 348
–, starvation stress response **43**, 325
–, stationary phase cells **43**, 325
Microbial control (*see also* Contamination) **39**, 119–124, 271–272
Microbial detachment **43**, 320, 349–351
–, attachment polymer oxidation **43**, 350–351
–, cell-directed **43**, 349–350
–, enzymatic release **43**, 350
–, physicochemical **43**, 351
Microbial flora, distribution **37**, 71
–, gastrointestinal tract, control **37**, 47–50
Microbial growth, scanning electron microscopic studies of **22**, 245–249
Microbial inactivation (*see also* Thermal processing, meat/poultry products), heat **44**, 147–186
–, pulsed electric field (PEF) processing **44**, 10–15
–, –, determinant factors **44**, 11–12
–, –, high-acid liquid foods (fruit juices) **44**, 12–15
–, –, temperature **44**, 11, 12
Microbial infections, gastrointestinal immune system **37**, 23–24
Microbial inhibition by ultraviolet and X-ray radiations **1**, 375

Microbial inhibition by ultraviolet and X-ray radiations (*cont'd*)
– by –, through interference with cell membrane **1**, 377–380
– by –, – with enzymes **1**, 380–385
– by –, – with genetic mechanism **1**, 374–377
Microbial inoculation, chocolate and **31**, 215
Microbial sources of protein **18**, 85–140
– of –, algae **18**, 116–128
– of –, bacteria **18**, 88–116
– of –, fungi **18**, 116
– of –, palatability and digestibility of **18**, 128–129
– of –, research needs for **18**, 128–131
– of –, yeasts **18**, 88–116
Microbiological assays, and ion-exchange chromatography **33**, 33
–, eluted folates **33**, 29–30
–, folate determination **33**, 21–22
–, modifications **33**, 22
Microbiological auditing (*see also* Sterilization tests) **32**, 14–15
Microbiological fermentation of fish **4**, 210–213, 219, 222, 224
Microbiological time–temperature integrators **44**, 179–180
–, endpoint procedure (quantal response) **44**, 179
Microbiology, meat processing **21**, 195–197, 199–206
–, scanning electron microscopy applied to **22**, 239–250
Micrococcus **45**, 198
–, as source of protein **18**, 91, 93
–, effect of nitrites on **3**, 295
–, enzyme action in **2**, 369
–, growth rate of **7**, 101, 102
–, halophilic **7**, 112
–, in fresh fish **2**, 350, 353
–, in pork **3**, 293
Micrococcus aureus, germicidal action of lauryldimethylbenzylammonium chloride **2**, 155
Micrococcus cerificans, propagation of **18**, 93
Micrococcus lipolyticus, in slime production in bacon **3**, 309
Micrococcus luteus **44**, 213
Microcrystalline cellulose/corn starch composite films **44**, 384
Microcystis sp., toxicity of **18**, 124
Microdialysis **40**, 183–190, 194–195
Microemulsions **34**, 84, 162–165
–, phase diagram **34**, 163
–, polar lipids **34**, 163–164
Microencapsulation **34**, 165–168
Microfibrils, components **31**, 120, 122, 123
–, dicotyledonous plants **31**, 126–128
–, dietary fiber and **31**, 136, 139, 158
Microflora, in dehydrated mashed potatoes **25**, 111–112
Microgravity **40**, 121
Micro-organisms, as affected by benzoic and salicylic acids **11**, 331–353
–, as target for thermal processes **23**, 76–77
–, cardiolipin **37**, 263
–, cloned gene expression **36**, 144–151
–, effect on carbohydrates **16**, 204
–, – on cheese ripening **16**, 232ff, 255ff, 282ff
–, – on food quality **16**, 161ff
–, – on meat emulsions **16**, 132
–, – on milk products **16**, 198ff
–, – on proteins **16**, 166ff
–, heat tolerance **12**, 73
–, in animal feeding **30**, 345
–, influence of freezing rate **6**, 169
–, – of freezing temperatures on **6**, 164
–, in frozen and chilled beef **12**, 169, 171–173
–, in frozen meat **6**, 188
–, in meat animals **6**, 115
–, in noncitrous fruit juices, chemical changes induced by **9**, 259–272
–, –, control of **9**, 247–257
–, –, effects on appearance **9**, 257–259
–, –, relation to climate **9**, 243–244
–, –, – to insects **9**, 244
–, –, – to season **9**, 242
–, –, sources **9**, 237–246
–, –, varieties **9**, 222–237
–, –, washing, effects on **9**, 245
–, metabolism, affected by acids **11**, 336–339
–, –, rates **12**, 75
–, morphology of, using scanning electron microscopy **22**, 240–242
–, pH influence on **11**, 333–336
–, phosphatidylglycerol **37**, 262
–, protein production from petroleum **30**, 345
–, proteins of **16**, 18
–, salt and sugar tolerance **12**, 58–59, 86
–, –, culture temperature **12**, 59
–, seed storage proteins expression **36**, 151–163
Microscopy **41**, 167
–, coalescence measurement **34**, 176–177
Microsomal enzymes, control **33**, 305–306
–, fish lipids **33**, 291–297
–, lipid oxidation, catalysis **33**, 256–259

Microsomes, endogenous proteolytic enzymes and **31**, 352, 366, 367
–, heart, peroxidation, α-tocopherol effects **33**, 213
–, liver **15**, 37
–, –, α-tocopherol, binding **33**, 196–197
–, –, –, concentrations **33**, 212
–, –, –, transfer factors **33**, 194–195
–, lung, peroxidation, α-tocopherol effects **33**, 213
Microsporum conis, germicidal action of CPCl on **2**, 152
Microsporum lanosum, germicidal action of ADBACl on **2**, 147
Microvilli **41**, 158
Microwave exposure effects, heating mechanism **43**, 68–78
–, –, absorbed microwave power calculation (power equation) **43**, 70–71
–, –, dielectric properties **43**, 69–74
–, –, dipolar water molecule rotation **43**, 68, 69
–, –, frozen foods **43**, 71, 73–74
–, –, ion movements **43**, 69, 70
–, microbiological **43**, 87–92
–, –, athermal **43**, 89–92
–, –, selective power absorption **43**, 89
–, –, spore growth **43**, 88
–, –, thermal **43**, 87–89
–, non-thermal **43**, 86–87, 89–92
–, –, adverse health effects **43**, 129
–, nutritional **43**, 92–93
–, safety aspects **43**, 88, 128–130
–, selective heating effects **43**, 74–78
–, –, concentration effects **43**, 76–78
–, –, in-depth heating **43**, 75–76
–, sensory **43**, 93–95
–, –, flavor compounds **43**, 94–95
–, spluttering/superheating **43**, 87, 99
–, temperature measurement methods **43**, 82–85
–, –, fiberoptic thermometry **43**, 84–85, 86
–, –, glass thermometers **43**, 83–84
–, –, infrared imaging **43**, 84
–, –, problems **43**, 83
–, –, thermocouple probes **43**, 83
Microwave foods **43**, 67, 102–105
–, chain of development **43**, 105
–, composition/formulation effects **43**, 104–105
–, dielectric properties **43**, 103–104
–, flavors **43**, 103, 104
–, geometry **43**, 103
–, packaging **43**, 67, 106–109, 131
–, –, active packaging **43**, 107–109
–, –, materials **43**, 106–107
–, –, metals **43**, 107
–, –, susceptors (receptors) **43**, 108–109
–, surface browning/crisping **43**, 105, 108
–, texture **43**, 103, 105
Microwave industrial equipment **43**, 109–128, 131
–, applicators **43**, 110–114
–, –, cavity **43**, 110–111
–, –, horn **43**, 111, 112
–, –, periodic structure **43**, 111, 112, 113
–, –, single mode **43**, 113–114, 115
–, –, travelling wave (Meander) **43**, 113
–, components **43**, 109–110
–, design **43**, 109–114
–, frequencies **43**, 109–110
–, heating applications **43**, 67, 114–128
–, –, advantages/disadvantages **43**, 116–117
–, –, basic requirements **43**, 116
–, –, blanching **43**, 117
–, –, cooking–coagulation **43**, 117–118
–, –, dehydration **43**, 122–124
–, –, killing insects/molds/bacteria **43**, 119
–, –, pasteurization/sterilization **43**, 125–128
–, –, preconditioning **43**, 119
–, –, tempering/thawing **43**, 119–122
–, –, volume expansion **43**, 118–119
Microwave oven **43**, 95–96, 130
–, IEC standard performance test **43**, 100
–, oven field distribution **43**, 96–100
–, –, computer simulations **43**, 100, 131
–, –, confined modes **43**, 97
–, –, mode stirrer **43**, 97
–, power ratings/rate of heating **43**, 100–102, 130
–, – of –, differential heating **43**, 102
–, – of –, spluttering/bumping **43**, 99
Microwave processing, of flexibly packaged foods **23**, 397–398
Microwaves **15**, 277ff
–, absorption into food **15**, 286
–, baking **15**, 292
–, cooking **15**, 290
–, definition **43**, 68
–, frequencies **15**, 279, 287
–, heating **15**, 278
–, process devices **15**, 282
–, reheating of baked products **38**, 220–221
–, sterilization **15**, 291
Microwave technology **43**, 65–131
–, domestic use, *see* Microwave oven
–, emission (leakage) standards **43**, 129
–, exposure limits **43**, 129

Microwave technology (*cont'd*)
–, historical development **43**, 66
–, industrial use, *see* Microwave industrial equipment
–, interference **43**, 130
–, vacuum drying **43**, 123, 124
Microwave treatment, proteins **35**, 336–337
Midazolam **44**, 308
Mildew, germination of **7**, 97
Milk (*see also* Cheese) **13**, 292–295; **14**, 242; **15**, 237; **16**, 139
–, alginates in chocolate milk **11**, 147
–, arsenic **36**, 238
–, as allergen **42**, 26–27
–, ascorbic acid content **4**, 395–401
–, aseptic **32**, 20–21
–, bacterial content during freezing storage **6**, 197
–, bacterial resistance to pasteurization **2**, 82
–, boron **36**, 238
–, calcium **36**, 213–218
–, carrageenan in stabilization **11**, 129–131
–, cheese quality **39**, 248–249
–, chemical forms **36**, 209
–, chloride **36**, 212–213
–, chocolate and **31**, 253–255, 330
–, chromium **36**, 237
–, citrate **39**, 200–201
–, cobalt **36**, 237
–, composition **10**, 43–45
–, composition (bovine, human) **33**, 421–423
–, conching **31**, 298
–, condensed **15**, 309; **31**, 256, 257
–, –, thixotropic gels in sweet-ened **8**, 21
–, –, viscosities of **8**, 24, 40
–, containers, sterilization of **3**, 187
–, contamination with pyrrolizidine alkaloids **45**, 70, 72, 91
–, conversion to cheese **39**, 164–165, 166, 169–195
–, copper **36**, 228–229
–, crumb, advantages **31**, 291
–, –, chocolate and **31**, 284–286, 330
–, –, conching **31**, 298
–, –, flavor **31**, 290, 291
–, –, processing **31**, 286–290
–, crystallization **39**, 117–118
–, curd tension of **8**, 19
–, DDT in **2**, 211–212, 214
–, dried **31**, 258–261
–, –, addition of alkaline compounds to **3**, 72
–, –, annual production of **3**, 46
–, –, ascorbic acid content **4**, 399–400
–, –, caramel flavor in **3**, 98, 99
–, –, chemical changes in flavor of **3**, 104, 105
–, –, clarification of **3**, 73
–, –, detection of neutralization in **3**, 72
–, –, deterioration of nonlipids in **3**, 97–105
–, –, effect of manufacturing procedures on **3**, 71–93
–, –, – of quality on sensory tests **2**, 230
–, –, – of storage on biological value of protein in **4**, 270
–, –, – of temperature on scoring of **2**, 247
–, –, flavor requirements for **3**, 65
–, –, heat coagulation of **3**, 79–80
–, –, heat processing of **3**, 71, 73–78
–, –, in diets **1**, 108
–, –, influence of oxygen on flavor of **3**, 102, 104
–, –, moisture equilibria in **3**, 55–60
–, –, need for trained judges for scoring **2**, 235
–, –, nonfat solids of **3**, 72, 80–83
–, –, nutritional value of **3**, 63–64
–, –, production, storage, and utility of **3**, 45–118
–, –, quality requirements for **3**, 64–69
–, –, solubility tests on **3**, 67–69
–, –, specific grading requirements for **3**, 66
–, –, vitamin content of **3**, 63
–, effect of heat treatment on nutritive value of protein value in **4**, 248, 254
–, enzymatic changes in dried product **11**, 270–272
–, enzymes **39**, 213–215, 249, 257–258
–, evaporated **15**, 309
–, –, ascorbic acid content **4**, 399
–, –, color of **6**, 30
–, –, –, in candies **6**, 30
–, –, –, in precooked frozen foods **6**, 199
–, fat **31**, 263, 264, 278
–, fermentation **39**, 164–165, 174–175
–, fermented, lactase in **38**, 14–17
–, flat sour bacteria spores in **18**, 173–174
–, fluoride **36**, 238
–, freeze-dried **7**, 205, 230–231
–, –, deterioration of **7**, 230
–, frozen storage, effect on folate content (human) **33**, 51
–, furcellaran in milk products **11**, 159
–, β-galactosidase stability in **38**, 36
–, gelation by pectinate mixtures **1**, 421
–, heat treatment **39**, 187
–, homogenization of **10**, 53
–, human, freeze-drying of **7**, 230–231
–, human and cow's **36**, 211–212

–, –, comparison **2**, 21
–, in diets **1**, 109–110
–, in muffins **6**, 272
–, in precooked frozen foods **6**, 199
–, iodine **36**, 233–236
–, iron **36**, 221–225
–, lactate **39**, 198–200
–, lactic acid in **16**, 191
–, lactose **31**, 255, 256, 263; **39**, 174–177, 198–200
–, liquid, composition of **19**, 154
–, –, heat treatment of **3**, 73–83
–, low-lactose **38**, 6–7
–, –, processing by consumers **38**, 7–9
–, lysine measurement **35**, 194–195
–, lysinoalanine in **35**, 205–206
–, magnesium **36**, 218–219
–, manganese **36**, 230–231
–, minerals and trace elements (*see also* Cow's milk, Human milk, *and specific minerals and trace elements*) **36**, 209–240
–, molybdenum **36**, 236
–, nickel **36**, 238
–, partial replacement by soy or peanut protein **30**, 357
–, pasteurization, effect on folate binding **33**, 76
–, –, ultrahigh-temperature methods, effects on folate activity **33**, 51
–, phosphorus **36**, 219–221
–, potassium **36**, 212–213
–, powder, effect of sonic vibrations on **3**, 131
–, –, electronic drying of **3**, 142
–, –, fat extraction in **3**, 51–52
–, –, manufacture of **3**, 83, 84
–, –, roller-dried, desorption in **3**, 60, 61
–, –, spray-dried, desorption in **3**, 61
–, –, –, fat extraction in **3**, 51–52
–, –, –, manufacture of **3**, 83
–, –, ultraviolet radiation in manufacture of **3**, 150
–, –, vapor pressure–moisture content curve for **3**, 56
–, powders (*see also* Buttermilk powder, Dry whole milk, Nonfat dry milk, Skim milk powder, Sweet whey powder, Whey powder), amino acids related to flavor in **19**, 195–197
–, –, bacterial plate count, analysis of variance **5**, 205
–, –, carbohydrates in **19**, 183–187
–, –, composition of **19**, 153–154
–, –, enzymes in **19**, 182–183
–, –, flow diagram **19**, 153
–, –, in breadmaking, functions **19**, 149–152
–, –, lipids in **19**, 187–191
–, –, off-flavors in **19**, 202–205
–, –, preparation of **19**, 152–153
–, –, production and utilization of **19**, 148–149, 150
–, –, quality of **19**, 202–206
–, –, research needs on **19**, 207
–, –, vitamins and minerals in **19**, 192–195
–, production and marketing in USA **30**, 347–348
–, products **13**, 292–295
–, –, ascorbic acid addition to **18**, 234–236, 291–292
–, –, folate bioavailability **33**, 75–76
–, –, folate stability in **33**, 51
–, –, in candies **6**, 30
–, –, scanning electron microscopy of **22**, 287–288
–, –, used by the candy industry **6**, 3
–, protection of bacteria during freezing by **6**, 169
–, protein-bound thiamine in **6**, 261
–, proteins **10**, 45–50; **16**, 24, 44, 237
–, –, compositional analysis **35**, 341
–, quality **16**, 198ff
–, raw, sterilization of by cathode rays **3**, 166, 175
–, research needs **36**, 240
–, roller- and spray-dried **35**, 200
–, *Salmonella* in **3**, 227
–, selenium **32**, 92, 96, 98; **36**, 231–233
–, silicon **36**, 238
–, skim, half-life in column reaction **38**, 47, 50
–, –, heat treatment of **3**, 80
–, –, lactase stability, effect of enzyme concentration **38**, 37–38
–, –, –, – of media and temperature **38**, 37
–, –, sorption **39**, 99
–, sodium **36**, 212–213
–, solids, addition to potatoes **6**, 234
–, –, combination of sugars and **6**, 2
–, –, in milk chocolate type candies **6**, 37
–, –, percent in candies **6**, 29
–, spray-dried, average conditions for **2**, 403
–, –, density of powders in Niro dryer **2**, 422, 423
–, –, effect of humidity on **2**, 496
–, –, heat and material balance in Swenson dryer of **2**, 504, 506, 512
–, –, photomicrographs of spray dried **2**, 516
–, –, precondensing **2**, 475

Milk, spray-dried (*cont'd*)
–, –, reconstitution of **7**, 230
–, –, secondary drying of **2**, 501
–, –, terminal velocity of **2**, 469
–, –, use of bag filters in **2**, 404–407
–, –, – of Bishop dryer for **2**, 410
–, –, – of direct fired furnace for **2**, 486
–, stabilization of evaporated **2**, 24
–, storage **35**, 199
–, sugar, malabsorption **38**, 2–4
–, thiamine loss in **6**, 293
–, tocopherol composition (human) **33**, 179
–, tryptophan in **16**, 196
–, ultrasonic analysis, aggregates **45**, 152
–, –, fat globule particle sizing **45**, 150
–, –, imaging for spoilage measurement **45**, 154
–, use of ascorbic acid in **4**, 395–401
–, – of cation exchanger in determination of copper in **2**, 38
–, viscosity **39**, 44–45
–, viscosity of **8**, 39, 41
–, whey **31**, 261–263
–, whipping agent from protein of **6**, 24
–, zeolite treatment of **2**, 21–24
–, –, effect of acidity on calcium and phosphorus removal **2**, 22
–, –, – of alkali chloride on mineral composition of milk **2**, 23
–, zinc **36**, 225–228
Milk-based composite films **44**, 383
Milkfat (*see also* Dairy products), cholesterol **37**, 150
–, composition, *n*-3 fatty acids **37**, 147–148
–, –, *trans* isomers **37**, 146–147
–, –, predominant fatty acids **37**, 144–146
–, consumption, disappearance data **37**, 133–136
–, –, intake data **37**, 136–143
–, effect on serum lipids, animal studies **37**, 200–203
–, – on –, human trials **37**, 194–200
–, in total diet, CHD and cancer risks **37**, 224–225
–, –, products meeting current recommendations, available products **37**, 229–232
–, –, –, modified products **37**, 232–236
–, –, research needs **37**, 237–238
–, overall impact on health **37**, 224–229
–, phospholipids **37**, 150
–, relationship to CHD risk **37**, 203–206
–, research needs **37**, 236–239
–, trace lipids **37**, 150, 223
–, triglyceride structure **37**, 148–149
Milking machines, sanitizing studies on **2**, 177
Milk proteins **19**, 154–163
–, amino acid composition of **19**, 156–159
–, breadmaking quality related to **19**, 170–181
–, –, peroxide-treated milks **19**, 174–175
–, –, preheating effects **19**, 170–174
–, –, protein composition fluctuations **19**, 174
–, –, protein functions in **19**, 175–180
–, composition of **19**, 154–159
–, heat effects on **19**, 163–170
–, β-lactoglobulin–κ-casein interaction in **19**, 168–170
–, non-nitrogenous components of **19**, 159–160
–, serum proteins of, *see* α-Lactalbumin *and* β-Lactoglobulin
–, sulfhydryl groups in **19**, 168
Milk solids nonfat, chocolate and **31**, 257
Millet **16**, 7, 27
Minamata disease, occurrence of **18**, 155
Mincing devices **14**, 95–97
Mineral bioavailability, inositol phosphate influences **45**, 32–36
Mineral content of plants, effect of fertilizers on **1**, 310–314
– of vegetables, effect of blanching on **1**, 68
Mineral nutrients, absorption, inulin effects **43**, 32–34
–, microwave exposure effects **43**, 92
Minerals (*see also specific minerals*), as nutritional stress factors **4**, 109
–, contribution to meat flavor **18**, 38–39
–, human essential **36**, 210
–, in honey **24**, 305
–, in milk powders **19**, 192–195
–, in muscle **19**, 6
–, in nutrition **16**, 33
–, in tea **17**, 247–248
–, in vegetables, effect of blanching on **8**, 67
–, in wheat germ **23**, 204, 207–208, 232–235
–, nutrition **39**, 280, 282–283
Mineral salts, in candies **6**, 30
–, in fruits **17**, 181
Mineral toxicity, of mechanically deboned red meat **27**, 53–56
Miniemulsions **34**, 83–84
Minihomogenizer **34**, 169
MIRINZ tenderometer **21**, 167
Miso **16**, 50
–, wheat germ use in **23**, 285
Miso isoflavones **44**, 213

Misoprostol **44**, 299
Missing values **40**, 271–272
Mitochondria **15**, 83
–, benzoic and salicylic acids, effect on oxidative phosphorylation in **11**, 347
–, cardiolipin content, ischemia effects **37**, 301–302
–, endogenous proteolytic enzymes and, exopeptidases **31**, 347
–, in ripening fruits **30**, 173–174
–, liver, α-tocopherol concentrations **33**, 212
–, meat technology **31**, 394, 408
–, membrane fluidity, cardiolipin effect **37**, 299
–, metabolism, lactate indicator **37**, 349
–, muscle physiology **31**, 373
–, oxidative metabolism disorders **37**, 379–381
–, proteinase distribution **31**, 366, 367
–, protein importation and translocation, cardiolipin role **37**, 275–277
–, SH groups in **24**, 42
–, thiaminepyrophosphate effects **30**, 173, 174
Mitochondrial folate **40**, 99, 100–101
Mixed emulsifier system, competitive adsorption **34**, 126–127
Mixed protein gels, complex **34**, 263
–, composite or multicomponent **34**, 262–263
–, filled **34**, 263
–, gelatin–egg white gels, *see* Gelatin–egg white gels
–, interpenetrating polymer network **34**, 263
–, selective mixing (*see also* Polymer mixtures) **34**, 264–272
–, –, anisotropic structure **34**, 264
–, Takayanagi equations **34**, 272–274
–, types **34**, 261–264
Mixing, non-Newtonian **11**, 423–429
Mixing of meat emulsions **16**, 116ff
Mixing power, calculating requirements, for Newtonian fluids **11**, 423–426
–, –, for non-Newtonian fluids **11**, 426–428
–, –, for pseudo-plastics **11**, 428
Mixograph **45**, 285
MM equation **38**, 202
Mobility, defined by WLF equation **38**, 179
–, diffusional, above and below glass transition temperature **38**, 173–174
–, water, in glassy materials **38**, 169–170
Mobilization, tocopherols **33**, 186–189
Modal matrix, identifiability **40**, 315–316
Modeling (*see also* Compartmental modeling, Parameter, Software), computational aspects, *see* Dynamic system, Graph theory, Identifiability problem, Kinetic parameter distribution, Linear integrator, Neural network
–, connectivity **40**, 27, 32, 43, 306, 315
–, constructs **40**, 282
–, dynamic systems **40**, 323–338
Modified essential amino acid index **35**, 219
Modulus, elastic **39**, 7
–, loss **39**, 23
–, molecular models **39**, 35–37
–, rigidity **39**, 8
–, shear **39**, 8, 56
–, storage **39**, 22–23
–, Young's **39**, 7, 254
Moisture, cheese **39**, 178, 198, 251–253
–, chocolate and, emulsifiers **31**, 281, 282
–, –, milk **31**, 259, 260
–, –, milk crumb **31**, 288, 289
–, –, packaging **31**, 318
–, –, refining **31**, 295
–, –, sweeteners **31**, 264, 266, 268, 269, 272
–, effects on fruit composition **9**, 301
–, IM meat (*see also* Dehydration control, IM meat) **39**, 73, 100–102, 105–106, 141–142
–, olive oil and **31**, 458
Moisture content, adjustment, proteins **35**, 335
Moisture equilibria determinations by radio-frequency waves **3**, 143
Mojonnier spray dryer, "air gun" orifice in **2**, 474–475
–, operation of **2**, 420–422, 501
Molal osmotic coefficient, calculation of **7**, 86–87
Molar surface tension increment, soy protein isolate **34**, 308
Molasses **17**, 124–125
–, analyses for SO_2 **5**, 121
–, citrus, composition of **17**, 92
–, –, –, production of **17**, 90
–, cooling after spray drying **2**, 486
–, flavor constituents of **2**, 277
–, production of **17**, 94
–, –, alcohol from **17**, 80
Molds (*see also specific molds and* Micro-organisms) **15**, 289
–, action of epoxides on **1**, 384
–, chocolate and **31**, 219, 229, 256, 268
–, destruction of by ultraviolet light **3**, 149
–, discolorations on meat **6**, 142
–, effects on malic acid **9**, 269
–, growth on cocoa **8**, 287
–, in noncitrus fruit juices **9**, 234–236

Molds (*cont'd*)
–, in soy sauce mash **10**, 113–115
–, koji cultivation **30**, 196–197, 220–221
–, olive oil and **31**, 461, 471
–, on refrigerated meats **6**, 139
–, sulfite effects **30**, 11
–, water requirements, germination and **7**, 94–97
–, –, growth rate and **7**, 97–100
–, xerophilic, water requirements and **7**, 115–117
Molecularity **14**, 291–292
Molecular mass, whey proteins, table **33**, 349
Molecular model **39**, 35–37
Molybdenum, in milk **36**, 236
–, in wines **8**, 137, 193
Molybdenum–inositol phosphate interactions **45**, 36
Moment curve **40**, 50–52
Monilia, survival of at low temperatures **3**, 446
Monilia albicans, germicidal action of ADBACl on **2**, 147
Monilinia fructicola **15**, 173
Monkey, essentiality of *n*-3 PUFA **35**, 115
–, storage of DDT in **2**, 211
–, toxicity of DDT on **2**, 208
Monoamine oxidase inhibitors, role in histamine toxicity **24**, 145
Monocalcium phosphate, gelatin clarification and **7**, 248
Monochloramine, germicidal agent in **7**, 135
Monocotyledons, dietary fiber and **31**, 124, 135–138
Monocrotaline **45**, 66, 67, 78, 79, 80, 88
Monoferric phytate, purification from wheat bran **28**, 34
Monoglutamyl folates, bioavailability, comparative **33**, 65–66
–, –, table **33**, 66
–, chiral stability **33**, 13
–, deuterated, synthesis **33**, 11–12
–, HPLC methods of separation and analysis **33**, 26–33
–, racemization of glutamate α-carbon product **33**, 13
–, stability in aqueous solution **33**, 45
Monoglycerides, type of emulsifier **6**, 12
Monoketosamines **14**, 179–183
–, derived from primary amines **12**, 26–28
–, – from secondary amines **12**, 28–35
–, hydrolytic decomposition **12**, 28
–, preparation **12**, 5–8
Monolayers, phospholipid, α-tocopherol effects **33**, 215
Monomeric proteins, genetic control **36**, 36–37
–, wheat proteins **36**, 27–29
Mononuclear killer cells, characterization **37**, 10
Monosaccharides, reaction with proteins **3**, 273–277
Monosaccharide unit, atom labeling **42**, 146–147
Monoses, in fresh cocoa bean juice **8**, 239
Monosodium glutamate **10**, 195
–, flavor profile and **7**, 13
Monotony, flagging appetite **21**, 16–17
Monounsaturated fatty acids (MUFAs) **36**, 264
–, effects on serum lipoproteins and apolipoproteins **37**, 159–170
–, *trans* fatty acids **37**, 175–178
–, *cis* monounsaturates **37**, 171–175
–, plasma lipid/lipoprotein responses **36**, 295–305
–, –, atherosclerosis **36**, 303–304
–, –, high-fat versus low-fat diets **36**, 296
–, –, LDL lowering mechanism **36**, 301–302
–, –, studies **36**, 298–299
–, –, trans fatty acids **36**, 304–305
Monte Carlo simulation **40**, 270–271
Monterpenes, Labiatae **42**, 249–250
Moray eel poisoning **10**, 138
Moricizine **44**, 306
Mormon cricket meal **40**, 160–163
Moromi, *see* Soy Sauce, Japanese, mash
Morphine **44**, 296, 323
Morpholine, *N*-nitroso compounds and **31**, 59–61, 92, 95
Morphology, carcinogen risk assessment and **31**, 25, 28, 43
Mortadella **39**, 78
Motion, equation of **32**, 42
Motor oil, calculated vs. experimental heat transfer in **11**, 419
Mott's procedure **20**, 247–251
Mouth-feel **41**, 165
Mozzarella cheese, contamination **39**, 287
–, flavor **39**, 235
–, proteolysis **39**, 211, 226
–, ultra filtration **39**, 194
mRNA (*see also* Messenger RNA), isolation, cDNA cloning **36**, 139–140
MSG, idiosyncratic reactions **42**, 30–31
–, role in food-borne illness **42**, 13
Mucilage, dietary fiber and **31**, 141, 169, 182

–, in cocoa beans **8**, 263
Mucopolysaccharides, collagen and **7**, 260
–, connective tissue, association with **28**, 261–262
–, endogenous proteolytic enzymes and **31**, 402, 403
–, gelatin and **7**, 271, 272
Mucor, effect of ultraviolet radiation on **3**, 148
–, in bacon **3**, 298
Mucor hiemalis **15**, 212
Mucor piriformis **45**, 181
Mucor stolonifer, control of by ozone **3**, 466
Mucosal cell **40**, 245, 246, 250
MUFAs, *see* Monounsaturated fatty acids
Muffins, thiamine retention in **6**, 272, 273
Mullet, aerobic bacteria in **2**, 350
–, poisoning, occurrence of **18**, 155
Multiple inositol polyphosphate phosphatase (MIPP) **45**, 11, 12
Multiple photon microscopy (MPM), fat crystal network microstructure **44**, 38
Multiple scattering theory **45**, 113–116
Multipoint attachment theory, sweeteners **42**, 215, 217
Mung bean, phytate (inositol hexakisphosphate) synthetic pathway **45**, 8
Munsell color system **9**, 165–168
Murexine, structure of **18**, 153
Murnong **43**, 6–7, 46
Murphree vapor efficiency equation **20**, 29
Muscle (*see also* Glycogen phosphorylase metabolism) **9**, 3; **14**, 37; **19**, 1–74
–, actin **26**, 65–66
–, actinins **26**, 67–68
–, actomyosin **26**, 66
–, amino acid content in aging **9**, 36–37
–, biochemistry **19**, 13–22
–, –, role in meat quality **21**, 99–113
–, bloody, spoilage of **7**, 52
–, bundle arrangement **19**, 7
–, bundle size **14**, 47–49
–, capillary system of **19**, 12–13
–, cells **26**, 62
–, characteristics **14**, 47–52
–, chemistry **26**, 58–74
–, collagen **26**, 59–61
–, collagen types **28**, 235–128
–, color chemistry **26**, 88–90
–, components **20**, 258–267
–, –, quantitative distribution **26**, 75–76
–, composition, variation in **26**, 74–75
–, compositional analysis **35**, 339–341
–, composition and morphology **19**, 3–13
–, –, general aspects **19**, 7–11
–, connective tissue of **20**, 264–267
–, contractile elements in **9**, 2
–, contractile process of **19**, 313–314; **20**, 262–263
–, –, active phase **9**, 12
–, –, actomyosin in **9**, 11–12
–, –, experimental models **9**, 13–14
–, –, relaxed phase **9**, 12
–, –, –, schematic of **9**, 12
–, –, –, theories of **9**, 10–13
–, –, sources of energy **28**, 206
–, –, speed of **19**, 23–24
–, –, water-holding capacity and **20**, 280–281
–, diseases and disorders, age effects **37**, 368–369
–, –, atrophy **37**, 363–364
–, –, clinical symptoms, muscle fatigue **37**, 342
–, –, –, muscle function, unusual **37**, 343
–, –, –, muscle weakness **37**, 341–342
–, –, –, myoglobinuria **37**, 342–343
–, –, connective tissue diseases, acquired disorders **37**, 401–405
–, –, –, genetic diseases **37**, 389–401
–, –, –, nutritional diseases **37**, 387–389
–, –, diagnosis, biopsies **37**, 345
–, –, –, blood chemistry **37**, 343–344
–, –, –, clinical examination **37**, 343
–, –, –, electrical stimulation tests **37**, 347–348
–, –, –, electromyography **37**, 344
–, –, –, nuclear magnetic resonance **37**, 345
–, –, –, protein turnover **37**, 350
–, –, –, provocation tests **37**, 348–349
–, –, exercise effects **37**, 368–369
–, –, glycolytic disorders **37**, 374–379
–, –, –, acquired diseases **37**, 379
–, –, –, lipid metabolism disorders **37**, 381–383
–, –, –, mitochondrial oxidation disorders **37**, 379–381
–, –, –, myotonic syndromes **37**, 383–387
–, –, hypertrophy **37**, 363–364
–, –, inflammatory myopathies **37**, 362
–, –, muscular dysgenesis **37**, 370–371
–, –, myoclonus **37**, 371–373
–, –, neuropathies **37**, 364–365
–, –, research needs **37**, 405–409
–, elastin **26**, 61
–, endogenous proteolytic enzymes and, *see* Endogenous proteolytic enzymes
–, enzyme activities of **19**, 14–16
–, –, neural regulation **19**, 54–56

Muscle (*cont'd*)
–, extracellular components **9**, 3; **26**, 58–62
–, fatigue **37**, 341–342
–, fibers **20**, 260–263
–, –, differentiation **19**, 29–50
–, –, –, biochemical **19**, 36–45
–, –, –, histochemical **19**, 30–36
–, –, –, physiological **19**, 45–50
–, –, isolation of **19**, 348–349
–, –, microstructure of **19**, 283–285
–, –, SH group role in **24**, 40
–, fibrous proteins **26**, 59–62
–, flavor chemistry **26**, 87–88
–, flavor precursors in extracts of **18**, 29
–, function, electrical stimulation **37**, 347–348
–, –, provocation tests **37**, 348–349
–, –, related quadriceps **37**, 348
–, –, unusual **37**, 343
–, glycogen **26**, 72–73
–, gross composition of **19**, 280–281
–, ground substance **26**, 62
–, growth **40**, 142
–, in meat science, importance **19**, 57–61
–, innervation in **19**, 24–25
–, in porcine stress syndrome **28**, 202–210
–, –, contractile proteins **28**, 200–202
–, –, neuromuscular junction **28**, 193–195
–, –, sarcoplasmic reticulum **28**, 195–200
–, intracellular material **9**, 3
–, intracellular proteins **26**, 62–69
–, ions **26**, 70–72
–, lipids **26**, 73
–, literature on **9**, 1–2
–, location **14**, 52–53
–, meat quality of **26**, 76–157
–, –, and chemistry **26**, 83–87
–, –, and elastin **26**, 85
–, –, and extracellular components **26**, 83–84
–, –, and fat **26**, 85–86
–, –, and intracellular components **26**, 86–87
–, –, and muscle biophysics **26**, 90–94
–, –, and proteins **26**, 86–87
–, –, and structure **26**, 82–83
–, –, ante-mortem factors affecting **26**, 94–95
–, –, evaluation **26**, 76–82
–, metabolism **19**, 16–19
–, –, halothane and **28**, 207–209
–, microstructure of **19**, 281–283
–, morphology, as related to meat quality **21**, 113–121
–, myofibrillar proteins **26**, 63–66
–, myosin **26**, 63–65
–, neural influence on **19**, 50–56
–, –, enzyme profiles **19**, 54–56
–, –, motor units **19**, 53–54
–, –, trophic **19**, 50–53
–, nonprotein components **9**, 5
–, nonprotein nitrogenous substances **26**, 74
–, nucleotides in **18**, 44
–, of abalone **23**, 152
–, –, amino acids of **23**, 154
–, pale, soft, exudative, biochemistry of **21**, 106–109, 111–113
–, –, –, –, endocrine interrelationship **21**, 87–98
–, –, –, –, occurrence and processing of **21**, 123–128
–, –, –, –, rigor mortis **21**, 80–81
–, –, –, –, thyroid role **21**, 96–98
–, pH **14**, 123–124
–, physiology **13**, 152–156
–, –, red and white **13**, 156
–, –, rigor mortis **13**, 152–154
–, –, rigor resolution **13**, 154–156
–, physiology of **19**, 23–25
–, post-mortem aging of **20**, 268–277
–, proteins *see* Muscle proteins
–, relaxants, taste sensation effects **44**, 309–310
–, relaxation **9**, 12, 26–28
–, –, chemical factors in **9**, 26–28
–, research needs for **19**, 61–63
–, resting potential of **19**, 25
–, reticulin **26**, 61–62
–, sarcoplasmic proteins **26**, 63
–, sarcoplasmic reticulum of **19**, 19–20
–, scanning electron microscopy of **22**, 288–289
–, shortening in thawing **9**, 23–26
–, skeletal, myofibrillar proteins of **19**, 279–360
–, structure **14**, 128–129; **26**, 54–58
–, sulfhydryl groups **14**, 123
–, synonyms for **19**, 2–3
–, thermal denaturation **35**, 344
–, tropomyosin **26**, 66–67
–, ultrafiltration **40**, 193
–, ultrastructure of **19**, 11–12
–, vitamin B6 metabolism **40**, 115–116, 120–121
–, vitamins **26**, 73–74
–, wasting **40**, 140–141
–, water content **26**, 69–70
–, weakness **37**, 341–342
–, –, in Duchenne and Becker's muscular dystrophies **37**, 352
Muscle area, cross-sectional **37**, 346

Muscle-meat conversion (*see also* Dehydration control, IM meat) **39**, 90–97
Muscle proteins **9**, 5–10; **10**, 55–59
–, free water in **10**, 860–362, 363
–, heating effects on **20**, 281–297
–, *C*-protein **26**, 68–69
–, *M*-protein **26**, 68
–, regulatory **26**, 66–69
–, SH groups in **24**, 31–40
–, thermal scanning rheological analysis **35**, 351–353
–, water-binding by **10**, 856–362
Muscovite, volume per oxygen atom in **2**, 3
Muscular dysgenesis **37**, 370–371
Muscular dystrophies, Becker's **37**, 351–359
–, Duchenne **37**, 351–359
–, endogenous proteolytic enzymes and **31**, 389–391
–, limb girdle **37**, 359
–, myotonic **37**, 359–361
–, ocular myopathies **37**, 361–362
–, Steinert's disease **37**, 359–361
Musculature, ante-mortem treatment **13**, 134–145
–, –, environment **13**, 134–140
–, –, nutrition **13**, 141–143
–, –, treatments **13**, 143–145
–, changes, biochemical **13**, 100–104
–, –, physiological **13**, 97–100
–, –, post-mortem **13**, 97–107
–, –, solubility **13**, 104–107
–, environment effect **13**, 134–140
–, –, cold **13**, 135–136
–, –, combination **13**, 139–140
–, –, warm **13**, 136–138
–, enzymes and metabolites **13**, 145–150
–, –, ATPase **13**, 149–150
–, –, dehydrogenase, lactic **13**, 147–148
–, –, glycolysis **13**, 148–149
–, –, phosphofructokinase **13**, 145–147
–, –, phosphorylase **13**, 145–147
–, histology **13**, 107–120
–, –, irregular band structure **13**, 114–120
–, –, muscle structure **13**, 107–114
–, incidence, breed of pig **13**, 125–128
–, –, geographical area **13**, 120–122
–, –, heritability **13**, 128–129
–, –, lean-to-fat ratio **13**, 125
–, –, season **13**, 124
–, –, sex **13**, 124–125
–, –, temperature **13**, 122–124
–, –, weight **13**, 124–125
–, nutrition effects **13**, 141–143
–, physical, chemical properties **13**, 94–97
–, post-mortem studies **13**, 132–134
–, –, biopsy and samples **13**, 132
–, –, glycogen structure **13**, 133–134
–, prevention **13**, 167
–, PSE porcine **13**, 89–178
–, tissue sensitivity **13**, 97
–, transformations, post-mortem **13**, 91–97
–, treatments **13**, 143–145
–, variations in a carcass **13**, 129–132
–, – in –, between muscles **13**, 129–130
–, – in –, semitendinosus **13**, 131–132
–, – in –, within muscles **13**, 130–131
Mushrooms **15**, 236
–, canned, nutrients in **1**, 43, 46–49
–, –, use of ascorbic acid in **4**, 369–370
–, composition of oil of **2**, 277
–, enzyme characteristics of **3**, 20
–, phenolase preparations obtained from **3**, 7
–, tyrosinase of **3**, 2
Mussels, ozone treatment **45**, 197
–, saxitoxin from **18**, 155
Mustard gas, chromosomal breaks produced by **1**, 376
Mutagen **32**, 169–170
–, antimutagenesis **32**, 165–166
–, from aqueous Maillard reactions **32**, 161–164
–, nitroso **32**, 164–165
–, pyrolysate **32**, 157–161
Mutagenesis, carcinogen risk assessment and **31**, 28
–, *N*-nitroso compounds and **31**, 74
Mutagenicity, by food cooking and processing **30**, 122–123
–, *in vivo* tests (*see also In vitro* mutagenicity tests) **34**, 397–399
–, of shoyu compounds **30**, 298–299
Mutation **34**, 389–390
–, carcinogen risk assessment and **31**, 25, 28
–, *N*-nitroso compounds and **31**, 64
–, of fungi **15**, 159
Mutton, processing **21**, 186–187, 193–194
–, thiamine loss in **6**, 275, 276
Mya arenaria **10**, 145
Myasthenia gravis **37**, 33, 366–367
Mycelium **15**, 153, 160
Mycobacterium, as source of protein **18**, 91
Mycobacterium fortuitum **45**, 173
Mycobacterium phlei, germicidal action of CPCl on **2**, 152
Mycobacterium tuberculosis in milk **2**, 82
Mycoderma, destruction of by heat **3**, 435
Mycoloxins, of *Byssochlamys* spp. **25**, 267–277

Mycostat **39**, 85
Mycotoxins **39**, 285–290
–, degradation by sulfiting agents **30**, 17
–, differing from aflatoxins, production by molds **30**, 297
–, irradiation effects on **24**, 186
Myelin proteolipid protein **45**, 30
Myoclonus **37**, 371–373
–, epilepsy **37**, 372
–, inherited, in Hereford Cattle **37**, 373
–, spastic mice **37**, 372–373
–, spontaneous **37**, 372
Myofiber **39**, 92, 94–96, 124, 125
Myofibrillar proteins (*see also individual proteins*) **19**, 279–360
–, actomyosin **34**, 252–254
–, definition and classification **34**, 249–250
–, denaturation effects on **19**, 321–322
–, heat-gelling and emulsification effects on **19**, 320–321
–, in a food system **19**, 314–322
–, –, intact myofibril **19**, 314–317
–, –, isolated proteins **19**, 319–322
–, metabolic activity in muscle **19**, 20–22
–, molecular biology of **19**, 285–313
–, –, individual proteins **19**, 288–313
–, –, review of developments in **19**, 285–288
–, myosin **34**, 250–252
–, –, gelation mechanism **34**, 250–251
–, –, gel properties **34**, 251–252
–, preparative procedures for **19**, 322–349
–, quality of muscle related to differences in **19**, 319–320
–, salt-soluble proteins **34**, 254–255
–, SH groups in **24**, 31–40
–, –, functional role **24**, 36
Myofibrils (*see also* Fibrils) **14**, 35, 51
–, endogenous proteolytic enzymes and **31**, 411–413
–, endopeptidases **31**, 353, 354
–, isolation of **19**, 348–349
–, meat technology **31**, 397, 399, 400, 404, 409
–, muscle physiology **31**, 370, 371, 373, 374, 379
–, proteinase activity **31**, 387, 391
–, proteinase distribution **31**, 367, 369
Myogen **9**, 5
–, enzymes in **9**, 5–6
Myoglobin **10**, 57–58; **13**, 101–102
–, and meat color **9**, 3
–, denaturation, cooked meat color change **44**, 167, 168, 169
–, effect on color of bacon **3**, 314
–, freeze-dried beef and **7**, 211–212
–, in meat during curing **29**, 10–12
–, –, nitrosochromogen production **29**, 10–12
–, in muscle **19**, 3–4, 8
–, *N*-nitroso compounds and **31**, 73
–, structure **22**, 4
–, structure and properties **29**, 8–11
–, warmed-over flavor development in cooked meat and **29**, 39–41
Myoglobinuria **37**, 342–343
Myo-inositol **45**, 3, 36
–, anticancer activity **45**, 37, 38
–, food sources **45**, 36–37
–, plasma lipid effects **45**, 40
Myopathies, atrophic **37**, 363–364
–, endogenous proteolytic enzymes and **31**, 391
–, inflammatory **37**, 362
–, ocular **37**, 361–362
Myosin **9**, 4, 6–7, 11–12; **10**, 55–57, 356–357, 375, 376, 389, 392; **16**, 114
–, action on adenosine triphosphate **1**, 6
–, aggregation **19**, 292–294
–, denaturation, pH dependent **35**, 336
–, endogenous proteolytic enzymes and, meat technology **31**, 394, 396, 397, 400, 404, 407, 409, 410
–, enzyme activity **19**, 291–292
–, fatty acid modification **35**, 330–331
–, fragments by proteolysis **19**, 290–291
–, function in contraction **9**, 6
–, "heavy" **9**, 6–7
–, in relation to meat structure **1**, 207–208
–, isolation of **19**, 288–289
–, "light" **9**, 6–7
–, molecular structure of **19**, 289–290
–, molecular weight **9**, 6
–, molecule schematic **9**, 7
–, muscle physiology **31**, 370, 371, 374
–, myofibrillar proteins **34**, 250–252
–, peptide chains in **9**, 6
–, proteinase activity **31**, 388
–, rod, melting process **35**, 322
–, salt effects **35**, 326
–, SH groups in **24**, 35
–, –, function **24**, 36–38
–, splitting of ATP **9**, 22–23
Myosin A, preparation of **19**, 343–345
Myosin B (*see also* Actomyosin), preparation of **19**, 345–348
Myosin-cleaving-protease, endogenous proteolytic enzymes and **31**, 353
Myositis, active **37**, 342
Myotomy, effect on meat quality **21**, 101–102

Myotonia congenita **37**, 383–384
Myotonic muscular dystrophy **37**, 359–361
Myricetin, lipoxygenase inhibition **33**, 317
–, structure **33**, 311
–, structure of **19**, 80
Myristic acid, in poultry fat **1**, 212
–, plasma lipid/lipoprotein response **36**, 269
Myristicin, in parsley oil **2**, 273
Mytilus californianus **10**, 144, 175
Mytilus edulis **10**, 144, 145

Na^+/K^+ ATPase, *n*-3 PUFA effects **35**, 131–132
Nabumetone **44**, 296
Nacconol NR, effect on tubercle bacilli **2**, 148
NAD, *see* Nicotinamide-adenine dinucleotide
NADH, *see* Reduced nicotinamide dinucleotide
NADP, *see* Nicotinamide-adenine dinucleotide phosphate
Naegeli starch **41**, 168
Na:K exchange **14**, 3
Nagaoka formula **20**, 246–247
Naive data pooling **40**, 273
Nalbuphine **44**, 296
Naphthaleneacetic acid, methyl ester of, use to inhibit sprouting in potatoes **1**, 284
β-Naphthol, microbial inhibition by **1**, 388
Naphthol sulfonates, microbial inhibition by **1**, 386
Naphthoresorcinol, glycyrrhizin assay and **7**, 370
Naphthylamine, effect of ion size on adsorption of **2**, 11–12
2-Naphthylamine, carcinogen risk assessment and **31**, 16
NARADCOM system, package durability in **23**, 400–401
Naringenin **44**, 197
Naringin in grapefruit **2**, 260
– in –, removal from citrus peel juice **2**, 30
Narrow-gap coaxial viscometers **11**, 374–377
Nasal potency meter **14**, 10
Nash pump **15**, 316
Natick–Swift retort packaging line, description of **23**, 338–340
National Academy of Sciences, carcinogen risk assessment and **31**, 8–10, 22
– of –, *N*-nitroso compounds and **31**, 72, 73, 98, 99
National Canners Association **32**, 6
National Food Processors Association **32**, 6
National Toxicology Program, carcinogen risk assessment and **31**, 25
Natrolite, volume per oxygen atom in **2**, 3
Natto **16**, 51
Natural fats, structure of **23**, 8
Natural killer cells, characterization **37**, 10
Na-yeast **12**, 64, 67
Near-infrared spectroscopy, meat endpoint temperature monitoring **44**, 175
Nebulin, endogenous proteolytic enzymes and **31**, 400, 401, 406
Necic acids **45**, 66
Nectarines, removal of gases from by vacuum **3**, 36
–, use of SO_2 **5**, 141
Nedocromil **44**, 302
Needleman–Wunsch algorithm **42**, 50–51
Neisseria catarrhalis, germicidal action of CPCl on **2**, 152
Nelfinavir **44**, 286
Nelson, P.E. **32**, 23
Nematodes, kiwifruit damage **29**, 284
Neomycin, effect on flat sour bacteria spores **18**, 185
Neoplasia, carcinogen risk assessment and **31**, 42, 43
Neosartorya fischeri **45**, 197
Neosugar **43**, 5–6
–, intestinal/hepatic enzyme response **43**, 23
–, intestinal microflora response **43**, 21
Neper (Np) **45**, 106
Nereistoxin, as marine toxin **18**, 157
Nerves, effect of fatigue in taste scoring **2**, 241
–, – of temperature on **2**, 247
–, effect on muscle **19**, 50–56
Nerve tissue, *n*-3 PUFA **35**, 120–127
Nervous disease, smell perception effects **44**, 270–271
–, taste perception effects **44**, 265
Nervous system, effect of DDT on **2**, 206, 212, 213
Neural network **40**, 333–337
Neuropathies, muscular **37**, 364–365
Neurospora, mutations due to X-rays **3**, 160
Neurosporene **15**, 206
Neutral detergent fiber, dietary fiber and **31**, 151–155, 180
Neutralization **41**, 95–96
–, chocolate and **31**, 246, 247
–, olive oil and **31**, 463
Neutral salts, effect on wheat proteins solubility **36**, 12–14
–, protein stability **35**, 294–301

Neutron activation analysis, for detecting selenium **32**, 87–88
Nevirapine **44**, 285
Newman's solution, of heat conduction problems **20**, 224, 239
Newtonian fluids **9**, 176–177; **39**, 4–6, 34
–, power requirements for mixing **11**, 423–426
Newtonian viscosity **39**, 5
Newtonian zone **39**, 34
Niacin **15**, 127
–, content, effect of storage on **1**, 92, 94–95, 97–98
–, –, of apples and pears **8**, 368
–, –, of canned foods, effect of heat sterilization on **1**, 87–89
–, –, of vegetables, effect of blanching on **1**, 80–81
–, counteraction of "pellagragenic" factor by **1**, 125
–, effect of cathode rays on **3**, 168, 169
–, – of X-rays on **3**, 158
–, in wheat germ **23**, 208
–, loss during blanching of vegetables **8**, 75
–, retention of during electronic cooking **3**, 142
Niacinamide **6**, 302
Niacin deficiency **1**, 118
Nib, chocolate and, alkalization **31**, 247–249
–, –, conching **31**, 307
–, –, processing **31**, 241, 243–245
Nickel, effect on low-ester pectins **1**, 414
–, in milk **36**, 238
–, in wines **8**, 137
Nickel–phytate (inositol hexakisphosphate) interactions **45**, 32, 36
Niclosamide **44**, 286
Nicotinamide-adenine dinucleotide (NAD) **17**, 19–20, 25
–, reactions with sulfites **30**, 25
Nicotinamide-adenine dinucleotide phosphate (NADP) **17**, 16, 19
Nicotine **44**, 317
Nicotinic acid, *see* Niacin
Nifedipine **44**, 306, 320
Niridazole **44**, 286
Niro rotor, description of **2**, 457–458
Niro spray dryer, operation of **2**, 422–423
Nisin **16**, 180, 282; **39**, 283
–, effect on flat sour bacteria spores **18**, 185–186
Nitratase, salt concentration and **7**, 112
Nitrates, carcinogen risk assessment and **31**, 24
–, effect on bacteria in bacon **3**, 294–295
–, in meat curing **29**, 7–17
–, –, bacteriostatic action **29**, 13–14
–, –, color stabilization **29**, 7–8, 10–12
–, –, flavor production **29**, 11–13
–, –, myoglobin conversion to nitrosochromogen **29**, 10–12
–, *N*-nitroso compounds and, cheese **31**, 85, 86
–, –, cured meats **31**, 84, 85
–, –, fish **31**, 86
–, –, fried bacon **31**, 74–84
–, –, function **31**, 72–74
–, –, fundamentals **31**, 66
–, –, indirect contamination **31**, 96
–, –, regulation **31**, 84
Nitration of pectins **11**, 25
Nitric acid, effect on cation exchangers **2**, 6
Nitric oxide, nitrite/nitrate addition **31**, 73, 79
–, *N*-nitroso compounds and, fundamentals **31**, 62–64, 68
–, processing **31**, 90
–, reaction with hemoglobin in bacon **3**, 314
Nitrite–ascorbate combination, reduction of *N*-nitrosamine formation in cured meat **29**, 61–62
Nitrite ions, reaction with folates **33**, 44–45
Nitrites, as *Clostridium botulinum* inhibitor **22**, 159
–, as meat preservants **22**, 2–3
–, bacon flavor and **29**, 24–26
–, carcinogen risk assessment and **31**, 24
–, chlorine demand and **7**, 142
–, effect on bacteria in bacon **3**, 294–295
–, – on color of bacon **3**, 315, 316
–, – on "warmed-over" flavor **23**, 54
–, frankfurter flavor and **29**, 29–30, 32–33
–, ham flavor and **29**, 26–29
–, inactivation of enzymes by **1**, 383
–, inhibition of warmed-over flavor development in cooked meat **29**, 41–44
–, in meat curing, bacteriostatic action **29**, 13–14, 46–48
–, –, color stabilization **29**, 7–8, 10–12
–, –, effect on volatile compounds **29**, 64–70
–, –, flavor production **29**, 11–13
–, –, –, comparison with sodium chloride **29**, 30–32
–, –, myoglobin conversion to nitrosochromogen **29**, 10–12
–, microbial control **39**, 121, 122–123, 124
–, microbial mutations caused by **1**, 376
–, nitrosation of **22**, 8–10, 11

–, substitution by, alternatives, evaluation **29**, 56
–, –, fumarate esters **29**, 52
–, –, lactic acid-producing bacteria **29**, 55–56
–, –, radiation **29**, 52–55
–, –, sodium hypophosphite **29**, 52
–, –, sorbic acid **29**, 49–52
–, toxicity of **22**, 6
Nitroanisole demethylase **15**, 37
p-Nitrobenzyl ester of acetic acid in coffee **2**, 282
Nitrocatechol in respiration of potatoes **3**, 14
Nitrogen, carcinogen risk assessment and **31**, 39
–, chocolate and **31**, 220, 223, 246, 258, 297
–, dietary fiber and **31**, 173
–, dose–response **40**, 157–160, 164–166
–, effect on ascorbic acid content of plants **1**, 308–309
–, – on calcium absorption by plants **1**, 311–312
–, endogenous proteolytic enzymes and **31**, 410
–, extractable **14**, 121–122
–, free amino **14**, 211–213
–, fundamentals **31**, 59, 60, 62–67
–, in biomass **32**, 205, 210, 211, 222, 223
–, in cheese ripening **16**, 235ff
–, in cocoa beans and nibs **6**, 38
–, in muscle **14**, 51
–, in passion fruit **12**, 262–263, 267
–, in pectins **11**, 48
–, in proteins **16**, 9ff
–, in quaternary ammonium compounds **2**, 119, 126
–, in tea **11**, 218–221
–, in wheat flour **16**, 343ff
–, nitrite/nitrate addition **31**, 78, 79
–, olive oil and **31**, 460
–, processing **31**, 89, 90, 93
–, protein quality **40**, 160–162
Nitrogen blanket, as oxidation preventive **10**, 196, 197
Nitrogen compounds, contribution to meat flavor **18**, 40–43
–, in cocoa **2**, 283
–, in coffee **2**, 280
–, in soy sauce **10**, 78–82
–, of spoiling fish **2**, 375–376
Nitrogen compounds in citrus fruits, amino acids **9**, 316–318
– in –, analytical applications **9**, 319–320
– in –, bases **9**, 316–318
– in –, containing sulfur **9**, 318–319
– in –, factors affecting **9**, 315–316
– in –, proteins **9**, 319
Nitrogen dioxide, *N*-nitroso compounds and **31**, 62, 79, 90
Nitrogen equilibria, in heat treatment test for dry milk **3**, 54
–, in milk products **3**, 60
–, in packaging of milk products **3**, 86, 88
Nitrogen gas, packaging dehydrated potatoes in **1**, 271–272
Nitrogen oxides, as nitrosamine precursors **22**, 11–12
Nitrogen supply, effects on fruit composition **9**, 298–299
Nitrogen trichloride, microbial inhibition by **1**, 386
Nitrogen trichloride in treatment of citrus fruits **3**, 465
Nitroglycerin patch **44**, 314
p-Nitrophenyl phosphate, β-lactoglobulin binding **33**, 409
Nitroprusside test in milk **3**, 75, 82
Nitroreductase, fecal, lactic culture effects **37**, 99–101
Nitrosamides **31**, 65
N-Nitrosamides **31**, 100
–, fundamentals **31**, 58, 60, 64, 68
–, nitrite/nitrate addition **31**, 76
Nitrosamines, carcinogen risk assessment and **31**, 24
N-Nitrosamines **22**, 1–71; **31**, 55–57, 98–100
–, adduct formation of **22**, 18–20
–, analysis of **22**, 33–55
–, –, methods **22**, 39–46
–, animal studies on **22**, 29–32
–, as carcinogens **22**, 27–32
–, biochemical changes caused by **22**, 32–33
–, biological properties of **22**, 27–33
–, biosynthesis of **22**, 13
–, chemistry of **22**, 8–27
–, –, reactions **22**, 17–27
–, colorimetric analysis **22**, 41–42
–, cyclization of **22**, 24–25
–, detectors for **22**, 43–45
–, epidemiological studies on **22**, 27–29
–, formation in cured meat, mechanism of **29**, 57–58
–, – in –, reduction by ascorbate and its isomeres **29**, 14–15, 59–60
–, – in –, – by ascorbic acid long-chain acetals **29**, 60
–, – in –, – by ascorbyl palmitate **29**, 60
–, – in –, – by nitrite–ascorbate combination **29**, 61–62

N-Nitrosamines, formation in cured meat, reduction (*cont'd*)
–, – in –, – by α-tocopherol **29**, 60–61
–, from nitrosation **22**, 8–10
–, fundamentals **31**, 58–60, 62, 64–69, 71, 72
–, gas–liquid chromatography of **22**, 42–43
–, hydrogen bonding of **22**, 18–20
–, hydrolysis of **22**, 17–18
–, indirect contamination **31**, 93, 94, 96
–, in foods **22**, 47–53
–, in tobacco **22**, 53–55
–, isolation of **22**, 34–39
–, mass spectrometry of **22**, 16–17, 45–46
–, nitrite/nitrate addition **31**, 74–76, 79–82, 84–86
–, nonvolatile **22**, 46–47
–, oxidation of **22**, 24
–, photochemistry of **22**, 25–27
–, polarographic analysis of **22**, 39–40
–, processing **31**, 86, 87, 89–93
–, properties of **22**, 13–14
–, reduction of **22**, 21–24
–, spectroscopy of **22**, 14–16, 40–41
–, structure of **22**, 14–17
–, synthetic routes for **22**, 10–13
–, toxicity of, acute **22**, 29–30
–, –, historical aspects, subacute **22**, 30–32
–, transnitrosation of **22**, 20–21
N-Nitrosamino acids **31**, 99, 100
–, nitrite/nitrate addition **31**, 74, 76, 83
–, processing **31**, 89
Nitrosation, fundamentals **31**, 58–60, 62, 64–69, 71, 72
–, indirect contamination **31**, 95, 96
–, nitrite/nitrate addition **31**, 77–79, 85
–, *N*-nitroso compounds and **31**, 55, 99
–, processing **31**, 90, 91
N-Nitrosation **31**, 99, 100
–, fundamentals **31**, 60, 61, 63
–, nitrite/nitrate addition **31**, 78–83
–, processing **31**, 89–91
Nitrosoamines **32**, 157, 169–170
Nitrosochloride of *a*-pinene in parsley oil **2**, 274
Nitrosochromogen, conversion from myoglobin during meat curing **29**, 10–12
N-Nitroso compounds **31**, 54–57
–, analytical methods **31**, 66–69
–, and cheese **31**, 85, 86
–, and cured meats **31**, 84, 85
–, and fish **31**, 86
–, and fried bacon **31**, 74–84
–, and function **31**, 72–74
–, and fundamentals **31**, 60, 61, 66, 68
–, and indirect contamination **31**, 94, 96
–, and processing **31**, 92
–, and regulation **31**, 84
–, biological activity **31**, 64–66
–, catalysis **31**, 60–64
–, chemistry **31**, 58–60
–, food surveys **31**, 69–72
–, indirect contamination **31**, 95, 96
–, –, microbial activity **31**, 97
–, –, packaging **31**, 95
–, –, rubber **31**, 93, 94
–, inhibition **31**, 60–64
–, nitrite/nitrate addition, cheese **31**, 85, 86
–, –, cured meats **31**, 84, 85
–, –, fish **31**, 86
–, –, fried bacon **31**, 74–84
–, –, function **31**, 72–74
–, –, regulation **31**, 84
–, processing, dried products **31**, 91, 92
–, –, fish **31**, 92, 93
–, –, malt **31**, 86–91
–, relative exposure **31**, 97–99
–, research trends **31**, 100
N-Nitrosodibutylamine **31**, 94
N-Nitrosodiethanolamine **31**, 64, 98
N-Nitrosodiethylamine **31**, 56, 78, 95
N-Nitrosodimethylamine **31**, 54, 55, 57, 98, 99
–, formation in malt, sulfites and **30**, 17
–, fundamentals **31**, 61, 65, 67, 70, 71
–, indirect contamination **31**, 93, 95, 96
–, nitrite/nitrate addition **31**, 78, 80, 85
–, processing **31**, 86, 87, 89–93
N-Nitrosodipropylamine **31**, 96
N-Nitrosoglycocholic acid **31**, 68
N-Nitrosoguanidine **31**, 68
Nitrosohemoglobin **7**, 212
N-Nitrosomorphiline **31**, 74, 92, 95, 98
Nitroso mutagens **32**, 164–165
Nitrosomyoglobin, structure of **22**, 4
Nitrosophenol, *N*-nitroso compounds and **31**, 61
N-Nitrosopiperidine **31**, 74
N-Nitrosoproline **31**, 76–79, 89, 99
N-Nitrosopyrrolidine fundamentals **31**, 70, 71
–, nitrite/nitrate addition **31**, 74, 76–78, 80, 82–85
–, processing **31**, 87, 92
N-Nitrososarcosine **31**, 78
N-Nitrosothiol **31**, 79
N-Nitrosothizolidine **31**, 74, 82–84
N-Nitrosureas **31**, 64, 65, 67
Nitrosylhemochrome **16**, 150

Nitrosyl radicals **31**, 67, 68, 79
Nitrous acid **31**, 59, 60, 73
Nixtamalization **43**, 236
NLMIX software **40**, 275
Nocardia, as source of protein **18**, 91
–, propagation of **18**, 94–95, 97
Nomenclature **41**, 29
Nomographs color **9**, 172–174
2,6 Nonadienal in cucumber oil **2**, 276
Non-digestible carbohydrate **43**, 2, 6
–, intestinal microflora response **43**, 16, 19
–, –, ENDO project **43**, 18
–, potential physiological effects **43**, 27
–, prebiotics **43**, 16
Nonenzymatic browning, activation energies **35**, 196–197
Nonfat dried milk solids, chocolate and **31**, 262, 263
Nonfat dry milk (NFDM), amino acid composition of **19**, 158
–, lipids in **19**, 187
–, preparation of **19**, 152–153
–, –, flow diagram **19**, 153
–, production and utilization of **19**, 150
–, use in bakery and confectionery products **19**, 151
Nonidentifiable parameter **40**, 311
Nonlinear system, advantages **40**, 158, 317, 337
–, chaos **40**, 324–326
–, dimensionality **40**, 325–328
–, identifiability **40**, 317
–, linear differential equations **40**, 285–289
–, neural networks **40**, 335–336
–, nutrient response analyses **40**, 157–166, 228–229
NONMEM software **40**, 275
Nonmuscle proteins, thermal scanning rheological analysis **35**, 354–357
Non-Newtonian fluids, classification of **32**, 45–47
–, heat transfer characteristics **11**, 416–423
–, –, heat transfer with turbulent flow **11**, 422
–, –, power requirements for mixing **11**, 426–428
–, –, time-dependent **11**, 393–394
Non-Newtonian materials **9**, 177–179
–, dilatants **9**, 187
–, plastics **9**, 178
–, pseudoplastics **9**, 177–178
Non-Newtonian mixing **11**, 423–429
n-Nonoic acid in cocoa **2**, 283
Nonpolar side chain, frequency, wheat proteins **36**, 8
Nonprotein ingredients and additives, proteins **35**, 336
Nonstarch polysaccharides, analysis **31**, 142–146
–, content **31**, 146–150
–, dietary fiber and **31**, 170
Nonstarter lactic acid bacteria **39**, 198, 199, 211, 219–220, 230
–, future research **39**, 295
–, quality **39**, 250–251
–, temperature **39**, 256–257
Nonvolatile constituents of citrus oils, coumarin derivatives **9**, 340–342
– of –, steroids **9**, 342
– of –, triterpenoids **9**, 342
n-Nonylic alcohol in orange peel oil **2**, 265
Nonylmethyl(methyl)-*a*-oxysulfide in coffee **2**, 281
Noodles, Chinese buckwheat **44**, 413
–, fried, nutritious, for developing countries **22**, 194
–, Japanese buckwheat **44**, 412–413
–, technology **44**, 410–411
Norbixin, *see* Annatto extract
Nordihydroguaiaretic acid **5**, 271
–, effect on growth **3**, 203, 204
–, – on mortality of rats **3**, 205
–, in dehydrated bacon **3**, 319, 320, 321
–, inhibition of lipoxygenase **33**, 307
–, pathologic effects of **3**, 207
–, toxicity of as an antioxidant **3**, 200
Norfloxacin **44**, 291
Normal stress **39**, 13–14, 23
North America, buckwheat products **44**, 415
–, IM meat **39**, 80–82
Nortriptyline **44**, 312
Nose, artificial **14**, 20–21
Nosean, volume per oxygen atom in **2**, 3
Nougats, chemical composition and properties of **6**, 10
–, improved by sorbitol **6**, 11
–, stability of fats in **6**, 12
–, toughening of **6**, 7
Noyes process **15**, 343
Nozzles, as atomizing devices for spray dryers **2**, 439–445
–, capacity and spray angle of pressure type **2**, 448
–, effect of size on bulk density **2**, 472–473
–, Hunkle type **2**, 452–454
–, rules for liquids atomized by **2**, 446
–, two-fluid nozzles **2**, 451–454
NPEM2 software **40**, 276
NSLAB, *see* Nonstarter lactic acid bacteria

Nuclear magnetic resonance (NMR) spectroscopy, deuterated folates **33**, 12–13
–, for muscle disease/disorders **37**, 345, 406
–, high-molecular-weight glutenin subunits **45**, 272–273, 279, 282
–, –, domain structures **45**, 236, 237, 239
–, inositol phosphates **45**, 6
–, –, whole raw seed studies **45**, 13
–, meat endpoint temperature monitoring **44**, 175, 176
Nucleation **13**, 224–247, 258–260
–, critical nuclei size **13**, 246–247
–, heterogeneous **13**, 244–245
–, homogeneous **13**, 244–245
Nucleic acids, content, of mechanically deboned red meat **27**, 65–68
–, effect of X-rays on **3**, 165
–, in wheat germ **23**, 220
–, synthesis **40**, 81
Nucleophiles, *N*-nitroso compounds and **31**, 59, 60, 65
5′-Nucleotidase, hepatic, *n*-3 PUFA effects **35**, 131
Nucleotides, contribution to meat flavor **18**, 43–45
–, of abalone **23**, 157–160
Nucleotide sugars, conversion to, cellulose **30**, 165
–, –, hemicelluloses **30**, 164
–, plant, biosynthesis **30**, 162–163
Nucleus of the solitary tract **44**, 252, 253
Nusselt number **32**, 57, 58, 64, 67–68, 72, 73, 75, 79
Nutrient-response curve **40**, 157–166, 227–241
–, biochemical systems theory **40**, 233, 236–238
–, data analysis **40**, 238–240
–, equation derivation **40**, 229–232
–, graded level intake **40**, 157–166
–, metabolic control theory **40**, 233–236
–, perturbation response **40**, 285–289
–, rational polynomials **40**, 228–229, 231
Nutrients, loss of **17**, 81
–, variability in reaction to **1**, 140
Nutrients in tea **11**, 224–226
Nutrition **13**, 141–143
–, effects on gastrointestinal immunity **37**, 44–45
–, improvements, new technologies and **30**, 378
–, in poorest countries, new protein food production **30**, 380
–, –, population growth limit and **30**, 380
–, –, protein-rich food shipment **30**, 378–379
–, in world, food products to improve **22**, 187–203
–, of peanut protein **26**, 239–244
–, undernutrition, and meat quality **26**, 116–119
–, water requirements and **7**, 107–109
Nutritional beverage models, industrialization and **30**, 358
–, milk partial replacement by soy or peanut protein **30**, 357
Nutritional diseases, of connective tissue **37**, 387–389
–, smell perception effects **44**, 271
–, taste perception effects **44**, 266
Nutritional labeling, *see* Food labeling
Nutritional quality, future research on **10**, 65
Nutritional stress factors, destruction by processing **4**, 122–123
–, effect on food acceptance **4**, 124–126
–, nature of **4**, 107–110
–, normally found in foods **4**, 110–114
–, not normally found in foods **4**, 114–117
–, nutrient imbalance as **4**, 117–119
–, produced in foods by processing and storage **4**, 120–122
Nutritional stress factors and food processing **4**, 105–132
Nutritional therapies, AIDS **37**, 51–52
–, immunosuppressed conditions **37**, 51–52
–, intestinal diseases **37**, 51
Nutritional value, of cheese **39**, 277–283
–, of heated proteins **4**, 233–280
–, of IM meat **39**, 136–138
–, of mechanically deboned fish **27**, 111–120
–, of mechanically deboned poultry **27**, 110–120
–, of mechanically deboned red meat **27**, 74–88
–, –, protein quality **27**, 74–78
–, of protein, chemical vs biological ratings **4**, 242
–, of tea **17**, 278–279
Nuts (*see also specific types*), in candies **6**, 29, 45, 47, 48
–, insects infesting **4**, 307
–, selenium in **32**, 95
–, used by the candy industry **6**, 3

Oak root fungus (*Armillaria mellea*), kiwifruit killing **29**, 284
Oat flour, extracts of **6**, 14

Oat globulin, denaturation kinetics 35, 344–345
–, thermal characteristics, heat treatment effect 35, 337
–, –, reducing agent effect 35, 329
–, –, sodium dodecyl sulfate effect 35, 327–328
–, –, succinylation effects 35, 330
–, –, urea effect 35, 327–328
Oat plants, ascorbic acid content of, effect of soil properties on 1, 308
–, carotene content of, effect of soil properties on 1, 309
Oats 16, 7
–, analysis 31, 142, 150, 152
–, bitterness in 11, 292–298
–, –, differentiation of bitter substances 11, 295–297
–, –, enzyme content and taste changes 11, 293
–, –, inhibition of bitterness in 11, 297–298
–, –, moisture content and lipase inactivation temperature 11, 294
–, dietary fiber and 31, 120, 140, 185
–, inositol phosphate degradation during processing 45, 21
–, properties 31, 168–171
–, zinc absorption influence 45, 33
Obesity, and taste preferences 32, 245
–, impairment of food intake regulation 21, 51–53
–, low-fat diet effects 37, 226–229
Occupational asthma, carmine reactions 43, 206–207
Occupational hazards 32, 215
Occupational sensitivities 42, 31
n-9-Octadecenyldimethylbenzylammonium chloride, germicidal activity of 2, 137
9-Octadecenyldimethylethylammonium bromide, germicidal activity of 2, 137
–, inhibitors of 2, 166
–, use as sanitizer for glasses 2, 180
–, use in brewing industry 2, 175
n-9-Octadecenyldimethylethylammonium bromide, germicidal activity of 2, 137, 156–157
9-Octadecenyldimethyl *y*-phenylpropyl-ammonium bromide, germicidal activity of 2, 137
9-Octadecenyldimethylpropylammonium bromide, germicidal activity of 2, 137
Octanol in Formosan black tea 2, 287
Octoic acid, in cocoa 2, 283
–, in tea 2, 286
Octopus 39, 344
Octyl alcohol, in tea 2, 288
n-Octyl alcohol in manufactured tea 2, 286
Octyl ester of *n*-butyric acid in parsnip seed oil 2, 274
Ocular myopathies 37, 361–362
Odor, basic studies on, landmarks of advances 19, 223–224
–, chlorine and 7, 165
–, classification 14, 26
–, control 14, 2
–, detection, theory 14, 2–5
–, development of, in onion and garlic 22, 73–133
–, effect on scoring foods 2, 243
–, enzyme role 22, 116–118
–, evaluation, physical, chemical 14, 18–22
–, –, sensory 14, 1–32
–, fish spoilage and 7, 44–45
–, food 14, 266–267
–, from browning 14, 235–245
–, measurement 14, 5–24
–, philosophy of 7, 35–37
–, primary 14, 3–4
–, research 14, 24–25
–, technique interrelations 14, 22–24
Odor perception test 7, 16
Odor recognition series 7, 16–17
Off-flavor (*see also under* Flavors), cheese 39, 236, 239–242
–, fish 39, 349
Ofloxacin 44, 291, 322
Oiling-off test 34, 180
Oil phase, emulsifier interaction with oil/water interface 34, 105–106
Oils, aldehyde 14, 225
–, ascorbic acid protection of 18, 241–248
–, autoxidation 17, 28–29
–, color of 5, 317–321
–, content of canned orange juice 2, 265
–, decomposition on distillation of radish 2, 274
–, enzymatic changes during storage 11, 278–280
–, essential, in tea 11, 228–231
–, for frying oriental noodles 43, 160
–, from cocoa beans 8, 279
–, Ω-gliadins 45, 222
–, in apples 2, 262
–, in coconut 6, 48
–, in nutmeats 6, 48
–, nutrition 12, 270–271
–, oxidized 14, 223–225
–, passion fruit seed 12, 268–271

Oils (*cont'd*)
–, peanut, mixtures of **8**, 26
–, percentage, in onion **2**, 273
–, –, in peach pulp **2**, 265
–, –, in tea **2**, 285, 287
–, physical and chemical constants **12**, 269–270
–, refining and bleaching **12**, 268
–, spoilage correlations **45**, 153
–, storage **12**, 270
–, structural studies **45**, 278
–, tests for rancidity in coffee **2**, 277–278
–, tocopherols in **33**, 159–164
–, ultrasonic analysis, particle sizing **45**, 150
–, used by the candy industry **6**, 3
–, vegetable, ascorbic acid as antioxidant synergist in **4**, 389
–, –, winterizing of **6**, 44
–, viscosity **39**, 45; **45**, 147
–, yellowness in **5**, 311
Oilseeds, antinutritional factors in preparations **30**, 371
–, – in –, control during processing **30**, 371, 376
–, chemistry and technology **30**, 376
–, cottonseed **30**, 338–339
–, genetics **30**, 376–377
–, high-protein residues, in animal flesh model **30**, 358–359
–, peanuts **30**, 339
–, production by major producers **30**, 337
–, proteins, amino acid content **30**, 360–362
–, –, cereal enrichment with **30**, 356
–, –, digestibility **30**, 363
–, –, effects on blood lipids **30**, 372–375, 376
–, rapeseed **30**, 339
–, scanning electron microscopy of **22**, 286–287
–, soybeans **30**, 336, 338
–, soy protein, *see* Proteins, soybean
–, sunflower seed **30**, 339
–, utilization of **17**, 106–115
Oil suspensions **15**, 261
Oil/water emulsions, droplet size distribution **34**, 152
Oil/water interface, interfacial tension, microemulsions **34**, 163
–, protein load **34**, 117–123
–, –, as function of concentration **34**, 117–118
–, –, multilayer adsorption **34**, 121–122
–, –, relation to emulsion droplet size **34**, 119
–, –, temperature dependence **34**, 119–120
–, SBA adsorption kinetics **34**, 114–116
–, small-molecule emulsifiers, adsorption thermodynamics **34**, 102–104
Oleanolic acid, glycyrrhetic acid and **7**, 363–364, 366
Oleate, by singlet oxygen **33**, 252
–, carbonyl compounds generated from, table **33**, 265
–, oxidation, autoxidation **33**, 241
–, –, free radical and photosensitized, distributions of isomeric hydroperoxides, table **33**, 254
Olefinic acid, olive oil and **31**, 472
Oleic acid, autoxidation **33**, 241–242
–, chocolate and, cocoa butter **31**, 250, 274, 278
–, –, milk **31**, 254
–, –, packaging **31**, 324, 325
–, desaturase activity, diet effects **35**, 35–36
–, Δ^6-desaturase inhibition **35**, 40
–, desaturation, unsaturated fatty acids effects **35**, 31, 33
–, in natural fats **23**, 8
–, in poultry fat **1**, 212, 216, 217
–, olive oil and **31**, 463, 464, 474, 479
–, rate of esterification of butanol and **2**, 37
Oleodipalmitin, in cocoa fats **6**, 39
Oleodistearin, in cocoa fats **6**, 39
–, use of **6**, 15
Oleopalmitostearin, in cocoa fat **6**, 39
Oleoresin, multicomponent film incorporation **44**, 385
Oleorosin **15**, 246
Oleuropein, olive oil and **31**, 469
Oleyldimethylethylammonium bromide, structure of **2**, 122
Olfaction, and food preferences **32**, 243
–, enzymic **14**, 4
–, loss of **32**, 245–246
–, theory **14**, 2–5, 26
Olfactometer **14**, 6–14
–, air dilution **14**, 11–13, 22
–, blast type **14**, 7–8, 22
–, electronic **14**, 9
Olfactometry **14**, 6–14
Olfactory bulb **44**, 254, 255
Olfactory mucosa **44**, 253–254, 255
Olfactory receptor cells **44**, 253, 254
Oligofructose **43**, 5
–, anticancer activity **43**, 37
–, food sources **43**, 7, 9
–, intake **43**, 8
–, lipid metabolism effects **43**, 28, 29, 30, 31, 41
–, nutritional labeling **43**, 48

–, soluble dietary fiber properties **43**, 27
Oligonucleotide-mediated mismatch mutagenesis **36**, 173–175
Oligonucleotide-mediated mutagenesis **36**, 180–181
Oligosaccharides **16**, 394
–, formed by *Kluyveromyces lactis* **38**, 77, 79
–, in apples and pears **8**, 312
–, in cocoa beans **8**, 262
–, in low-lactose milk and whey products **38**, 84–85
–, production by transgalactosidation, lactose concentration **38**, 74–76
Olive oil **31**, 453, 454, 478, 479
–, adulteration **31**, 473, 474
–, composition **31**, 463
–, –, fatty acids **31**, 463, 464
–, –, glycerides **31**, 464, 465
–, –, nonglycerides **31**, 465–470
–, constituents **31**, 458–460
–, consumption **31**, 477, 478
–, development **31**, 457, 458
–, extraction **31**, 461–463
–, fishy flavors in **4**, 191
–, harvesting **31**, 460–461
–, in diet of rats **1**, 112
–, olive fruit **31**, 455, 456
–, olive tree **31**, 454, 455
–, packing **31**, 470, 471
–, production **31**, 456, 457
–, quality **31**, 474–477
–, rancidity **31**, 471–473
–, storage **31**, 461
–, toxicity of DDT solution to man **2**, 212
Olives, canned, use of ascorbic acid in **4**, 371
–, effect of heat on peroxidase in **3**, 28
–, – of salts and inhibitors on **3**, 30
–, extract, catalytic effect of **3**, 8
–, "oxidase," effect of temperature on **3**, 27
–, preparations from **3**, 25
Omeprazole **44**, 299
Oncorhynchus mykiss, *see* Rainbow trout
Onion oil, components of **22**, 110–111
Onions (*see also Allium*), ascorbic acid content of, effect of fertilizers on **1**, 309
–, composition and distillation of **2**, 272, 273
–, dehydrated **6**, 315
–, dicotyledonous plants **31**, 126, 127, 129, 131, 132
–, dietary fiber and **31**, 146, 164
–, flavones **5**, 270–283
–, flavor and odor development in **22**, 73–133
–, inositol phosphates content **45**, 23
–, inulin **43**, 9
–, lachrymatory factor in **22**, 96–97
–, loss of thiamine **6**, 288
–, ozone treatment **45**, 198
–, parenchyma cells in **2**, 299
–, threshold values of compounds of **22**, 113
–, F value for industrial processing of **2**, 102
–, volatile organic sulfur compounds **5**, 120
Oöspora lactis in pickle spoilage **3**, 458
Opiates, smell sensation effects **44**, 323
–, taste sensation effects **44**, 296
Opportunistic infection, probiotics in prevention **43**, 44–45
Optical microscopes **34**, 171
Optimal harvest time (O.H.T.) **9**, 63, 64, 69, 70, 114–116
Optimization, IM meat processing **39**, 138–143
Optimum frequency, of microwaves **15**, 292
Oral allergy syndrome **42**, 5, 7
Oral cavity, anatomy **29**, 163–164
–, food responses **29**, 170–175
–, sensitivity to pain **29**, 167–168
–, – to temperature **29**, 168–169
–, – to temperomandibular joint position **29**, 169–170
–, – to touch pressure **29**, 166–167
–, somesthetic receptors **29**, 164–166
Oral immunization, for IgA responses **37**, 21–22
Oral leukoplakia **40**, 57
Oral sensitivities, flavors or flavoring substances **42**, 24–25
Oral tolerance, as specific response **37**, 22
–, induction, autoimmune therapy by **37**, 50–51
Orange-G, collagen degradation and **7**, 256–257
Oranges **10**, 298, 305, 308, 313–314, 317, 322, 328, 331; **15**, 218, 350; **16**, 208
–, ascorbic oxidase in **3**, 16
–, cathode ray experiments with **3**, 170–174
–, concentrate, minimizing browning in **1**, 362, 364, 366
–, cytochrome oxidase in **3**, 16
–, effect of temperature on **3**, 17
–, iodine wrappings for **3**, 465
–, juice, ascorbic acid content **4**, 373, 380–381
–, –, browning in **1**, 328–329, 332–334, 336–341, 362, 365
–, –, canned **2**, 265
–, –, –, ascorbic acid content of **1**, 55
–, –, –, composition and distillation of **2**, 264–265

Oranges, juice, canned (*cont'd*)
–, –, –, nutrients in **1**, 43, 46–50
–, –, –, tin vs. glass containers for **1**, 98–100
–, –, chemical changes in during browning **1**, 331, 346, 349–350, 352–359
–, –, discoloration of **5**, 54
–, –, drum-drying of **7**, 227
–, –, effect of sound waves on **3**, 131
–, –, effects of sulfur dioxide addition to **5**, 77
–, –, fermentation in **3**, 452
–, –, flavor/vitamin C content retention **44**, 17–20
–, –, –, packaging materials influence **44**, 18–20
–, –, folate bioavailability **33**, 74–75
–, –, freeze-dried **7**, 174, 186, 189, 226–227
–, –, –, stabilization of **7**, 228
–, –, frozen **6**, 169
–, –, –, bacterial count of **6**, 181
–, –, germicidal effect **6**, 202
–, –, infrared dehydration of **3**, 146
–, –, iodine-reducing substances in **5**, 63
–, –, lactose-fermenting yeast occurring in **6**, 182
–, –, loss of thiamine **6**, 295, 304
–, –, microbial inactivation **44**, 12–13
–, –, pectin in **1**, 398
–, –, puff-drying of **7**, 227
–, –, pulsed electric field (PEF) processing **44**, 26, 27
–, –, shelf-life **44**, 15–16
–, –, spray-drying of **7**, 227
–, –, sterilization of by cathode rays **3**, 166, 167
–, –, survival of bacteria in **6**, 164
–, –, use of SO_2 for inhibiting browning **5**, 85
–, juice concentrate, SO_2 binding power **5**, 126
–, –, yeast infections **5**, 79
–, marine transport **12**, 185–187
–, oil, use of ascorbic acid in **4**, 405–406
–, ozone/carbon dioxide/argon mixed gas treatment **45**, 201
–, peel, brining **5**, 144
–, –, pectin in **1**, 400
–, pH of **3**, 432
–, pulp, pectin in **1**, 400
–, soft rot of **6**, 181
–, sour, astringency **5**, 273
–, temperature **12**, 187
–, treatment of, with 2-amino pyridine **3**, 464
–, –, with sodium orthophenylphenate **3**, 464
–, X-ray fluoroscopy of **3**, 159
Orbitort **32**, 60–65
Oregano, health implications **42**, 264–267
Organelles, expression specific to **41**, 128–129
–, transporting **41**, 143–144
Organic acids **15**, 128
–, in kiwifruit, composition **29**, 296
–, –, during growth and ripening **29**, 291–292
–, –, fresh, frozen, canned **29**, 294
–, –, seasonal changes **29**, 295–297
–, shoyu flavor and **30**, 264–265
Organic bases, in soy sauce **10**, 81–82
Organic matter, chlorination and **7**, 152–156
Organisms, competing **13**, 357–358
–, food poisoning **13**, 349–396
Organoleptic spoilage of fishes **2**, 373–375, 377
Organs, SH content of **24**, 52–55
Oriental noodles **43**, 141–189
–, alkaline salt content **43**, 143, 146, 148, 158–159, 187
–, antioxidants **43**, 160
–, buckwheat **43**, 159
–, classification **43**, 143–148
–, color **43**, 162
–, –, evaluation **43**, 173–175
–, –, factors affecting **43**, 178–183
–, differences from pasta **43**, 143
–, egg content **43**, 161
–, emulsifiers **43**, 162
–, flour, color deterininants **43**, 178–180, 181
–, –, protein quantity/quality **43**, 181, 187
–, –, specification **43**, 154–156
–, formulation **43**, 148, 149
–, historical aspects **43**, 142–143
–, ingredients **43**, 156–162, 187–188
–, oil content **43**, 160
–, polyphosphates **43**, 161
–, preparation procedure **43**, 143
–, preservatives **43**, 161–162
–, processing **43**, 146, 147, 148, 188
–, –, evaluation **43**, 172
–, production **43**, 162–171
–, –, air drying **43**, 168–170
–, –, compounding/sheeting **43**, 165–166
–, –, cooking **43**, 167
–, –, deep frying **43**, 170
–, –, dough resting **43**, 165
–, –, drying **43**, 168–171
–, –, mixing **43**, 162, 164–165
–, –, slitting/waving **43**, 166
–, quality evaluation **43**, 171–178
–, –, scoring factors **43**, 172, 173, 175–181

–, raw materials **43**, 143, 146
–, salt (white; common salt) content **43**, 143, 146, 157–158
–, size (width) **43**, 146, 147, 166
–, stabilizers **43**, 161
–, starch **43**, 159, 183–186, 187–188
–, –, amylose content **43**, 185
–, –, pasting properties **43**, 156, 184–185
–, –, swelling power/volume **43**, 185–187
–, texture, evaluation **43**, 175–178
–, –, factors affecting **43**, 183–188
–, vital gluten powder **43**, 161
–, water content **43**, 157
–, wheat **43**, 150–156
–, –, ash **43**, 154, 155
–, –, color **43**, 154, 156
–, –, millable wheat value index (MWVI) **43**, 152–153
–, –, protein content **43**, 153–154, 155, 159
–, –, single kernel characteristics **43**, 153
–, –, soundness **43**, 153
–, –, source **43**, 150–151
–, –, test weight **43**, 152
–, –, thousand-kernel weight **43**, 152
Ormer, *see* Abalone
Orotidine-5-phosphate pyrophosphorylase, in wheat germ **23**, 240
Orthoclase, volume per oxygen atom in **2**, 3
Orthophosphates **39**, 268–269
–, effect on appetite **1**, 133
Ortho-(*a*)-selinene in celery seed oil **2**, 272
Osazone, crystalline **12**, 25
Osborne classification, proteins **34**, 267–269
Osborne procedure **36**, 17–18
Oscillating can, heat transfer to **32**, 73–74
Oscillation of molecules **15**, 280
Oscillatory shearing **39**, 20–23
Osmoregulatory capacity **39**, 119
Osmosis of living plant cells **2**, 307
Osmotic dehydration, as food technological method, for developing countries **22**, 200
Osmotic pressure, calculation of **7**, 87
Osmotic treatment **39**, 96–97, 101, 110–113, 149–150
Osones, *cis* **12**, 25–26
–, *trans* **12**, 25–20
Ossein, acid processing of **7**, 242
–, gelatin manufacture and **7**, 238
–, liming of **7**, 240
Osteogenesis imperfecta **37**, 394–396
–, classification system **37**, 395
Osteophagia caused by phosphorus deficiency **1**, 119
Osteoporosis, calcium intake and **36**, 217–218
–, calcium supplements and **33**, 144–145
–, phytoestrogen health protective effects **44**, 227–229
–, prevalence in women on low-cholesterol diets **37**, 225–226
–, prevention, inulin **43**, 43–44
–, risk factors **33**, 104
Ostwald ripening **34**, 145–146
Ouabain resistance assay **34**, 395–396
Outer membrane polymers **43**, 322–323
Ovalbumin **1**, 150; **10**, 35, 40, 41–42
–, egg proteins **34**, 255–257
–, gels, degree of aggregation **34**, 209–210
–, Maillard reactions **35**, 199
Ovarian cancer, carcinogen risk assessment and **31**, 17
Ovoglobulins **1**, 150
Ovomucin **10**, 36, 39–41, 42
Ovomucoid **1**, 150; **10**, 36
Ovomucoidase in egg albumen **1**, 183
Oxalacetic carboxylase, in wheat germ **23**, 241
Oxalate, deposition of, from xylitol infusion **25**, 172
–, inhibition of enzymes by **1**, 384, 388
Oxalic acid, cathode ray experiments on **3**, 170
–, effect on adhesive properties of pea coats **2**, 315
–, – on browning in fruit products **1**, 358
–, – on calcium absorption **33**, 142–143
–, in rhubarb **3**, 346
–, in wheat germ **23**, 237
–, reaction with tin **3**, 340
Oxaprozin **44**, 297
Oxazoline compound, in meaty aroma **18**, 60
Oxidants, dough development and **29**, 237–238
Oxidases **16**, 431
–, amine **17**, 13
–, ascorbate **17**, 13, 17
–, cytochrome **17**, 10–11, 20, 258
–, *o*-diphenol **17**, 12, 17
–, –, reactions of **17**, 11–12
–, –, thermal inactivation **17**, 43
–, *p*-diphenol **17**, 12
–, glycollate **17**, 13–14
–, in food deterioration **17**, 18
–, in tea **17**, 256
–, in wheat germ **23**, 239, 240
–, polyphenol **17**, 239, 244
–, –, chromatography of **17**, 257
–, –, in fermentation **17**, 265
–, –, in oxidation **17**, 267

Oxidases, polyphenol (*cont'd*)
–, –, in tea **17**, 229, 256, 258–259
Oxidation **14**, 9–10
–, antioxidants, ascorbic acid **33**, 15, 310
–, –, butylated hydroxyanisole **33**, 309–310
–, –, butylated hydroxytoluene **33**, 309–310
–, –, classes **33**, 309
–, –, flavonoids **33**, 311–314
–, –, inhibitory effects on fish gill 12-lipoxygenase, table **33**, 308
–, –, naturally occurring **33**, 310
–, –, tocopherols **33**, 310
–, cardiolipin **37**, 275
–, during meat storage **23**, 51–53
–, effect on "off-flavor" of oranges **2**, 265
–, – on stability of DDT **2**, 205
–, – on staleness of coffee **2**, 277–278
–, fish lipids, enzyme-catalyzed **33**, 291–297
–, –, factors affecting **33**, 287–289
–, –, metal catalysis of **33**, 289–291
–, –, volatile compound generation **33**, 298–302
–, folate resistance to **33**, 45
–, folates, energies of activation, table **33**, 50
–, 10-formyl-tetrahydrofolate **33**, 46
–, freeze-dried beef and **7**, 211–213
–, 4α-hydroxy-5-methyl-tetrahydrofolate **33**, 46
–, IM meat **39**, 133–136
–, in fermentation of tea **11**, 240, 241
–, lactate **39**, 199
–, 5-methyl-tetrahydrofolate **33**, 45–47
–, of lipids **23**, 39–48
–, of phospholipids **23**, 45–46
–, olive oil and **31**, 467, 469–473
–, periodate **12**, 13
–, plant substrates **3**, 18–22
–, –, pigment formation in **3**, 22–24
–, polyunsaturated fatty acids, acid-catalyzed decomposition **33**, 278–280
–, –, autoxidation **33**, 239–249
–, –, control, antioxidants **33**, 309–310
–, –, –, flavonoids **33**, 311–319
–, –, –, lipoxygenase **33**, 306–309
–, –, –, microsomal enzymes **33**, 305–306
–, –, –, peroxidase **33**, 306
–, –, decomposition of acyl hydroperoxides **33**, 270–273
–, –, enzyme-initiated **33**, 256–270
–, –, oxygen activation **33**, 234–238
–, –, peroxidation *in vivo* effects on DNA **33**, 285–286
–, –, – on membranes **33**, 283–285
–, –, – on proteins **33**, 282–283
–, –, photosensitized singlet oxygen **33**, 249–256
–, –, reactants and inhibitors, active oxygen species **33**, 302–303
–, –, –, metals **33**, 303–405
–, –, –, oxygen **33**, 302
–, –, secondary products **33**, 276–278
–, –, volatile compounds from acyl hydroperoxides **33**, 273–275
–, –, volatile compounds in food **33**, 280–281
–, role in meat off-flavors **23**, 38
–, sugars **14**, 252–253
–, tetrahydrofolic acid, mechanism **33**, 42–43
–, α-tocopherol antioxidant functions in membranes **33**, 207–211
–, unsaturated fatty acids **35**, 23
N-Oxidation, meat mutagens **34**, 409–410
α-Oxidation **17**, 25–26
β-Oxidation **17**, 25
–, dietary fatty acids **35**, 5
–, α-linolenic acid **35**, 34
Oxidation potentials, folates, electrochemical detection in reversed-phase HPCL systems **33**, 30–32
Oxidative metabolism, mitochondrial disorders **37**, 379–381
Oxides, carcinogen risk assessment and **31**, 39
–, *N*-nitroso compounds and, nitrite/nitrate addition **31**, 78–80
–, –, processing **31**, 89, 90, 93
Oxidizers, carcinogen risk assessment and **31**, 24
Oxidizing agents, for SH groups **24**, 8
–, inhibition of enzymes by **1**, 381–382
Oxy acid in rye bread **2**, 276
Oxybutynin **44**, 298
Oxyfedrine **44**, 314
Oxygen **14**, 190
–, carcinogen risk assessment and **31**, 24
–, chlorination and **7**, 133
–, chocolate and, alkalization **31**, 247
–, –, cocoa butter **31**, 251, 252
–, –, milk **31**, 260
–, –, milk crumb **31**, 291
–, –, packaging **31**, 314, 316–319
–, effect on canned foods **3**, 345, 346
–, – on carotenoids **15**, 257
–, – on dough **16**, 418
–, endogenous proteolytic enzymes and **31**, 344
–, equilibria in milk powder **3**, 60
–, in wines **8**, 153
–, levels, control **33**, 302

–, microbial control **39**, 121
–, *N*-nitroso compounds and **31**, 62, 79, 89
–, olive oil and **31**, 467
–, on fruits **15**, 155
–, relation to sugar–protein reaction **3**, 102
–, removal of to prevent tallowiness in dried milk **3**, 93
–, role in browning reaction **32**, 133
–, uptake in lipid deterioration **3**, 93, 94
–, water requirements and **7**, 109
Oxygen-18, energy metabolism **40**, 173–178
Oxygen absorption by dehydrated potatoes **1**, 275–276
Oxygenase in plant tissues **3**, 3, 4
Oxygen scavengers, for lipid oxidation control **33**, 302
Oxyhemoglobin in poultry meat **1**, 209
Oxytetracycline **16**, 180
Oysters, decomposition **16**, 175
–, loss of thiamine in **6**, 280
–, use of ascorbic acid on **4**, 391
Ozone **45**, 167–208
–, analytical methods **45**, 204–205
–, as banana preservative **12**, 190
–, atmospheric **45**, 170–171
–, biological oxygen demand (BOD) of water **45**, 170
–, carcinogen risk assessment and **31**, 7, 39, 40
–, chemical oxygen demand (COD) of water **45**, 170
–, chemistry/physics **45**, 170–177
–, cycloaddition reactions **45**, 175
–, decomposition **45**, 176–177
–, –, catalysis by inorganic compounds **45**, 177
–, –, free radical species generation **45**, 176
–, –, inhibition **45**, 177
–, –, initiation **45**, 177
–, –, promotion **45**, 177
–, effect on fruits **15**, 68, 134, 156
–, electrophilic reactions **45**, 175
–, in storage atmosphere **12**, 101
–, microbial inactivation **45**, 170
–, –, biofilms **45**, 187, 198–199
–, –, effect of oxygen demand of medium **45**, 181, 182
–, –, food characteristics influencing efficacy **45**, 190, 191
–, –, food sanitizing applications **45**, 189
–, –, kinetics **45**, 187–188
–, –, mechanisms **45**, 187–188
–, –, pulsed electric field combined treatment **45**, 188, 203–204
–, –, relative humidity/microbial cell hydration **45**, 179
–, –, residual ozone values **45**, 180–181
–, –, spores **45**, 186, 187
–, –, targeted micro-organisms **45**, 186–187
–, *N*-nitroso compounds and **31**, 67
–, nucleophilic reactions **45**, 175
–, oxidation of sulfhydryl enzymes by **1**, 381
–, oxidation–reduction potential **45**, 171
–, pesticide residue reduction **45**, 170, 189, 199
–, physical properties **45**, 171
–, processing equipment interactions **45**, 183–185
–, –, materials compatibility **45**, 184
–, –, metals **45**, 184–185
–, –, plastics **45**, 185
–, –, rubber **45**, 185
–, production methods **45**, 204
–, reactivity **45**, 175–177
–, –, inorganic compounds oxidation **45**, 177
–, –, molecular ozone **45**, 175
–, solubility **45**, 172–173
–, stability **45**, 173–175
–, structure **45**, 171
–, toxicity **45**, 206–207
–, transfer from gas to liquid phase (contacting systems) **45**, 182–183
–, treatment chambers **45**, 182
–, treatment medium **45**, 178–181
–, –, oxygen demand **45**, 170, 181, 182
–, –, relative humidity **45**, 178–180
–, –, residual ozone **45**, 180–181
–, –, temperature **45**, 178
–, treatment of molds with **3**, 465, 466
–, water requirements and **7**, 110
–, workplace exposure thresholds **45**, 207–208
Ozone sanitization, combination treatments **45**, 200–204
–, –, carbon dioxide **45**, 201–202
–, –, chlorine **45**, 201
–, –, heat **45**, 202
–, –, hydrogen peroxide **45**, 200–201
–, –, pulsed electric field **45**, 188, 203–204
–, –, ultraviolet radiation **45**, 202–203
–, dry foods/ingredients **45**, 198
–, equipment treatment **45**, 192
–, filtration of treatment water **45**, 183
–, fish **45**, 197–198
–, food processing applications **45**, 186–199
–, –, chlorine treatment alternative **45**, 188–189

Ozone sanitization, food processing applications (*cont'd*)
–, –, environmental contaminants reduction **45**, 192
–, –, food characteristics influencing ozone-demand **45**, 190–191
–, –, food surface structure **45**, 190–191
–, –, limitations **45**, 206
–, –, safety issues **45**, 207
–, fruit **45**, 190, 191, 192, 194–195
–, meat **45**, 186, 189, 190, 191, 192, 193–194
–, metal contaminants removal from drinking water **45**, 177
–, packaging materials **45**, 192, 198–199
–, pesticide residue reduction **45**, 170, 189, 199
–, poultry carcasses **45**, 183, 190, 192, 193–194, 201
–, raw products/ingredients **45**, 191–192
–, regulatory status **45**, 206
–, shelf-life extension **45**, 193
–, storage applications (ozone gas) **45**, 178
–, surface decontamination **45**, 178
–, –, food contact surfaces **45**, 198–199
–, vegetables **45**, 190, 191, 194, 195–196

p53 **44**, 251
pl ester transfer protein, activity, *n*-3 PUFAs **36**, 326
–, –, *n*-6 PUFAs **36**, 293–295
pABG, *see para*-Aminobenzoylglutamate
Packaging **15**, 182
–, chocolate and **31**, 313, 314
–, dried milk products **3**, 85
–, evaluation **31**, 319, 320
–, flavor and **7**, 25
–, mango fruits for shipment **21**, 285–286
–, materials, insect penetration by **4**, 314–315
–, –, ozone treatment **45**, 192, 198–199
–, –, PEF treated orange juice flavor/vitamin C retention **44**, 18–20
–, meats **5**, 38, 39
–, microwave foods **43**, 67, 106–109, 131
–, requirements **31**, 314–319
–, role in chlorophyll formation in potato **21**, 328, 332
–, sorghum brewed products **43**, 245–246
–, systems **32**, 27–30
Packeria candidissima **45**, 77–78
PAGE, *see* Electrophoresis
PAH, *see* Polycyclic aromatic hydrocarbons
Pahutoxin, properties and pharmacology of **18**, 151–154
Pain, oral cavity sensitivity to **29**, 167–168
Paired sensory difference tests **2**, 222–224
Palatability, of mechanically deboned red meat **27**, 88–93
Pale, soft, and exudative pork, *see* Pork
Palmitic acid, chocolate and **31**, 250, 254, 275, 324, 325
–, in carrot seed oil **2**, 271
–, in celery seed oil **2**, 271
–, in cocoa fat **6**, 39
–, in coffee **2**, 279, 281
–, in natural fats **23**, 8
–, in parsley oil **2**, 273
–, in poultry fat **1**, 212
–, in tea leaves **2**, 286, 287
–, olive oil and **31**, 463, 464
–, plasma lipid/lipoprotein response **36**, 269
Palmitoleic acid, in natural fats **23**, 8
–, olive oil and **31**, 463, 464
Palmitostearin, in cocoa fats **6**, 39
Palm kernels **16**, 15
Palm oil, lauric fats in **6**, 32
–, tocopherol losses due to processing **33**, 160
–, tocotrienols in **33**, 160
Panama, Incaparina use in **22**, 198
Pancreas, dietary fiber and **31**, 170, 171
–, endogenous proteolytic enzymes and **31**, 345
Pancreatic amylase **41**, 158
–, effect on starch **2**, 328
–, inhibition by antienzymes **1**, 385
Pancreatic cancer, carcinogen risk assessment and **31**, 14
Pancreatin, digestion **35**, 220
Panels, formal sessions of **7**, 28–30
–, operation of **7**, 20–22
–, orientation of **7**, 23
–, scheduling of **7**, 21
–, selection of **7**, 15–18
Panel tests **14**, 69–73
–, consumer **14**, 135–136
–, laboratory **14**, 130–133
–, texture profile **14**, 133–135
Pantothenic acid, effect of cathode rays on **3**, 168
–, in apples and pears **8**, 368
–, in wheat germ **23**, 209
Pantothenic acid content, inability of rats to recognize **1**, 118
–, in eggs **1**, 153
–, inhibition of enzyme functioning in synthesis of **1**, 387
–, of canned foods **1**, 41–47

–, –, effect of storage on **1**, 93–95, 97–98
–, of foods, effect of heat sterilization on **1**, 87–88
Papain, as allergen **42**, 7–8
–, endogenous proteolytic enzymes and **31**, 345, 355
–, freeze-dried beef and **7**, 211
–, in papaya **17**, 184, 188
–, in poultry meat **1**, 210
Papaw, juice of **8**, 233
Papaya, flavor of **17**, 176
–, juice, in preparation of fish paste **4**, 219
Paper, licorice root and **7**, 346–347
Paphia stamina **10**, 145
Paprika **15**, 246
–, color range for **5**, 320
Paraffin, solubility of DDT in **2**, 204
Parallel-plate viscometers **11**, 371, 374
Paramagnetism **10**, 325
Paramecium phytase **45**, 11
Parameter (*see also* Kinetic parameter distribution), classification **40**, 310–311
–, definition **40**, 34
–, estimation **40**, 311–312
–, evaluation **40**, 40–43
–, identifiable **40**, 311
–, insensible **40**, 311, 319
–, nonidentifiable **40**, 311
–, sensible **40**, 311, 320
Parameter sharing **40**, 159–160
Paramyosin, melting **35**, 322
Paramyotonia congenita **37**, 384
Parasites, gastroenteritis-producing **37**, 39
–, radiation disinfestation of **24**, 198–199
Parathyroidectomy, effect on rats **1**, 123
Parenchymal cell **40**, 15–17, 40
Parenchymatous tissues, cellulose **31**, 126–128
–, components **31**, 120, 122, 124–126
–, dietary fiber and **31**, 151, 190
–, hemicellulosic polymers **31**, 128, 129
–, intestinal bacteria **31**, 181, 184
–, in vegetable matter, effect of blanching on **2**, 301
–, –, in white potato **2**, 323
–, –, method and rate of killing, effects of **2**, 301, 309
–, –, protoplasm in **2**, 309
–, –, size and shape of **2**, 298–301
–, –, turgidity of **2**, 307–309
–, monocotyledonous plants **31**, 136–138
–, pectic substances **31**, 129–132
–, properties **31**, 159, 161–166
–, seeds **31**, 135
Parenteral fat emulsions, ultrasonic particle sizing **45**, 150
"Parent gelatin", structure of **7**, 260–261
Parmesan cheese, contamination **39**, 287
–, flavor **39**, 243, 245
–, lipolysis **39**, 205
–, peptides **39**, 230–231
–, ripening **39**, 255
–, texture **39**, 254
Paroxetine **44**, 312
Parsley, constituents of oil of **2**, 273
Parsnips, blanching of **2**, 323
–, constituents of seed oil from **2**, 274
–, effect of blanching on **1**, 68
–, – of steaming on pectic substances of **2**, 311
–, inositol phosphates content **45**, 23
–, loss of thiamine on processing **6**, 288
Particles in dried milk, action of glycerol on **3**, 50
– in –, form and appearance of **3**, 49
– in –, size distribution and air cell volume of **3**, 48
Particle-streak method **32**, 50
Particulate matter, and heat transfer **32**, 74–76
Particulate products, aseptic processing of **32**, 30–32
Passiflora edulis forma flavicarpa **12**, 204, 207
Passiflora edulis Sims. **12**, 203, 207
Passiflora quandrangularis **12**, 207
Passion fruit, flavor of **17**, 176
–, iodine wrappings for **3**, 465
Passion fruit juice, composition **27**, 259–265
–, –, acids **27**, 262–263
–, –, alkaloids **27**, 263–264
–, –, amino acids **27**, 264
–, –, carotenoid pigments **27**, 264
–, –, cyanogenic constituents **27**, 265
–, –, enzymes **27**, 265
–, –, sugars **27**, 262
–, concentration of **27**, 265–267
–, –, by reverse osmosis **27**, 268
–, –, evaporators, selection of **27**, 265–266
–, –, powders **27**, 268–269
–, –, quality **27**, 267
–, –, volatile flavoring, recovery of **27**, 267–268
–, development, research needs **27**, 288–290
–, from pulp **27**, 251–252
–, preservation **27**, 257–259
–, starch, properties of **27**, 255–257
–, –, removal of **27**, 252–255

Passion fruit juice (*cont'd*)
–, volatile flavors **27**, 269–281
–, –, carotenoids **27**, 277–281
–, –, –, edulans **27**, 277–279
–, –, –, ionone derivatives **27**, 281
–, –, –, megastigmatrienes **27**, 279–281
–, –, effect of fruit maturity **27**, 287
–, –, – of fruit variety **27**, 285–287
–, –, – of processing **27**, 287–288
–, –, esters **27**, 277
–, –, flavor impact values **27**, 282–287
–, –, sulfur compounds **27**, 281–282
Passion fruit pulp, extraction **27**, 247–251
–, –, by centrifugal extractor **27**, 247
–, –, by converging cone extractor **27**, 247–250
–, –, by passypress extractor **27**, 250–251
–, preservation **27**, 257–259
Passive diffusion **40**, 248–251
Pasta-making **44**, 411
–, buckwheat products **44**, 415
Pasta products, nutritious, for developing countries **22**, 195
Pastes, choline content **11**, 300
–, lecithin reversion in **11**, 298–301
Pasteurization (*see also* Heat treatment) **10**, 50, 79, 115–119
–, by ultrahigh-temperature methods, effects on folate activity **33**, 51
–, cheese products **39**, 259–277
–, effect of cathode rays in **3**, 165
–, effect on enzymes in milk **3**, 53, 54
–, IM meat **39**, 121
–, in spray-drying **3**, 73
–, microwave heating **43**, 125–126
–, milk, effect on folate binding **33**, 76
–, of wine and beer by radio-frequency waves **3**, 133
Pasting behavior **41**, 165–166
Pastirma **39**, 74–75, 123
Pastries, flavor scores with different fats **5**, 181–183
–, reverted fats used in **4**, 194, 199
–, toughness of **8**, 35
–, wheat germ use in **23**, 284
Patch tests **42**, 36
Pathogens **15**, 135
–, effect of radiation on **15**, 150
–, microbial, control **37**, 47–48
–, postharvest **15**, 168
Patterson's Curse (*Echium plantagineum*) **45**, 72
Patulin, degradation by sulfiting agents **30**, 17
–, from *Byssochlamys* spp. **25**, 272–276
PC, *see* Parenchymal cell
PCPs, *see* Cheese, processed products
PDS index **35**, 215, 218
Peaches **15**, 223
–, air spaces in **2**, 333
–, barrelling **5**, 144
–, brandled, cost reduction report for preparing **4**, 62
–, browning of **3**, 26
–, canned, corrosion characteristics of **3**, 336
–, –, nutrients in **1**, 43, 46–50
–, –, use of ascorbic acid in **4**, 367
–, –, vitamin retention in **1**, 83, 92
–, –, with added sulfur **3**, 352
–, carbon dioxide in transportation of **3**, 468
–, composition and distillation of **2**, 265
–, dehydrated **6**, 316
–, dried, chemical changes during browning in **1**, 351
–, –, effect of temperature on browning in **1**, 329, 334
–, –, enzymic changes in **11**, 290
–, effect of pH on phenolase activity of **3**, 24, 26
–, – of sound waves on enzymes in **3**, 36
–, Elberta **3**, 29
–, firming agent **5**, 145
–, freestone, blanching of **3**, 136
–, –, canned with added sulfur **3**, 354
–, frozen, ascorbic acid content **4**, 384
–, –, discoloration of **5**, 87
–, –, removal of gases from **3**, 36
–, –, retarding enzymic browning in **3**, 31
–, –, thiourea in **3**, 32
–, hair cells in **2**, 304
–, inactivation of polyphenol oxidase in **3**, 29
–, iodine wrappings for **3**, 465
–, loss of thiamine in canned **6**, 296
–, lye *vs.* steam peeling, effect on ascorbic acid content of **1**, 83
–, micro-organisms in frozen **6**, 179
–, pH of **3**, 432
–, polyphenols and enzymic browning in **19**, 116–117
–, substrate activity in **3**, 16
–, Sunbeam **3**, 16, 36
–, tannin **5**, 281
–, test for "organic peroxide" in **3**, 31
–, use of SO_2 in dried **5**, 141
–, vitamin B in **1**, 42, 44, 45
Peach juice, ascorbic acid loss in bottling **1**, 63

Peach nectar, canned, ascorbic acid content **4**, 375
Pea flour, inositol phosphate degradation during processing **45**, 21
Peak temperature dynamic method **35**, 343–344
Pea legumin, expression in micro-organisms **36**, 160–161
Peanut aflatoxin, chemical inactivation **26**, 251–256
–, criteria for **26**, 252
–, in concentrates **26**, 254–256
–, in isolates **26**, 254–256
–, in meal **26**, 253–254
–, ozone treatment reduction **45**, 198
–, reagents **26**, 252–253
Peanut butter, in candy **6**, 45
–, use of ascorbic acid in **4**, 389
Peanut concentrates **26**, 224–226, 232–233
–, beverages **26**, 259–260
–, cereal foods **26**, 257–258
–, enriched bread and pasta **26**, 258–259
–, flour, defatted and grits **26**, 220–223
–, foods containing **26**, 257–260
–, full-fat **26**, 219–220
–, quality specifications **26**, 223
–, textured proteins **26**, 260
–, types of **26**, 218–219
Peanut foods in India **26**, 260–264
– in –, Bal Ahar **26**, 262
– in –, fortified atta **26**, 262
– in –, multipurpose food **26**, 262
– in –, peanut butter **26**, 264
– in –, protein beverages **26**, 263
– in –, protein-enriched biscuits **26**, 263
– in –, tapioca macaroni **26**, 263–264
Peanut leuco-anthocyanins **5**, 288
Peanut meal, deficiencies of **17**, 107
Peanut protein **40**, 231–232, 238–240
Peanuts **16**, 11, 52ff
–, antinutritional properties **26**, 239–242
–, as allergens **42**, 27
–, effect of storage on biological value of protein in **4**, 269
–, functional properties **26**, 244–251
–, –, baking properties **26**, 248–249
–, –, flavor and color **26**, 249–250
–, –, solubility **26**, 246–247
–, –, viscosity **26**, 247–248
–, globoid composition **28**, 9
–, in candies **6**, 29, 45
–, isolates **26**, 226–228
–, isolation of **26**, 223–224
–, nutritional properties **26**, 239–244
–, oils, mixtures of **8**, 26
–, oleic–linolenic fats in **6**, 32
–, phytate content **45**, 13
–, processing by-products **26**, 234
–, production **26**, 217–228
–, –, forms of **26**, 217–218
–, products, acylated **26**, 238–239
–, –, coisolates **26**, 239
–, –, hydrolyzates **26**, 237
–, –, partially defatted **26**, 236–237
–, –, succinylated **26**, 238
–, –, texturized **26**, 237–239
–, protein quality **26**, 242–244
–, –, amino acid composition **26**, 243–244
–, –, nutrient composition **26**, 242–243
–, research needs **26**, 264–267
–, roasted, Maillard reactions **30**, 112
–, thiamine content of **6**, 293, 299, 304
–, toxic properties **26**, 239–242
–, –, aflatoxin **26**, 239–240
–, –, goitrogens **26**, 240
–, –, hemagglutinin **26**, 240
–, –, phytic acid **26**, 241–242
–, –, protease inhibitors **26**, 240
–, –, saponins **26**, 241
–, used by the candy industry **6**, 3
–, volatiles, identification **30**, 112
–, wet-milling **26**, 228–232
–, –, advantages and disadvantages of **26**, 233–234
–, –, Berg process **26**, 230
–, –, C.F.T.R.I. process **26**, 230
–, –, Chayen process **26**, 231
–, –, commercial operations **26**, 234
Peanut starch, gelatinization of **2**, 327
Pear juice, canned, use of ascorbic acid in **4**, 378
–, combining with sulfur dioxide **5**, 79
–, pectin in **1**, 398
–, preparation of **17**, 94
–, wastes **17**, 94–95
Pears, canned, corrosion characteristics of **3**, 336
–, –, nutrients in **1**, 43, 48–49
–, –, use of ascorbic acid in **4**, 367
–, color in stewed **5**, 272
–, composition of **8**, 300
–, dehydrated **6**, 316
–, dietary fiber and **31**, 127, 139, 187
–, dried, browning **1**, 335, 365
–, –, –, effect of temperature **1**, 329
–, –, influence of oxygen on deterioration of **1**, 342

Pears (*cont'd*)
–, effect of temperature on sensory difference tests **2**, 248
–, frozen, retarding enzymic browning in **3**, 31
–, fruit, biochemistry of **8**, 297
–, gas storage of **3**, 468
–, mineral elements in **8**, 369
–, nitrogen content of **8**, 299
–, oxidase activity in **3**, 18
–, oxidizing enzymes in **8**, 354
–, pH of **3**, 432
–, polyphenols and enzymic browning in **19**, 115–116
–, respiration in **3**, 17
–, stone cells of **2**, 300
–, test for "organic peroxide" in **3**, 31
–, treatment against storage rots in **3**, 464
–, treatment of by radio waves **3**, 144
–, use of SO_2 in dried **5**, 141
–, vitamin content of **8**, 360
–, X-ray use in grafting **3**, 159
Peas (*see also* Carrots and Peas) **16**, 9, 67
–, ascorbic acid content of, effect of fertilizers on **1**, 310
–, –, – of sunlight on **1**, 310
–, bacterial counts during preparation for freezing **6**, 186
–, –, decrease in bacterial content by blanching **6**, 184
–, –, frozen **6**, 175
–, –, micro-organisms in **6**, 179, 186
–, –, thiamine destruction in **6**, 258, 285, 288, 296
–, blanching of **8**, 66
–, branching enzymes **41**, 100–101
–, canned **8**, 63
–, –, anaerobic bacteria in **2**, 71, 88
–, –, brine-packed **3**, 441
–, –, corrosion characteristics of **3**, 336
–, –, dielectric constant of **3**, 125
–, –, nutrients in **1**, 43, 46–50
–, –, pH of **3**, 432
–, catalase activity in **8**, 84
–, changes affecting color and flavor **8**, 64
–, –, in chlorophyll during blanching of **8**, 82
–, –, in unblanched frozen **8**, 96
–, changes of cellular adhesion in **2**, 315
–, dietary fiber and **31**, 133, 154, 170, 181
–, dried, enzymatic changes in **11**, 288, 289
–, dry, insects infesting **4**, 308
–, dry storage **9**, 62
–, effect of blanching on vitamin content **1**, 68–72
–, – of calcium, potassium on skins of **2**, 310
–, freeze-dried, storage stability of **7**, 229
–, freezing of **8**, 64
–, gelatinization of starch in **2**, 323
–, green, blanching **9**, 65, 70, 71, 73, 75, 76, 81, 83, 88, 91, 93, 132–134
–, –, chemical composition **9**, 62–92
–, –, –, relation to maturity **9**, 62–63
–, –, cleaning **9**, 128–129
–, –, color **9**, 75–76
–, –, drying **9**, 139–141
–, –, effect of heat processing on protein value in **4**, 247
–, –, field transport **9**, 126–128
–, –, flavor **9**, 73–74, 75, 87
–, –, freezing **9**, 90, 92, 93, 138–139
–, –, grade standards **9**, 111–113
–, –, harvesting methods **9**, 122–126
–, –, maturity **9**, 95–122
–, –, –, measurement of **9**, 96–122
–, –, –, prediction of **9**, 113–122
–, –, nutritive value **9**, 93–95
–, –, research needs **9**, 141–142
–, –, scheduled planting **9**, 121–122
–, –, size grading **9**, 129–130
–, –, specific gravity **9**, 99–101, 134–138
–, –, texture **9**, 72–73, 75, 78, 87
–, –, water content **9**, 63–67
–, –, yield prediction **9**, 122
–, greenness of **5**, 326–328
–, leucoplasts in **2**, 306
–, loss of ascorbic acid during blanching of **8**, 76, 89
–, – of carotene during blanching of **8**, 72
–, – of riboflavin during blanching of **8**, 75
–, – of thiamine during blanching of **8**, 74
–, parenchyma tissue in **2**, 300
–, pectic material in coats of **2**, 310
–, phytic acid content, effect of cooking **28**, 42–43
–, sampling for flat sour contamination of **18**, 191
–, schlereids in **2**, 304
–, spore counts of **8**, 92
–, SSS in **41**, 84–85
–, sugar content of frozen **8**, 102
–, thermal resistance of spares in **2**, 71
–, thiamine content of **1**, 66
–, F value for industrial processing of **2**, 102
–, vitamin B in **1**, 42, 44, 45
Pea vicilin **36**, 114
–, expression in micro-organisms **36**, 161
Pecans **16**, 16

Pecan trees, mineral composition of foliage **5**, 197
Pectase, deesterification of pectinic acids by **1**, 411–412
–, use of cation exchanger for removal of **2**, 37
Pectates, use in gelling reactions **1**, 421
Pectic acid, molecular shapes and interactions **42**, 169, 171
–, possible formula for **11**, 5
Pectic compounds, effect of changes on softening plant tissue **2**, 310
–, effects of blanching on **2**, 322
–, – of steaming on **2**, 311
–, in collenchyma **2**, 304
–, in pea coats **2**, 315
–, in vegetable tissue, effect on parenchyma tissue **2**, 301
Pectic polysaccharides, arabinogalactans **30**, 145
–, binding to xyloglucan **30**, 150–151
–, galactans **30**, 144–145
–, homogalacturonan **30**, 143
–, links between fractions **30**, 149–150
–, plant cell wall, arabinans **30**, 143–144
–, rhamnogalacturonan I **30**, 142–143
–, rhamnogalacturonan II **30**, 143
Pectic substances, changes during ripening of apples and pears **8**, 347
–, in apples **8**, 337
–, in dehydrated mashed potatoes **25**, 73–79
–, in fruits **17**, 182
–, in tea **17**, 233–234
–, reviews of chemistry of **11**, 5
Pectinases, of *Byssochlamys* spp. **25**, 264–266
Pectinates, composition of **1**, 402
–, mixtures, use of to gel milk **1**, 421
–, rate of demethylation of **1**, 409–410
–, use in freezing fruits **1**, 421
Pectinesterase **17**, 22
–, in fruits **17**, 184
Pectinic acids, commercial production of **11**, 29–30
–, –, extraction **11**, 13–15
–, –, sugars liberated by partial acid hydrolysis **11**, 13
–, composition of **1**, 397, 399
–, molecular shapes and interactions **42**, 169–172
Pectin methylesterase **17**, 52
–, during ripening **30**, 175
–, in bananas **17**, 50
–, in fruits, galacturonosyl residue deesterification **30**, 175
–, multiple forms **30**, 175
–, of tea **24**, 236
–, role in potato tubers **25**, 79
Pectins **12**, 264–265; **15**, 80, 118
–, acetylated **1**, 398
–, action in gelation **8**, 35
–, analysis and characterization **11**, 45–61
–, apple, molecular weight of **1**, 398
–, araban content **11**, 73–80
–, ash and nitrogen contents **11**, 48
–, beet, molecular weight of **1**, 398
–, bulk density in drying **2**, 473, 500
–, changes in, during storage of fruit pulps **1**, 401
–, changes in growing fruit **1**, 402
–, – in softening pickles **2**, 315
–, chemistry **6**, 26; **10**, 10–11; **11**, 12–61
–, choice of plant tissue to use **11**, 12–13
–, chromatographic fractionation **11**, 47
–, citrus, effect on calcium absorption **33**, 141–142
–, –, molecular weight of **1**, 398
–, combination with lignins **11**, 82
–, content of apples and pears **8**, 300
–, deesterification of **1**, 406–412
–, dietary fiber and **31**, 118, 190, 191
–, –, analysis **31**, 142, 146, 148, 150, 152, 153
–, –, components **31**, 121–124, 140, 141
–, –, dicotyledonous plants **31**, 124, 126, 129–133, 135
–, –, intestinal bacteria **31**, 172, 175, 176, 182, 185–187
–, –, monocotyledonous plants **31**, 136, 137
–, –, properties **31**, 154, 155, 158, 163–171
–, effect of steaming on **2**, 311
–, effects on tocopherol bioavailability **33**, 171–172
–, enzymes in extraction **11**, 38–45
–, ester formation, between cellulose and **11**, 66–70
–, –, between hemicelluloses and **11**, 70–80
–, extent of acetylation **11**, 61
–, extracted from cocoa **8**, 263
–, extraction for study of **11**, 9–12
–, extraction procedures for analysis **11**, 11
–, extractives and extraction procedures **11**, 21–45
–, fractional extraction **11**, 26–36
–, fruit, substitution for animal gelatins **1**, 418
–, gelation, by low-ester pectins **1**, 416–420
–, –, high-solids, preparation of **1**, 415–416

Pectins, gelation (*cont'd*)
–, –, low-solids, calcium requirement for **1**, 416–418, 419–420
–, –, –, changes in, with aging **1**, 420
–, –, –, pectinate requirement for **1**, 418–419
–, –, optimum pH of **1**, 413, 415, 416
–, –, speed of **1**, 413, 415, 416
–, grades of, in relation to deesterification **1**, 413, 415
–, high and low methoxyl **6**, 28
–, highly polymerized **1**, 399–405
–, –, composition of **1**, 396–399
–, histological and histochemical studies **11**, 9
–, in cocoa beans and nibs **6**, 38
–, in gels **17**, 195–196
–, in gum drops **6**, 29
–, in inhibition of corrosion **3**, 343
–, in kiwifruit after storage and canning **29**, 295
–, in plant tissues **11**, 61–93
–, in tea **11**, 222–223
–, jelly grade, and arabinose content **11**, 76
–, –, and galactose content **11**, 75
–, –, and galacturonic acid content **11**, 74
–, jellying power of **1**, 407
–, low-ester, effect of acidity changes on viscosity of **1**, 413–414
–, –, – of heavy metal ions on viscosity of **1**, 414–415
–, –, properties of **1**, 413–420
–, –, uses of **1**, 420–421
–, manufacture of **17**, 95
–, methods of drying **1**, 405
–, mineral constituents **11**, 49–50
–, molecular shapes and interactions **42**, 167, 169–172
–, –, calcium pectate **42**, 169–172
–, –, pectic acid **42**, 169, 171
–, –, pectinic acid **42**, 169–172
–, –, sodium pectate **42**, 169–170
–, molecular sizes **11**, 63–66
–, nitration **1**, 398; **11**, 25
–, nomenclature for **1**, 395–396, 397
–, non-uronide constituents associated with **11**, 47–52
–, non-uronide contents **11**, 50–52
–, olive oil and **31**, 460, 463
–, orange, molecular weight of **1**, 398
–, photomicrograph of spray-dried **2**, 515
–, plant tissues for investigations **11**, 12–21
–, polymerization of in commercial products **1**, 401
–, polyvalent ion bridges in **11**, 83–93
–, possible enmeshing linkages between molecules **11**, 7
–, precipitation of **1**, 399, 416–418
–, preparation of apple marc for **11**, 17–21
–, – of plant materials for extraction **11**, 16–21
–, purification of **11**, 52–56
–, reference books on **11**, 6
–, role in fruit firmness **11**, 30–33
–, salt linkages with protein **11**, 80–82
–, sequestering agents **11**, 36
–, spectroscopic characterization **11**, 60–61
–, starch in **11**, 52
–, transformation to pectic acid **1**, 406
–, uronide contents **11**, 50, 58
–, use of enzymes in analyzing **11**, 38–45
–, – of Swenson dryer for **2**, 420
–, variation in water solubility **11**, 63
–, viscosity **1**, 405–406
–, viscosity and arabinose content **11**, 77
Pectolytic enzymes **17**, 52
Pediatrics, effects of lactic cultures on diarrhea **37**, 87–89
Pedicularis (betony) **45**, 77
Pediococcus, heat destruction of **3**, 436
–, salt-tolerant, in mash **30**, 230, 232
Peebles atomizer, operation of **2**, 455
Peebles spray dryer, operation of **2**, 423–425, 498
Peeling, *see* Casings, removal of
Pegaso near isogenic line **45**, 252–253
Pelagic fish **39**, 351
Pelargonidin, structure of **19**, 79
Pemmican **39**, 81
Penetration devices **14**, 81–86
Penetrometer **14**, 85–86
D-Penicillamine **44**, 297
Penicillin, as food allergen **42**, 8
–, cathode ray sterilization of **3**, 187
–, in control of *Salmonella* infection **3**, 231
–, in foods **37**, 43
–, inhibition of cell division by **1**, 375
–, ribonucleic acid dissimilation by **1**, 375
–, therapeutic action of **2**, 143
–, treatment of by radio-frequency radiations **3**, 143, 144
Penicillium, ascospores, destruction rate curve for **3**, 434
–, effect of ultraviolet radiation on **3**, 148
–, exposure to radio waves **3**, 144
–, germination of **7**, 95
–, growth rate of **7**, 98
–, heat resistance **3**, 436, 456
–, –, curves for **3**, 438

–, in bacon **3**, 298
–, in canned blueberries **3**, 443
–, inhibition of by carbon dioxide **3**, 444
–, sterilization of **3**, 134
–, survival of at low temperatures **3**, 446
–, thermal death time curves for **3**, 439
–, X-ray mutations in **3**, 160
Penicillium digitatum **15**, 176
–, control of by ammonia **3**, 465
–, ethylene production **12**, 126, 189–190
–, in lemons **12**, 107
–, in oranges **12**, 107
Penicillium expansum **15**, 178; **45**, 191
Penicillium glaucum **12**, 110
–, control of by ozone **3**, 466
–, in rancidification of fats **3**, 311
Penicillium italicum **15**, 176
Penicillium sclerotia, destruction rate curve for **3**, 434
Peniophora lycii phytase **45**, 10, 11
Pentachlorophenols (PCPs), carcinogen risk assessment and **31**, 19, 20
–, fish preservation and **7**, 67
Pentamidine **44**, 292, 322
Pentanol in potato oil **2**, 275
Pentazocine **44**, 297
Pentosans **16**, 389ff
–, in cocoa beans and nibs **6**, 38
–, in mash, shoyu color formation and **30**, 245
–, in mature peas **2**, 310, 314
–, –, effect of cooking on **2**, 311
Pentose, dietary fiber and **31**, 172, 175
–, shoyu color intensity and **30**, 248
Pentoxifylline **44**, 317
Peppergrass, composition of oil of **2**, 275
Pepperoni **39**, 78
Peppers **15**, 234
–, ascorbic acid content of, effect of light on **1**, 299
–, bacterial contamination of pork sausage by **6**, 189
–, canned, nutrients in **1**, 43, 46–49
–, dehydrated **6**, 315
–, ozone treatment **45**, 198
–, red Hungarian, in capillary resistance **5**, 276
–, Spanish, in fish paste **4**, 221
Pepsin, endogenous proteolytic enzymes and **31**, 345
–, inactivation of **1**, 383
Pepsin digest-dialysate method **35**, 215
Pepsin digest residue method **35**, 214–215, 218
Pepsin inhibitor, effect on enzyme **1**, 385
Pepsin in poultry meat **1**, 210–211, 251
Pepsin pancreatin digest-dialysate method **35**, 214–215, 218
Pepsin-pancreatin digest method **35**, 214–215, 218
Peptidases **16**, 291ff; **39**, 215, 216–218, 220, 223–225
–, endogenous proteolytic enzymes and **31**, 387, 389
–, in tea **24**, 234–235
Peptide bonds, endogenous proteolytic enzymes and **31**, 344
–, endopeptidases **31**, 353, 354, 356, 357, 360–362
–, exopeptidases **31**, 346–348
–, hydrolysis, measurement **35**, 223
–, meat technology **31**, 410, 411
–, thermal inactivation **35**, 247
Peptides (*see also* Emulsification peptides) **16**, 239ff, 270
–, amphiphilic design **42**, 99–100
–, –, graphical representations **42**, 99–102
–, chocolate and **31**, 224, 226, 270, 297
–, collagen hydrolysates and **7**, 270
–, computer-aided design **42**, 103–104
–, endogenous proteolytic enzymes and, endopeptidases **31**, 352, 360
–, –, exopeptidases **31**, 350
–, –, meat technology **31**, 410–413
–, gelatin hydrolysates and **7**, 267–270
–, *N*-nitroso compounds and **31**, 79
–, reaction with glucose **3**, 255
–, secondary structure **42**, 95–99
–, –, aliphatic side chains **42**, 98–99
–, –, amino acid sequences **42**, 96–97
–, –, helix formation **42**, 97–99
–, –, hydrophobic and hydrophilic residues **42**, 96
–, –, β-sheet formation **42**, 98
Peptidyl lysyl hydroxylase defect, in Ehlers–Danlos syndrome **37**, 392–393
Peptidyl lysyl oxidase defect, in Ehlers–Danlos syndrome **37**, 392–393
Peptization **39**, 265
Peptone solutions, use in testing thermal bacterial resistance in foods **2**, 66
PER, *see* Protein efficiency ratio
Peracetic acid food sanitization **45**, 189
Perch **39**, 340
Perchlorethylene, carcinogen risk assessment and **31**, 20
Perennial buckwheat (*Fagopyrum cymosum*) **44**, 396, 397

Pergolide mesylate **44**, 310
Perhydroxyl radical, formation **33**, 237
Periandra dulcis, glycyrrhizin and **7**, 343
Peridinium polonicum, toxin from **18**, 158
Perilla oil, DHA levels in brain phosphoglycerides **35**, 125–126
Perimysium **9**, 3; **14**, 35
Periodic paralysis, hyperkalemic **37**, 385–386
–, hypokalemic **37**, 384–385
Periodontal disease, in Ehlers–Danlos syndrome **37**, 392–393
–, xylitol and **25**, 152–153
Permanganate, dietary fiber and **31**, 153
–, oxidation of sulfhydryl enzymes by **1**, 381
Permanganate reduction, fish freshness and **7**, 61–62
Permeability, evaluation **31**, 315–318
–, membranes to ions/small molecules, α-tocopherol effects **33**, 218
Permeability coefficient **39**, 185–186
Permittivity **43**, 69, 78
Peroxidase **16**, 432; **17**, 59
–, biological role **10**, 7–8
–, control of oxidative activities **33**, 306
–, effect of temperature on **3**, 27–29
–, fish lipid oxidation **33**, 293
–, inactivation, time–temperature relationships **3**, 53
–, in eggs **1**, 183
–, –, microbial inhibition by **1**, 386
–, in food deterioration **17**, 18
–, in milk, effect of cathode rays on **3**, 175
–, in papaya **17**, 183
–, in plant tissues **3**, 3–8
–, in processing **17**, 5
–, in tea **17**, 231, 256; **24**, 234
–, in wheat germ **23**, 240
–, lipid oxidation **33**, 259–261
–, oxidation mechanisms **17**, 14–16
–, oxidation of pyrogallol by **3**, 22
–, properties of **17**, 8–9
–, pseudo- **17**, 9
–, regeneration of **17**, 53–56
–, test for in fruits **3**, 31
–, thermal inactivation of **17**, 39–42
–, time–temperature indicator **44**, 180, 181
–, with H_2O_2, meat mutagen modulation **34**, 429
Peroxidase activity, as blanching index **17**, 3, 5
Peroxidation, lung and heart microsomes, α-tocopherol effects **33**, 213
–, membrane, inhibition by α-tocopherol **33**, 210
–, membrane lipids, α-tocopherol role **33**, 213
Peroxides **14**, 305–307
–, conversion from unsaturated fat **3**, 96
–, determination of in dry milk **3**, 94, 95
–, formation of **17**, 27
–, –, in yellowing of bacon **3**, 312, 316
–, linolenate and linoleate **17**, 29
–, olive oil and **31**, 467
Perphenazine **44**, 312
Persimmon **15**, 226
Perturbation response **40**, 285–289
Pesticide residues, in foods **37**, 43
–, reduction by ozone treatment **45**, 170, 189, 199
Pesticides **14**, 310–311
–, carcinogen risk assessment and **31**, 6
–, chocolate and **31**, 225, 226
–, *N*-nitroso compounds and **31**, 95–97
Petasitenine **45**, 66, 67
Petasites officinalis **45**, 76
Pet food production **39**, 83–85, 118, 126
Petroleum ether, solubility of DDT in **2**, 203, 204
Petunia seeds, transgenic **36**, 171
Petzholdt conche, chocolate and **31**, 304
Petzold integrator **40**, 297, 299–303
Peyer's patches, accessory cells **37**, 15
–, characterization **37**, 15
–, components **37**, 10
–, gut antigen uptake **37**, 14–15
PGE, *see* Pregastric esterase
PGE_2, immunological function effects **35**, 99–100
PGSR response **14**, 21–22
pH **14**, 123–124, 100–191
–, adjustment, proteins **35**, 335–336
–, changes, during storage of apples **8**, 327
–, changes in value in fish muscle **2**, 362–363, 372, 373
–, cheese, *see* Cheese, pH
–, chlorination and **7**, 148–149
–, coalescence stability and **34**, 143, 145
–, effect of cation exchanger on sugar beet juice **2**, 25–26
–, – of fish fatigue on **2**, 361
–, effect on bacterial growth in fish **2**, 361
–, – on browning in potato powder **1**, 272
–, – on calcium binding by fiber **33**, 136
–, – on cocoa seeds **8**, 249
–, – on discoloration of meat **5**, 30
–, – on dissociation of sulfurous acid **8**, 167
–, – on enzymes **17**, 47–48
–, – on folate absorption **33**, 53–54

–, – on folates, behavior **33**, 5–6
–, – on –, intestinal absorption **33**, 67
–, – on –, stability during extraction **33**, 15–16
–, – on galactose and glucose bisulfite equilibrium constants **5**, 67–71
–, – on gelatin **8**, 35
–, – on germicidal activity **2**, 133–134, 136, 149
–, – on glucose–alanine reaction **3**, 253
–, – on growth of micro-organisms **3**, 431
–, – on heat destruction values **3**, 437–440
–, – on metabolism of micro-organisms **11**, 333–336
–, – on micro-organisms in fruit juices **9**, 226–228, 252–257
–, – on phenolase activity in fruits **3**, 24–26, 27–30
–, – on preservative action of SO_2 **5**, 124
–, – on protein thermal behavior **35**, 323–325
–, – on rancidity **5**, 30
–, – on relief from stomach ulcers **2**, 32
–, – on salt tolerant yeasts **3**, 453
–, – on sugar–amino acid reaction **3**, 250
–, – on thermal death point of micro-organisms **3**, 438–440
–, – on thermal resistance of bacteria **2**, 67
–, – on thiamine destruction **6**, 259, 272
–, – on whey proteins, binding of flavor compounds to **33**, 411–412
–, – on –, film-forming properties **33**, 394
–, – on –, foams **33**, 401, 403
–, – on –, functional properties **33**, 369
–, – on –, gelling properties **33**, 386–387
–, – on –, gelling time **33**, 387
–, – on –, heat treatment **33**, 376–378
–, – on –, solubility **33**, 375
–, – on –, thermal denaturation behavior **33**, 379–381
–, emulsifying activity index and **34**, 154
–, emulsion coalescence **34**, 136
–, fish freshness and **7**, 62
–, for adsorption of citrulline **2**, 38
–, – of pectase **2**, 37
–, IM meat **39**, 121, 123, 124, 126, 148
–, in cheese ripening **16**, 234, 251
–, in eggs **10**, 39
–, in fermenting cocoa **8**, 245, 273
–, in fresh cocoa bean pulp **8**, 241
–, inhibition of enzymes by **1**, 380–381
–, in water-holding capacity of meat **10**, 368–373, 375, 379–380, 381, 386, 391–392, 393–395, 424, 431
–, isoelectric, whey proteins, table **33**, 349
–, lactase **38**, 65, 69–71
–, β-lactoglobulin changes as function of **33**, 351
–, of apples and pears **8**, 300, 372
–, of buffer in thermal resistance tests **2**, 81
–, of canned foods, relative to vitamin losses **1**, 92
–, of dehydrated potatoes, relation to fluorescence **1**, 276
–, of grape juice **8**, 145
–, of limed pineapple juice **2**, 18
–, of muscle of meat animals **6**, 122
–, of must and wine **8**, 157, 158
–, of phemerol **2**, 154
–, of wines **5**, 416; **6**, 83; **8**, 187
–, primary plant cell wall growth and **30**, 160, 166–167
–, protein emulsifier modification **34**, 150
–, relation to IQ-like compound formation **34**, 435
–, – to pectin extraction **1**, 402–406
–, selection and **38**, 33
–, SO_2 liberation and **30**, 21
–, sulfite antimicrobial efficacy and **30**, 11–12
–, test for quality **2**, 381–382
–, values, in canned foods **3**, 337–340
–, –, in fresh fruits **3**, 432
–, –, in fresh vegetables **3**, 432
–, –, in soy sauce **10**, 80, 112, 114
–, –, in sugar–sulfur dioxide reaction **3**, 461
–, water requirements and **7**, 109–110
Phage vectors, gene cloning **36**, 138–139
Pharmacokinetics, graph theory **40**, 339
–, population analysis **40**, 265–278
Phase inversion temperature (PIT), emulsifiers **22**, 326
–, small-molecule emulsifiers **34**, 101–102
Phaseolin (see *also* French bean phaseolin) **36**, 114–115
Phaseolus vulgaris L., iron availability of low-phytic acid varieties **45**, 34–35
Phase transition, at superlow temperatures **27**, 344–349
–, –, recrystallization **27**, 348–349
–, –, vitrification **27**, 344–348
–, during freezing and rewarming of foods **27**, 326–343
–, – of –, conditions during freezing **27**, 329–343
–, – of –, eutectic temperature **27**, 326–329
–, during freezing and thawing of model systems **27**, 315–326
–, – of –, antemelting and recrystallization **27**, 324–326

Phase transition, during freezing and thawing of model systems (*cont'd*)
–, – of –, eutectic freezing **27**, 316–320
–, – of –, vitreous structures **27**, 320–324
Phase transition temperature, in fruit and vegetable juices **27**, 339
Phase–volume ratio **34**, 84
pH-drop initial rate assay **35**, 221
Phemerol, effect on influenza virus **2**, 138
–, film formation of **2**, 144
–, neutralization by anion agent **2**, 132
–, structure of **2**, 121, 154–155
–, therapeutic action of **2**, 143
–, toxicity of **2**, 130, 131
Phendimetrazine **44**, 314
Phenformin **44**, 307
Phenindione **44**, 288
Phenmetrazine theovalate **44**, 324
Phenobarbital **44**, 298
Phenolases, *see* Oxidase, *o*-diphenol *and* Polyphenol oxidase
Phenolic acids **44**, 196
–, chocolate and **31**, 233
–, cinnamic acid based **42**, 252
–, olive oil and **31**, 467
Phenolic esters, analysis **31**, 148, 152, 153
–, dietary fiber and **31**, 119, 122, 190
–, intestinal bacteria **31**, 175, 182, 187, 189
–, monocotyledonous plants **31**, 137, 138
Phenolics, chocolate and **31**, 297
–, dietary fiber and **31**, 140, 148
–, –, components **31**, 121, 123
–, –, dicotyledonous plants **31**, 127, 129, 130
–, –, intestinal bacteria **31**, 178, 186, 188
–, –, monocotyledonous plants **31**, 137, 138
–, olive oil and **31**, 467, 469
Phenolic substances, in apples and pears **8**, 352
–, in tea **17**, 220–231
–, in wheat germ **23**, 237
–, non-phenolic substances, in tea **17**, 231–248
Phenolic substrates, chemical investigations of **3**, 11
Phenols (*see also* Ellagic acid, Flavonoid, Gallic acid, Hydroxycinnamate, Lignin, Tannin), activity as surface-active agents **1**, 378, 385–386
–, and fruit astringency **13**, 179–227
–, –, hydroxylation pattern change **13**, 208
–, animal adaptation to **27**, 157–158
–, animal consumption of **27**, 162–210
–, –, ellagic acid **27**, 170–172
–, –, flavonoids **27**, 173–191
–, –, gallic acid **27**, 170–172
–, –, hydroxycinnamate **27**, 167–170
–, –, lignins **27**, 208–210
–, –, tannins **27**, 191–208
–, animal metabolism of **27**, 158–162
–, as nutrients **27**, 166–167
–, biosynthesis **27**, 151–153
–, chlorine and **7**, 165
–, chocolate and **31**, 221
–, classification and structure **29**, 118–121
–, coefficient test for germicidal action of quaternary ammonium compounds **2**, 158–159
–, compounds, in bread **2**, 276
–, –, in coffee **2**, 280, 281
–, –, in maple syrup **2**, 277
–, –, in tea **2**, 286
–, concentration to destroy staphylococci **2**, 135
–, effect on mortality of rats **3**, 206
–, evolution **27**, 153–154
–, formation in curing smoke, from cellulose pyrolysis **29**, 123
–, – in –, from lignin pyrolysis **29**, 121–123
–, – in –, temperature effects **29**, 124–125, 140
–, from plants **27**, 154–157
–, gel-rigidity and **7**, 297
–, in beech smoke **29**, 124–127
–, –, temperature effect **29**, 124–125
–, in celery seed oil **2**, 271
–, in cherries **2**, 264
–, in curing smoke, antimicrobial effect as antioxidants **29**, 144–146
–, –, content **29**, 123–127
–, –, effect on flavor **29**, 140–144
–, –, mutagenic activity **29**, 150
–, inhibition of lipoxygenase **33**, 307
–, inhibitory effects on fish gill 12-lipoxygenase, table **33**, 308
–, in liquid smoke preparations **29**, 127–130
–, in parsley oil **2**, 274
–, in primary plant cell wall **30**, 152
–, in smoke and smoked ham **29**, 133
–, in smoked products **29**, 130–132
–, in solid smoke preparations **29**, 130
–, *N*-nitroso compounds and **31**, 60, 61
–, of plant origin, in foods **27**, 149–221
–, olive oil and **31**, 466, 467, 469
–, pathologic effects of **3**, 207
–, pyrolysis products **27**, 163–166
–, shoyu flavor and **30**, 278–280
–, simple type, in food browning **19**, 81–82
–, therapeutic action of **2**, 144

–, toxicity, carcinogenicity **27**, 216–218
–, –, mimic-interaction with metabolism **27**, 211–212
–, –, mutagenicity **27**, 216–218
–, –, nutritional load **27**, 212–214
–, –, penetration effects **27**, 214–215
–, –, protein binding **27**, 215
–, –, uncoupling of oxidative phosphorylation **27**, 216
–, –, when used as antioxidants **3**, 201
Phenoxyl radical, α-tocopherol **33**, 208–210
Phentermine **44**, 314
Phenylacetic acids, flavor profile and **7**, 12
–, in Formosan black tea oil **2**, 297
–, in seisin-oolong black tea oil **2**, 287
Phenylalanine ammonia lyase, of tea **24**, 234
Phenylbutazone **44**, 297
Phenylenediamine, combination with *o*-quinone **3**, 20
–, oxidation by oranges **3**, 16
Phenylethyl alcohol, in Formosan black tea **2**, 287, 288
–, in manufactured tea **2**, 286
–, in oranges **2**, 264
–, in raspberries **2**, 269
Phenylethyl isothiocyanate, in water cress **2**, 285
Phenylethyl thiocyanate, in mushroom oil **2**, 277
Phenylphenol in fruit wrappings **3**, 465
Phenylpropionic acid nitrile in water cress **2**, 275
Phenylpropyl alcohol, in Formosan black tea **2**, 288
Phenytoin **44**, 312
Pheophytin, formation of **17**, 32
Pheophytin *a* **17**, 242
–, olive oil and **31**, 460, 469
Pheophytin *b* **17**, 242
–, olive oil and **31**, 460, 469
Phloem, desirability in foods **2**, 306
–, dietary fiber and **31**, 122
–, fibers in **2**, 304–305
Phloretin **40**, 208–209, 211; **44**, 197
Phlorizin **40**, 208–209
Phloroglucinol, condensation of **17**, 258–259
–, in tannin formation **17**, 225
Phonons **45**, 103
Phosphatases **16**, 294; **45**, 24
–, inactivation of **17**, 36–37
–, in egg yolk **1**, 184
–, in honey **24**, 330
–, in wheat germ **23**, 239
–, time–temperature relationships for inactivation of in milk **3**, 53, 54
Phosphate buffer, use in blanching carrots **2**, 330
Phosphate carrier protein, cardiolipin association **37**, 280–281
Phosphate changes in fish muscle **2**, 363–364
Phosphate esters, appearance in destruction of cell membrane **1**, 378
–, role in carbohydrate metabolism **1**, 131–133
Phosphate groups, effect on salting-out and salting-in **34**, 316–320
Phosphates **39**, 269
–, absorption, inulin effects **43**, 32
–, effect on calcium absorption **33**, 143–144
–, – on "warmed-over" flavor **23**, 54–55
–, inhibition of warmed-over flavor development in cooked meat **29**, 41, 44
–, in meat curing, color improvement **29**, 16
–, –, flavor development **29**, 32
–, –, water binding increase **29**, 15–16
–, inorganic, determination of **19**, 324–325
–, in wines **8**, 137, 153
–, loss of in blanching **8**, 65
Phosphate solutions, use in testing thermal resistance of bacteria in foods **2**, 65, 66, 81
Phosphatides, in nonenzymic browning **17**, 33
–, structure of **23**, 6
–, –, in wheat germ, effect on baking quality **23**, 274
Phosphatidylcholine liposomes, α-tocopherol transfer to rat liver mitochondria **33**, 194
Phosphatidylglycerol, degradation **37**, 274–275
–, in animals **37**, 263
–, in micro-organisms **37**, 262
–, in plants **37**, 262–263
–, synthesis, intracellular location **37**, 267–270
–, –, pathway **37**, 265–266
Phosphoarginine, in abalone **23**, 157
Phosphoglucomutase, in wheat germ **23**, 240, 241
6-Phosphogluconate isocitric dehydrogenase, in wheat germ **23**, 240
Phosphoglucose isomerase mutants **41**, 146
3-Phosphoglycerate **41**, 145–148
Phosphoglycerate mutase as endpoint cooking temperature indicator **44**, 172
Phosphoglycerides, platelet, fatty acid composition **35**, 55–56

Phosphoglycerol phosphatase, in wheat germ **23**, 241
Phosphoinositide transduction pathway, role in taste induced by saccharin and SC45647 sweeteners **42**, 224–227
Phospholipase A_2, cardiolipin association **37**, 284–285
–, platelet, α-tocopherol effects **33**, 219–220
Phospholipase C **45**, 27
–, activity, sweetener-induced taste **42**, 224–226
Phospholipases, eicosanoids synthesis **35**, 93–94
Phospholipid bilayers, α-tocopherol effects **33**, 215–216
Phospholipid fraction of dried egg yolk, effect of storage on **2**, 249
Phospholipid-hydrolytic activity in barley malt flour as a function of relative humidity **11**, 305
Phospholipid monolayers, α-tocopherol effects **33**, 215
Phospholipids **15**, 33
–, as factors in fat reversion **4**, 197
–, biosynthesis of **23**, 12–13
–, brain, DHA levels **35**, 124–126
–, breakdown of **17**, 25, 32
–, chocolate and **31**, 283, 324
–, effects on quaternary ammonium compounds **2**, 131–132
–, – on wheat germ **23**, 280
–, endogenous proteolytic enzymes and **31**, 380
–, fatty acid changes **35**, 56–58
–, in abalone **23**, 162
–, in egg yolk **1**, 150–151
–, in milkfat **37**, 150
–, in off-flavor production **17**, 33
–, in oxidation **17**, 32–33
–, interconversion of **23**, 14
–, in wheat flours, breadmaking and **29**, 253, 257
–, –, cookie quality and **29**, 259
–, in wheat germ **23**, 223, 224
–, olive oil and **31**, 466, 469
–, oxidation of **23**, 45–46
–, *n*-3 PUFA effects **35**, 149
–, structure of **23**, 9–15
–, warmed-over flavor development in cooked meat and **29**, 39–41
Phosphomonoesterase, inhibition of **1**, 388
–, in wheat germ **23**, 210–211
Phosphopeptides, calcium absorption and **36**, 217
Phosphoric acid, in grape waste **2**, 16
–, in rye bread **2**, 276
Phosphorus **16**, 239ff
–, content of apples and pears **8**, 371, 386
–, determination in phosphate rock **2**, 39
–, in tea **17**, 247
–, radioactive **3**, 156
–, removal from milk **2**, 35
Phosphorus and phosphorus compounds, in wheat germ **23**, 233, 234
Phosphorus compounds, in peas, loss in processing **9**, 72–73
–, –, relation to maturity **9**, 71–72
–, –, – to texture **9**, 72–73
Phosphorus content, deficiency in rats **1**, 119–120
–, of canned foods **1**, 44, 48, 49
–, of plants, effect of fertilizers on **1**, 312–313
Phosphorus starch granules **41**, 30
Phosphorus supply, effects on fruit composition **9**, 299
Phosphorylase (*see also* Glycogen phosphorylase metabolism), endogenous proteolytic enzymes and **31**, 379
–, mechanisms **41**, 159–160
–, starch degradation **41**, 135–136, 153–154
Phosphorylase-stimulation assay **41**, 89
Phosphorylation, endogenous proteolytic enzymes and **31**, 359, 374
–, fruit ripening and **30**, 173
–, protein emulsifier modification **34**, 153–155
–, whey protein modification by **33**, 419
Phospohexonate, acceleration of trimethylamine oxide reduction by **2**, 369
Photooxidation, polyunsaturated fatty acids **33**, 249–251
–, products **33**, 251–256
Photosynthesis cells **41**, 139–140
pH-stat assay **35**, 221
o-Phthalaldehyde, reactive lysine measurement **35**, 193
Phthalein value, fish freshness and **7**, 64
Phycin **17**, 184
Phycoerythrin as time–temperature integrator **44**, 184–185
Phycomyces blakesleeanus **15**, 212
Phycomycetes **15**, 167
Phylase, in wheat germ **23**, 210–211
Physiologic rhythm (*see also* Bioperiodicity) **40**, 217
Physiology, of normal vegetable tissues, effect of death on **2**, 308–309
–, –, normal cells turgidity **2**, 307–308

–, post-harvest **12**, 116–127
Phytases **45**, 8–9
–, activation in seeds/grains before cooking **45**, 9
–, animal cell lines **45**, 24
–, animal digestive tract **45**, 24
–, cell/tissue activity **45**, 9–10
–, classification **45**, 11
–, phytate degradation during food processing **45**, 16, 20, 21
–, purified enzymes activity **45**, 10
Phytate, *see* Inositol hexakisphosphate *and* Phytic acid
Phytic acid, activity, cereal **28**, 63
–, –, wheat **28**, 62
–, autolysis of, effect of pH **28**, 64
–, –, – of temperature **28**, 64
–, beans, cooking and canning, effect of **28**, 46–47
–, bioavailability of **28**, 23–28
–, –, calcium **28**, 30–31
–, –, copper **28**, 41–42
–, –, iron **28**, 33–36
–, –, magnesium **28**, 31–33
–, –, manganese **28**, 41–42
–, –, zinc **28**, 36–41
–, biological function **28**, 7
–, biological value, in laying hens **28**, 26
–, –, in swine **28**, 25
–, breadmaking and **28**, 55–60
–, characterization of **28**, 21–23
–, content, bran **28**, 14
–, –, bread **28**, 15
–, –, flour **28**, 14
–, –, soybean **28**, 60
–, –, tempeh **28**, 60
–, –, whole grain **28**, 14
–, cooking, effect on **28**, 42–48
–, destruction during breadmaking **28**, 55–60
–, –, fermentation **28**, 55–60
–, determination analytical methods **28**, 15–18
–, digestion of **28**, 23–28
–, effect on calcium absorption **33**, 134–142
–, – on mineral bioavailability **28**, 29–42
–, – on retention of ingested phosphorus **28**, 27
–, fermentation and **28**, 55–60
–, germination and **28**, 48–54
–, –, in cereals **28**, 49–50
–, –, in legumes **28**, 51–52
–, –, phytase activity changes **28**, 53–54
–, –, phytate phosphorus changes **28**, 53–54
–, globoid composition **28**, 9
–, historical background **28**, 1–4
–, hydrolysis **28**, 24–28, 65–67
–, –, and baking **28**, 57
–, –, effect of preheating **28**, 65
–, –, – of soaking **28**, 66
–, –, in calves and steers **28**, 24
–, –, in chicks and laying hens **28**, 27
–, –, in rats **28**, 28
–, in Iranian flat breads **28**, 37
–, in legumes **28**, 1–91
–, in rice, effect of cooking **28**, 48
–, in seeds, effect of soaking **28**, 66
–, in sesame meal effect of autoclaving **28**, 45
–, in soy isolates **28**, 70
–, interference with calcium absorption **1**, 124
–, monoferric, purification from wheat bran **28**, 34
–, occurrence **28**, 7–12
–, pH and protein–mineral interactions **28**, 18–21
–, phytase and, in wheat **28**, 62
–, phytate–protein–mineral interactions **28**, 18–21
–, phytin–protein complex, dissociation of **28**, 73
–, processing effect of **28**, 42–48
–, removal **28**, 67–74
–, –, from soybean meal **28**, 68
–, –, from soy protein **28**, 68–74
–, –, –, at pilot plant **28**, 69
–, –, –, by diafiltration **28**, 72–74
–, –, –, by dialysis and anion exchange **28**, 72
–, –, –, by ultrafiltration **28**, 74
–, –, with calcium and barium ions **28**, 68
–, research needs **28**, 75
–, structure **28**, 4–6
Phytic acid phosphorus, content in cereals and legumes **28**, 10–13
Phytin, dietary fiber and **31**, 165
–, in bread, adaptation of man to **1**, 129
–, in cocoa beans **8**, 262
Phytoene **15**, 206
Phytoestrogens **44**, 195–234
–, analytical methods **44**, 201–203
–, antioxidant activity **44**, 225–226
–, assays **44**, 196
–, bioavailability/metabolism **44**, 218–222
–, chemistry **44**, 197–199
–, definition **44**, 196–197
–, effects of processing **44**, 212–218
–, estrogen receptor actions **44**, 222–223
–, estrogen-related effects, *in vitro* **44**, 223

Phytoestrogens, estrogen-related effects (*cont'd*)
–, –, *in vivo* **44**, 224–225
–, health protective effects **44**, 227–234
–, –, bone **44**, 227–229
–, –, cancer **44**, 229–232
–, –, cardiovascular **44**, 232–234
–, metabolism prior to absorption **44**, 199, 207
–, physiological effects **44**, 222–227
–, role in plants **44**, 200
–, sources **44**, 203–212
–, structural aspects **44**, 197, 198
–, toxicity **44**, 226–227
Phytofluene **15**, 126, 132, 206
Phytohemagglutinin, *see* Lectin
Phytohormones **15**, 85
Phytomonas phaseoli, effect of pH on thermal death point of **3**, 438
Phytophthora **15**, 176, 180
Phytophthora parasitica **45**, 181
Phytosterols **44**, 196
Pichia miso, for polyalcohol production **12**, 77, 80–83
Pickles, brine (gherkins), corrosion characteristics of **3**, 336
–, –, *Oöspora lactis* in **3**, 458
–, –, study of yeasts in **3**, 453
–, –, tests on during pasteurization **3**, 437
–, softening by hydrolysis **2**, 315
Pickling, use for developing countries **22**, 201
Picolines in cyclic type of quaternary ammonium **2**, 125, 128
Pies, alginates in fillings **11**, 152
–, carrageenan in fillings **11**, 128–129
–, gelatin and **7**, 324
–, gum tragacanth in fillings **11**, 185
Pigmentation **15**, 132
Pigments **14**, 185–191
–, aspects of formation of in fruit products **3**, 22–24
–, brown **12**, 39–45
–, derivatives of myoglobin **5**, 20
–, formation **12**, 42–45
–, –, factors affecting **12**, 43–45; **14**, 189–191
–, –, intermediates **12**, 42–43; **14**, 186–189
–, from model systems **12**, 39–41
–, –, absorption **12**, 41
–, –, dialyzable **12**, 39
–, –, insoluble **12**, 40–41
–, –, nondialyzable **12**, 40
–, –, soluble **12**, 40–41
–, from natural systems **12**, 41–42
–, –, darkened dried apricots **12**, 41–42
–, –, isolated by dialysis **12**, 42
–, –, maple syrup **12**, 42
–, heme **5**, 2, 14
–, hemoglobin, oxidation of **5**, 22
–, in abalone **23**, 163–164
–, in apples and pears **8**, 379
–, in citrus fruits, blood oranges **9**, 328
–, –, –, grapefruit **9**, 328
–, –, –, limes **9**, 328–329
–, –, –, oranges and tangerines **9**, 324–328
–, in cocoa beans and nibs **6**, 38
–, in cured meats **5**, 17
–, infrared spectra **14**, 185
–, in fruits **17**, 174
–, in meat **5**, 12, 13
–, in passion fruit **12**, 212–213, 228, 239, 259–260
–, in tea **11**, 226–227; **17**, 241–243
–, in wheat germ **23**, 237
–, oxidation products of heme pigments **5**, 13
–, oxyhemoglobin, absorption spectrum **5**, 28
–, preparation **14**, 185–186
Pigmenturia **37**, 3–44
Pig protein and amino acid **35**, 212–213
Pigskins, acid processing of **7**, 242
Pimentos, canned, nutrients in **1**, 43, 46–49
–, distribution of pH measurements **5**, 168
Pimozide **44**, 312
Pineapple, adsorbability on cation exchangers **2**, 12
–, ascorbic acid content of, effect of iron on **1**, 308
–, bran, as animal feed **17**, 95–96
–, bromelin in **17**, 188
–, calcium content of, effect of fertilizers on **1**, 311–312
–, canned, corrosion characteristics of **3**, 336, 338, 346
–, –, nutrients in **1**, 46–49
–, –, vitamins in winter vs. summer packs **1**, 82
–, –, – in –, retention during storage **1**, 92
–, comparison of summer and winter fruits **2**, 265
–, composition and distillation of **2**, 265–269
–, flavor **17**, 176–177
–, –, components **1**, 135–136
–, fractionation of volatile oil of **2**, 266–267
–, industry, use of ion exchange resins in **2**, 18–20
–, iron content of, effect of fertilizers on **1**, 313–314

–, juice, ascorbic acid content of, correlation of total acidity with **1**, 303–304
–, –, –, effect of light on **1**, 303, 305
–, –, –, – of temperature on **1**, 303
–, –, canned, ascorbic acid content **4**, 375, 380
–, –, –, nutrients in **1**, 43, 46–50
–, –, effect of headspace on shelf-life of **3**, 348
–, –, in control of browning **3**, 24, 33
–, –, in preparation of fish sauce **4**, 216, 219
–, –, usage of **17**, 95
–, –, vitamin retention during storage **1**, 92
–, loss of thiamine in **6**, 296
–, percentage of volatile oil in **2**, 266
–, phosphorus content of, effect of fertilizers on **1**, 313
–, wastes **17**, 95–96
Pinene, in carrot seed oil **2**, 271
–, in parsley oil **2**, 274
Pink discoloration, in foods **19**, 128–129
Pipe fouling, ultrasonic detection **45**, 153
Piperacillin **44**, 292
Piperidine **12**, 29–30
–, fish spoilage and **7**, 45
–, maltose or maltulose **12**, 34
Pirbuterol acetate **44**, 302, 322
Piroxicam **44**, 297
Piston pump, for thermoprocessed food filling **23**, 367
Pi theorem **32**, 49
Pitting, in fruit **10**, 319–320, 336
Pituitary, glycyrrhizin and **7**, 258
Pituitary hormone, effect on appetite **1**, 122
Placeable filler, for thermoprocessed food **23**, 368–369
Plaice, aerobic bacteria in **2**, 350
–, rigor mortis in **2**, 366
Planck's constant **17**, 38
Plank's formula **20**, 237
Plant cell, primary wall, components, cellulose **30**, 147
–, –, –, glycoproteins **30**, 147–149
–, –, –, hemicellulose **30**, 145–147
–, –, –, pectic polysaccharides **30**, 141–145
–, –, models (*see also* Cell wall, plant, models) **30**, 152–168
–, –, structure, glucuronoarabinoxylan and **30**, 151
–, –, –, hydroxyproline-rich glycoproteins and **30**, 151–152
–, –, –, links between, pectic fractions **30**, 149–150
–, –, –, –, xyloglucan and cellulose **30**, 150–151
–, –, –, –, xyloglucan and pectin **30**, 151
–, –, –, phenols and **30**, 152
–, structure **30**, 140–141
–, walls (*see also* Acid phosphatase) **34**, 344
–, –, isolation **34**, 345–346
Plant-derived food, selenium in **32**, 91–95
Plant extracts, meat mutagen modulation **34**, 429
Plant flavonoids, effect on "warmed-over" flavor **23**, 55–56
Plant foods, contents of linoleic and linolenic acids **35**, 16–17
Plant products **13**, 306–311
Plant proteins (*see also* Dietary fatty acids), future research on **10**, 67
–, versus animal proteins **36**, 91
Plant pyrrolizidine alkaloid sources **45**, 62–65
Plant residues, utilization of **17**, 96–106
Plants (*see also specific species*), C_4 **41**, 148–150
–, acyl composition of phosphatidylglycerol **37**, 299
–, aquatic, consumption of **20**, 193
–, ascorbic acid as spray for **18**, 295–296
–, as protein food, cereals **30**, 335–336
–, cardiolipin **37**, 263–264
–, chilling requirement of **25**, 199–202
–, chilling sensitivity of **25**, 194–199
–, legumes **30**, 336
–, new forms, *see* Protein foods, new, based on plant sources
–, oilseeds (*see also* Oilseeds) **30**, 336–339
–, parts used as food **25**, 212
–, phosphatidylglycerol **37**, 262–263
–, regeneration **36**, 165; **41**, 128
–, scanning electron microscopic studies on **22**, 250–252
–, starch degradation pathway **41**, 155–156
–, survival of, at low temperatures **25**, 193–211
–, transformation **41**, 131–134
–, winter hardiness of **25**, 202–208
Plant seed oils, fatty acid composition **35**, 18
Plant tissues, confocal scanning laser microscopy **43**, 355
–, microbial attachment **43**, 344–347
–, moisture distribution **27**, 303–307
–, surface structural aspects **43**, 344
–, water content **27**, 299
Plaque, dental, biochemistry of **25**, 140–141
–, –, xylitol effects on **25**, 149
Plasma, calcium concentrations **33**, 112–114

Plasma (*cont'd*)
–, folate concentrations **33**, 60
–, gelatin and **7**, 326–327
Plasma lipids (*see also n*-3 Polyunsaturated fatty acids *and n*-6 Polyunsaturated fatty acids), dietary fat quantity and **36**, 306–307
–, α-linolenic acid conversion **35**, 66–72
–, monounsaturated fatty acids **36**, 295–305
–, *n*-3 PUFA effects **35**, 133–134
–, response to saturated fatty acids **36**, 266, 268–271
Plasma lipoproteins (*see also n*-3 Polyunsaturated fatty acids *and n*-6 Polyunsaturated fatty acids) **36**, 256–260
–, apoproteins **36**, 258
–, cardiovascular disease risk **36**, 260–261
–, characteristics and function **36**, 256–257
–, chylomicrons **36**, 258
–, dietary fat, quantity versus quality **36**, 305–315
–, genetics and **36**, 328–331
–, HDL **36**, 259–260
–, intravascular processing, *n*-6 PUFA effects **36**, 291–295
–, LDL **36**, 259
–, monounsaturated fatty acids **36**, 295–305
–, response to saturated fatty acids **36**, 266, 268–271
–, tocopherol distribution **33**, 174–177
–, VLDL **36**, 259
Plasmalogens, structure of **23**, 10
Plasma membrane, sweet taste receptors **42**, 217–219
Plasma proteins, blood proteins **34**, 260–261
Plasmid vectors, gene cloning **36**, 137–138
Plasmin **39**, 213–214
Plasmolysis of plant tissue, theory of **2**, 308
Plastein, synthetic, effect of sound waves on **3**, 131
Plasticization, by sugars **38**, 156–159
–, by water **38**, 150–159, 187–188
–, –, breakfast cereals, crispness and **38**, 185
–, –, distinguished from presence of water **38**, 156–157
–, –, unfreezability **38**, 170
–, effect on glass transition temperature **38**, 118, 120–125
Plasticizer, effect on curing and vitrification **38**, 214
Plastic pouches, ultrasonic leak detection **45**, 154
Plastids, amylase in **2**, 328
–, types in parenchyma vegetable tissue **2**, 306
Plate heat exchanger **32**, 15
Platelets, aggregability, EPA effects **35**, 85
–, –, linoleic acid **35**, 89–90
–, –, linseed oil **35**, 136
–, –, *n*-3 PUFA **35**, 137
–, –, thromboxane and **35**, 97
–, anti-cardiolipin antibody binding **37**, 307
–, function **35**, 97
–, membrane fluidity, α-tocopherol effects **33**, 217–218
–, phospholipase A_2 activity, α-tocopherol effects **33**, 219–220
–, tocopherol association with **33**, 177
–, α-tocopherol concentrations **33**, 212
–, α-tocopherol content, vitamin E status and **33**, 189–190
Plate–plate geometry **39**, 29–31
Pleospora herbarum **15**, 177
Plexiglas, use in nozzles for spray-drying **2**, 452
PLP, *see* Pyridoxal phosphate
Plug flow, temperature distribution for **11**, 422
Plum juice, pectin in **1**, 398
Plums, canned with added sulfur **3**, 353
–, – with citric acid **3**, 342
–, effect of pectin in spray-drying of **2**, 500
–, egg, storage of **3**, 468
–, pH of **3**, 432
Poisoning, fish sausage and ham **12**, 414–415
–, food **13**, 349–396
–, –, effect of nitrofurazone **12**, 415
Poisson flow **40**, 247
Polarimetry **41**, 167
Polarity index, of emulsifiers **22**, 325
Polarity ratio, wheat proteins **36**, 8
Polarized light microscopy, anhydrous milkfat **44**, 61, 65
–, fat crystal network microstructure **44**, 75–80
–, –, crystallization process **44**, 80, 81, 82
–, palm oil **44**, 62–63, 65
Polarizing microscope **34**, 170
Polar lipids, in microemulsions **34**, 163–164
Pollen, of tea, chemistry of **11**, 232
Pollinators, passion fruit **12**, 208
Pollock, correlation between pH and spoilage of **2**, 381
–, organoleptic spoilage of **2**, 377
Pollution, and corn production **32**, 188, 201, 221–224
Polyacrylamide gel electrophoresis, cheddar cheese ripening **34**, 363

–, meat endpoint temperature monitoring **44**, 175
Polyalcohol production by osmophilic yeasts **12**, 76–83
– by –, by *Pichia miso* **12**, 77, 80–83
– by –, by *Saccharomyces rouxii* **12**, 82
Polyarthritis **37**, 398–399
Polychlorinated biphenyls, carcinogen risk assessment and **31**, 20
–, in foods **37**, 43
Polycyclic aromatic hydrocarbons (PAH), in curing smoke **29**, 99, 101, 104–106, 110, 112, 113, 117, 134–136, 140, 147–148, 150
–, smoked meat product contamination **29**, 147–149
Polycycline **16**, 180
Polydextrose, chocolate and **31**, 272
Polyethenoxyethers **14**, 354–355
Polyethylene **12**, 232
Polyethylene film, bacterial rot of mango **21**, 273
–, chlorophyll development in potato **21**, 328–329
Polyethylene glycol, preferential hydration and thermal stability **35**, 293
Polygalacturonase **17**, 22
Polygalacturonic acids, in pectin **1**, 399
–, in pectinic acid **1**, 399
Polyglutamate **40**, 97, 99
Polyglutamylation **40**, 91, 103
Polyglutamyl folates, affinity chromatography **33**, 38
–, bioavailability **33**, 64–65
–, C-9–N-10 bond **33**, 34–38
–, chain length determination with HPLC methods **33**, 34–38
–, chiral stability **33**, 13
–, deuteration **33**, 11–12
–, dietary, deconjugation **33**, 54–55
–, enzymatic deconjugation **33**, 18
–, HPLC methods **33**, 34–38
–, ion-exchange separations **33**, 33–34
–, long-chain reduced (6S), biological synthesis **33**, 11–12
–, separation by gel filtration chromatography **33**, 33
–, synthesis **33**, 6–8
–, –, liquid-phase methods **33**, 7
–, –, pteroic acid preparation **33**, 7–8
–, –, solid-phase methods **33**, 6–7
Polyglycerol polyricinoleate, chocolate and **31**, 283
Polyglycerophospholipids, abundance **37**, 261–262
–, degradation **37**, 274–275
–, discovery **37**, 261
–, synthesis, intracellular location **37**, 267–270
–, –, pathways **37**, 264–267
Poly(α-L-guluronic acid), molecular shapes and interactions **42**, 173–175
Polyhydric alcohols, protein stability effects **35**, 290–294
Polyisobutylene, local viscosity **38**, 192
Poly(β-D-mannuronic acid), molecular shapes and interactions **42**, 172–173
Polymer hydration, ultrasonic analysis **45**, 151–152
Polymeric proteins, genetic control **36**, 32–37
–, glutenins **36**, 22–25
–, HMW albumins **36**, 26–27
–, peak I, composition **36**, 52, 54
–, structure in native state **36**, 39–44
–, – in –, experimental measurements **36**, 41–43
–, – in –, glutenin subunit arrangement **36**, 42, 44
–, – in –, molecular weight distribution **36**, 40–41
–, triticins **36**, 24, 26
–, wheat proteins **36**, 22–27
Polymerization, by transglutaminase **34**, 160
–, gelatin and **7**, 328
Polymer mixtures, compatibility and molecular weight **34**, 271
–, Flory–Huggins expression **34**, 265
–, in solution, thermodynamics **34**, 265–272, 266
–, Osborne classification **34**, 267–269
–, polymer–polymer interaction parameters **34**, 266
–, polymer–solvent interaction parameters **34**, 265–266
–, protein compatibility **34**, 267–272
–, proteins belonging to different classes **34**, 269–271
–, ternary systems **34**, 266–268
Polymer–plasticizer blends, glass transition temperature **38**, 145–147, 149–150
Polymer–polymer blends, diffusional motion **38**, 174–175
–, glass transition temperature **38**, 145–147, 149–150
Polymers, amorphous, curing **38**, 213–214
–, –, thermosetting **38**, 212–226
–, –, wheat gluten, *see* Gluten
–, chocolate and, cocoa bean chemistry **31**, 229

Polymers, chocolate and (*cont'd*)
–, –, cocoa butter **31**, 252
–, –, packaging **31**, 317, 319
–, –, processing **31**, 215, 222
–, –, sweeteners **31**, 272
–, crystalline melting enthalpies **38**, 190
–, dietary fiber and **31**, 190, 191
–, –, analysis **31**, 142, 146, 148, 150
–, –, components **31**, 120–124, 138–141
–, –, dicotyledonous plants **31**, 124, 126–129, 131–133
–, –, intestinal bacteria **31**, 172, 182, 186, 189
–, –, monocotyledonous plants **31**, 136–138
–, –, properties **31**, 155, 157, 158, 160, 163, 164, 166–168, 170, 171
–, glass-forming, T_m/T_g ratio **38**, 191–192
–, highly flexible, equation of state **34**, 56
–, junction zone **39**, 42
–, partially crystalline, fringed micelle model of crystalline–amorphous structure **38**, 129, 133
–, –, viscoelastic behavior **38**, 183–184
–, rheological properties **39**, 48–53
Polymethylgalacturonase, in ripening fruits, pectin degradation and **30**, 179
Polymorphonuclear leukocytes **35**, 103, 108–109
Polymyositis **37**, 362
Polyols, in apples and pears **8**, 312
–, protein thermal behavior effects **35**, 327
–, stabilizing effect, α-amylase **35**, 293
–, –, chymotrypsinogen **35**, 291–292
Polyox **12**, 349–357
–, applications **12**, 353–357
–, –, cosmetics **12**, 355–356
–, –, pharmaceuticals **12**, 356–357
–, –, water soluble films **12**, 354–355
–, background **12**, 349–350
–, preparation **12**, 350–351
–, properties **12**, 351–353
–, –, plasticity **12**, 352–353
–, –, toxicology **12**, 353
–, –, viscosity **12**, 351
Polyoxyethylene sorbitan monostearate, in chocolate bars **6**, 44
Polypeptide chain, configurations **34**, 55–56
Polypeptide fraction, adsorption of by cation exchangers **2**, 12
Polypeptides, chocolate and **31**, 222–224
–, endogenous proteolytic enzymes and, endopeptidases **31**, 352, 358, 359
–, –, exopeptidases **31**, 349, 351, 352
–, –, meat technology **31**, 397, 399–401, 406
–, –, nonmuscle cathepsins **31**, 364
–, *N*-nitroso compounds and **31**, 79
Polyphenolase, activity in ripe apples and pears **8**, 367
–, spraying potatoes with **8**, 356
Polyphenolic compounds, *N*-nitroso compounds and **31**, 60, 61
Polyphenolics, analysis **31**, 150, 151
–, dicotyledonous plants **31**, 124, 126, 128
–, dietary fiber and **31**, 119, 123
–, intestinal bacteria **31**, 182, 188
–, monocotyledonous plants **31**, 138
Polyphenol oxidases (*see also* Oxidase, polyphenol), activation of **19**, 108–109
–, catecholase activity of **19**, 90–91
–, copper role in **19**, 91–94
–, cresolase activity of **19**, 88–90
–, inactivation of **19**, 104–108
–, –, by heat **19**, 105
–, –, by miscellaneous chemicals **19**, 107–108
–, –, by sulfur dioxide **19**, 106–107
–, in enzymic food browning **19**, 82–97
–, –, individual foods **19**, 109–123
–, in fruit products **3**, 7–8
–, –, effect of temperature on activity of **3**, 26, 30
–, inhibition by sulfiting agents **30**, 10
–, isolation and assay of **19**, 84–88
–, of tea **24**, 233–234
–, substrate specificity of **19**, 94–97
Polyphenols **12**, 240, 259
–, bactericidal activity of **17**, 218
–, changes during fermentation and drying of cocoa **8**, 269, 270
–, chocolate and, cocoa bean chemistry **31**, 226, 229, 233
–, –, processing **31**, 215, 221, 222
–, –, *Theobroma cacao* L. **31**, 325, 326
–, in enzymic browning (of), apples **19**, 114–115
–, –, apricots **19**, 119
–, –, bananas **19**, 118–119
–, –, beets **19**, 121–122
–, –, cocoa **19**, 112–114
–, –, dates **19**, 119–120
–, –, grapes and wine **19**, 117–118
–, –, pears **19**, 115–116
–, –, potatoes **19**, 120–121
–, –, tea **19**, 109–112
–, –, tomatoes **19**, 120
–, in food browning **19**, 75–145
–, in fresh cocoa cotyledons **8**, 264
–, in nonenzymic food browning **19**, 123–131
–, –, leucoanthocyanidins and **19**, 128–130

–, –, metal–polyphenol complexing **19**, 123–127
–, –, turbidity in beer **19**, 131
–, in tea **17**, 218; **24**, 236–240
–, olive oil and **31**, 467, 479
–, polymerization in enzymic food browning **19**, 102–104
–, precursors of aroma **8**, 279
–, radioprotective effects of **17**, 218
Polyphenols in tea **2**, 284, 285, 286
Polyphosphates **39**, 267–269; **43**, 161
–, making gels from pectic acid **1**, 415
–, pectin extraction **1**, 400, 404–405
–, use in gelling reactions with pectic acid and pectates **1**, 421
Polypodium, glycyrrhizin and **7**, 343
Polysaccharide dispersion **39**, 46
Polysaccharide–lipid edible films **44**, 351–371
–, applications **44**, 369–371
–, –, fruit ripening retardation **44**, 370
–, oxygen barrier properties **44**, 364–365, 366–367
–, –, relative humidity effects **44**, 365
–, –, temperature effects **44**, 365, 368
–, solute barrier properties **44**, 368–369
–, –, relative humidity effects **44**, 369
–, –, temperature effects **44**, 369
–, water barrier properties **44**, 351–359, 360–362
–, –, relative humidity effects **44**, 363–364
–, –, surfactant effects **44**, 359, 363
–, –, temperature effects **44**, 364
Polysaccharides (*see also specific types*) **42**, 131–204
–, chocolate and **31**, 221
–, collagen and **28**, 261–265
–, crystal systems **42**, 136
–, degradation **41**, 160
–, dietary fiber and **31**, 118–120, 191
–, –, analysis **31**, 142, 150–152
–, –, components **31**, 122–124, 139–141
–, –, dicotyledonous plants **31**, 124, 126, 128, 129, 131–135
–, –, intestinal bacteria **31**, 172, 174–182, 186, 187, 189
–, –, monocotyledonous plants **31**, 136
–, –, properties **31**, 154, 155, 158, 167, 168, 171
–, electron density **42**, 143
–, endogenous proteolytic enzymes and **31**, 403
–, equator and meridian **42**, 142
–, for production of gums **12**, 285
–, helical **42**, 144
–, importance **42**, 131–132
–, in apples and pears **8**, 330
–, in cocoa bean pulp **8**, 240
–, in spoiled table wines **6**, 78
–, in tea **11**, 221–222
–, mixed **42**, 200, 202
–, model building and refinement techniques **42**, 145–146
–, molecular shapes and interactions **42**, 146–201
–, –, alternating (1 → 3) and (1 → 4)-linked polysaccharides **42**, 180–185
–, –, –, agarose **42**, 184–185
–, –, –, carrageenans **42**, 180–184
–, –, arabinan **42**, 198–201
–, –, branched polysaccharides **42**, 194–199
–, –, –, *Rhizobium trifolii* CPS **42**, 194–197
–, –, –, xanthan **42**, 196–199
–, –, gellan family **42**, 185–194
–, –, –, potassium native gellan **42**, 186–188
–, –, –, welan **42**, 191–194
–, –, (1 → 3)-linked polysaccharides **42**, 175–180
–, –, –, β-glucan **42**, 175–179
–, –, –, scleroglucan **42**, 179–180
–, –, (1 → 4)-linked polysaccharides **42**, 147–175
–, –, –, alginic acid **42**, 172–175
–, –, –, amylose **42**, 156–168
–, –, –, cellulose **42**, 148–153
–, –, –, galactomannans **42**, 155–156
–, –, –, mannan **42**, 152–155
–, –, –, pectin **42**, 167, 169–172
–, –, potassium gellan **42**, 187–191
–, morphology to macroscopic properties **42**, 202–203
–, natural **12**, 287
–, ordered molecules **42**, 137–144
–, plant cell wall, synthesis from nucleotide sugars **30**, 162–165
–, reactions with proteins **3**, 277–278
–, reserve **41**, 4–6
–, single crystals, oriented fibers, and powder specimens **42**, 134–137
–, structure factor **42**, 143
–, structure–function–property correlations **42**, 132–133
–, unit cell **42**, 135–136, 138
–, utilization by spoilage bacteria in wine **6**, 91
–, X-ray diffraction **42**, 133–146
Polysorbate 20, *N*-nitroso compounds and **31**, 81
Polysorbate 60, chocolate and **31**, 312

Polystyrene **12**, 156
n-3 Polyunsaturated fatty acids **35**, 132–148
–, atherogenesis **36**, 327–328
–, atherosclerosis and heart disease **35**, 133–138
–, Ca^{2+}/Mg^{2+} ATPase **35**, 129–131
–, cancer **35**, 143–146
–, CETP **36**, 326
–, chylomicron metabolism **36**, 318–319
–, deficiency **35**, 114
–, –, irreversible visual defects **35**, 118–119
–, –, learning ability effects **35**, 122
–, desaturation rates **35**, 78–81
–, dietary **35**, 107–109
–, –, requirements **35**, 151–155
–, encephalomalacia **35**, 127–128
–, essentiality, humans **35**, 113–115
–, –, marine species **35**, 112–113
–, –, monkeys **35**, 115
–, –, rodents **35**, 115–116
–, HDL, metabolism **36**, 324
–, –, receptor expression **36**, 327
–, hepatic 5′-nucleotidase **35**, 131
–, HTGL **36**, 325
–, immune cell effects **35**, 109–111
–, inflammation **35**, 139–143
–, insulin receptor **35**, 132
–, intravascular lipoprotein metabolism and lipoprotein receptors **36**, 325–327
–, LCAT **36**, 325–326
–, LDL, metabolism **36**, 322–324
–, –, receptor **36**, 326–327
–, LPL **36**, 325
–, macrophages and immune function **35**, 146–148
–, mechanisms **35**, 148–151
–, –, cyclooxygenase **35**, 150–151
–, –, desaturases **35**, 148–150
–, –, lipoxygenase **35**, 151
–, membranes and enzymes **35**, 129
–, Na^+/K^+ ATPase **35**, 131–132
–, nerve tissue and learning ability **35**, 120–127
–, patients with hyperlipidemia **36**, 316–317
–, plasma lipid/lipoprotein responses **36**, 315–328
–, plasma triacylglycerol response **36**, 316–317
–, reproduction **35**, 128–129
–, studies **36**, 315–316
–, tissue composition effects **35**, 122–123
–, VLDL metabolism **36**, 319–322
n-6 Polyunsaturated fatty acids, chylomicron metabolism effects **36**, 273–275
–, desaturation rates **35**, 78–81
–, dietary **35**, 106–107
–, equations to estimate effects **36**, 271–272
–, HDL metabolism effects **36**, 285–291
–, hypocholesterolemic effect mechanisms **36**, 272–273
–, intravascular processing of lipoproteins **36**, 291–295
–, LDL metabolism effects **36**, 278–285
–, plasma lipid/lipoprotein response **36**, 271–295
–, VLDL metabolism effects **36**, 275–278
Polyunsaturated fatty acids (PUFAs) **35**, 5–6; **36**, 265
–, *n*-3 **37**, 178–179
–, *n*-6 and *n*-3 ratios **35**, 157–159
–, biosynthesis **35**, 79
–, desaturation **35**, 26, 35–36
–, dietary, eicosanoids and **35**, 105–111
–, effects of linolenate and linoleate **35**, 38–39
–, effects on serum lipoproteins and apolipoproteins **37**, 159–170
–, elongation **35**, 26
–, incorporation into cardiolipin **37**, 291–294
–, in fish lipids **33**, 286
–, in milk **37**, 146
–, membrane roles **35**, 9–10
–, –, metabolism **35**, 22–23
–, olive oil and **31**, 477
–, oxidation control, antioxidants **33**, 309–310
–, –, flavonoids **33**, 311–314
–, –, –, antioxidant action **33**, 314–316
–, –, –, effects on lipoxygenase **33**, 316–317
–, –, lipoxygenase **33**, 306–309
–, –, microsomal enzymes **33**, 305–306
–, –, peroxidase **33**, 306
–, oxidation mechanisms, enzyme-initiated **33**, 256–270
–, –, free radical oxidation **33**, 239–249
–, –, oxygen activation **33**, 234–238
–, –, photosensitized singlet oxygen **33**, 249–256
–, oxidation of fish lipids, enzyme-catalzyed **33**, 291–297
–, – of –, factors affecting **33**, 287–289
–, – of –, metal catalysis of **33**, 289–291
–, – of –, volatile compound generation **33**, 298–302
–, oxidation products, acid-catalyzed decomposition **33**, 278–280
–, –, decomposition of acyl hydroperoxides **33**, 270–273

–, –, secondary products **33**, 276–278
–, –, volatile compounds from acyl hydroperoxides **33**, 273–275
–, –, volatile compounds in food **33**, 280–281
–, oxidation reactants and inhibitors, active oxygen species **33**, 302–303
–, –, metals **33**, 303–305
–, –, oxygen **33**, 302
–, peroxidation *in vivo* effects, on DNA **33**, 285–286
–, –, on membranes **33**, 283–285
–, –, on proteins **33**, 282–283
–, prostanoid-mediated mechanism **35**, 145–146
–, retina and visual function **35**, 117–120
Polyvinylamine **14**, 221
Polyvinylpyrrolidone (PVP) **12**, 333–340
–, applications **12**, 336–340
–, –, beer **12**, 336–338
–, –, dehydrated foods **12**, 339–340
–, –, fruit juices **12**, 339
–, –, low-calory sweeteners **12**, 340
–, –, oil-soluble vitamins **12**, 340
–, –, sausage casings **12**, 340
–, –, wines **12**, 338–339
–, background **12**, 333–334
–, properties **12**, 334–336
–, –, film forming **12**, 335
–, –, solubility **12**, 335
–, –, toxicology **12**, 335
Pome fruits **15**, 177
Pomegranate, anatomy of **17**, 169
Pompe's disease **37**, 377
Popov–Belevitch–Hautus tests **40**, 350–351
Population kinetics, *see* Kinetic parameter distribution
Porcine stress syndrome **37**, 379, 408
–, characterization **28**, 169–173
–, classification **28**, 170–171
–, etiology of, catecholamines **28**, 187–189
–, –, –, corticosteroids **28**, 190–192
–, –, –, thyroid **28**, 189–190
–, –, hormones **28**, 187–192
–, –, lactate production **28**, 215
–, –, muscle metabolism **28**, 192–211
–, –, –, contractile proteins **28**, 200–202
–, –, –, mitochondria **28**, 202–210
–, –, –, neuromuscular junction **28**, 193–195
–, –, –, sarcoplasmic reticulum **28**, 195–200
–, malignant hyperthermia **28**, 173–175
–, –, blood gases **28**, 174
–, –, electrolytes during epidodes **28**, 174
–, –, rectal temperature changes **28**, 175
–, pale, soft, exudative syndrome **28**, 175–177
–, predictive tests, genetics **28**, 178–179
–, –, halothane exposure **28**, 182–186
–, –, hematological test **28**, 181–182
–, –, muscle biopsies **28**, 182–186
–, –, post-mortem glycolysis **28**, 185–186
–, –, serological tests **28**, 179–181
Porin **41**, 144
Pork (*see also* Meat quality) **14**, 41; **39**, 75, 76, 79, 83
–, age **14**, 48
–, animal physiology and meat quality **21**, 71–155
–, canned, effect of storage on vitamin B content **1**, 97–98
–, dark, firm, and dry (DFD) **37**, 379, 408
–, dehydrated **7**, 218
–, –, thiamine destruction **6**, 261, 263
–, effect of heat treatment on nutritive value of protein in **4**, 249–250, 253
–, – of pH during curing **5**, 31
–, energy costs **39**, 145
–, extract, effect on fat **5**, 22
–, fat rancidity **5**, 4, 5
–, fatty acids **5**, 6
–, – in fat of **23**, 23
–, freeze-dried **7**, 218–220
–, –, rehydration of **7**, 220
–, –, storage stability of **7**, 219
–, grain **14**, 49
–, ground, effect of ascorbic acid on storage life **4**, 394
–, heat processing **2**, 82; **39**, 107
–, loss of thiamine **6**, 275, 281, 282, 304
–, luncheon meat, retention of vitamin B in **1**, 86–98
–, meat mutagens **34**, 423
–, microbial control **39**, 123–124
–, microbial count of frozen **6**, 188
–, pale, soft, and exudative (PSE) **37**, 379, 408
–, process techniques **39**, 90
–, sausage, rancidity **5**, 23
–, "sex odor" in **23**, 39
–, shear testing **14**, 77–78
–, structural alteration **39**, 93
–, texture **39**, 125
–, thiamine **6**, 300
–, –, decomposition in **6**, 258
–, –, retention in frozen **6**, 294
Pork and beans, frozen, bacterial count of **6**, 199
Porosity, friction-factor factor as a function of **11**, 430
–, IM meat **39**, 110

Porosity (*cont'd*)
–, Reynolds number factor as a function of **11**, 430
Position on tree, effects on fruit composition **9**, 296–298
Posterior distribution **40**, 268
Postharvest diseases **15**, 147ff
–, cause **15**, 166
–, control of **15**, 170ff
–, in berries **15**, 171
–, in fruits **15**, 173, 176
–, in tomatoes **15**, 180
–, in vegetables **15**, 179
Post-mortem factor and muscle composition **26**, 129–151
–, biochemical changes **26**, 132–135
–, cold shortening phenomenon **26**, 137–138
–, influence of aging **26**, 140–142
–, – of carcass characteristics **26**, 131–132
–, – of cooking methods **26**, 146–151
–, – of slaughtering methods **26**, 129–130
–, – of tenderization **26**, 142–146
–, ultrastructural changes **26**, 135–136
Postprandial changes, in tocopherol content of lipoprotein fractions **33**, 176
Potash, alcoholic, dehydrochlorination of DDT by **2**, 203
Potassium, chocolate and **31**, 246, 271
–, content of apples and pears **8**, 371, 386
–, deficiency of **17**, 247
–, dietary fiber and **31**, 140, 141, 153
–, effect on ascorbic acid content of plants **1**, 308, 310
–, – on calcium absorption by plants **1**, 311–312
–, endogenous proteolytic enzymes and **31**, 380
–, in ion exchange reactions **2**, 10
–, in milk **36**, 212–213
–, in wines **8**, 137, 138, 139, 193
–, loss of, in blanching **8**, 65
–, olive oil and **31**, 459
Potassium chloride, in diet of rats **1**, 112
–, use in regeneration of zeolite in milk industry **2**, 23
Potassium deficiency **1**, 120–121
Potassium gellan, molecular shapes and interactions **42**, 187–191
Potassium iodide, combination with *o*-quinone in fruit products **3**, 20
Potassium iodine **44**, 317
Potassium ions, effects on β-galactosidase **38**, 82
Potassium native gellan, molecular shapes and interactions **42**, 186–188
Potassium salts, use of to form pectic acid **1**, 406
Potassium supplements, for hypokalemic periodic paralysis **37**, 385
Potassium supply, effects on fruit composition **9**, 299–300
Potassium thiocyanate, gelatin manufacture and **7**, 240
Potato chips **15**, 293
–, deterioration in **1**, 259, 273, 286
Potatoes **14**, 268; **15**, 231
–, ADPGlc PPase **41**, 48–49
–, analyses for SO_2 **5**, 59
–, ascorbic acid content of, effect of location and season on **1**, 296–297
–, –, – of nitrogen on **1**, 309
–, –, – of rainfall on **1**, 304
–, –, – of sunlight on **1**, 302
–, as starch model **41**, 9–10
–, black heart in **3**, 6
–, branching enzymes in **41**, 93, 98–99
–, browning in during drying **1**, 259–263
–, calcium content **10**, 183, 194
–, calories per pound **6**, 233
–, canned, calories per pound **6**, 233
–, –, deterioration in **1**, 259, 286
–, characteristics **41**, 164
–, chlorophyll formation and glyco-alkaloid toxicity **21**, 307–354
–, constituents of oil of **2**, 275
–, consumer preferences for **3**, 401, 402, 409
–, consumer survey study of **3**, 422
–, cooked, freezing of **6**, 237
–, cooking quality in relation to reducing sugars **1**, 283
–, cortex of **10**, 182
–, culture **10**, 201–202
–, cytochrome oxidase in **3**, 15
–, decrease in bacterial content by blanching **6**, 184
–, dehydrated, as food staple **6**, 232
–, –, browning during storage **1**, 263–272, 273–279, 286
–, –, browning in, effect of raw material factors on **1**, 261–263
–, –, –, – of sulfiting on **1**, 260–261
–, –, calories per pound **6**, 233
–, –, chemical changes during storage **1**, 273–279
–, –, compression of **1**, 271–272, 281
–, –, defects in **1**, 257–286

–, –, development of defects in during storage **1**, 263–272
–, –, effect of moisture content on **1**, 263–266, 276, 280–281
–, –, – of packaging on storage life of **1**, 271–272
–, –, – of raw material factors on storage life of **1**, 268–271
–, –, – of sugars on **1**, 280–284
–, –, – of sulfiting on **1**, 266–268, 278–280
–, –, – of temperature on **1**, 263–266
–, –, factors influencing deterioration of **1**, 259–273
–, –, mashed **25**, 55–136
–, –, "off-flavors" developed in during storage **1**, 276
–, –, thiamine in **6**, 300
–, –, vitamin losses in **1**, 261
–, –, weight, space requirement **6**, 233
–, dehydration of **3**, 143
–, dicotyledonous plants **31**, 126, 127, 131, 132
–, dietary fiber and, analysis **31**, 142, 146, 150
–, discoloration during dehydration **5**, 89
–, dried, enzymic changes in **11**, 288
–, drying of **8**, 32
–, effect of blanching on **1**, 68, 77
–, – of dehydration on **2**, 324
–, – of salts on tensile strength of **2**, 315–316
–, – of temperature and moisture content on browning in **1**, 259–260
–, – of variation on sensory tests **2**, 22
–, flavonoids **5**, 282
–, freezing, effects on **10**, 183
–, French fried, deterioration in **1**, 259, 273, 286
–, gelation in **10**, 182
–, histological changes in processing **10**, 182–183
–, in beef stew, thiamine retention **6**, 284
–, in diet **1**, 109–110
–, inhibition of sprouting in **1**, 284
–, inositol phosphate content **45**, 23
–, leucoplasts in **2**, 306
–, life cycle **41**, 10
–, loss in blanching **8**, 66
–, loss of thiamine on processing **6**, 289
–, mashed, thiamine in **6**, 292
–, maturation **10**, 188
–, modification **41**, 129
–, non-waxy type **6**, 243
–, nutritional stress factor in **4**, 111–113
–, oxidation of phenol in **3**, 6
–, pectic materials in **10**, 183, 194
–, periderm **10**, 187, 202
–, phenolase obtained from **3**, 7
–, phosphorus content of, effect of fertilizers on **1**, 313
–, polyphenolase, spraying with **8**, 356
–, polyphenolase in **3**, 14
–, polyphenols and enzymic browning in **19**, 120–121, 124–125
–, preparation of prepeeled **5**, 128, 146
–, preservation of **6**, 231
–, processing for chipping **10**, 205–208
–, properties **31**, 155, 157–159, 170
–, protein crystals **10**, 185, 187
–, radio-frequency heating of **3**, 136
–, rate of oxidation in **3**, 14
–, raw, nutritive value of **2**, 327
–, reducing sugar content of **1**, 281–284; **10**, 187, 191
–, –, in relation to cooking quality **1**, 283
–, respiration of **3**, 9
–, riced, development of **6**, 233
–, silage made from **1**, 272
–, solamine in **1**, 124
–, specific gravity **10**, 185, 186, 187, 188–190, 200
–, spray-drying **2**, 454; **6**, 234
–, sprouting, inhibition of **10**, 203–204
–, starch in **41**, 3
–, –, gelatinization **2**, 317, 319
–, storage **10**, 204–205
–, sulfiting for drying **5**, 142, 143
–, sweet, canned, nutrients in **1**, 43, 46–50
–, –, loss of thiamine **6**, 290
–, –, processing of **6**, 290, 292
–, synthetic chips, alginates in **11**, 155
–, test for mealiness of **2**, 250
–, textural changes during cooking **2**, 311–314
–, texture **10**, 182–183
–, varieties **10**, 182–183, 202
–, vitamin C content of **6**, 249
–, weight, space requirement **6**, 233
Potato flour, rate of darkening of **1**, 264
Potato granules, add-back method of drying **6**, 238
–, calories per pound **6**, 233
–, characteristics of **6**, 232
–, color of **6**, 248
–, drying methods and equipment **6**, 245
–, effect of conveying system on quality of **6**, 240
–, – of specific gravity of **6**, 243

Potato granules, effect (*cont'd*)
–, – of temperature of mixing and tempering on **6**, 242
–, nutritive value of **6**, 249
–, processes for manufacture **6**, 236
–, product quality of **6**, 247
–, quality evaluation of **6**, 249
–, weight, space requirement **6**, 233
Potato products, ascorbic acid addition to **18**, 236–237
–, Maillard reactions **30**, 113
–, volatiles, identification **30**, 113
Potato pulp, composition of **17**, 121
–, protein enriched **17**, 122
Potato shreds **6**, 234
Potato starch **17**, 121–122
Potato wastes **17**, 87–88
Potency, carcinogen risk assessment and **31**, 36, 37
Potential, action **40**, 331–332
Potential energy, excess **34**, 31–32
Poultry (*see also* Mechanically deboned poultry) **13**, 164, 305–306, 321–322; **14**, 96
–, bacterial flora on **6**, 192
–, by-products **17**, 133–134
–, carrageenan in **11**, 133–135
–, chemical composition of edible portion of **1**, 206–207
–, cooking for sensory tests **2**, 229
–, disintegration of fibers during aging of **1**, 247–251
–, effect of temperature **5**, 38
–, factors influencing flavor of **1**, 219–224
–, factors influencing juiciness of **1**, 225–230
–, factors influencing tenderness of **1**, 230–232
–, fat, changes in during storage **1**, 213
–, –, composition of **1**, 211–212
–, –, effect of diet on composition of **1**, 213
–, –, iodine value of **1**, 212–213
–, –, rancidity in **1**, 214–215; **5**, 4, 5
–, –, stability of, *in-situ* **1**, 214–218
–, fatty acids **5**, 6
–, frozen, factors influencing flavor of **1**, 222–224
–, histological changes in during aging of **1**, 236–251
–, infrared radiation in rearing of **3**, 147
–, meat, post-mortem changes in **1**, 232–234
–, muscle, glycogen content of **1**, 233, 253
–, –, histology of **1**, 209–211, 234–253
–, –, proteins of **1**, 207–211
–, –, tenderness and histological changes during aging **1**, 251–253
–, radurization of **24**, 189–192
–, rigor mortis in **1**, 232–234
–, –, nodes in **1**, 245–247
–, *Salmonella* infection in **3**, 222–224
–, skin fat **5**, 7
–, storage of DDT in **2**, 211
–, temperature use for sensory tests **2**, 247
–, toughness and tenderness of **8**, 13
–, turbulence in fibers of **1**, 244
–, use of antioxidant **5**, 26
–, "warmed-over" flavor in **23**, 1–74
Poultry carcasses, hydrogen peroxide combined treatment **45**, 201
–, ozone treatment **45**, 190, 192, 193–194
–, prefiltration of treatment water **45**, 183
–, residual ozone values **45**, 180
Poultry products, thermal processing, *see* Thermal processing
Poultry skin, confocal scanning laser microscopy **43**, 355
–, inhibition methods **43**, 353
–, mechanisms **43**, 341, 342, 399
–, microbial attachment **43**, 339–343
–, physical entrapment **43**, 341, 347
–, physicochemical detachment **43**, 351
–, process treatment effects **43**, 341, 343
–, properties of attached bacteria **43**, 348
–, structural aspects **43**, 339, 340
Power consumption of agitators **11**, 424–425
Power law, rheology **39**, 5–6, 34, 46, 56
Power-law model **32**, 47, 48
PPD index **35**, 215, 218
Prandtl number **32**, 49, 64, 68, 69, 70, 72, 73, 75, 76, 79, 80
Pravastatin **44**, 288
Prebiotics **43**, 16, 18, 20, 21, 35
–, dose–response relations **43**, 21
–, estrogen recyling enhacement **43**, 44
Preblending **16**, 136
Precipitation, fish freshness and **7**, 62
–, versus gelation **39**, 183–184
Prefabrication **14**, 71
Preferential hydration, glycerol **35**, 291
–, proteins, neutral salts **35**, 298–299
Prefreezing **13**, 320–322, 330
–, freeze-drying and **7**, 217
–, methods of **7**, 175
Pregastric esterase **39**, 202
Pregnancy **40**, 86, 91, 112–113
Prepacking, passion fruit **12**, 232–233
Prepared foods **41**, 165
Prephenic acid, in catechin synthesis **17**, 225
Prepyriform cortex **44**, 255
Prerigor processing, IM meat **39**, 93

Preripening in cheese **16**, 238
Prescott, Samuel Cate **27**, 1–20
–, –, books written by **27**, 15, 17–18
–, –, Boston Bacteriological Club and **27**, 15
–, –, career, early **27**, 5–7
–, –, contemporaries **27**, 12–13
–, –, contributions, to chemistry of coffee **27**, 10–11
–, –, –, to refrigeration and freezing of foods **27**, 8–10
–, –, –, to thermal processing **27**, 7–8
–, –, education **27**, 3–5
–, –, honors, awards, and public service **27**, 14–16
–, –, Institute of Food Technologists, and **27**, 11–12
–, –, Massachusetts Institute of Technology, and **27**, 16–18
–, –, Underwood, William Lyman, work with **27**, 7–8
–, –, –, World War I, during and after **27**, 8
Preservation, additives, chemical **13**, 288–289
–, by use of CMC **12**, 312–313
–, – of –, coatings **12**, 313
–, – of –, fresh fish **12**, 312–313
–, commercial **13**, 317–329
–, –, methods **13**, 318–319
–, –, prefreezing **13**, 320–322
–, –, quality **13**, 322–323
–, –, selection **13**, 319
–, –, storage **13**, 323–327
–, –, thawing **13**, 327–329
–, concentration nonaqueous constituents **13**, 270–271
–, crystallization **13**, 244–259
–, –, growth **13**, 247–252
–, –, location **13**, 257–259
–, –, nucleation **13**, 244–247
–, –, re- **13**, 253–257
–, –, size **13**, 252–253
–, deterioration causes **13**, 311–317
–, –, during freezing **13**, 311–315
–, –, during storage **13**, 315–316
–, –, during thawing **13**, 317
–, effect on food **13**, 289–311
–, freezing, diagrams **13**, 259–269
–, –, rate **13**, 274–287
–, IM meat **39**, 85–88, 93, 118–119
–, low-temperature **13**, 219–347
–, of abalone **23**, 168–173
–, of passion fruit **12**, 245–252
–, –, blends **12**, 251–252
–, –, freezing **12**, 249
–, –, microbiological aspects **12**, 250–251
–, –, storage **12**, 249–250
–, –, thermal processing **12**, 245–249
–, of soy sauce **12**, 85–86
–, water, and ice **13**, 221–235, 238–244
–, –, pure, phase diagram **13**, 236–238
–, –, volume changes **13**, 272–274
Preservatives, effects of sterilization **12**, 407–410
–, fish sausage and ham in combination **12**, 408–410
–, – in –, germicidal effects **12**, 409
–, oriental noodles **43**, 161–162
–, permissible **12**, 407–408
Preserves **15**, 342
–, electronic cooking of **3**, 142
Press-fluid determination **14**, 106–109
–, Grau and Hamm **14**, 107–108
Press method of measuring water in meat **10**, 365–377
Pressometers **14**, 106–107
Pressure, gas-flow and **7**, 193–194
–, limiting for yeast growth **12**, 62–63
–, –, tolerance of soy yeasts **12**, 62–63
–, osmotic **12**, 53, 59, 61–63
–, sugar concentration of **12**, 61
–, vapor transport and **7**, 196–198
Pressure drops, flow rate at various **11**, 388–393
Primethamine, effects on folate absorption and metabolism **33**, 70
Prion diseases (*see also* Bovine spongiform encephalopathy) **43**, 275–285
–, genetics **43**, 285–287
–, species barriers to transmission **43**, 290–292, 293
Prion precursor protein (PrP) **43**, 272
–, infective conformation (PrP{S}sc{s}) **43**, 272, 273, 274, 279
–, –, nervous tissue damage **43**, 274–275
–, –, pre-clinical detection **43**, 300, 301
–, –, strains **43**, 288
Prion precursor protein (PrP) gene **43**, 272–273, 285
–, CJD susceptibility-associated polymorphism **43**, 282, 293
–, knockout mice **43**, 273
–, mutation **43**, 273, 274
–, –, inherited human spongiform encephalopathies **43**, 280, 281, 285, 287
–, –, spontaneous PrP^{sc} formation **43**, 287
–, scrapie susceptibility **43**, 286, 287
Prions **43**, 272–275
–, infectivity **43**, 294–295
Prior distribution **40**, 268, 269–271, 273–276

PROALCOOL **32**, 211–215
Probes, radioactive, cardiolipin-derived **37**, 316–317
–, sampling **40**, 183–184, 185–186, 188, 190
Probiotic cultures, adherence in human intestine **37**, 74–77
–, ingestion **37**, 48–49
–, lactic acid bacterial strains **37**, 115–116
Probiotics **43**, 15, 21
–, anticarcinogenic properties **43**, 34
–, colonic survival **43**, 16
–, opportunistic infection prevention **43**, 44–45
Probucol **44**, 288, 320
Procainamide **44**, 306
Procaine **44**, 287
Procainesterase in eggs **1**, 183
Processed cheese products **39**, 259–277
Processed foods, effect on nitrogen metabolism **21**, 24
Processing, effect on chlorophyll **17**, 5
–, – on proteins **16**, 27
–, high-temperature short-time **17**, 3–4
–, of bread **16**, 335ff
–, of cheese **16**, 231ff
–, of emulsions **16**, 145ff
–, of ham, fish **12**, 391
–, sausage, crushing **12**, 379–380
–, –, cutting finely **12**, 379
–, –, fish **12**, 379–484
–, –, grinding **12**, 379, 381–382
–, –, mixing in pork fat **12**, 384–385
–, –, seasoning **12**, 382–384
–, time calculation **12**, 403–407
–, –, heat penetration **12**, 404–405
–, –, lethality **12**, 406–407
–, –, safety factor **12**, 406
Processing support, modeling **40**, 282–283
Prochlorperazine **44**, 308
Procollagen, *see* Collagen
Procollagen endopeptidase, in Ehlers–Danlos syndrome **37**, 392–393
Product holding tube **32**, 16
Product inhibition, lactase **38**, 9–13
Progressive myoclonus epilepsy **37**, 372
Prolamins (*see also* Zeins) **36**, 93, 95
–, classification **36**, 95
–, corn **38**, 275, 277
–, HMW **36**, 100–101
–, relationship among prolamins **36**, 103
–, sequences and positions of prolamin box **36**, 97, 99
–, solubility **36**, 103
–, sulfur-poor **36**, 100
–, sulfur-rich **36**, 100
–, wheat **38**, 216
–, with sequenced cDNA and genes **36**, 97–98
Prolidase, endogenous proteolytic enzymes and **31**, 349
Proliferation, carcinogen risk assessment and **31**, 26
Prolinase, endogenous proteolytic enzymes and **31**, 349
Proline, endogenous proteolytic enzymes and, exopeptidases **31**, 348–350, 352
–, –, meat technology **31**, 410
–, gelatin structure and **7**, 268–270
–, *N*-nitroso compounds and **31**, 76–78, 80
Promethazine **44**, 308
Promoters **41**, 128–129
–, carcinogen risk assessment and **31**, 28
Proosdij cheese **39**, 243
Prooxidants, heme compounds as **23**, 45
Propafenone **44**, 306, 321
Propagation, olive oil and **31**, 471, 472
–, passion fruit **12**, 208, 272–273
Propanal, as flavor component in onions **22**, 101
Propanol, soybean protein denaturation **30**, 213
Propantheline bromide **44**, 299
S-(1-Propenyl)-L-cysteine sulfoxide, as alliinase substrate **22**, 96–97
–, as odor principle in onion **22**, 91
–, structure of **22**, 96
1-Propenylsulfenic acid, structure of **22**, 97
Propionaldehyde in onion oil **2**, 273
Propionibacter in bacon **3**, 308
Propionic acid **16**, 185, 253
–, fish spoilage and **7**, 48
–, in decomposing salmon **2**, 371
–, microbial inhibition by **1**, 387, 390
Propionic acid esters, in cocoa **2**, 283
–, in molasses **2**, 277
–, in parsnip seed oil **2**, 274
–, in tea leaves **2**, 285, 287
Propofol **44**, 287
n-Proponol in apples **2**, 263
Propranolol **44**, 306
Propylaldehyde in black tea **2**, 287
Propylallyl sulfides in *Allium scorodoprasum* L. **2**, 273
Propylene oxide, esterification of carboxyl groups by **1**, 383
–, hydrolysis in foods **1**, 389
–, sterilization of dried fruits with **3**, 466

Propyl gallate, effect of, on blood constituents 3, 204
–, –, on growth **3**, 203
–, –, on mortality of rats **3**, 205
–, inhibition of, lipid oxidation by microsomes **33**, 306
–, lipoxygenases **33**, 307
–, pathologic effects of **3**, 207
–, toxicity of as an antioxidant **3**, 200
Propylthiouracil **44**, 299, 322
Prosciutti **39**, 79
Prostacyclin **35**, 97–98
Prostaglandins **35**, 98–101
–, elevated synthesis, inflammation **35**, 140
–, endogenous proteolytic enzymes and **31**, 380, 382
Prostaglandin H synthase, eicosanoids synthesis **35**, 94–97
Prostanoids, inflammation and **35**, 141
–, synthesis **35**, 91
–, –, α-LNA effects **35**, 151
Prostate cancer, carcinogen risk assessment and **31**, 14, 17, 22
Prosthetic group, of enzymes **17**, 7, 34
–, protohematin IX, properties of **17**, 8, 10
Protease inhibitors, composition **28**, 134–139
–, distribution in plants **28**, 133
–, from beans **28**, 128–141
–, medical importance **28**, 139–141
–, nomenclature **28**, 129–133
–, occurrence **28**, 129–133
–, physicochemical properties **28**, 134–139
–, significance in plants **28**, 133
Proteases **16**, 430
–, amino acid sequence in **10**, 7
–, endogenous proteolytic enzymes and **31**, 344, 345, 412
–, in eggs **1**, 183
–, meat technology **31**, 401, 404, 406–410
–, muscle physiology **31**, 379, 381
–, proteinase activity **31**, 384–387, 390, 392
Pro-Teen, use in developing countries **22**, 196–197
Δ-Protein, precipitation from muscle **19**, 326–328
Proteinases **16**, 288; **39**, 211–225, 257–258
–, activity **31**, 383
–, –, animal age **31**, 387
–, –, endocrines **31**, 388, 389
–, –, endogenous inhibitors **31**, 383–385
–, –, muscle type **31**, 385, 386
–, –, muscular dystrophies **31**, 389–391
–, –, nerve system **31**, 387, 388
–, –, nutrition **31**, 386, 387
–, –, physical exercise **31**, 391–393
–, –, weightlessness **31**, 393
–, distribution **31**, 366–369
–, endogenous proteolytic enzymes and **31**, 344, 346, 411–414
–, in wheat germ **23**, 210, 239
–, muscle physiology **31**, 369
–, –, conflicting results **31**, 381, 382
–, –, protein **31**, 369–373
–, –, protein catabolism **31**, 377–381
–, –, protein turnover **31**, 373–376, 382, 383
–, of *Byssochlamys* spp. **25**, 266–267
Protein beverages, for developing countries **22**, 195
Protein catabolism, calcium **31**, 380, 381
–, endogenous proteolytic enzymes and **31**, 377, 383
–, lysosomes **31**, 377–379
–, meat technology **31**, 410
–, nonlysosomal proteinases **31**, 379, 380
–, proteinase activity **31**, 388, 391, 392
Protein concentrate, from soybeans **17**, 108
Protein-containing conditioning films **43**, 326–327
Protein content of foods as affected by preparation and cooking **4**, 245
– of vegetables, effect of blanching **1**, 68
Protein deficiency, effects on connective tissue **37**, 388–389
Protein efficiency ratio (PER) **16**, 37; **17**, 115; **39**, 137
Protein emulsifiers, acylation **34**, 151–152
–, chemical modification **34**, 150–151
–, covalent attachment of hydrophobic groups **34**, 156
–, deamidation **34**, 155–156
–, disulfide bond reduction **34**, 158
–, enzymatic modification **34**, 158–159
–, esterification **34**, 152–153
–, glycosylation **34**, 156–157
–, heat **34**, 147–150
–, hydrophobic ligands **34**, 160–162
–, modification **34**, 146–162
–, partial hydrolysis **34**, 159–160
–, pH **34**, 150
–, phosphorylation **34**, 153–155
–, polymerization, by transglutaminase **34**, 160
–, reductive alkylation **34**, 158
–, salt effect **34**, 161–162
Protein films, interfacial rheology **34**, 124–126
Protein food products, textured, for improved world nutrition **22**, 187–203

Protein foods, consumption per capita, worldwide **30**, 334–335
–, interaction with energy foods **30**, 332–334
–, land animals (*see also* Animals, land) **30**, 339–349
–, marine animals (*see also* Animals, marine) **30**, 349–352
–, new, based on plant sources, animal flesh model **30**, 358–360
–, –, cereal–legume model **30**, 355–357
–, –, government regulations **30**, 377
–, –, nutritious beverage models **30**, 357–358
–, plants **30**, 335–339
Protein gels, *see* Mixed protein gels
Protein hydrolyzates **10**, 195
Protein kinase C, cardiolipin association **37**, 285
Protein–lipid edible films **44**, 371–382
–, applications **44**, 381–382
–, oxygen barrier properties **44**, 378
–, relative humidity effects **44**, 381
–, water barrier properties **44**, 372–378, 379–380
Protein–lipid interaction, effect on baking quality **29**, 263–264
Protein malnutrition **16**, 1ff
Protein matrix **39**, 124, 125, 266–267
Protein–propyleneglycol alginate composite films **44**, 383
Protein–protein associations, thermal stability **35**, 266
Protein–protein interactions, gel **34**, 208
–, protein thermal behavior effects **35**, 331–333
Proteins (*see also* Amino acid sequence alignments, Casein, Food proteins, Glycogen phosphorylase metabolism, Retinol-binding protein, Seed storage proteins, Thermal analysis, Transthyretin metabolism) **36**, 91
–, adsorption at air–water interface **34**, 11–13
–, adsorption at fluid interfaces **34**, 1–2
–, affinity of surface-active ions for **1**, 379
–, aldoses and derivatives **14**, 219–220
–, aliphatic indices **35**, 258, 260
–, amino acid sequences **42**, 47–48
–, amyloid **40**, 150
–, and fructose **14**, 221–222
–, and oxidized lipids **14**, 225–226
–, animal, digestibility **30**, 363
–, –, effects on humans, blood lipids and **30**, 372–375
–, artificial fibers, carrageenan in **11**, 135
–, as cryostabilizers **35**, 345–348
–, as "dough softening factor" in milk **3**, 81–83
–, as emulsifiers **34**, 109–128
–, –, adsorption kinetics **34**, 114–117
–, –, competitive adsorption in mixed emulsifier system **34**, 126–127
–, –, equation of state, proteins at interfaces **34**, 111–113
–, –, hydrocarbon/water interface **34**, 121
–, –, interfacial pressure **34**, 123
–, –, interfacial properties **34**, 110–111
–, –, interfacial rheology of films **34**, 124–126
–, –, limiting interfacial area **34**, 113
–, –, load at oil/water interface **34**, 117–123
–, –, reversibility and thermodynamic consideration **34**, 123–124
–, –, surface pressures **34**, 112
–, –, surface viscosity **34**, 124–126
–, –, unfolding at interface **34**, 113–114
–, as emulsion stabilizers **22**, 339–340
–, as food allergens **42**, 6–7, 46, 64
–, binding **40**, 117, 122–127
–, biological utilization **35**, 185–186
–, bound carbohydrates **14**, 215–218
–, bread enriched with glycolipid–wheat flour interaction in baking of **20**, 178–184
–, cereal enrichment with **30**, 356
–, chocolate and, alkalization **31**, 220–225
–, –, milk **31**, 253–255, 257, 259–261, 263
–, –, milk crumb **31**, 285
–, –, sweeteners **31**, 271, 275
–, –, *Theobroma cacao* L. **31**, 323, 325
–, configuration and conformation at interfaces **34**, 55–60
–, –, adsorbed state **34**, 59
–, –, fibrinogen and factor XII **34**, 59
–, –, flexible polypeptides **34**, 55–56
–, –, highly flexible polymers **34**, 56
–, –, π–a plots **34**, 57–58
–, –, synthetic polypeptides **34**, 59–60
–, –, transferred monolayer **34**, 60
–, conformation, effect on functional properties of whey proteins **33**, 367–369
–, conformation role on adsorption **34**, 22–38
–, – on –, abnormalities in apparent diffusion coefficient **34**, 29–30
–, – on –, alcohols **34**, 30–31
–, – on –, apparent diffusion coefficients **34**, 27–29
–, – on –, attractive hydrophobic potential **34**, 32
–, – on –, BSA intermediates **34**, 30–31

–, – on –, correlation of molecular and conformational properties **34**, 23–24
–, – on –, electrostatic potential energy **34**, 32
–, – on –, excess potential energy **34**, 31–32
–, – on –, first-order kinetics **34**, 24–25
–, – on –, frictional coefficient **34**, 29
–, – on –, kinetics **34**, 22–34
–, – on –, ln(dπ/dt) versus π plots **34**, 34–35
–, – on –, molecular rearrangement **34**, 34–38
–, – on –, optimum conformation **34**, 36–37
–, – on –, protein as surfactant, molecular properties **34**, 25
–, – on –, solute–solvent interaction **34**, 31
–, – on –, solution conformation **34**, 26–27
–, – on –, surface area cleared by surface penetration and molecular rearrangement **34**, 34–36
–, – on –, surface hydrophobic patches **34**, 33
–, – on –, surface pressure versus concentration **34**, 37–38
–, – on –, surfactants **34**, 33–34
–, – on –, time-dependent changes in surface pressure and concentration **34**, 22–23, 26–27
–, connective tissue **14**, 38
–, content, increasing in wheat **36**, 75
–, decomposition **16**, 163ff
–, denaturants, microbial inhibition by **1**, 380
–, denaturation **17**, 36, 45; **39**, 100
–, –, agents **5**, 19
–, –, by freezing **6**, 164, 167
–, –, in fish flesh, during frozen storage **26**, 275–307
–, –, in frozen fish, dehydration **26**, 283–284
–, –, –, factors causing **26**, 281–306
–, –, –, ice crystal formation **26**, 281–283
–, –, –, lipid hydrolysis **26**, 294–295
–, –, interaction between factors **26**, 304–306
–, –, in water and sugar solutions **35**, 291
–, –, lipid oxidation **26**, 296–297
–, –, lipids **26**, 290–294
–, –, –, solute concentration **26**, 285–290
–, –, –, –, divalent cations **26**, 289–290
–, –, –, –, salt **26**, 286–287
–, –, –, TMAOase activity **26**, 298–304
–, –, research needs **26**, 306–307
–, desorption from air–water interface **34**, 52
–, desorption rates and surface pressures **34**, 53–54
–, dietary, effect on calcium absorption **33**, 143–144
–, dietary fiber and **31**, 119, 182
–, –, analysis **31**, 143, 150, 152, 153
–, –, components **31**, 122, 123, 141
–, –, dicotyledonous plants **31**, 124, 129, 132
–, –, monocotyledonous plants **31**, 137, 138
–, –, properties **31**, 155, 165, 169
–, diffusion coefficients **34**, 19–20
–, diffusion-controlled adsorption **34**, 16–20
–, digestibility **35**, 185–226
–, –, animal bioassays **35**, 211–213
–, –, carbonyl-amine reactions **35**, 189–201
–, –, change in melting temperature **35**, 286–287
–, –, decrease in Maillard reaction **30**, 121
–, –, future directions **35**, 226
–, –, immobilized digestive enzyme assay **35**, 222–225
–, –, in oilseeds **30**, 363
–, –, in roasted wheat **30**, 218–219
–, –, loss and LAL content **35**, 209–210
–, –, lysine loss and **35**, 224–225
–, –, Maillard reaction **35**, 200–201
–, –, optimal thermal processing **35**, 189
–, –, proteolysis **35**, 186–188
–, –, racemization and cross-linking **35**, 201–211
–, –, soluble enzyme assays **35**, 213–222
–, –, –, characteristics **35**, 216–217
–, –, –, classification **35**, 214
–, –, –, enzymatic digestion-dialysis technique **35**, 218–220
–, –, –, multienzyme, initial rate methods **35**, 220–221
–, –, –, pepsin digest-dialysate method **35**, 215
–, –, –, pepsin digest residue method **35**, 214–215, 218
–, –, –, pepsin pancreatin digest-dialysate method **35**, 214–215, 218
–, –, –, pepsin-pancreatin digest method **35**, 214–215, 218
–, –, –, pH drop assays **35**, 221
–, –, thermal unfolding and aggregation **35**, 189
–, dry processing **35**, 333–334
–, effect of heat on nutritive value **4**, 233–280
–, efficiency ratio **35**, 221
–, electrostatic effects **34**, 38–47
–, –, concentration versus surface pressure **34**, 41
–, –, ionic strength and rate of change of surface pressure **34**, 42–44
–, –, ln(dπ/dt) versus π plots **34**, 43, 45

Proteins, electrostatic effects (*cont'd*)
–, –, net change and steady-state surface pressure **34**, 42–43
–, –, potential barriers **34**, 39
–, –, π–a relationship of β-caseins **34**, 40–41
–, –, steady-state surface pressure and ionic strength **34**, 43, 45
–, –, surface-active properties **34**, 42
–, –, surface area cleared during surface penetration and molecular rearrangement **34**, 45–46
–, –, surface pressure variation with time **34**, 42
–, endogenous proteolytic enzymes and, endopeptidases **31**, 353, 354, 357, 362
–, –, extracellular **31**, 371–373
–, –, intracellular **31**, 370, 371
–, –, meat technology **31**, 398, 406, 409–411
–, –, muscle physiology **31**, 369, 370
–, –, proteinase activity **31**, 385–387
–, energy barrier theory **34**, 20–22
–, engineering **36**, 91–92
–, –, thermal stability **35**, 280
–, expression **41**, 128–129
–, extraction **17**, 101–102
–, fish spoilage and **7**, 43–44
–, flavoring substance content **42**, 17–20
–, from tomato wastes **17**, 103–104
–, functional domains **42**, 65
–, functional properties **34**, 300
–, gel-forming **39**, 186–187
–, gels, thermal scanning rheological analysis **35**, 350–357
–, glucose reaction **14**, 218–219
–, heat transfer treatments **35**, 336–337
–, hydration, ultrasonic analysis **45**, 151–152
–, hydrophilic side chains **42**, 94
–, hydrophobic interactions **35**, 239–240
–, in abalone **23**, 151–156
–, in algae **16**, 16, 73
–, in aquatic food **20**, 189–216
–, in bread **16**, 340, 387, 421
–, in candies **6**, 30
–, in cereal grains **16**, 6ff, 19
–, in cheese **16**, 237ff
–, in cocoa beans and nibs **6**, 38
–, in connective tissue **20**, 264
–, in corn by-products **17**, 119
–, in cow's milk **2**, 21, 22
–, in dehydrated mashed potatoes **25**, 79–84
–, in dough **16**, 421
–, in dried milk products, chemical changes in **3**, 53–55
–, –, chemical treatment of **3**, 51
–, –, denaturation of **3**, 53–55
–, in foods, chemical properties **10**, 26–27
–, –, dehydration, effects on **10**, 30, 59
–, –, freezing, effects on **10**, 28–29, 52
–, –, heat, effects on **10**, 27–28, 48–49, 50–52
–, –, physical properties **10**, 26
–, –, radiation, effects on **10**, 49, 59, 66–67
–, –, role of **10**, 24, 25
–, –, salts, effects on **10**, 30
–, –, shear force, effects on **10**, 29–30, 41, 53
–, –, solvents, effects on **10**, 30
–, –, surface action, effects on **10**, 9–9
–, in fruits **17**, 183
–, in honey **24**, 305–308
–, injurious compounds in **1**, 127
–, in leaves **16**, 16, 72
–, in legumes **16**, 9ff, 24, 66ff
–, in meat emulsions **16**, 111ff, 133ff
–, –, denaturation **16**, 117ff
–, –, extraction **16**, 122ff
–, –, freezing **16**, 135
–, –, rigor **16**, 135
–, –, salt solubility **16**, 111
–, –, texture **16**, 149
–, in micro-organisms **16**, 18
–, in milk, *see* Milk proteins
–, in muscle **19**, 3–4
–, in nutmeats **6**, 48
–, in olive oil **31**, 458, 460, 463
–, in pears **8**, 392
–, in peas, loss in processing **9**, 71
–, –, relation to maturity **9**, 70–71
–, in plants, winter hardiness and **25**, 205–206
–, in seeds **16**, 11, 21, 44, 52
–, insolubilization of in milk **3**, 101
–, in tea **11**, 218–221; **17**, 236–241
–, in tomato seed **17**, 84
–, in vegetables **16**, 1ff
–, –, consumption **16**, 1ff
–, –, digestibility **16**, 26, 75
–, –, isolates **16**, 20, 53
–, –, production **16**, 22ff
–, –, supplemented **16**, 34, 44, 53, 66
–, –, toxicity **16**, 32
–, –, utilization **16**, 23, 43, 74
–, –, value **16**, 21, 74
–, in wheat **16**, 343
–, –, interaction with glycolipids in breadmaking **20**, 165–166
–, in wheat flours, breadmaking and **29**, 246–251
–, –, composition **29**, 241–243
–, –, dough properties and **29**, 243–246

–, –, gluten, *see* Gluten
–, in wheat germ **23**, 203, 205, 213–216
–, in yeast **16**, 18
–, lipid oxidation effects **33**, 282–283
–, loss in blanching of vegetables **8**, 71
–, lysinoalanine content **35**, 209
–, melting points **35**, 258, 260
–, mesophilic and thermophilic, amino acid exchanges **35**, 259, 261
–, –, substitutions **35**, 267
–, microbial sources of **18**, 85–140
–, milk, loss in browning **6**, 31
–, modifications of sugar properties produced by **6**, 53
–, moisture content adjustment **35**, 335
–, muscle **35**, 339–341
–, –, and meat quality **26**, 86–87
–, myofibrillar (*see also* Myofibrillar proteins) **13**, 115–120
–, nitrogen content, of apples and pears **8**, 300
–, –, of cocoa cotyledons **8**, 263
–, *N*-nitroso compounds and **31**, 65, 73, 92
–, nongluten **29**, 242
–, nonprotein ingredients and additives **35**, 336
–, nutrient-response **40**, 231–232, 238–240
–, nutrition **39**, 277
–, Osborne classification **34**, 267–269
–, oxidation, freeze-dried beef and **7**, 212–213
–, partial thermal denaturation, foaming properties **34**, 71
–, peanut **40**, 231–232, 238–240
–, –, milk partial replacement by **30**, 357
–, pH adjustment **35**, 335–336
–, preferential hydration, neutral salts **35**, 298–299
–, quality **40**, 160–162, 165–166
–, –, effect of storage on **4**, 267
–, –, IM meat **39**, 136–137
–, –, methods for determining **4**, 234–237
–, –, microwave exposure effects **43**, 92
–, –, of mechanically deboned fish **27**, 117
–, –, of mechanically deboned poultry **27**, 117
–, –, of mechanically deboned red meat **27**, 74–78
–, –, oriental noodle flours/wheat **43**, 153–154, 155, 159, 181, 187
–, –, sorghum **43**, 223, 239
–, *o*-quinone complexing with, in enzymic browning **19**, 98–102
–, radiation effects on **24**, 169–170
–, reactions **14**, 210–223
–, – with monosaccharides **3**, 273–277
–, – with polysaccharides **3**, 277–278
–, – with sulfites **30**, 23–24
–, recombinant **40**, 8
–, reversibility of adsorption **34**, 52–55
–, role as flavor precursor in cocoa bean **8**, 281
–, sarcoplasmic **13**, 115–120
–, skeletal muscle **14**, 37
–, solubility **34**, 15–16
–, –, measurement, meat endpoint temperature monitoring **44**, 175
–, solubility-related parameters **36**, 7
–, solvent treatments **35**, 334
–, source of **17**, 100–104
–, soy, whipping agent **6**, 22
–, soybean, denaturation for shoyu preparation **30**, 211–217
–, –, digestibility after denaturation **30**, 214–215
–, –, hydrolysate, sulfur-containing volatile compounds **30**, 283
–, –, iron absorption, human, and **30**, 364–368
–, –, iron metabolism, human, and **30**, 364–368
–, –, meat product partial replacement by **30**, 359–360
–, –, milk partial replacement by **30**, 357
–, –, zinc absorption, human, and **30**, 369–370
–, –, zinc metabolism, human, and **30**, 369–370
–, stability **35**, 239–249
–, –, acetamidation **35**, 272–273
–, –, acylation **35**, 270–271
–, –, aliphatic amino acids **35**, 258–259, 261
–, –, amino acid, composition **35**, 266–269
–, –, Arg residues **35**, 266–268
–, –, correlation with α-helix and β-structure **35**, 253
–, –, cross-linking **35**, 274–276
–, –, Cys residues **35**, 268
–, –, disulfide bonds **35**, 284–290
–, –, flexibility indices **35**, 262
–, –, Gibbs free energy, enthalpy, and entropy **35**, 242
–, –, guanidination **35**, 273–274
–, –, hydrogen bonds **35**, 252–253
–, –, hydrophobic amino acids **35**, 265
–, –, –, Leu content **35**, 261
–, –, –, mutant proteins **35**, 262–264
–, –, hydrophobic interactions **35**, 257–266

Proteins, stability (*cont'd*)
–, –, immobilization **35**, 276–277
–, –, ligand binding **35**, 253–257
–, –, modification of functional groups **35**, 269–274
–, –, neutral salts **35**, 294–301
–, –, pyromellitic dianhydride effect **35**, 271–272
–, –, salt bridges **35**, 250–252
–, –, salt effects **35**, 325–326
–, –, site-directed mutagenesis **35**, 277–284
–, –, succinylation **35**, 272
–, –, sugars and polyhydric alcohols effects **35**, 290–294
–, –, thermal inactivation, irreversible **35**, 246–249
–, –, thermal stability curve **35**, 243–245
–, –, thermal unfolding, reversible **35**, 240–246
–, –, tritium–hydrogen isotope exchange measurement **35**, 274
–, –, two-state thermal transition **35**, 241
–, starch granules **41**, 31–32
–, storage **35**, 338–339
–, structure **34**, 13–16
–, –, disulfide bond **34**, 14
–, –, folding **34**, 13, 15
–, –, hydrophobic and hydrophilic amino acid ration **34**, 14–15
–, –, polypeptide backbone **34**, 14
–, –, secondary and tertiary **34**, 14
–, –, thermodynamic stability **34**, 13–14
–, structure-modifying agents, thermal behavior effects **35**, 327–329
–, sulfited, metabolism, rat **30**, 37
–, surface activity **34**, 2–3
–, surface area-to-volume ratio **39**, 195
–, surface hydrophobicity **34**, 127–128
–, surface pressure **34**, 16
–, synthesis **19**, 19
–, –, fruit ripening and **30**, 171
–, synthesis in apples **8**, 391
–, thermal characteristics, low-temperature **35**, 346–347
–, thermal denaturation **35**, 244
–, transferred **42**, 45–46
–, two-state model **35**, 240–241
–, unfolding **35**, 239
–, utilization, relationship of growth to **1**, 130
–, water structure role **34**, 47–52
–, –, alterations in structure **34**, 47–49
–, –, β-casein behavior **34**, 48–52
–, whipping agents **6**, 20, 53
–, with acetaldehyde **14**, 220
Protein–solvent interactions, gel **34**, 208
Protein-stabilized foams **34**, 60–71
–, factors affecting foamability and stability **34**, 70–71
–, stability **34**, 62–67
–, –, disjoining pressure **34**, 64–65
–, –, elasticity **34**, 65–66
–, –, equation of state method **34**, 68
–, –, film drainage rate **34**, 63
–, –, foam collapse rate **34**, 68
–, –, liquid drainage method **34**, 67–68
–, –, measurement methods **34**, 67–70
–, –, polyhedron-shaped cell **34**, 62–63
–, –, rheological properties **34**, 66–67
–, volume increase rate **34**, 61
Protein–starch interaction **16**, 384
Protein–sulfhydryl groups **16**, 363
Protein turnover, endogenous proteolytic enzymes and **31**, 345, 411, 413
–, for myopathy diagnosis **37**, 350
–, in atrophic muscle **37**, 364
–, muscle physiology **31**, 369, 373–377, 379–381
–, proteinase activity **31**, 386–388, 390, 392
–, research needs **37**, 406–407
Protein vacuoles, chocolate and **31**, 220, 221
Proteoglycans, dietary fiber and **31**, 121, 124, 128, 129, 132
–, endogenous proteolytic enzymes and **31**, 403, 406
Proteolysis **10**, 31
–, as structural probe **35**, 186–188
–, cheese **39**, 176–177, 209–234, 236, 255
–, chocolate and **31**, 222, 223
–, fish **39**, 337
–, –, effect of storage temperature **2**, 361, 371
–, –, spoilage **7**, 49
–, IM meat **39**, 131
–, tyrosine color test for **2**, 371, 382
Proteolytic activity, in soy sauce production **10**, 108–111
Proteolytic enzymes **17**, 22, 184
–, rote in meat tenderness **20**, 273–274
Proteose–peptones, bovine milk, structure **33**, 358
Proteus, in bacon **3**, 308, 309
–, in pork **3**, 293
Proteus in Canadian haddock **2**, 350
Proteus vulgaris, germicidal action of CPCl on **2**, 152
–, salicylic acid effect on oxidation of gluconate by **11**, 339–341

–, uptake of benzoic acid as function of pH **11**, 335
Protocatechuic acids, in respiration experiments with potatoes **3**, 14
–, olive oil and **31**, 467
Protohematin IX, molecular properties of **17**, 8
Protomyosin **9**, 6
Proton-induced X-ray emission method of selenium detection **32**, 88
Protopectin, chemistry of **11**, 1–107
–, early evidence for **11**, 21–23
–, effects of steaming on **2**, 311
–, hydrolysis products of **11**, 4
–, in growing tissue **1**, 401
–, insolubility of **11**, 61–93
–, model of **11**, 5
–, penetrating tissue to reach it **11**, 62
–, possible linkages in **11**, 3
–, reviews on **11**, 3
–, structure **11**, 4
–, theories on its nature **11**, 2
Protoplasm in parenchyma vegetable cells **2**, 306
– in –, during osmosis **2**, 307
– in –, effect of quantity on water retention **2**, 308
– in –, effect on product of permeability change of **2**, 308
Protoplast transformation **41**, 127–128
Protozoa, hunger in **1**, 133
Protriptyline **44**, 3 12
Provitamin A **15**, 209
–, value in foods **15**, 216
Provitamins D, ultraviolet activation of **3**, 153
Prunes **15**, 225
–, air spaces in **2**, 333
–, corrosion characteristics of **3**, 336–339
–, dried, enzymic changes in **11**, 290
–, effect of sugar solutions on phenolase activity in **3**, 34–35
–, Italian, canned, nutrients in **1**, 43, 46–49
–, juice, canned, ascorbic acid content **4**, 375, 377
–, –, fresh, use of ascorbic acid in **4**, 377
–, –, irradiation of by cathode rays **3**, 181
–, –, spectra of **3**, 178
–, oxidase activity in **3**, 10
–, polyphenolase and peroxidase activity in **3**, 29
Prymnesin, as marine toxin **18**, 157
PSE pork, *see* Pork
Pseudoephedrine **44**, 289
Pseudomonas **32**, 19
–, as sources of protein **18**, 91
–, attachment, confocal scanning laser microscopy **43**, 355
–, –, detachment **43**, 349, 350
–, –, excreted substances **43**, 323, 327, 329
–, –, glass surfaces in milk **43**, 332
–, –, growth condition influences **43**, 324
–, –, inhibition methods **43**, 353
–, –, S layers **43**, 323
–, –, meat tissue **43**, 334, 335, 336
–, –, plant surfaces **43**, 345, 346
–, –, stainless steel surfaces **43**, 330, 331, 333
–, –, –, transfer from meat **43**, 339
–, effect of nitrites on **3**, 295
–, green discoloration of **7**, 56
–, growth rate of **7**, 101–103
–, in fresh fish **2**, 350, 353
–, –, enzyme action in **2**, 369
–, propagation of **18**, 94
Pseudomonas aeruginosa **45**, 180
–, germicidal action of CPCl on **2**, 152
Pseudomonas fluorescens **45**, 180, 188, 199
–, effect of benzoic acid **11**, 346–347
–, – of – on oxidation of acetate **11**, 344
–, in eggs **1**, 186
–, influence of temperature on growth **2**, 360
–, in pork **3**, 293
–, survival of at low temperatures **3**, 446
–, ultraviolet detection of in eggs **3**, 154
Pseudomonas putida **45**, 180
Pseudoplastic behavior **39**, 5, 6
Pseudoplastic fluids **39**, 56
–, calculating mixing-power requirements **11**, 428
–, estimating turbulence onset in **11**, 413–416
–, heat-transfer coefficients in tubes **11**, 417–420
Pseudo-(*B*)-selinene in celery seed oil **2**, 272
Psilocybin **44**, 312
Psoriasis, EPA effects **35**, 143
Psychopharmacologic agents, smell sensation effects **44**, 323
–, taste sensation effects **44**, 310–313
Psychrometry, use in spray-drying **2**, 497
Psychrophiles **13**, 349–350, 360–370, 382
–, lowest growth temperatures **13**, 362–370
–, –, at ⩽–10°C **13**, 365–368
–, –, in storage **13**, 365–368
–, –, on foods **13**, 363–364
–, –, on microbiological media **13**, 366–367
Psychrotroph **13**, 361–362
Pt, *see* Phloretin
PTEN **45**, 29

Pterin **40**, 86, 91
Pteroic acid, for polyglutamyl folate synthesis **33**, 7–8
Pteroylglutamate (*see also* Folate metabolism) **40**, 81–82, 97, 99, 103
Pteroylglutamic acid (*see also* Folic acid) **40**, 82
Pteroylpolyglutamate hydrolases, identification and properties **33**, 55–56
–, in folate deconjugation **33**, 17
Pteroyltriglutamate, determination in conjugase assay by reversed-phase HPLC **33**, 31
Puddings, bag-in-box aseptic **32**, 20–23
–, carrageenan in **11**, 128–129
–, milk alginates in **11**, 144–145
Puerarin **44**, 205
Puff drying **10**, 16, 17
–, advantages of **7**, 174
Puffer fish, intoxication from **18**, 147–151
Puffer poisoning **10**, 157–138
Pulp, passion fruit **12**, 234–258
Pulsed electric field (PEF) processing **44**, 1–28
–, current flow **44**, 10
–, electric field strength **44**, 10, 11
–, engineering aspects **44**, 2–10
–, fluid handling system **44**, 6, 8–10
–, high-acid liquid foods, *see* Fruit juices
–, microbial inactivation **44**, 10–15
–, –, determinant factors **44**, 11–12
–, ozone-combined sanitization procedures **45**, 188, 203–204
–, PEF Consortium for Technology Commercialization **44**, 25, 26
–, physical properties of processed products **44**, 21–25
–, – of –, density **44**, 24
–, – of –, electrical conductivity **44**, 22–23
–, – of –, specific heat **44**, 24
–, – of –, viscosity **44**, 23
–, pulse generator **44**, 2–3
–, –, system diagrams **44**, 3, 4, 5
–, system components **44**, 2, 3
–, temperature control **44**, 11, 12, 22, 23, 24, 25
–, total treatment time **44**, 10, 11
–, treatment chambers **44**, 4–6
–, –, co-axial **44**, 5
–, –, co-field **44**, 5, 7
–, treatment parameters **44**, 10
Pulsed mode ultrasonic measurements **45**, 123–124
Pulse generator **44**, 2–3
–, bench-top scale **44**, 4, 5
–, plant scale system diagram **44**, 3, 4
Pulses **16**, 9ff, 67
Pumping requirements, contraction and expansion losses **11**, 409–412
–, friction factor **11**, 409
–, generalized Reynolds number **11**, 409
–, kinetic, potential, and flow energy losses **11**, 409–412
–, mechanical energy balance **11**, 408
–, rheology **11**, 406–413
Pumping systems, for applesauce **11**, 407
Pumpkin, canned, corrosiveness of **3**, 340
–, –, in enameled cans **3**, 374
–, loss of thiamine on processing **6**, 290
–, protection of ascorbic acid in **5**, 87
–, F value for industrial processing of **2**, 102
Pumps, freeze-drying and **7**, 176–177, 209
–, in aseptic processing **32**, 16
–, water removal and **7**, 177–178
Punctanecine **45**, 77
Puncture, in flexible-package leak studies **23**, 414
Pungency, development of, in onion and garlic **22**, 73–133
–, enzyme role **22**, 116–118
Purées, frozen fruit **5**, 87
Purines **17**, 234
–, in tea **11**, 217–218
Purothionin, characterization of **20**, 154–156
Purpurogallin, formation of **3**, 22–23
–, structure of **19**, 103
Putrefaction, black spot **12**, 395
–, detection **12**, 395–396
–, –, discoloration **12**, 395
–, –, keeping quality **12**, 392
–, –, prevention **12**, 410–414
–, –, relation to processing temperature **12**, 392
–, –, signs of **12**, 393
–, –, types of **12**, 394–395
–, fish sausage and ham bacteria **12**, 396
Putrefactive anaerobe No. 3679, destruction rate curve for **3**, 434
Putrescine, cheese **39**, 234
–, fish **39**, 337–339, 341–346, 349–351, 353–356, 358
–, fish spoilage and **7**, 46, 47
–, in putrid abalone **23**, 166
–, *N*-nitroso compounds and **31**, 76, 77
Pyrazines, chocolate and **31**, 235, 236, 251, 297
–, derivatives **32**, 126–127, 135
–, formation in sugar–amine model system **30**, 108

–, – in –, sugar role **30**, 108
–, in coffee **2**, 281
–, in potato products **25**, 105–108
–, meat flavor and **18**, 60
–, *N*-nitroso compounds and **31**, 56
–, shoyu flavor and **30**, 281–282
–, –, pasteurization and **30**, 282
Pyridine, derivatives **32**, 135
–, in coffee gases **2**, 279
–, in cyclic type of quaternary ammonium **2**, 125, 128
–, in food and meat flavor **18**, 60
–, solubility of DDT in **2**, 203
–, use in separation of basic amino acids from cation exchanger **2**, 34
Pyridinols **32**, 138–140
Pyridoxal phosphate (*see also* Vitamin B6 metabolism) **40**, 121–122, 123, 135; **41**, 53–55
–, as phosphorylase cofactor **40**, 136–140, 142–145
–, reactions catalyzed by **22**, 98–99
Pyridoxamine metabolism (*see also* Vitamin B6 metabolism) **40**, 121–122, 123
Pyridoxic acid **40**, 112, 116, 117, 120–125, 127
Pyridoxine, adsorption by anion exchanger **2**, 38
–, content of canned foods **1**, 42, 45, 47
–, effect of cathode rays on **3**, 168
–, in wheat germ **23**, 209
–, metabolism (*see also* Vitamin B6 metabolism) **40**, 121–122, 123
Pyridoxine deficiency **1**, 117–118
Pyrimethamine **44**, 292
Pyrocatechol in coffee **2**, 281
Pyrodinium phoneus **10**, 140, 174
Pyrogallol, inhibition of lipoxygenase **33**, 307
Pyrolysate mutagens **32**, 157–161
Pyrolysis, in wood during curing smoke generation **29**, 93–98
–, of cellulose, phenol formation **29**, 123
–, of lignin, phenol formation **29**, 121–123
–, products, genotoxicity, *in vivo* **34**, 399
–, –, IQ-like compound formation role **34**, 434–435
γ-Pyrones, shoyu flavor and **30**, 272
Pyrophosphatase **41**, 130
–, thermal stability **35**, 255–256
Pyrophosphates, effect on appetite **1**, 133
Pyrrole compounds, in food flavor **18**, 61
Pyrrole pigments, meat mutagen modulation **34**, 431–432
Pyrroles **32**, 138–140
–, effect on oil stability of coffee bean **2**, 278
–, in coffee **2**, 279
Pyrrolidine, in carrot leaf **2**, 271
–, *N*-nitroso compounds and **31**, 61, 76, 77
Pyrrolizidine alkaloids **45**, 61–93
–, carcinogenic potential **45**, 62, 66, 78, 81
–, chemical structure **45**, 65–66, 67, 71
–, consumer protection measures **45**, 69, 73–74, 91–93
–, food contamination **45**, 66, 68–73
–, –, cereal grains contaminated with weeds **45**, 68, 69–70, 91
–, –, eggs **45**, 73, 91
–, –, honey **45**, 72, 91
–, –, meat **45**, 73
–, –, milk **45**, 70, 72, 91
–, –, preventive measures **45**, 91
–, herbal medicine sources **45**, 66, 68, 73–78
–, –, adverse health effects awareness **45**, 91, 93
–, metabolism **45**, 81–83, 84–85, 86–87
–, –, dehydrogenation **45**, 82
–, –, detoxification **45**, 83
–, –, *N*-oxidation **45**, 82–83
–, plant sources **45**, 62–65
–, toxicity **45**, 62, 78–81
–, –, acute **45**, 78
–, –, cardiopulmonary **45**, 80–81
–, –, diagnostic problems **45**, 81
–, –, DNA cross-links formation **45**, 83, 88–90
–, –, DNA–protein cross-links **45**, 90, 92
–, –, hepatic veno-occlusive disease **45**, 69–70, 72, 75–76, 77, 79–80, 91
–, –, hepatotoxic synergism with copper **45**, 79
–, –, human poisoning incidents **45**, 62, 68, 73, 75–77
–, –, mechanism **45**, 83, 88–91
–, –, megalocytosis **45**, 88, 89
–, –, progressive nature **45**, 79–80
–, –, species differences in susceptibility **45**, 78–79
–, –, structural determinants **45**, 65
–, transplacental transmission **45**, 76
Pyruvate decarboxylase **17**, 20–21
Pyruvate dehydrogenase deficiency, in muscle **37**, 380
Pyruvate kinase as endpoint cooking temperature indicator **44**, 171
Pyruvic acid **16**, 216
–, abnormal metabolization of **1**, 113, 131
Pythium debaryanum **15**, 180
PZ, *see* Phlorizin

Quadriceps muscle, testing **37**, 347
Quadruple-effect evaporation, cost of **20**, 90
Quality, assurance of, in flexibly packaged foods **23**, 404–417
–, cheese **39**, 184–193, 246–254
–, fish **39**, 350–352
–, food, appearance **9**, 157–197
–, –, control methods **9**, 156
–, –, flavor **9**, 209–212
–, –, –, correlated measurements **9**, 212
–, –, –, odor **9**, 211–212
–, –, –, taste **9**, 210–211
–, –, human evaluation **9**, 154–155
–, –, instrumentation **9**, 155–157
–, –, –, sampling **9**, 156
–, –, kinesthetics **9**, 197–209
–, –, –, classification **9**, 198–199
–, –, –, instrumental measurement **9**, 201–209
–, –, –, principles of measurement **9**, 199–201
–, –, methodology **9**, 213–214
–, –, principles of measurement and control **9**, 154–457
–, –, – of –, significant correlations **9**, 155
–, –, terminology **9**, 213
–, IM meat **39**, 114–138
Quantal response (endpoint procedure) **44**, 179
Quarg cheese **39**, 178
–, citrate **39**, 201
–, syneresis **39**, 190
–, ultrafiltration **39**, 193
Quasi-identifiability **40**, 314
Quaternary ammonium compounds, bacterial action **2**, 137
–, basic principles of application **2**, 170–171
–, commercially available compounds **2**, 146–157
–, commercial preparations **2**, 145
–, commercial products **2**, 120–122
–, compatabilities of **2**, 133
–, factors affecting germicidal activity **2**, 133–137
–, –, concentration **2**, 136
–, –, organic matter **2**, 136
–, –, pH **2**, 133–134
–, –, potentiation **2**, 136
–, –, temperature **2**, 135–136
–, film formation of **2**, 144
–, fungicidal action **2**, 138
–, general chemical structure of **2**, 119–125
–, general properties of **2**, 129–130
–, incompatability of **2**, 131–133
–, industrial application of **2**, 171–184
–, mechanism of action **2**, 144
–, methods of estimating concentration of **2**, 167–170
–, – of evaluating germicidal action and toxicity of **2**, 157–167
–, – of –, inactivators in **2**, 166
–, relationship of chemical structure to germicidal activity **2**, 138–143
–, studies concerning structure **2**, 125–129
–, therapeutic effectiveness **2**, 143
–, toxicity of **2**, 130–131
–, virucidal action **2**, 138
Quazepam **44**, 308
Quenching, by α-tocopherol, oxygen- or carbon-centered fatty acyl radicals or active oxygen **33**, 208–211
–, singlet oxygen **33**, 210, 303
Quercetin, in browning **3**, 12
–, inhibition of soybean lipoxygenase-dependent linoleate peroxidation **33**, 317
–, percentage in green tea **2**, 284
–, structure **19**, 80; **33**, 311
Quinine sulfate, temperature effect on taste intensity tests **2**, 246
Quinoa floor, inositol phosphates degradation during processing **45**, 22
Quinoline, in cyclic type of quaternary ammonium **2**, 125
–, in Formosan black tea **2**, 287
Quinone, formation of **17**, 267–269, 273
–, –, in oxidative deamination **17**, 239
–, –, in tea **17**, 217
–, in respiration experiments with potatoes **3**, 14
o-Quinone, complexing with amino acids and proteins **19**, 98–102
–, coupled oxidation **19**, 97–98
–, polymerization of polyphenols **19**, 102–104
–, secondary reductions of in enzymic food browning **19**, 97–104
p-Quinone, estimation of fish freshness and **7**, 63

r gene **41**, 100–101
Rabbit muscle, rigor in **9**, 19–20, 21
Rabbits, distribution of DDT in **2**, 210
–, effects of DDT on skin of **2**, 207
–, stability of fat **5**, 7
–, toxicity of DDT to **2**, 208
–, use in toxicity tests for quaternary ammonium compounds **2**, 130, 153

Race, and food selection **32**, 258–260
Racemization and cross-linking **35**, 201–211
–, chemistry **35**, 201–204
–, essential amino acids **35**, 208
–, factors affecting extent of **35**, 204–208
–, mechanism **35**, 201–203
–, protein digestibility and biological value effects **35**, 208–211
–, protein stability **35**, 274–276
–, protein structure effect **35**, 205–207
–, rate constants **35**, 202–203
Racks, for retorting **23**, 388–390
Radiation (*see also* Irradiation) **15**, 71, 241
–, application rates **15**, 156
–, carcinogen risk assessment and **31**, 41
–, dose rates **15**, 67
–, in meat curing as alternative to nitrite **29**, 52–55
–, ionizing (*see also* Proteins in foods), on peroxidase activity **17**, 40
–, laboratory data **31**, 33
–, mechanisms **15**, 63
–, sources **15**, 87
–, statistics **31**, 13, 16, 24
–, units **15**, 58
γ-Radiation, mango fruit storage and preservation **21**, 280–281
–, potato storage **21**, 340–342
Radiation-convection **13**, 253–257
–, accretive **13**, 254, 256
–, irruptive **13**, 254–255
–, migratory **13**, 254–256
Radiation disease, prophylaxis of **17**, 218
Radiation preservation, of fishery products **22**, 166–167
Radical exchange, computation **40**, 248
Radicals **15**, 65
–, free **17**, 17, 28–29
–, in peroxidase oxidation **17**, 16
–, peroxy **17**, 31
Radioactive isotopes, application in agriculture **3**, 156
–, germicidal action of **3**, 155, 156
–, use in foods **3**, 155, 156
Radioactive probes, cardiolipin-derived **37**, 316–317
Radioactive tracer (*see also* Stable isotope tracer) **40**, 64
–, by vitamin B6 **40**, 137–138
–, for vitamin B6 **40**, 114–116
–, glycogen phosphorylase **40**, 137–138
–, membrane vesicles **40**, 200, 203
–, transthyretin **40**, 150–152
Radioactivity, carcinogen risk assessment and **31**, 15, 47
Radiochemical yields **15**, 68
Radio-frequency waves, economics of using **3**, 144–146
–, heating **3**, 132–145
–, illustration of **3**, 124
–, in dielectric and induction heating **3**, 123–125
–, miscellaneous uses for **3**, 143–144
–, sterilization by **3**, 132–133
–, –, thermal requirements of **3**, 144
Radioimmunoassays, for folate determination **33**, 26
–, phytoestrogens **44**, 202–203
Radioisotope techniques **17**, 225
Radiolabeling, calcium bioavailability **33**, 123–124
–, folate bioavailability **33**, 61–64
–, folates **33**, 11–12
Radiometric testing **32**, 15
Radiotherapy, smell/taste perception changes **44**, 275, 276, 277, 278, 279, 323
Radish, composition and distillation of **2**, 274
–, loss of thiamine in **6**, 296
–, oil extraction by ether **2**, 274
Radish juice, loss of thiamine **6**, 295
Radium, in Russian wines **8**, 195
Radurization, of food **24**, 188–197
Raffinose, in cocoa beans **8**, 262
Rainbow trout (*Oncorhynchus mykiss*) **39**, 349
–, culture, ozone water treatment **45**, 181, 190
Raisins, chlorophyll in **5**, 104
–, use of SO_2 in golden bleach **5**, 141
–, – of – in sulfur bleach **5**, 141
Raleigh waves **45**, 104–105
Raloxifene **44**, 223
Ramifying aggregates, three types illustrated **11**, 6
Ramipril **44**, 307
Rancidity, effect of light **5**, 36
–, – of meat constituents **5**, 30
–, effect on metals **5**, 33
–, – on oxygen **5**, 36
–, – on pH **5**, 30
–, – on physical factors **5**, 36
–, – on salts **5**, 31
–, – on smoke **5**, 34
–, – on spices **5**, 35
–, – on temperature **5**, 37
–, in dehydrated mashed potatoes **25**, 112–122

Rancidity (*cont'd*)
–, in fats **5**, 1, 4
–, –, as stress factor **4**, 116
–, in meats **5**, 3
–, in olive oil **31**, 471–473
–, of candies **6**, 12
–, oxidative **5**, 4; **6**, 13
Ranking tests, applications of **7**, 8–9
–, use in sensory difference tests **2**, 227
Raoult's law **39**, 99
Rapeseed meal **17**, 107
Rapeseed oil, incorporation into cardiolipin **37**, 295–297
–, reversion problems in **4**, 192
Raphanol in radish **2**, 274
Raspberries, ascorbic acid content of, effect of sunlight on **1**, 301
–, composition and distillation of **2**, 269
–, influence of oxygen on deterioration of **1**, 341
Raspberry juice, ascorbic acid loss in bottling **1**, 63
–, canned, use of ascorbic acid in **4**, 373
–, deterioration of **1**, 328, 333, 341
–, effect of temperature on changes in **1**, 333
Rat, acute toxicity of DDT on **2**, 208
–, chronic toxicity of DDT on **2**, 209
–, – of –, effect on reproduction **2**, 210
–, distribution of DDT in **2**, 210, 211
–, effects of DDT on kidney and liver of **2**, 213
–, – of – on skin of **2**, 207
–, secretion of DDT in milk of **2**, 211
–, storage of DDT in **2**, 211
–, use in toxicity tests for quaternary ammonium compounds **2**, 130, 153
Rate bioassays, compared with IDEA digestibility **35**, 223–224
Rate of shear, in fluid consistency **11**, 368–371
Rat granuloma pouch assay, 2-amino-3-methylimidazo[4,5-*f*]quinoline **34**, 407
Rat liver, salicylic acid effect on incorporation of C^{14} by **11**, 345
Rausing, Ruben **32**, 17
Ravo-Rapid spray dryer, operation of **2**, 429–430
Rayleigh number **32**, 80
*rbc*S gene **41**, 13232
RBE (Relative biological efficiency) **15**, 60, 70
RBP, *see* Retinol-binding protein
RDAs, iodine **36**, 234
–, iron **36**, 221
Reactions, classes **14**, 293–301
–, mechanisms **14**, 287–301
–, order of **14**, 292–293
–, thermal unimolecular **14**, 301–315
–, –, catalysis **14**, 318
–, –, diagnostic tests **14**, 316–318
–, –, heterogeneous **14**, 318
–, –, homogeneous **14**, 318
–, –, theory **14**, 315–318
–, thermo-reorganization **14**, 300–301
Reactive epitope, cardiolipin **37**, 312–314
Rec assay system **32**, 156
Receptors, olfactory **14**, 2–3
Recombinant protein **40**, 8
Recommended daily allowance, folate **40**, 83
Recommended Dietary Allowance, calcium **33**, 105, 108–112
–, folate **33**, 52
–, tocopherols **33**, 167
Recommended Dietary Intake, folates **33**, 52
–, tocopherols **33**, 166
Recovery, analyte **40**, 187–190
Recovery response, creep test **39**, 20
Recrystallization **38**, 211–212
Rectilinear approach (*see also* Linear system) **40**, 157–158
–, REDUCE software **40**, 330
Red blood cells, anti-cardiolipin antibody binding **37**, 308
Red char, aerobic bacteria in **2**, 350
Redisposition, anti- **14**, 358–359
Red meat, mechanical deboning of (*see also* Mechanically deboned red meat) **27**, 23–95
Red muscle, *see* Muscle
Redoxases **16**, 309
Redox potential, effects on whey protein foams **33**, 401
Red tide **10**, 139, 141
–, ciguatera and **18**, 147
–, saxitoxin and **18**, 155
Reduced nicotinamide dinucleotide (NADH) **17**, 18–20
–, ubiquinone oxidoreductase, cardiolipin association **37**, 286
Reducing agents, inhibition of enzyme activity by **1**, 382–383
Reducing sugars, boiled with aqueous ammonia, mutagenicity **30**, 122
–, browning reactions with, HVP, artificial meat flavor **30**, 106–109
–, browning reactions with alkylamines **30**, 81
–, – with amino acids **30**, 89
–, – with *N*-glycoside formation **30**, 81

–, – with nitrogen compounds, chemical sequences **30**, 82–84
–, reactions with sulfites **30**, 23
Reduction methods, chemical, for (6-ambo)-5,6,7,8-tetrahydrofolate **33**, 8
–, electrochemical, for (6-ambo)-5,6,7,8-tetrahydrofolate **33**, 9
–, enzymatic, for (6S)-5,6,7,8-tetrahydrofolate **33**, 9
Reductive alkylation, whey proteins **33**, 421
Reductive pentose phosphate pathway **41**, 140–141, 143
Reductones **12**, 28–35; **14**, 181–183
–, amino-hexose **12**, 33
–, freeze-dried beef and **7**, 213
–, gelatin and **7**, 271
–, piperidino-hexose, radioactivity **12**, 32–33
–, shoyu oxidative browning during storage and **30**, 252–253
Ree–Eyring equation **39**, 34, 46
Refining, chocolate and **31**, 330
–, –, amorphous sugar production **31**, 295, 296
–, –, conching **31**, 307
–, –, operation **31**, 292–295
–, –, purpose **31**, 291, 292
–, olive oil and **31**, 463
Refractive index, gelatin testing and **7**, 249–250
Refrigerants, secondary **12**, 165–166
Refrigerated foods, processing of **25**, 211–228
Refrigeration, effect on folate in human milk **33**, 51
–, on ships, automatic controls **12**, 192–193
–, –, distribution **12**, 165–166
–, –, research **12**, 193
–, plants, designing of **20**, 128–150
–, –, efficiency factors **20**, 129–130
–, –, evaporators in **20**, 130–138
Regeneration **41**, 128
Regulatory proteins, endogenous proteolytic enzymes and **31**, 395, 398–400
Reindeer meat, life sustained by **1**, 109
Relative humidity (*see also* Water activity) **39**, 98, 108, 109
–, and phospholipid-hydrolytic activity in barley, malt flour **11**, 305
–, equilibrium **39**, 115–116
Relaxation, diffusion-limited, rate defined by WLF equation and Arrhenius equation **38**, 205–206
–, enthalpic **38**, 172–173
α Relaxation **38**, 199
β Relaxation **38**, 199–200
Relaxation test, rheology **39**, 19–20, 58
Relishes, carrageenan in **11**, 135–136
Renal solute load, cow's milk **36**, 213
Rendering practices **43**, 270, 271
–, tallow production **43**, 297
Rennet **16**, 237, 289
–, addition **39**, 188
–, coagulation **39**, 169–178, 249–250, 293
–, inactivation **39**, 197
–, lipases **39**, 202
–, substitutes **39**, 172
Rennin **10**, 48–50
–, induced clotting of casein **34**, 334–337
Repair, membrane proteins by α-tocopherol **33**, 210–211
Replacement therapy, for Duchenne and Becker's muscular dystrophies **37**, 358
Reproduction, effects of DDT on **2**, 210
–, *n*-3 PUFA effects **35**, 128–129
Reptation **39**, 39–40
Reptiles, *Salmonella* in **3**, 228
Repulsion forces **14**, 370–371
–, potential energies in colloidal suspensions **11**, 368
Resazurin, fish freshness and **7**, 63–64
–, reduction test for egg pulp **1**, 186–187
Reserve glucans **41**, 5
Reserve polysaccharides **41**, 4–6
Residence time, β-carotene **40**, 44–46, 61
–, folate **40**, 88–89, 90
–, transthyretin **40**, 152–155
Resinous cation exchangers, chemical constitution **2**, 4–6
–, effect of acidic group on **2**, 5
–, flow rate through **2**, 11
–, physical structure of **2**, 6
–, titration curves for **2**, 5
Resins, chocolate and **31**, 247
–, dietary fiber and **31**, 161
–, endogenous proteolytic enzymes and **31**, 345
–, olive oil and **31**, 463
–, polyox **12**, 290
Resistant starch, dietary fiber and **31**, 148, 150, 155, 170, 186
Resource Conservation and Recovery Act, carcinogen risk assessment and **31**, 6
Respiration **15**, 78, 83; **17**, 19–20
–, carbon dioxide **12**, 116–119
–, climacteric rise **12**, 116–118
–, –, reduced oxygen **12**, 117–118
–, –, temperature **12**, 117
–, fruits **17**, 186–187

Respiration (*cont'd*)
–, fruits and vegetables **12**, 116–119
–, in cheese ripening **16**, 311ff
–, in fruit maturation, carbon dioxide tension **10**, 324–329
–, in kiwifruit during growth and ripening **29**, 288, 290–291
–, in relation to composition **10**, 307–308
–, – to temperature **10**, 316–320
–, molds and fungi, effects on **10**, 332–333
–, oxygen tension **10**, 320–424
–, passion fruit **12**, 223–229
–, patterns of **10**, 296, 297, 298
–, rates of **10**, 298–300, 312–313
–, role of ethylene in **10**, 334–335
–, zymasic in apples **12**, 124
Respiratory chromogenes **17**, 227
Respiratory infections, licorice and **7**, 353
Respiratory quotient **40**, 175
Response curve, *see* Nutrient-response curve
Restriction enzymes, gene cloning and manipulation **36**, 134, 136
Retention, folates, after cooking or thermal processing, table **33**, 48
–, –, ascorbate/ferrous sulfate effects **33**, 49–50
–, –, folic acid in fortified food **33**, 52
Reticulin **9**, 3, 10
–, endogenous proteolytic enzymes and **31**, 371, 372, 374
Reticulocytes, endogenous proteolytic enzymes and **31**, 354, 380
Retina, desaturase activity **35**, 83
–, *n*-3 PUFA **35**, 117–120
Retinal outer rod segments, α-tocopherol concentrations **33**, 212
Retinal pigment epithelium, tocopherols in **33**, 180
Retinoids **40**, 38–39, 44, 47–49
–, carcinogen risk assessment and **31**, 22, 24
Retinol, β-carotene **40**, 30, 31, 33, 66
–, –, empirical data **40**, 50–52
–, –, final model **40**, 43–47
–, –, intermediate models **40**, 39
–, vitamin A **40**, 3, 9, 11, 14, 15–16
–, –, pool size **40**, 21–22
–, –, turnover **40**, 12–13, 14, 19, 21
Retinol-binding protein, β-carotene **40**, 32–33, 38, 46
–, vitamin A **40**, 4, 8, 9, 11, 14, 16–17
–, –, kidneys **40**, 21
Retinyl ester, β-carotene **40**, 32, 59, 66, 69
–, –, intermediate models **40**, 38–40
–, –, turnover **40**, 47
–, vitamin A **40**, 4, 11, 16
Retorting of flexible-packaged foods **23**, 375–399
Retort pouches, materials for **23**, 313, 326
–, production systems for **23**, 335
Retrogradation **41**, 20, 166
Retrograde dialysis **40**, 190
Retronecine **45**, 66, 67
Retrorsine **45**, 78, 79, 80, 88
Reverse micellar solution **34**, 164
Reverse osmosis **15**, 356
–, aroma recovery in **20**, 45–50
–, cost of **20**, 92–93
–, whey protein preparation with **33**, 361
Reverse osmosis–ultrafiltration, whey protein preparation with **33**, 361
Reverse phase HPLC/UV absorbance detection, phytoestrogens **44**, 201, 202
Reversion, in fats, characterization of **4**, 186–187
–, –, flavor characteristics **4**, 187–190
–, in fats and oils, chemical changes associated with **4**, 190–201
–, –, control of by processing **4**, 201
Rework, processed cheese **39**, 273
Reynold's equation, film drainage rate **34**, 63
Reynolds metals' system, for flexible packaging **23**, 337–338
Reynolds number **32**, 49, 57, 58, 64, 67–68, 69, 70, 72, 73, 75, 79, 80
–, as a function of porosity and sphericity **11**, 430
–, vs. friction factor **11**, 410, 414
Rhabdomyoma **37**, 342–343
Rhamnogalacturonans, dietary fiber and **31**, 130, 135, 146, 164
–, endopolygalacturonase and **30**, 176–177, 179
–, pectic, degradation during fruit ripening **30**, 176–177, 179
Rhamnose, chocolate and **31**, 272
–, dietary fiber and **31**, 131, 188
Rheem Manufacturing Company **32**, 10
Rheological properties, protein-stabilized foams **34**, 66–67
Rheology, application to chocolate coating **11**, 394–399
–, – to determining pumping requirements **11**, 406–413
–, background information **39**, 2–3
–, basic concepts **39**, 3–12
–, –, ideal elastic behavior **39**, 7–8
–, –, shear rate **39**, 4–6
–, –, shear stress **39**, 4–6

–, –, time effects **39**, 8–9
–, –, viscoelasticity **39**, 9–12
–, –, viscous flow **39**, 4–6
–, constitutive models **39**, 33–44
–, –, Bird–Carreau **39**, 37–39, 49–52, 54
–, –, Casson **39**, 34, 46
–, –, concentrated solution/melt theories **39**, 37–41
–, –, Cross equation **39**, 34, 46
–, –, dilute solution molecular theories **39**, 35–37
–, –, Doi–Edwards **39**, 39–41, 52–53
–, –, Herschel–Bulkley **39**, 6, 34, 46
–, –, Leonov **39**, 59
–, –, Maxwell **39**, 9–10, 43, 58
–, –, power law **39**, 5–6, 34, 46, 56
–, –, Ree–Eyring equation **39**, 34, 46
–, –, rigid rod **39**, 36–37
–, –, solid foods **39**, 41–44
–, –, steady shear flow **39**, 33–35
–, –, usefulness **39**, 62
–, definition **39**, 2, 3
–, engineering properties **39**, 44–61
–, –, dough **39**, 53–55, 58–59
–, –, emulsions **39**, 55–58
–, –, entanglement **39**, 48–53
–, –, extensional flow **39**, 58–59
–, –, formulations development **39**, 59–61
–, –, polymers **39**, 48–53
–, –, steady shear viscosity **39**, 44–46
–, –, yield stress **39**, 6, 46, 48
–, experimental methods **39**, 12–23
–, –, biaxial extension **39**, 16–17, 58, 59
–, –, creep test **39**, 20, 43, 56–57
–, –, extensional flow **39**, 14–17
–, –, linear viscoelasticity **39**, 10, 18–23
–, –, sinusoidal oscillatory shearing **39**, 20–23
–, –, steady shear measurement **39**, 12–14
–, –, stress relaxation test **39**, 19–20, 58
–, –, transient flow **39**, 17
–, –, uniaxial extension **39**, 14–16
–, gelation **39**, 41–43, 60–61
–, instrumentation **39**, 23–33
–, –, capillary tube geometry **39**, 24–26
–, –, concentric cylinder geometry **39**, 31–33
–, –, cone–plate geometry **39**, 27–28
–, –, error sources **39**, 26, 28, 33
–, –, plate–plate geometry **39**, 29–31
–, of bread dough **11**, 401–406
–, of cheese (*see also* Cheese, texture) **39**, 186, 254–255, 273
–, of semiliquid foods **39**, 1–69
–, research needs **39**, 62
Rheometer **39**, 23–24, 48
–, capillary **39**, 26, 59
–, cylinder **39**, 33
Rheopectic fluids **11**, 394; **32**, 46
Rheumatoid arthritis **37**, 398–399
–, EPA effects **35**, 141–142
Rhizobium trifolii CPS, molecular shapes and interactions **42**, 194–197
Rhizopus **44**, 213
–, effect of carbon dioxide **12**, 109
–, food fermentation **30**, 221
–, growth rate of **7**, 98
–, in bacon **3**, 298
–, innoculated fruit **12**, 106
–, water requirement of **7**, 110
Rhizopus stolonifer **15**, 167, 173
Rhodamine 3GO, glycyrrhizin assay and **7**, 369
Rhodobacter spheroides **41**, 44
Rhodospirillum rubrum **41**, 43
Rhubarb, as a browning preventive **3**, 33
–, corrosiveness of **3**, 341, 346
–, nutritional stress factor in **4**, 111–113
Rhubarb juice, canned, use of ascorbic acid in **4**, 377
Rhythm, biological, *see* Bioperiodicity
Riboflavin **6**, 261, 302; **15**, 128
–, content of apples and pears **8**, 368
–, effect of cathode rays on **3**, 168, 170, 171
–, – of spray-drying on **2**, 401
–, – of X-rays on **3**, 158
–, loss during blanching of vegetables **8**, 75
–, retention of, in electronic cooking **3**, 139, 140, 142
–, –, in infrared-treated wheat germ **3**, 146
–, ultraviolet examination for **3**, 153
Riboflavin content, deficiency **1**, 117–118
–, efficiency of food utilization increased by **1**, 117
–, of canned foods **1**, 41–47
–, –, effect of heat sterilization on **1**, 87–89
–, –, – of storage on **1**, 93–95, 97–98
–, of eggs **1**, 153
–, of plants, effect of climate on **1**, 307
–, of vegetables, effect of blanching on **1**, 80–81
–, –, – of storage on **1**, 64–65
–, retention in canned tomato products **1**, 93–95
Ribonuclease, in tea **24**, 236
–, in wheat germ **23**, 241
–, succinylation **35**, 272
–, thermal inactivation, irreversible **35**, 248–249

Ribonuclease (*cont'd*)
–, thermal unfolding **35**, 188
Ribonucleic acid (RNA) (*see also* Messenger RNA) **17**, 52
–, inhibiting dissimilation by penicillin **1**, 376
–, reactions with sulfites **30**, 26
Ribose, in apples and pears **8**, 313
Rice **16**, 6, 27
–, artificial drying of **8**, 121
–, *Aspergillus fumigatus* phytase transgenic expression **45**, 34
–, branching enzymes **41**, 99–100
–, dietary fiber and **31**, 122, 136–138, 140, 169
–, food protein engineering **36**, 187
–, globoid composition **28**, 9
–, home frozen **6**, 207
–, inspection of **8**, 121
–, phosphorus content of, effect of fertilizers on **1**, 313
–, phytate (inositol hexakisphosphate) content **45**, 12, 13, 16
–, phytic acid, effect of cooking on **28**, 48
–, polished, deficiencies caused by **1**, 109
–, polychlorinated biphenyl-contaminated **37**, 43
–, protein bodies **36**, 124
–, reduced phytate gene mutations **45**, 34
–, SSS in **41**, 78
–, thiamine loss in **6**, 274
Rice bran **17**, 107–108
Rice-mill feeds **17**, 114
Rice polish extracts **5**, 103
–, destruction of antineuritic activity by SO_2 **5**, 103
Rice Starch, gelatinization temperature of **2**, 319
Ricotta cheese **39**, 178, 193
Riddelliine **45**, 80, 88
Rifabutin **44**, 292
Rigidity, modulus **39**, 8
Rigidity factor, gelation **34**, 222
Rigid rod model **39**, 36–37
Rigor, effect on meat emulsions **16**, 135
–, – on protein extraction **16**, 123
Rigor mortis **14**, 58–59; **39**, 91–93
–, ammonia liberation in **9**, 18–19
–, ATP decrease in **9**, 14–26
–, changes following **20**, 269–277
–, characteristics of fish in **2**, 347
–, description of **20**, 268–269
–, differences from muscle contraction **9**, 11
–, effects of glucose on **9**, 21
–, – of preslaughter conditions on **9**, 20–21
–, enzyme changes in **20**, 273–277
–, fish preservation and **7**, 71–72
–, glycogen content of muscle **9**, 15–23
–, glycolosis in **9**, 14–22
–, influence of species, temperature, and treatment of fish on **2**, 364–367
–, insulin injections and **9**, 21
–, Marsh–Bendall factor **9**, 18, 28
–, microstructure changes after **20**, 271–272
–, onset of **9**, 14–23
–, pH in **9**, 11
–, pH of fish during **2**, 361
–, relation to hydration in meat **10**, 385–491
–, resolution of **9**, 26–37
–, –, chemical changes in **9**, 26–28
–, –, connective tissues **9**, 30–31
–, –, dissolution of actomyosin **9**, 31–32
–, –, histology of **9**, 29–30
–, temperature in **9**, 11
–, theory of **1**, 8–10
–, work done in **9**, 11
Rigorometer **14**, 103–104
Rimantadine **44**, 300
Rind, chemical aspects **12**, 258–263
–, –, carbohydrates **12**, 258
–, –, composition **12**, 258–259
–, –, nitrogenous substances **12**, 262
–, –, organic acids **12**, 258
–, –, pectic substances **12**, 260–262
–, –, pigments **12**, 259–260
–, –, polyphenols **12**, 259
–, manure **12**, 266
–, passion fruit **12**, 258–266
–, stock feed **12**, 265–266
–, utilization **12**, 264–266
–, –, commercial recovery of pectin **12**, 264
Ripening (*see also* Climacteric), cheese, *see* Cheese, ripening
–, chemical changes in **10**, 300–301, 310–313
–, control of **10**, 315–336
–, IM meat **39**, 108–110, 122, 130–131
–, oxidative phosphorylations in **10**, 340–342
–, role of ethylene in **10**, 329–334, 335
Risk factors, cancer, animal studies **37**, 219–223
–, –, breast cancer **37**, 211–212
–, –, colon cancer **37**, 212–213
–, –, milkfat relationship **37**, 224–225
–, –, research needs **37**, 237
–, coronary heart disease, effects of milk and dairy products **37**, 203–206
–, –, milkfat relationship **37**, 224–225
–, –, research needs **37**, 237

–, osteoporosis **33**, 104
Risperidone **44**, 312
Ritonavir **44**, 286
RK integrator, *see* Runge Kutta integrator
RNA, *see* Messenger RNA *and* Ribonucleic acid
Roasting, chocolate and **31**, 237–241, 329, 330
–, –, cocoa butter **31**, 249, 250
–, –, conching **31**, 298, 307
–, –, liquor preparation **31**, 243–246
Roccal, bacterial reduction in milk by **2**, 136
–, effect on influenza virus **2**, 138
–, use in brewing industry **2**, 175
–, – in dairy industry **2**, 178
Rockfish **39**, 355
–, ozone treatment **45**, 197
Rodents, essentiality of *n*-3 PUFA **35**, 115–116, 152
–, *Salmonella* in **3**, 227
Rod outer segments, DHA and **35**, 117–118
Rogers spray dryer, operation of **2**, 404
Rolling, in tea manufacture **17**, 263–264
Romano cheese **39**, 199, 205
Room calorimetry **40**, 171, 172
Roots **15**, 179; **41**, 3
Rootstock, effects on fruit composition **9**, 292–294
Rosemary, antioxidant activity **42**, 248, 258
–, compounds, isolation and identification **42**, 254–256
–, –, relative antioxidant activity levels **42**, 257
–, extracts, antioxidant activity **42**, 251–254
–, –, heat stability **42**, 262–263
–, health implications **42**, 264–267
–, monterpenes **42**, 250
–, oleoresin **42**, 253–254
–, synergisms and heat stabilities **42**, 258–263
Rosmariquinone **42**, 262
–, chemoprevention **42**, 266
Rotary filler-sealer machine **23**, 341
Rotational diffusion **38**, 196–197
Rotational viscometers, fluid with a yield stress in **11**, 381–384
–, wide-gap **11**, 378–381
Roto-Cut machine **16**, 127
Rotting, fungal, delay by carbon dioxides **12**, 109–111
–, –, *Gloeosporium album* **12**, 111
–, –, *Gloeosporium perennans* **12**, 111
Rouse-segmented chain model **39**, 40
RP-HPLC, *see* Chromatography
RPPP, *see* Reductive pentose phosphate pathway
rr gene **41**, 13434
Rubber products, *N*-nitroso compounds and **31**, 93, 94, 97
Rubidium, in French white wine **8**, 195
Rubus fruticosus (blackberry) **44**, 207, 211
Rumen, phospholipids in **23**, 36
Ruminants, fatty acids in fats of **23**, 25, 28
Runge Kutta integrator **40**, 290, 291, 297, 299–303
Russian buckwheat products **44**, 414–415
Russian comfrey (*Symphytum uplandicum*) **45**, 74–75
Rutabagas, *see* Swedes
Rutin **44**, 408
Rye **16**, 7
–, effect on chicks **1**, 124
–, phytase **45**, 9, 21
–, phytate (inositol hexakisphosphate) **45**, 9
–, –, degradation during processing **45**, 21
–, prolamins **36**, 95
Ryegrass, fatty acids in, comparison with depot fats of grazing animals **23**, 28, 38
Rye plants, carotene content of, effect of fertilizers on **1**, 309
Rye starch, gelatinization temperature of **2**, 319
–, swelling of **2**, 319–320

S/M, *see* Salt-in-moisture
S layers **43**, 323
SAAM software **40**, 6, 9, 31, 61, 126–127, 274
–, linear integrator **40**, 290, 296, 303
–, modeling construct **40**, 282
p-Saccharic acid, glycyrrhizin and **7**, 359
Saccharides, chocolate and **31**, 266, 267
Saccharin (*o*-sulfobenzimide), carcinogen risk assessment and **31**, 23, 26, 27
–, chocolate and **31**, 269
–, preference for in relation to blood glucose **1**, 138
–, sweetener-induced taste, phosphoinositide transduction pathway **42**, 224–227
–, sweet taste of **2**, 261
Saccharomyces, as sources of protein **18**, 90–116
–, effect of pH on thermal death point of **3**, 438
–, heat destruction of **3**, 435
–, lethal effect of acetic acid on **3**, 458
–, lethal temperature of **3**, 437

Saccharomyces (*cont'd*)
–, pH in frozen cells of **3**, 449
Saccharomyces cerevisiae, benzoic and salicylic acids effects on **11**, 334–336
–, expression in french bean phaseolin **36**, 161–162
–, α-gliadin **36**, 162
–, γ-gliadin **36**, 162–163
–, growth in molasses **17**, 124
–, maize zein **36**, 163
–, pea legumin **36**, 160–161
–, pea vicilin **36**, 161
–, pulsed electric field (PEF) inactivation **44**, 13
–, soybean glycinin **36**, 158–160
Saccharomyces cerevisiae phytase **45**, 11
Saccharomyces ellipsoideus, growth inhibition by SO_2 **5**, 125
–, production of 2,3-butylene glycol in wine **5**, 379
–, – of citric acid **5**, 399
Saccharomyces rouxii, K and Na of cells **12**, 65–66
–, cellular potassium loss **12**, 67
–, culture temperature **12**, 73–74
–, growth **12**, 70
–, in mash, salt-tolerant **30**, 230, 232
–, permeability of cell membranes **12**, 67
–, – of –, in ripening soy mashes **12**, 57
–, – of –, salt tolerance **12**, 71–73
–, – of –, sugar tolerance **12**, 72–73
–, – of –, viability **12**, 66
–, strong fermentation **30**, 270
Safety (*see also* Contamination *and* Food poisoning) **39**, 283–292
–, lactic acid bacteria consumption **37**, 114–115
Safflower meal, composition **17**, 112–113
–, for human consumption **17**, 113
Safflower oil, brain phosphoglyceride effects **35**, 77
–, DHA levels in brain phosphoglycerides **35**, 124–126
Saffron **43**, 196, 211
–, adverse reactions **43**, 211–212
Safranin-O, collagen degradation and **7**, 257–258
Sage, antioxidant activity **42**, 248, 258
–, antioxidant compounds **42**, 257–258
–, health implications **42**, 264–267
–, monterpenes **42**, 250
Sago starch, gelatinization temperature of **2**, 319
–, swelling of **2**, 320
Sailfish **39**, 352
Salad dressings **39**, 56–58
–, alginates in **11**, 154
–, carrageenan in **11**, 135–136
–, guar gum in **11**, 169
–, gum tragacanth in **11**, 182–184
–, ultrasonic particle sizing **45**, 150
–, use of ascorbic acid in **4**, 389
Salami **39**, 77–78, 85, 118, 122
Salchichon **39**, 83
Salfasalazine, antifolate effects **33**, 71
Salicylase in eggs **1**, 183
Salicylates **44**, 297
Salicylazosulfapyridine, antifolate effects **33**, 70–71
Salicylic acid, effect on metabolism of micro-organisms **11**, 331–353
–, – on oxidation of glucose by *Proteus vulgaris* **11**, 339–341
–, – on oxidative phosphorylation in isolated mitochondria **11**, 347
–, – on processes of intact cells **11**, 339–347
–, – on rat-liver incorporation of C^{14} **11**, 345
–, – on *Saccharomyces cerevisiae* **11**, 334–336
–, effects on micro-organisms, assimilatory processes **11**, 343–347
–, – on –, oxidation of TCA-cycle intermediates **11**, 342–343
–, – on –, – of the acetyl group **11**, 341–342
–, in Formosan black tea oil **2**, 287
–, inhibition of cell-free enzymes **11**, 348
–, in seisin-oolong tea oil **2**, 287
–, metabolic pathways in micro-organisms **11**, 338
–, microbial inhibition by **1**, 387–388, 390
–, research needs on metabolic inhibition in micro-organisms **11**, 349–351
Saliva, human, meat mutagen modulation **34**, 432
Salivary α-amylase **41**, 158
Salivation, physiology, food texture effect **29**, 173–175
Salmon **39**, 355
–, bacterial count of stored **2**, 357
–, comparison of aerobic bacterial flora in fresh and spoiling **2**, 353
–, fat spoilage in **2**, 373
–, ingestion, urinary mutagenicity and **34**, 412–413
–, ozone treatment **45**, 192
–, Pacific, anaerobic bacteria in **2**, 351
–, –, bacterial attack on stored **2**, 356

–, predominate acid formation in decomposing 2, 371
–, tests for quality of **2**, 380
–, B vitamins in **1**, 42, 44, 45
Salmonella **13**, 353, 357–358, 381–382; **45**, 169, 183, 193, 194
–, attachment, confocal scanning laser microscopy **43**, 355
–, –, inhibition methods **43**, 353
–, –, meat tissue **43**, 336, 337
–, –, plant surfaces **43**, 345
–, –, poultry skin **43**, 341, 342, 343
–, –, properties of attached cells **43**, 347, 348
–, –, stainless steel **43**, 331, 333
–, –, –, transfer from chicken skin **43**, 339
–, –, starvation stress **43**, 325
–, carcinogen risk assessment and **31**, 28
–, definition of **3**, 210–215
–, fever, symptoms of **3**, 215
–, foodborne illness **44**, 153
–, gastroenteritus, symptoms of **3**, 215
–, growth rate of **7**, 104–105
–, in arthropods **3**, 228, 229
–, in dust **3**, 229
–, in eggs **1**, 188; **3**, 224–226
–, infection as a food industry problem **3**, 209–240
–, –, elimination of animal reservoirs of **3**, 230–231
–, –, miscellaneous preventive procedures **3**, 233–234
–, –, prevention and control of **3**, 229–235
–, –, prevention of transmission by humans **3**, 231–232
–, in food storage and refrigeration **3**, 232–233
–, in frozen foods **6**, 201
–, in frozen poultry **6**, 193
–, in household pets **3**, 227
–, in human carriers **3**, 231
–, in meat **3**, 220–222
–, in milk **3**, 227
–, in poultry **3**, 222–223
–, in rodents **3**, 228
–, in vegetables **3**, 219
–, in water **3**, 229
–, isolation and identification technics for **3**, 217–219
–, lethal effect of acetic acid on **3**, 458
–, lowest growth temperature **13**, 355–356
–, modes of infection **3**, 219–229
–, pulsed electric field (PEF) inactivation **44**, 12
–, septicemia, symptoms of **3**, 215
–, serological types of **3**, 212–214
–, survival of during storage **3**, 232
–, thermal inactivation, kinetics **44**, 153–158, 163, 164
–, –, mathematical models **44**, 165
–, –, sample variables **44**, 166
–, –, time–temperature integrator **44**, 177–178
–, –, USA meat processor regulations **44**, 150, 151, 152
–, viable counts of **7**, 106
–, water requirements, nutrition and **7**, 107
–, –, stability of **7**, 110–111
Salmonella aertrycke, effect of pH on thermal death point of **3**, 438
Salmonella choleraesuis, isolation of **3**, 210
Salmonella enterica ser. Enteritidis **45**, 193, 194
Salmonella enteritidis, antigenic formula for **3**, 214
–, effect of ultraviolet radiation on **3**, 151
Salmonella kentucky, isolation of **3**, 214
Salmonella lexington, isolation of **3**, 214
Salmonella miami **3**, 219
Salmonella pullorum, elimination of infection in turkeys **3**, 230
–, isolation technic for **3**, 217
Salmonella sandiego, isolation of **3**, 214
Salmonella typhimurium **45**, 180, 203
–, antigenic formula for **3**, 214
–, elimination of infection in turkeys **3**, 230
–, mutation induced by, boiled sugar–ammonia mixture **30**, 122
–, –, shoyu ingredients **30**, 298–299
Salmonella typhosa, isolation procedure for **3**, 218
Salmonellosis, clinical manifestations of **3**, 215–216
–, incidence of **3**, 216–217
Salsify, pH of **3**, 432
Salt (*see also* Sodium chloride *and* Sodium compounds) **15**, 305, 343
–, bacterial contamination of pork sausage by **6**, 189
–, effect on β-galactosidase stability **38**, 36
–, – on meat tenderness **9**, 32–35
–, emulsifying **39**, 263, 267–272
–, emulsion stability effect **34**, 161–162
–, linkages with protein in pectins **11**, 80–82
–, olive oil and **31**, 460
–, tolerance by wine spoilage bacteria **6**, 91
Salt balance, licorice and **7**, 356–358
Salt bridges, protein stability **35**, 250–252
Saltiness, ionic composition of **2**, 260

Salting, cheese **39**, 166, 177–178
Salt-in-moisture, cheese **39**, 198, 251–253
Salt preservation, botulism and **22**, 165
–, of abalone **23**, 170–171
Salts, and inhibitors, effect on oxidase activity **3**, 30–34
–, as corrosion inhibitors **3**, 343
–, calcium, solubility, table **33**, 145
–, effect on whey protein gel structure **33**, 387–388
–, gelatin and, melting point **7**, 302–303
–, –, rigidity **7**, 296
–, –, swelling **7**, 299
–, in soy sauce **10**, 83–87
–, osmophilic yeasts and **7**, 114–115
–, protein thermal behavior effects **35**, 325–326
Salt-soluble proteins, myofibrillar proteins **34**, 254–255
Salvation Jane (*Echium plantagineum*) **45**, 72
Samples, preparation of **7**, 24
–, presentation of **7**, 23–27
Sampling probe **40**, 183–184, 185–186, 188, 190
Sanitation, scanning electron microscopic studies on **22**, 292
Sanitization methods, ozone applications, *see* Ozone sanitization
–, requirements for food safety **45**, 169–170
Sanitizers **14**, 430–442
–, chemical **14**, 434–442
–, heat **14**, 431–434
Sapodilla, anatomy of **17**, 169
Sapogenin, licorice root and **7**, 342, 360
Saponification, olive oil and **31**, 473
Saponin, licorice root and **7**, 342
Sapotalin, glycyrrhizin and **7**, 360
Saquinavir **44**, 286
Sarcina, growth rate of **7**, 102
Sarcolemma **9**, 3; **14**, 35–41
–, SH groups in **24**, 41–42
Sarcomere **9**, 3–4
Sarcoplasm, endogenous proteolytic enzymes and **31**, 347, 380
Sarcoplasmic matrix, SH groups in **24**, 42–43
Sarcoplasmic proteins **20**, 263
–, endogenous proteolytic enzymes and **31**, 411
–, heat effects on **20**, 294–295
–, meat technology **31**, 395, 406, 410
–, muscle physiology **31**, 370, 373
Sarcoplasmic reticulum **21**, 86–87, 105–106, 169
–, endogenous proteolytic enzymes and **31**, 367, 369, 380
–, lipid and protein contents **35**, 130
–, of muscle **19**, 19–20
–, SH groups in **24**, 41
Sarcosine, *N*-nitroso compounds and **31**, 78
Sardine **39**, 339, 346, 352
"Sashimi", abalone as **23**, 146
SAS software **40**, 50, 160
Saturability, membrane transport **40**, 251, 261
Saturated fatty acids **36**, 263–264
–, effects on serum lipoproteins and apolipoproteins **37**, 159–170
–, incorporation into cardiolipin **37**, 295–297
–, plasma lipid/lipoprotein responses **36**, 266, 268–271
–, –, lauric acid **36**, 268
–, –, medium-chain fatty acids **36**, 270–271
–, –, myristic acid **36**, 269
–, –, palmitic acid **36**, 269
–, –, stearic **36**, 269–270
Saturation, olive oil and **31**, 454, 473, 477
Sauces, carrageenan in **11**, 135–136
–, flexible packaging for **23**, 325
–, guar gum in **11**, 169
–, gums in **11**, 115
–, gum tragacanth in **11**, 182–184
Sauerkraut, ascorbic acid in **10**, 236–239, 263, 275
–, canned, nutrients in **1**, 43, 46–50
–, –, use of ascorbic acid in **4**, 369–370
–, chemical changes in **10**, 246–250
–, chemical constituents of **10**, 269–273
–, color changes in **10**, 238, 252, 254–255, 262–263, 264, 265, 266, 271–273, 278
–, corrosion characteristics of **3**, 336
–, history **10**, 235, 240–241
–, inoculation of **10**, 250–253
–, manufacturing methods **10**, 240–246, 253–259, 273–278
–, nutritional qualities **10**, 235–240
–, quality characteristics **10**, 259–266
–, sulfur compounds in **10**, 266–269
Saurine, fish spoilage and **7**, 47
–, histamine toxicity and **24**, 129
Sausages **39**, 76–79, 83
–, aging **12**, 418–420
–, casings **6**, 134
–, curing, methods **29**, 21
–, differences from fish paste **12**, 370–371
–, effects of preserves **12**, 407–416
–, energy costs **39**, 146
–, fermentation **39**, 95, 109–110, 122, 125

–, fish **12**, 367–424
–, food poisoning **12**, 414–415
–, history of **12**, 368–369
–, –, production statistics **12**, 369
–, manufacture **12**, 376–392
–, origins of bacteria **12**, 396–403
–, pork, organisms in **6**, 188
–, preparation **12**, 369–371
–, preservation **39**, 118–119
–, processing **12**, 369–370, 403–407
–, –, time calculations **12**, 403–407
–, production problems **39**, 88–89
–, putrefaction **12**, 392–396, 410–414
–, –, prevention **12**, 410–414
–, quality standards **12**, 420–422
–, rancidity in cooked **5**, 23
–, – in raw **5**, 23
–, raw materials **12**, 371–376
–, ripening of effects on SH groups **24**, 80
–, sanitary measures **12**, 414–417
–, storage **12**, 417–418
–, synthetic casings, alginates in **11**, 150
Saxidomus giganteus **10**, 145, 156, 175
Saxidomus nuttallii **10**, 144
Saxitoxin, structure and pharmacology of **18**, 155–157
SC, *see* Stellate cell
Scald **15**, 179
–, soft **12**, 114
–, superficial **12**, 115–116, 182
Scale invariance **44**, 45
Scaling theory, colloidal gels **44**, 45–54
–, fat crystal networks **44**, 55–58
Scallops **39**, 345, 349
–, saxitoxin from **18**, 155
Scanning acoustic microscopy **45**, 156
Scanning electron microscopy (SEM) **22**, 205–307
–, ancillary techniques for **22**, 237
–, anhydrous milkfat **44**, 61, 62
–, applications of **22**, 217–222
–, –, in microbiology **22**, 239–250
–, –, in plant studies **22**, 250–252
–, –, miscellaneous biological **22**, 252–258
–, chemically interesterified milkfat **44**, 61, 63, 64
–, contrast mechanisms in **22**, 215–217
–, dietary fiber and **31**, 183–185
–, electron probe microanalysis by **22**, 223–229
–, elemental analyses by **22**, 222–231
–, historical aspects of **22**, 206
–, information sources on **22**, 207–208
–, in sanitation studies **22**, 292
–, instrumentation for **22**, 209–217
–, of antibiotic effects **22**, 249–250
–, of cereal grains **22**, 259–274
–, –, processing studies **22**, 275–278
–, of cereal storage **22**, 242–245
–, of foods and food products **22**, 258–292
–, of malting and brewing **22**, 278–281
–, of milk products **22**, 287–288
–, of oilseeds **22**, 286–287
–, of starches **22**, 281–286
–, polysaccharide–lipid edible films **44**, 357
–, principles of **22**, 208–217
–, sample preparation for **22**, 200, 231–240
–, specimen manipulation in **22**, 238–239
–, transmission electron microscopy (TEM), compared to **22**, 210–211
–, use as transmission electron microscopy **22**, 220
Scenedesmus **16**, 74
–, as sources of protein **18**, 117–128
Schiff's base **12**, 16–19
Schiff's glucose derivative **12**, 19
Schizosaccharomyces pombe, phytate (inositol hexakisphosphate) synthetic pathway **45**, 7
–, wine deacidification by **25**, 32–38
Scholle Corporation **32**, 20, 21, 30
Scleroderma **37**, 402
Scleroglucan, molecular shapes and interactions **42**, 179–180
Sclerotinia sclerotium **15**, 177
Scombroid poisoning (*see also* Histamine, toxicity from) **10**, 188
–, fish **42**, 10
–, occurrence of **18**, 154–155
Scombrotoxicosis **39**, 337, 346–348
Scones, losses of thiamine in baking **6**, 271
Scopolamine **44**, 298
Scoring, applications of **7**, 6–7
Scoring test, use in sensory difference tests **2**, 225–226
Scott spray dryer, operation of **2**, 428
Scraped-surface heat exchanger **32**, 15–16
Scrapie **43**, 272, 275–277
–, endemic infection **43**, 296
–, genetic susceptibility **43**, 285–286
–, infectivity **43**, 295, 298
–, –, mouse bioassay **43**, 300
–, prion inactivation **43**, 295, 296
–, strains **43**, 288
SC45647 sweeteners, sweetener-induced taste, phosphoinositide transduction pathway **42**, 224–227
Scurvy **10**, 235, 236–237; **37**, 387–388
Scutellum, of wheat germ **23**, 194–195

Scyllo-inositol **45**, 37
SDS, *see* Sodium dodecyl sulfate
SDS-PAGE, ripening cheddar cheese **34**, 368–369
Seafood (*see also* Biogenic amines, fish and shellfish), heart disease and **35**, 134
–, irradiation of **24**, 174–182
–, radurization of **24**, 192–194
Sealing, in flexible packaging **23**, 346–363
–, of retort pouches **23**, 355–359
Sea perch, aerobic bacterial flora of **2**, 350
–, dimethylamine production in **2**, 371, 381
Searle cylinder geometry **39**, 31
Seasonal variation, in plasma α-tocopherol concentration **33**, 176
Sea water **15**, 343
Secoisolariciresinol **44**, 199, 201, 207, 218
–, antioxidant activity **44**, 226
–, *in vivo* antiestrogenic effects **44**, 225
–, metabolism **44**, 221
–, toxicity **44**, 226
Secondary electron emission, in scanning electron microscopy **22**, 215
Sedanoloid, percentage in celery seed oil **2**, 271
Sedanonic acid anhydride in celery seed oil **2**, 271
Sedatives, taste sensation effects **44**, 307–308
Seeds **41**, 1–2
–, analysis **31**, 146, 148
–, chemical aspects **12**, 266–268
–, chilling sensitivity of **25**, 194–196
–, dicotyledonous plants **31**, 133–135
–, dietary fiber and **31**, 119, 120
–, inositol phosphates content **45**, 12–15
–, intestinal bacteria **31**, 181, 182
–, mucilage **31**, 141
–, nutritional aspects **12**, 270–271
–, of cereals **16**, 6ff
–, of legumes **16**, 9ff, 66ff
–, of palms **16**, 15ff
–, of passion fruit **12**, 266–271
–, oil, enzymatic changes during storage **11**, 278–280
–, oilseeds **16**, 11ff, 44ff
–, production **16**, 12
–, properties **31**, 155, 157, 169
–, proteins in **16**, 12, 21, 24
–, selenium in **32**, 95
–, technological aspects **12**, 268–270
–, –, meal **12**, 270
–, –, oil **12**, 268–270
Seed storage proteins (*see also* Food protein engineering, Food proteins, Legumes) **36**, 89–188
–, biosynthesis **36**, 123–125
–, biscuitmaking quality **36**, 133
–, breadmaking quality **36**, 131–133
–, cereal storage proteins **36**, 93, 95–103
–, cloned gene expression in micro-organisms **36**, 144–151
–, – in –, *Escherichia coli* **36**, 145–149
–, – in –, expressed proteins, characterization of **36**, 151
–, – in –, –, detection of **36**, 150–151
–, – in –, yeast **36**, 150
–, emulsification **36**, 131
–, expression **36**, 151–163
–, –, *Escherichia* coli **36**, 151, 153–158
–, –, french bean phaseolin **36**, 161–162
–, –, in transgenic plants **36**, 163–172
–, –, –, *Agrobacterium tumefaciens*-mediated transformation system **36**, 164
–, –, –, chimeric genes **36**, 169
–, –, –, direct transformation system **36**, 164–165
–, –, –, 7S globulins **36**, 166, 168
–, –, –, 11S globulins **36**, 168–169
–, –, –, HMW glutenin **36**, 170–171
–, –, –, plant regeneration **36**, 165
–, –, –, processing, modification and assembly of expressed proteins **36**, 171–172
–, –, –, required DNA element for gene expression regulation **36**, 165–171
–, –, –, zeins **36**, 169–170
–, –, maize zein **36**, 163
–, –, pea legumin **36**, 160–161
–, –, pea vicilin **36**, 161
–, –, *Saccharomyces cerevisiae* **36**, 158–160
–, –, soybean glycinin **36**, 151, 153–160
–, –, wheat α-gliadin **36**, 162
–, –, wheat γ-gliadin **36**, 162–163
–, –, wheat HMW glutenin **36**, 162
–, functional properties **36**, 125–127
–, gelation **36**, 126, 128–131
–, –, soybean glycinin **36**, 126, 128–130
–, –, *Vicia faba* legumin **36**, 129, 131
–, gene cloning **36**, 134–144
–, –, cDNA cloning **36**, 139–142
–, –, cosmid vectors **36**, 139
–, –, DNA/RNA-modifying enzymes **36**, 136–137
–, –, DNA sequencing **36**, 143–144
–, –, genomic DNA cloning **36**, 142–143
–, –, mRNA isolation **36**, 139–140
–, –, phage vectors **36**, 138–139

–, –, plasmid vectors **36**, 137–138
–, –, restriction enzymes **36**, 134, 136
–, –, RNA sources **36**, 140
–, –, screening of cDNA and genomic DNA libraries **36**, 143
–, –, synthesis and cloning of cDNA **36**, 140–142
–, nutritional properties **36**, 92–94
–, pasta cooking quality **36**, 133–134
–, properties conferred to food systems **36**, 127
–, research needs **36**, 187–188
Selectins **45**, 30
Selegiline **44**, 310
Selenium, analysis in foods, methods for **32**, 86–88
–, and cooking techniques **32**, 94, 96
–, as a nutritional stress factor **4**, 114
–, bioavailability of **32**, 99–102
–, carcinogen risk assessment and **31**, 22, 24
–, chemical speciation in foods **32**, 88–89
–, counteraction of toxicity of **1**, 128
–, daily requirement for humans **32**, 105
–, deficiency **36**, 231–232
–, effect in diets **1**, 121–122
–, geographical distribution in foods **32**, 89–91
–, in animal-derived foods **32**, 95–98
–, in human diets **32**, 102–105
–, in liquid formula diet **32**, 98–99
–, in milk **36**, 231–233
–, in plant-derived foods **32**, 91–95
–, toxicity **32**, 108
Selenium absorption, phytate (inositol hexakisphosphate) effects **45**, 32, 35
Selenocysteine **32**, 89
Selenomethionine **32**, 88–89
Self-association phenomenon, concentration-dependent, of folates **33**, 6
Self-similarity **44**, 43, 44, 71
–, fat crystal network microstructure **44**, 71, 72, 73, 74
d-Selinen, percentage in celery seed oil **2**, 271
Semidry meat production, *see* Dehydration control, IM meat
"Semi-micro" method of testing quaternary ammonium disinfectants **2**, 160
Semiquinone, reaction in oxidation **3**, 21, 22
Semisolid food, heat processing of **23**, 106
Semorelin **44**, 318
Semperfresh **44**, 370
Senecio **45**, 80
–, contamination of staple foods **45**, 68, 69–70
–, – of –, prevention **45**, 91
Senecio burchelli **45**, 69
Senecio disease **45**, 69
Senecio ilicifolius **45**, 69
Senecio jacobaea (tansy ragwort) **45**, 70, 72
Senecio longilobus **45**, 77
Senecionine **45**, 66–67, 72, 76–78, 80, 88
–, metabolism **45**, 82, 84–85
Senecio riddellii **45**, 65
Senecio triangularis **45**, 77
Seneciphylline **45**, 71–72, 76, 78, 80, 88
Senescence, in fruit **10**, 297
–, radiation inhibition of **24**, 201–204
Senkirkine **45**, 66, 67
Sensible parameter **40**, 311, 320
Sensitivity analysis **40**, 7, 234–235, 238–240
Sensory analysis **19**, 215–277
–, applied studies in, landmarks **19**, 224–228
–, approaches to **19**, 216–217
–, basic advances in, landmarks **19**, 217–224
–, –, odor studies **19**, 223
–, –, problems **19**, 222–223
–, educational and extension work **19**, 240–245
–, –, sensory courses **19**, 244–245
–, –, sensory training **19**, 243–244
–, objectivized quality evaluation studies **19**, 248–261
–, –, color assessment **19**, 254–259
–, –, national committees **19**, 260–261
–, –, preparation factors **19**, 259–260
–, –, visual assessment **19**, 253–254
–, problems in **19**, 261–262
–, research needs in **19**, 264–266
–, specialized research **19**, 228–240
–, –, flavor studies **19**, 231–240
–, –, texture studies **19**, 229–231
–, stimulation phenomena in **19**, 245–248
–, –, increasing sensory potentials **19**, 247–248
Sensory stimulus, food **21**, 39–43
Sensory system, for food texture perception **29**, 160–162
Separation technique, *see* Microdialysis *and* Ultrafiltration
Sequestering agents **14**, 355–358
–, in pectins **11**, 363
Serine **16**, 247
Serine protease, endogenous proteolytic enzymes and **31**, 381, 382, 385
Serine proteinase, activity **31**, 383, 384, 388, 390, 391

Serine proteinase (*cont'd*)
–, endogenous proteolytic enzymes and **31**, 345, 411
–, endopeptidases **31**, 352–354, 362
–, exopeptidases **31**, 348
–, meat technology **31**, 409, 410
–, muscle physiology **31**, 380
–, nonmuscle cathepsins **31**, 364, 365
Serratia, in bacon **3**, 308
–, in pork **3**, 293
Serratia marcescens, excreted substances **43**, 323
Sertraline **44**, 312
Serum albumin, blood proteins **34**, 259–260
Serum proteins of milk, heat effects on **19**, 165–168
Sesame **16**, 12, 72ff
Sesame meal, phytic acid content, effect of autoclaving **28**, 45
Sesame oil, solubility of DDT in **2**, 203
Sesame seed meal **17**, 107
Sesquiterpenes, percentage, in carrot seed oil **2**, 271
–, –, in celery seed oil **2**, 271
Sesquiterpene selinene in celery seed oil **2**, 271
Sex, carcinogen risk assessment and **31**, 13, 14
Sex factors, effect on composition of depot fat **23**, 32
"Sex odor", in pork **23**, 39
Shallenberger/Acree AH–B model **42**, 215
Shannon criterion **40**, 224
Shaping, cheese **39**, 166
Shark, spoilage of **7**, 52–54, 61
Shear, oscillatory **39**, 20–23
–, steady **39**, 12–14, 33–35, 44–48
Shear force **39**, 103
Shear history **39**, 59–60
Shearing devices **14**, 66–81
Shear modulus **39**, 8, 56
–, dependence on gelation concentration **34**, 229–230
–, equilibrium elastic **34**, 217
–, gelation, pH dependence **34**, 230–231
–, soy proteins **34**, 236–237
Shear press **9**, 104–105
Shear rate **39**, 4–6, 12–14
–, relations with shear stress, for ammonium alginate solution **11**, 373, 375, 376, 377
–, – with –, for applesauce **11**, 375
–, – with –, for banana purée **11**, 376
–, – with –, for various fluids **11**, 372
–, rheological instrumentation **39**, 24–33
Shear resistance **39**, 95–96
Shear strain **39**, 10–12
Shear stress **39**, 4–6, 24–33, 28
–, in fluid consistency **11**, 368
–, relations with shear rate, for ammonium alginate solution **11**, 373, 375, 376, 377
–, – with –, for applesauce **11**, 375
–, – with –, for banana purée **11**, 376
–, – with –, for various fluids **11**, 372
Shear thickening **32**, 45–46; **39**, 5–6
Shear thinning **32**, 45–46; **39**, 5–6; **41**, 165
Sheep, digestive process of **6**, 116
–, skinning **6**, 152
–, slaughter of **6**, 125
Sheep casings, sterilization of **3**, 163
Sheeting rolls, in dough development **29**, 238–241
Shelf life (*see also* Preservation) **39**, 90, 118, 164
–, extension by ozone treatment **45**, 193
–, of meats, SH group effects on **24**, 84
Shellfish, biogenic amines, *see* Biogenic amines, fish and shellfish
–, frozen **6**, 213
–, selenium in **32**, 96, 97
–, toxins from **18**, 155–157
Shellfish poison, animal lethal dose **10**, 150–151
–, commercial processing, effects on **10**, 159–160
–, domestic cooking, effects on **10**, 158–159
–, human lethal dose **10**, 148–149
–, ionizing radiation, effects on **10**, 160–161
–, isolation **10**, 153–156
–, occurrence and distribution **10**, 149–146
–, pharmacology **10**, 151–153
–, prevention and control **10**, 161–173
–, properties **10**, 156–158
–, research needs **10**, 173–176
–, sources **10**, 138–142
–, symptoms **10**, 146–148
Shell of abalone **23**, 164, 178
Sherbets, alginates in **11**, 147
–, gum karaya in **11**, 187
–, gum tragacanth in **11**, 184
Sherry wine, Spanish-type **6**, 88
Shigella spp., germicidal action of CPCl on **2**, 152
Shijoka **15**, 306
Shikimic acid, in catechin synthesis **17**, 225
Shipping tests, of flexible packages **23**, 403–404
Ships, refrigerated **12**, 150–167
–, –, cargo space **12**, 150–151

–, –, for bananas **12**, 150
–, –, for chilled beef **12**, 150–151
Shoanin **44**, 207
Shock avoidance, α-LNA and **35**, 126
Shoot organogenesis, chocolate and **31**, 320
Short chain fatty acids, dietary fiber and **31**, 173–175, 182, 183, 185
–, inulin effects **43**, 32
Shortening, effect on flour–water bread doughs **38**, 220
–, reversion problems in **4**, 202
Shoyu, bactericidal action **30**, 299–300
–, browning during brewing **30**, 244–251
–, –, amino–caronyl reactions and **30**, 250
–, –, components related to **30**, 245–248
–, –, 3-deoxy-D-glucosone and **30**, 249–250
–, –, formyl nitrogen and **30**, 248
–, –, pentosan content and **30**, 245
–, –, pentose and **30**, 248
–, –, soybean/wheat ratio and **30**, 246–249
–, –, temperature and **30**, 251–252
–, –, xylose consumption and **30**, 245–246
–, browning during storage, cationic fractions and **30**, 253–254
–, –, iron and **30**, 257
–, –, melanoidins and **30**, 255–256
–, –, oxidative reactions, Amadori compounds and **30**, 254–255
–, –, reductones and **30**, 252–253
–, –, temperature and **30**, 256–257
–, carcinogenicity, negative results **30**, 300–301
–, chemical analysis **30**, 199
–, –, comparison with protein hydrolysate **30**, 201
–, color, browning compounds **30**, 242–243
–, –, importance **30**, 241–242
–, –, measurement during browning reactions **30**, 243–244
–, flavor components **30**, 305–313
–, future research, color preservation **30**, 304
–, –, enzyme supplement **30**, 303
–, –, flavor improvements **30**, 304
–, –, koji molds **30**, 301–302
–, –, mash fermentation period reduction **30**, 302–303
–, –, raw materials **30**, 301
–, –, refining and pasteurization **30**, 303–304
–, koikuchi type, *see* Koikuchi shoyu
–, mutagenic substance production **30**, 298–299
–, –, nitrosable premutagens from **30**, 299
–, preparation **30**, 197–201
–, –, history **30**, 198
–, production and sales **30**, 199
–, saishikomi type, preparation **30**, 208
–, shiro type, preparation **30**, 207–208
–, tamari type, preparation **30**, 206–208
–, usukuchi type, preparation **30**, 206
Shrimp **39**, 346, 355
–, bacteria species in **6**, 191
–, in fish sauce **4**, 217, 220
–, –, salted and dried **4**, 226
–, –, use of ascorbic acid on **4**, 391
–, meat, ozone treatment **45**, 197–198
–, –, residual ozone values **45**, 180
Sialomacromolecules, xylitol effects on **25**, 150–152
Sicco near isogenic line **45**, 251–252
–, dough properties **45**, 259–261
Side groups, in proteins **10**, 27, 35
Sideroxylon richardii, glycyrrhizin and **7**, 343
Sieve analysis, of wheat germ **23**, 201
Sieve tubes in vegetable tissue **2**, 301
sIgA, *see* IgA, secretory
Silage preparation **17**, 99–100
Silica, dietary fiber and **31**, 140
Silicate exchangers, use to separate arginine **2**, 38
–, volume per oxygen atom in **2**, 3
Silicon, in milk **36**, 238
–, in wines **8**, 139, 156
Siliqua patula **10**, 144, 145
Silver, in wines **8**, 196
Silver ions, inhibition of enzymes by **1**, 382
Silver nitrate, use in test for ascorbic acid **2**, 334
Similarity transformation, identifiability **40**, 315, 317
Simple extension **39**, 15
Simpson's formula **23**, 94
Simulation (*see also* Bioperiodicity, Membrane transport, Nutrient-response curve), graph model **40**, 348
–, population kinetics **40**, 270–271
Simvastatin **44**, 288
Sinc (Scrapie Incubation Period) **43**, 286, 291
Singer's equation **34**, 56–57
Single-cell protein, cell yield **26**, 7–23
–, –, and heat load **26**, 18–22
–, –, and oxygen demand **26**, 13–18
–, –, dilution rate **26**, 9–13
–, concentrates **26**, 39–45
–, –, coagulation **26**, 42–43
–, –, hydration properties **26**, 40
–, –, mechanical properties **26**, 43
–, –, microstructure **26**, 43
–, –, physical properties **26**, 39–40

Single-cell protein, concentrates (*cont'd*)
–, –, structure potential **26**, 43–45
–, –, theological properties **26**, 40–42
–, economic potential **26**, 6–23
–, engineering problems **26**, 6–23
–, in foods, utilization **26**, 23
–, interaction with other compounds **26**, 45–46
–, organisms **26**, 5–6
–, production, economic determinants **26**, 22–23
–, purification **26**, 33–39
–, raw materials **26**, 3–5
–, –, alcohols **26**, 4
–, –, carbohydrates **26**, 4–5
–, –, methane **26**, 4
–, –, paraffin hydrocarbons **26**, 3–4
–, yeast **26**, 23–33
–, –, cell surface **26**, 26
–, –, colloidal properties of **26**, 26–29
–, –, flavor **26**, 32–33
–, –, physicochemical properties **26**, 29–32
–, –, texturization of **26**, 33
Single-piston valve homogenizer **34**, 169
Singlet oxygen, formation **33**, 235
–, oxidation, inhibition **33**, 255–256
–, –, linoleate **33**, 253
–, –, oleate **33**, 252
–, photosensitized lipid oxidation **33**, 249–256
–, quenching by α-tocopherol **33**, 210, 303
Sinusoidal oscillatory tests **35**, 351
Sip (Scrapie Incubation Period) **43**, 286
Sister chromatid exchanges **34**, 396
Site-directed mutagenesis **35**, 277
–, enthalpy–entropy compensation effect **35**, 283
–, protein stability **35**, 277–284
β-Sitosterol, olive oil and **31**, 467, 473
Size, effects on fruit composition **9**, 298
Size and shape, measurement of **9**, 187–192
Skeletal muscle, myofibrillar proteins in **19**, 279–360; **24**, 31
Skeletal muscle protein, endogenous proteolytic enzymes and **31**, 405
Skim milk, liquid, composition of **19**, 154
–, powder, composition of **19**, 154
–, –, minerals and salts in **19**, 194
–, –, vitamins in **19**, 192
Skin **40**, 9, 49
–, chemical composition **28**, 323
Skin cancer, carcinogen risk assessment and **31**, 15, 19
Skin pick test **42**, 35
Skins for sausages, *see* Casings
Skin tests, food allergy **42**, 35
Skipjack tuna **39**, 350, 351, 354
Slaughter, future research on **10**, 65–66
–, post- **14**, 58–64
–, pre- **14**, 39–57
Slice-cured meat **39**, 75
Sliding friction, factor in consistency **11**, 357
Slimectins **43**, 323
Slippage, rheological instrumentation **39**, 26, 30–31
Slovenian buckwheat products **44**, 414
Slowest heating zone **32**, 56
Slurries, cheese **39**, 259
Small-molecule emulsifiers **34**, 97–109
–, choice **34**, 97–102
–, Gibbs adsorption equation **34**, 102
–, hydrophilic–lipophilic balance **34**, 99–100
–, in food productions **34**, 108–109
–, interfacial properties of surfactants **34**, 104–106
–, liquid crystalline phase formation **34**, 106–108
–, Lissant method **34**, 100–101
–, oil/water interface, adsorption thermodynamics **34**, 102–104
–, phase inversion temperature **34**, 101–102
Small surface-active molecule additives, coalescence and **34**, 144–145
Smell perception, disease-related losses **44**, 264, 270–274
–, –, Alzheimer's disease **44**, 280–282
–, –, cancer **44**, 275–280
–, –, endocrine disease **44**, 272
–, –, head trauma **44**, 275
–, –, local conditions **44**, 273
–, –, nervous disease **44**, 270–271
–, –, nutritional/metabolic disease **44**, 271
–, –, viral infections **44**, 274, 275
–, elderly people **44**, 248–249, 262–264
–, –, suprathreshold perceptual losses **44**, 263–264
–, –, threshold detection elevation **44**, 263
–, –, trigeminal stimulants **44**, 264
–, learned associations **44**, 248
–, medication effects **44**, 248, 249, 283–284, 319, 320–324
–, neural pathway **44**, 254–255
–, physiology **44**, 253–256
–, –, age-related changes **44**, 255–256
–, role in food intake/digestion **44**, 248
–, transduction pathways **44**, 254
Smoke, effect on rancidity **5**, 34
Smoke curing, *see* Curing smoke

Smoke-curing concentrates, flavor studies on **19**, 235–236
Smoked food products, botulism from **22**, 164–165, 166
Smoked foods, carcinogen risk assessment and **31**, 24
Smoked meat, flavor of **18**, 21
Smoked products, chemical composition **29**, 104–135
–, –, analytical methods **29**, 109–112
–, –, bologna layers **29**, 109
–, –, compounds identified from smoke, *see* Curing smoke, identified compounds
–, –, phenol content **29**, 130–132
Smoke generators, fluidization **29**, 97
–, friction **29**, 96
–, laboratory, according to Tóth **29**, 98
–, –, for isothermal smoke development **29**, 97–98
–, –, two-stage **29**, 97
–, steam **29**, 96
–, with heat supply **29**, 95–96
Smoking, carcinogen risk assessment and **31**, 3
–, –, epidemiology **31**, 38, 39
–, –, laboratory data **31**, 25, 29
–, –, statistics **31**, 13–16, 19
–, flavor testing and **7**, 18
–, nitrosamines and **22**, 53–55
–, *N*-nitroso compounds and **31**, 82, 83, 92, 98, 99
–, of meats, effects on SH groups **24**, 80–81
Smoldering sawdust, steam-volatile and -nonvolatile fractions **29**, 107–108
Smooth muscle spasmogens, leukotrienes as **35**, 103–104
Snack foods, of high nutritive quality, for developing countries **22**, 196–197
Snapdragons **41**, 10–11
Sniff methods **14**, 14–18
–, scaling **14**, 16
Snorkel technique, for package air removal **23**, 371
Soap **14**, 351
–, amine **14**, 351–352
–, cation **12**, 410
–, spray dryers for **2**, 431–433
–, –, relation of bulk density to speed of dryer **2**, 472, 476
–, –, sphere formation during drying **2**, 474
Soba (buckwheat noodles) (*see also* Buckweat *and* Oriental noodles) **43**, 146, 159
Sobrasada **39**, 79
Social forestry **32**, 204–205
Sockeye salmon, ozone treatment **45**, 197
Soda ash, use in sugar beet industry **2**, 27
–, – in synthetic aluminosilicate **2**, 4
Sodium, chocolate and **31**, 246, 270
–, dietary fiber and **31**, 161, 162
–, in ion exchange reactions **2**, 8, 10, 11
–, in milk **36**, 212–213
–, in wines **8**, 135, 137, 139, 196
–, radioactive **3**, 155
–, ratio of, to potassium in fruit **8**, 374
Sodium ascorbate, *N*-nitroso compounds and **31**, 80, 84
Sodium benzene-sulfinate, combination with *o*-benzoquinone **3**, 19
Sodium bicarbonate, effect on blue mold **3**, 464
Sodium bisulfite, combination with *o*-quinone **3**, 20
–, purity definition, Food Chemical Codex **30**, 6
Sodium carbonate, effect on canned foods **2**, 315
–, regeneration of anion exchanger by **2**, 17
–, use of to form pectic acid **1**, 406
Sodium carboxymethylcellulose **12**, 294–314
–, bakery applications **12**, 302–305
–, –, breads and cakes **12**, 304–305
–, –, icings **12**, 303–304
–, confectionery **12**, 307–308
–, dairy applications **12**, 297–302
–, development **12**, 294–295
–, dietetic foods **12**, 308–309
–, dry package mixes **12**, 311–312
–, food preservation **12**, 312–313
–, meringues **12**, 304
–, –, pie fillings **12**, 302–303
–, processed foods **12**, 310–311
–, properties **12**, 295–297
–, –, pH **12**, 295–296
–, –, storage of solutions **12**, 297
–, –, viscosity **12**, 296
–, –, water solubility **12**, 295
–, salad dressings, sauces, gravies **12**, 305–306
–, use in spray-drying **2**, 496
Sodium chloride, added in canning **3**, 351, 352
–, chocolate and **31**, 218
–, effect of temperature in taste intensity tests **2**, 246
–, – of treating potatoes with before blanching **1**, 272
–, effects on "warmed-over" flavor **23**, 56–57

Sodium chloride, effects (*cont'd*)
–, – on water-holding capacity of meat **10**, 372, 413–420, 423–425
–, in determining undenatured serum protein **3**, 83
–, in diet of rats **1**, 112
–, influence on bacterial resistance to heat **2**, 67
–, inhibition of microbial growth by **3**, 293–294
–, – of proteinases by **1**, 380
–, in meat curing **29**, 3–5
–, –, flavor development, comparison with nitrite **29**, 30–32
–, in soy sauce **10**, 77–78, 112, 114–115
–, *N*-nitroso compounds and **31**, 80
–, photomicrographs of spray-dried **2**, 514
–, regeneration of ion exchangers by **2**, 16, 19
–, use in regeneration of zeolite in milk industry **2**, 23
Sodium-chloro-2-phenylphenate, treatment of fruit molds by **3**, 464
Sodium cholate, dietary fiber and **31**, 160–163
Sodium citrate added to milk **3**, 69
– to –, in inhibition of corrosion **3**, 342
Sodium compounds, in cheese ripening **16**, 233
–, in protein extraction **16**, 123
Sodium decyl sulfate, neutralization or germicidal activity by **2**, 132
Sodium deficiency **1**, 120
Sodium deoxycholate, dietary fiber and **31**, 161
Sodium diethyl dithiocarbamate, effect on plant respiration **3**, 16
Sodium dithionite, reaction with folic acid **33**, 8
Sodium dodecyl sulfate (SDS), gel electrophoresis, ripening cheddar cheese **34**, 366–368
–, oat globulin thermal characteristics effect **35**, 327–328
–, sedimentation baking test **29**, 213–214
Sodium erythorbate, *see* Erythorbic acid
Sodium fluoride **44**, 300
Sodium hexametaphosphate, effect on adhesive properties of pea coats **2**, 315
–, relation to gelation pH of pectin **1**, 415
Sodium hydroxide, gelatin manufacture and **7**, 240
–, in detection of "remade" milk **3**, 70
–, regenerated resin in grape industry **2**, 16
–, use as regenerator of anion exchanger in pineapple industry **2**, 20
–, use in regeneration of zeolite in milk industry **2**, 23
–, use of to form pectic acid **1**, 406
Sodium hypophosphite, antibotulinal activity in cured meat **29**, 52
Sodium ion, ionophoretic capability of cardiolipin **37**, 273–274
Sodium lauryl sulfate **44**, 301
–, effects on whey protein foams **33**, 401
–, germicidal action of **2**, 132
–, use as wetting agent on zeolite **2**, 23
–, virucidal action of **2**, 138
Sodium metabisulfite, dough development and **29**, 234, 238
Sodium myristyl sulfate, virucidal action of **2**, 138
Sodium naphthuride, inactivator of quaternary ammonium compounds **2**, 166
Sodium nitrate, in bacterial destruction in bacon curing **3**, 295
–, influence on bacterial resistance to heat **2**, 67
Sodium nitrite, fish preservation and **7**, 69
–, in bacterial destruction in bacon curing **3**, 295
Sodium orthophenylphenate, treatment of citrus fruits by **3**, 464
Sodium pectate, molecular shapes and interactions **42**, 169–170
Sodium phosphate in diet of rats **1**, 112
Sodium salts, age-related taste threshold **44**, 257, 258
Sodium silicate, effect of spray-drying on **2**, 476
–, effect on molds **3**, 464
–, regeneration of zeolite by **2**, 24
Sodium sulfate, effect on cetyltrimethyl-ammonium bromide **2**, 136
–, gelatin manufacture and **7**, 240–241
Sodium sulfite, microbial inhibition by **1**, 386
Sodium taurocholate, dietary fiber and **31**, 160, 161, 163
Sodium tetraborate, treatment of citrus fruits by **3**, 463–464
Sodium thiosulfate in inhibition of corrosion **3**, 343
Sodium tripolyphosphate, control of microsomal-enzyme-associated lipid oxidation **33**, 305–306
Software (*see also* Linear integrator) **40**, 281–283
–, MAPLE **40**, 330

–, MATHEMATICA **40**, 330
–, REDUCE **40**, 330
–, CONSAM **40**, 6, 9, 21, 32, 274, 290
–, IDENT **40**, 318
–, MESOSAUR **40**, 221, 223
–, NLMIX **40**, 275
–, NONMEM **40**, 275
–, NPEM2 **40**, 276
–, SAAM, *see* SAAM software
–, SAS **40**, 50, 160
–, SYSTAT **40**, 221
–, USC*PACL **40**, 276
Softwood, lignin pyrolysis **29**, 121–122
–, phenol composition **29**, 127
Soil, and substrates **14**, 394–404
–, –, separation from **14**, 329–330
–, dispersion, in solution **14**, 330–332
–, –, stabilization of **14**, 332–334
–, erosion **32**, 188, 216–221, 225–226
–, flat sour bacteria spores in **18**, 169–173
–, nutrient loss **32**, 221–223
–, oily **14**, 376–379, 380–383
–, –, heterogeneous **14**, 384–385
–, –, removal **14**, 379–385
–, particulate **14**, 371–375
–, –, solid **14**, 383–384
–, passion fruit **12**, 208
–, removal, detergent type **14**, 407–409
–, –, time **14**, 406–407
–, –, variables **14**, 404–419
–, selenium in **32**, 89–91
–, type **14**, 345
Sojourn time, β-carotene **40**, 44–46, 49, 51–52, 61
–, vitamin A **40**, 12–13
Solanine **21**, 309
–, in potatoes **1**, 124
–, –, distribution **21**, 310–312
–, toxicology of **21**, 342–348
Solar energy use **32**, 193, 197
Solar ponds **15**, 305
Solid fat content, ultrasonic sensing, isothermal scanning **45**, 139–140
–, –, temperature scanning **45**, 141
Solid fat index, chocolate and **31**, 231
Solid foods, rheology model **39**, 41–44
Solid-phase methods, for polyglutamyl tolate synthesis **33**, 6–7
Solids, evaporation from **7**, 191–192
Solka floc, dietary fiber and **31**, 178–180
Solubility (*see also* Wheat proteins), calcium, effect on bioavailability **33**, 145–147
–, calcium salts, table **33**, 145
–, prolamins **36**, 103
–, whey proteins **33**, 374–375
Soluble dietary fiber, inulin/fructooligo-saccharide **43**, 26–27
–, –, nutritional labeling **43**, 48, 49
–, physiological definition **43**, 27
Soluble enzyme assays, protein digestibility **35**, 213–222
Soluble starch synthases, characterization **41**, 76
–, classification **41**, 80–81
–, forms **41**, 75–78
–, granule bound, *see* Granule-bound starch synthase
–, starch biosynthesis **41**, 111–113
–, waxy gene **41**, 81–82, 84–85
Solutes, diffusion in aqueous food glasses **38**, 169–177
–, humidity and **7**, 93–94
Solutions, vapor pressure of **7**, 85–86
–, viscosity, three types of flow **29**, 180
Solvent treatments, proteins **35**, 334
Somatic embryogenesis, chocolate and **31**, 320
So-men **43**, 146
Somesthetic receptors, in oral cavity **29**, 164–166
Sonic and ultrasonic vibrations **3**, 123
–, use of **3**, 130–132
Sonication, wheat proteins **36**, 15–17
Sorbic acid, antibotulinal activity in cured meat **29**, 49–52
–, – in –, mixtures with nitrite **29**, 51–52
Sorbitan monostearate, in chocolate bars **6**, 44
Sorbitol, chocolate and **31**, 267, 268, 272, 274
–, fudge and nougat improved by **6**, 11
–, in apples and pears **8**, 314
–, use of ion exchangers in dimineralizing of **2**, 30
Sorbose, chocolate and **31**, 267, 268, 272
Sorghum **15**, 235; **16**, 6; **43**, 217–255
–, breadmaking **43**, 228–233
–, –, custard/batter process **43**, 232
–, –, wheat composite bread **43**, 229–231
–, –, wheatless bread **43**, 231–233
–, brewing **43**, 243–250
–, –, conventional beer **43**, 247–250
–, –, packaging **43**, 245–246
–, –, sorghum beer **43**, 243–247
–, cakes **43**, 233
–, condensed tannins (proanthocyanins) **43**, 222
–, –, inactivation for malting **43**, 241

Sorghum, condensed tannins (proanthocyanins) (*cont'd*)
–, –, reduction during decortication **43**, 224
–, cookies **43**, 233–234
–, –, texture **43**, 234
–, endosperm anti-fungal proteins **43**, 241–242
–, enzymatic modification of flour **43**, 235
–, fermentation **43**, 250–254
–, –, alcoholic **43**, 250–252
–, –, fusel oils **43**, 251
–, –, lactic acid **43**, 252–254
–, flour, phytate content **45**, 16
–, grain chemistry **43**, 219, 222–223
–, grain structure **43**, 219, 220–221
–, granolas **43**, 237–238
–, importance in semi-arid areas **43**, 218–219
–, instant/ready-to-eat products **43**, 236–218
–, leuco-anthocyanin **5**, 288
–, malt **43**, 223, 238, 249–250, 251
–, malting **43**, 221, 238–243
–, –, applications **43**, 238–239
–, –, floor malting **43**, 242, 243
–, –, free amino nitrogen (FAN) content **43**, 240, 241, 250, 251–252
–, –, outdoor system **43**, 243
–, –, pneumatic malting **43**, 242, 243
–, –, steeping conditions **43**, 240–241
–, –, technologies **43**, 239–243
–, milling **43**, 221, 224–228
–, –, dehulling (decortication) **43**, 224–226
–, –, dry **43**, 224–228
–, –, roller mills **43**, 226–228
–, –, wet **43**, 228
–, pasta/noodles **43**, 235–236
–, pigments **43**, 223
–, production **43**, 218
–, protein quality **43**, 223, 239
–, rice substitutes **43**, 235
–, starch gelatinization temperature **43**, 223
–, tortillas **43**, 236
–, water-insoluble glucuronoarabinoxylans **43**, 223, 250
–, weaning porridges **43**, 237
–, –, critical control points in fermented products **43**, 253, 254
–, –, malt addition (power flour) **43**, 238–239
Sorption **39**, 99–100, 125
Sorption isotherms, for barley malt flour and lecithin **11**, 305, 307, 312
–, for predicting storage stability **11**, 313–314
–, of water and aroma components in foods **20**, 63–64
Sounds, crushing, role in food fracturability perception **29**, 192–194
Soups, bacterial content of frozen **6**, 199
–, consistency of **8**, 28
–, flexible packaging for **23**, 327
–, gelatin and **7**, 325
Sour dough breads, phytate content **45**, 20
Souring, in cereals and cereal products **11**, 301–302
Soy, use in candy **6**, 32
Soya flakes, in dehydrated pork loaves **6**, 300
Soybean albumin, use of Bishop spray dryer for **2**, 410
Soybean glycinin, expression in *Escherichia coli* **36**, 151, 153–158
–, – in –, expression plasmid construction **36**, 154–155
–, – in –, proglycinin homologue proteins in JM105 cells **36**, 154–156
–, – in –, N-terminal amino acid sequence **36**, 156–158
–, – in *Saccharomyces cerevisiae* **36**, 158–160
–, – in –, food protein engineering **36**, 176–184
–, β-Spiral **36**, 132–133
Soybean meal, effect of heat on nutritive value **4**, 246, 251–253, 254–262
–, phytate removal **28**, 68
–, toxic **10**, 32
Soybean oil, avoiding fatigue during judging **2**, 242
–, brain phosphoglyceride effects **35**, 77
–, color of **5**, 321
–, DHA levels in brain phosphoglycerides **35**, 124–125
–, fishy flavors in **4**, 191
–, α-linolenic acid **35**, 19
–, oxidation of **4**, 190
–, reversion problems in **4**, 187, 190, 195–203
–, steam refining, tocopherol losses due to **33**, 160, 162
–, tests for rancidity **2**, 250
–, training judges for tests on **2**, 235
–, use of ranking sensory difference test on judging of **2**, 227
Soybean oil meal, effect of storage on biological value of protein in **4**, 268–269
Soybean phytoestrogens **44**, 197, 200
–, coumestans **44**, 211, 214
–, health protective effects **44**, 227
–, –, bone **44**, 228–229
–, –, cancer **44**, 229–230

–, –, cardiovascular **44**, 232–234
–, isoflavones **44**, 203, 205
–, –, assays **44**, 202, 203
–, –, effects of processing **44**, 212–217
–, –, low-fat products **44**, 215–217
Soybean production, and erosion **32**, 218
Soybean protein, mutagenicity of derivatives of **32**, 166
Soybeans **16**, 11ff, 44ff, 50ff; **17**, 108
–, antitrypsin in **1**, 385
–, chemical composition **10**, 104–105
–, chocolate and **31**, 278
–, dietary fiber and **31**, 160
–, injurious substances in **1**, 108–109, 125–126
–, inositol phosphates, calcium absorption influence **45**, 35
–, –, degradation during malting **45**, 22
–, loss of thiamine on processing **6**, 290
–, phytate (inositol hexakisphosphate) **45**, 12
–, –, reduced content gene mutations **45**, 34
–, –, synthetic pathway **45**, 8
–, phytic acid content **28**, 60
–, protein hydrolysate, sulfur-containing compounds **30**, 283
–, selenium in **32**, 92–94
–, shoyu preparation, ethanol and propanol treatment **30**, 213
–, –, methanol treatment **30**, 213
–, –, protein denaturation by, cooker construction **30**, 214–215
–, –, –, cooking **30**, 211–217
–, –, –, improved method **30**, 215–217
–, –, –, NK method **30**, 212–214
–, –, –, protein digestibility and **30**, 214–215
–, –, –, steaming pressure **30**, 214–217
–, thiamine retention in **6**, 285
–, whole and defatted, comparison **30**, 209–211
Soybean/wheat ratio, for shoyu, browning reactions during brewing and **30**, 248–249
–, koji cultivation and **30**, 224
Soy cake, composition of **10**, 116
Soy flour, insects attacking **4**, 327–328
Soymilk, edible films **44**, 374
–, isoflavones **44**, 212, 213, 216
Soy products, allergenicity **42**, 7
Soy protein composite films **44**, 382
–, protein–lipid water barrier properties **44**, 374–375
–, protein–propyleneglycol alginate **44**, 383
Soy protein–dextran conjugate, emulsifying activity **34**, 157
Soy protein enteropathy **37**, 31
Soy protein isolate, binding constants **34**, 305–306
–, denatured soy isolate **34**, 304–307
–, molar surface tension **34**, 308
–, native soy isolate **34**, 303–304, 306–307
–, salt anion binding **34**, 308–310
–, salt-induced solubility profiles **34**, 301–310
–, theory **34**, 302–303
Soy proteins (*see also* Proteins, soybean), alkali treatments **35**, 209
–, classification **34**, 231–232
–, concentrate, meat mutagen modulation **34**, 432
–, denaturation **34**, 234–235
–, gel formation mechanism **34**, 232–236
–, gels, rheology **34**, 236–237
–, globulin fraction amounts and composition **34**, 231–232
–, phytic acid removal **28**, 68–74
–, residues, racemization rate constants **35**, 202–203
–, subunits **34**, 235–236
–, tryptic digestion, emulsifying capacity and stability **34**, 159–160
Soy sauce **14**, 239; **44**, 214
–, color **10**, 87, 111
–, composition **10**, 77–87
–, flavor, chemical components of **10**, 87–104
–, –, sources of **10**, 104–114
–, fractional distillation of **10**, 95–100
–, in Korea **30**, 202
–, in Taiwan **30**, 202
–, Japanese (*see also* Shoyu), aroma, sources of **10**, 104–114
–, mash **10**, 111–115
–, mutagenicity **32**, 164–165
–, preservatives in **10**, 119–123
–, processing methods **10**, 106–107
–, production and consumption, in China **30**, 202
–, salt for, from salted fish **4**, 223
–, types **10**, 76
Spaghetti, alginates in **11**, 157
Spaghetti and meat balls, home frozen **6**, 207
–, F value for industrial processing of **2**, 102
Spanish mackerel **39**, 337
Sparse data situation (*see also* Kinetic parameter distribution) **40**, 265–266, 272
Spastic mice **37**, 372–373
Species differences, cardiolipin acyl composition **37**, 290
Spectrometers, mass (*see also* Mass spectrometry) **14**, 235

Spectrophotometry, in color measurement **9**, 161–162
–, in flavor chemistry **9**, 211–212
Spectroscopy, infrared **14**, 192
–, of nitrosamines **22**, 14–16
Spectroturbidimetric methods **34**, 172
Spectrum, electromagnetic, illustrative chart of **3**, 121
Spermidine **39**, 337, 341–343, 350, 352
–, analytical techniques **39**, 354–356
–, *N*-nitroso compounds and **31**, 76, 77
Spermine **39**, 337–339, 341–343, 350, 352
–, analytical techniques **39**, 354–356
Sphericity, friction-factor factor as a function of **11**, 430
–, Reynolds number factor as a function of **11**, 430
Spheroidine, toxic properties of **18**, 148
Sphingolipids, structure and biosynthesis of **23**, 15–17
Sphingomyelins, structure of **23**, 16
Sphingosine, biosynthesis of **23**, 17
–, structure of **23**, 16
Spices, as allergens **42**, 27–28
–, capsicum, color of **5**, 319
–, contact dermatitis **42**, 29
–, effect on rancidity **5**, 35
–, irradiation of **24**, 183–139
–, sterilization of by cathode rays **3**, 163
Spinach, ascorbic acid content of **1**, 52
–, –, effect of fertilizers on **1**, 308
–, –, – of light on **1**, 299
–, ascorbic acid oxidase in **3**, 15
–, bacterial count of **6**, 186
–, blanching of **3**, 136
–, calcium content of, effect of location on **1**, 310–311
–, canned, corrosiveness of **3**, 341
–, –, nutrients in **1**, 43, 46–50
–, –, sterilization of **3**, 441
–, carotene in **8**, 104
–, changes in chlorophyll during blanching **8**, 81
–, chloroplasts in **2**, 306
–, crude lipid from **8**, 100
–, effect of blanching on vitamin content of **1**, 67–68, 73, 77, 81
–, – of storage on vitamin content of **1**, 65
–, frozen, bacterial count of **6**, 186
–, greenness of **5**, 326–328
–, heating and cooling curves for processed **2**, 50, 54
–, losses during blanching **8**, 66
–, –, ascorbic acid **8**, 89
–, –, carotene **8**, 72
–, –, riboflavin **8**, 75
–, –, thiamine **8**, 74
–, loss of thiamine on processing **6**, 290, 295
–, nutritional stress factor in **4**, 111–113
–, pH of **3**, 432
–, phosphorus content of, effect of fertilizers on **1**, 313
–, polyphenolase in **3**, 15
–, raw and cooked, carotene concentration **5**, 223–225
–, total folate content, table **33**, 40
–, B vitamins in **1**, 42, 44, 45
Spinach beet, distribution of oxidase in **3**, 11
Spinach leaf enzyme **41**, 47–48
Spin cooker, heat transfer in **32**, 69–70
Spirodela polyrhiza **45**, 8, 23
Spironolactone **44**, 307
Spirulina spp., as sources of protein **18**, 117–128
Spleen, distribution of DDT in **2**, 210
–, endogenous proteolytic enzymes and **31**, 353, 361, 362, 365, 368
Split-pea soup **32**, 9
Splits, gelatin manufacture and **7**, 238
Spoilage (*see also* Contamination *and* Decomposition), of fish, histamine role in **24**, 135–139
Sponge cake, freeze-dried egg and **7**, 225
Sponges, gelatin and **7**, 327
Spore count **15**, 161
Sporendonema sebi, water requirements of **7**, 116
Spores, bacterial **32**, 6–9, 18–19, 25, 26, 32
–, resistance, chlorine and **7**, 156–158
–, –, heat and **7**, 121
Sporotrichum, survival at low temperatures **3**, 446
Sporozoa, jellied meat effect and **7**, 57
"Spray Dehydration" dryer, operation of **2**, 410
Spray devices **14**, 426–427
Spray dryer, atomizing devices of **2**, 439
–, –, bulk density **2**, 471–477
–, –, centrifugal type **2**, 454, 465
–, –, dispersion **2**, 465–471
–, –, nozzles used as **2**, 439–454
–, co-current dryers, horizontal **2**, 402–407
–, –, simple vertical downward **2**, 407–414
–, –, vertical upward **2**, 425–430
–, complex vertical co-current dryers **2**, 414, 425
–, control of product accumulation inside **2**, 492–494

–, counter-current dryers, vertical **2**, 430–433
–, economics of **2**, 491
–, evaporative capacity of **2**, 502
–, heat supply **2**, 486–490
–, –, industrial burner types **2**, 488
–, –, safety devices **2**, 489–490
–, humidity problems **2**, 496–502
–, laboratory spray dryers **2**, 433–439
–, materials of construction **2**, 490
–, principal designs of **2**, 401–439
–, product cooling devices **2**, 486
–, product recovery and handling **2**, 477–485
–, thermal efficiency of **2**, 503–513
Spray-drying, aroma retention in **20**, 65–73
–, chocolate and **31**, 287, 288, 291, 311
–, cost of **20**, 94–96
–, microencapsulation by **34**, 165–166
–, preconcentration effects on **20**, 98
Sprays, copper **9**, 301
–, effects on fruit composition **9**, 300–301
–, hormonal **9**, 301
–, lead arsenate **9**, 300–301
–, oil **9**, 300
Spreadability **39**, 275
Spreading coefficient **11**, 400
Sprouting, radiation inhibition of sprouting of **24**, 201–204
Squalene, olive oil and **31**, 466, 473
–, structure of **23**, 18, 19
Squash **15**, 233
–, effect of cold storage on **2**, 331, 334
–, loss of thiamine on processing **6**, 290
–, F value for industrial processing of **2**, 102
Squid **39**, 344
SSS, *see* Soluble starch synthase
Stability, films, protein structure and **33**, 394–395
–, foams, overrun **33**, 400–401
–, –, protein structure and **33**, 398–400
–, folates, during cooking or thermal processing **33**, 47–51
–, –, effects of aqueous extraction **33**, 49
–, –, in milk products **33**, 51
–, –, intrinsic **33**, 40–47
–, –, monoglutamyl folates in aqueous solution at room temperature **33**, 45
–, β-galactosidase **38**, 35–39
Stabilization, IM meat preservation **39**, 85–88
Stabilizers, foam **12**, 324
–, ice cream **12**, 297–300
–, –, concentrations of carboxymethylcellulose **12**, 299
–, –, in HTST systems **12**, 299–300
–, ice pops and sherbets **12**, 300–301, 326
–, milk **12**, 301–302
–, oriental noodles **43**, 161
Stable isotope tracer (*see also* Radioactive tracer), by vitamin B6 **40**, 138–140
–, β-carotene **40**, 64, 72, 74
–, folate **40**, 86–90
–, for vitamin B6 **40**, 116
–, glycogen phosphorylase **40**, 138–140
–, total energy expenditure **40**, 175–176
Stachydrine in fruit products, relationship to browning **1**, 353
Stachyose, in cocoa beans **8**, 262
Stainless steel surfaces, microbial attachment **43**, 330–331
Staling of flavor in milk products **3**, 97
Standard deviation, fractional **40**, 29, 41
Stanton number **32**, 80
Staphylococcal enterotoxin, effects on gastrointestinal immunity **37**, 35
Staphylococcal nuclease, site-directed mutagenesis **35**, 283
Staphylococci, concentration of disinfectants destroying **2**, 135
–, in bakery products **2**, 82
–, in frozen food **6**, 200
–, toxin formation by **6**, 210
Staphylococcus albus, germicidal action of CPCl on **2**, 152
Staphylococcus aureus **13**, 253, 357–358, 381–382; **45**, 180
–, attachment **43**, 324, 328, 333, 335
–, canned food and **7**, 121
–, destruction of **3**, 130
–, effect of cathode rays on **3**, 163
–, – of concentration on germicidal power of cationic detergents **2**, 134, 135, 137, 140, 141, 147, 148, 152, 153, 162, 164
–, – of pH on thermal death point of **3**, 438
–, – of ultraviolet radiation on **3**, 151
–, growth rate of **7**, 103–104
–, lowest growth temperature **13**, 355–356
–, viable counts of **7**, 106
–, water requirements, nutrition and **7**, 107
–, –, oxygen and **7**, 109
–, –, stability of **7**, 110
Staphylococcus epidermidis, attachment **43**, 324, 328
Starch (*see also* Amylose *and* Amylopectin) **15**, 118; **39**, 60
–, acid-modified **38**, 294
–, biosynthesis, ADPglucose **41**, 34–37
–, –, alternative pathways **41**, 37–38
–, –, CAM plants **41**, 150–152
–, –, complete pathway **41**, 111–113

Starch, biosynthesis (*cont'd*)
–, –, enzymes, limiting **41**, 134–135
–, –, *glg* C and **41**, 131–134
–, –, initiation **41**, 107–110
–, –, leaves **41**, 148
–, –, manipulation **41**, 135–136
–, –, C_4 plants **41**, 148–150
–, –, rate **41**, 38–39
–, –, studies **41**, 33–34
–, caryposis **41**, 1–2
–, characterization **41**, 1
–, chocolate and **31**, 236, 247, 248, 296
–, content, of apples and pears **8**, 300
–, –, of fruits, changes in **8**, 331
–, corn and wheat **6**, 12
–, crosslinked **38**, 293
–, degradation **41**, 135–136
–, –, amylase **41**, 153–154
–, –, debranching enzymes **41**, 154–155
–, –, outside chloroplast **41**, 156–157
–, –, pathway **41**, 155–156
–, –, phosphorylase **41**, 153–154
–, dextrins **41**, 158
–, dietary fiber and **31**, 118–120, 140, 141, 190
–, –, analysis **31**, 142–146, 150, 152
–, –, intestinal bacteria **31**, 181, 183
–, –, properties **31**, 154–156, 158, 159, 165, 169, 170
–, digestion, human **41**, 157–158
–, dust explosions **6**, 37
–, flat sour bacteria spores in **18**, 174–178
–, gelatinization and retrogradation studies **38**, 123, 128–129
–, glassy state **38**, 123, 126–127
–, grains, effect of blanching on **2**, 322–327
–, –, – of heat and chemical on **2**, 318–321
–, –, – of milling on **2**, 321–322
–, –, gelatinization and nutritive value of **2**, 327–328
–, –, structure of **2**, 316–318
–, granules, amylopectin **41**, 13, 16, 20–23
–, –, amylose **41**, 13, 16, 20–23
–, –, dried **41**, 165
–, –, formation **41**, 110–111
–, –, lipids in **41**, 30
–, –, minor constituents **41**, 30
–, –, orientation **41**, 27–29
–, –, phosphorus in **41**, 30
–, –, proteins in **41**, 31–32
–, –, structure **41**, 13
–, green algae **41**, 4
–, in apples **8**, 318
–, –, trends in **8**, 391
–, in candies **6**, 29, 33
–, in cocoa beans and nibs **6**, 38
–, in dehydrated mashed potatoes **25**, 85–96
–, industrial, analysis **41**, 167–168
–, –, applications **41**, 163–164
–, in fish sausage and ham **12**, 411–412, 418, 421
–, in fruits **17**, 182
–, in kiwifruit during growth and ripening **29**, 291–292
–, in passion fruit **12**, 236–237
–, in peas **9**, 65–68
–, in pectins **11**, 52
–, in ripening fruits, hydrolysis **30**, 172
–, in roasted wheat, digestibility **30**, 218–219
–, in tea **17**, 231
–, in wheat flours, breadmaking and **29**, 262
–, –, fractionation **29**, 227–228
–, –, interchanging between two samples **29**, 228–230
–, –, separation **29**, 222–224
–, jellies, ingredients in **6**, 29
–, –, made by **6**, 33
–, –, molding of **6**, 36
–, –, tenderness of **6**, 12
–, leaves **41**, 3–4
–, licorice root and **7**, 343
–, lintnerized **41**, 168
–, manufacturing **41**, 164–166
–, measurement of **9**, 67–68
–, metabolism, *Arabidopsis thaliana* model **41**, 10
–, –, *Chlamydomonas reinhardtii* model **41**, 11
–, –, maize model **41**, 7–9
–, –, model comparisons **41**, 6–7
–, –, potato model **41**, 9–10
–, –, snapdragon model **41**, 10–11
–, –, wheat model **41**, 6–7
–, methodology **41**, 29
–, modification **41**, 168–169
–, modified, products from **38**, 293–294
–, molds in **6**, 12
–, molecules, crosslinking **41**, 168
–, Naegeli **41**, 168
–, native, products from **38**, 292–293
–, nomenclature **41**, 29
–, photosynthesis cells **41**, 139–140
–, polymers, biodegradable **41**, 169–170
–, potato **17**, 121–122
–, –, physical characteristics of **6**, 242
–, –, rehydration of **6**, 234
–, production wastes **17**, 115–122
–, properties **41**, 164–166

–, relation to maturity **9**, 67–68
–, – to texture **9**, 67
–, roots **41**, 3
–, scanning electron microscopy of **22**, 281–286
–, seeds **41**, 1–2
–, soluble (*see also* Soluble starch), in reconstituted potato granules **6**, 251
–, –, protective action on thiamine **6**, 261, 284
–, stabilized **38**, 293
–, storage tissues **41**, 117
–, sweetener conversion **41**, 169
–, swelling of granules **11**, 8
–, synthesis, genetic engineering **41**, 125–126, 130–131
–, –, vectors **41**, 126–127
–, trioses in hydrolysates **6**, 19
–, tubers **41**, 3
Starch–protein complex, in corn **17**, 117
Starch–water system, gelatinized, glass transition temperature as function of mass fraction **38**, 152–153
STAR (Italian) system, durability of **23**, 399–400
–, for retort packaging of processed foods **23**, 341–342
Starter bacteria **39**, 196, 201, 203, 215–225, 250
–, modified **39**, 258–259
Starters, in sauerkraut production **10**, 250–253
Starvation, effects on connective tissue **37**, 388–389
State diagrams **38**, 135–143
–, glass transition temperature, as function of mass fraction **38**, 152–153
–, –, location **38**, 199
–, references **38**, 137–138
Staudinger's viscosity "law" in food engineering applications **11**, 367
Stavudine **44**, 285
Steady shear flow **39**, 33–35, 44–48
Steady shear measurement **39**, 12–14
Steam-air cooks, for retorting **23**, 392–395
Steam coil heater, used in spray-drying **2**, 486
Steam ejector, freeze-drying and **7**, 176–177, 208
–, water removal and **7**, 178
Steam flush, for package air removal **23**, 373
Steam recompression **15**, 334
Steam refining, effect on tocopherol content of soybean oil **33**, 160, 162
Steam sterilization **32**, 4–9, 14, 20, 27
Stearates, polyoxyethylene **6**, 12
Stearic acid, chocolate and **31**, 250, 254, 275, 324, 325
–, hypolipidemic effect **35**, 4–5
–, olive oil and **31**, 463, 464
–, plasma lipid/lipoprotein response **36**, 269–270
Stearic acid in poultry fat **1**, 212
Stearyldimethylbenzylammonium chloride, structure of **2**, 121
Stearyltrimethylammonium bromide, structure of **2**, 121
–, therapeutic action of **2**, 143
Steel, use in spray dryers **2**, 490
Steel as a base for tin plate **3**, 363–366
Steeping, corn **38**, 278–280
–, wheat germ **23**, 276–277
Steepwater, absorption by corn **38**, 280–281
Steers **14**, 40
Stefan's problem **20**, 224
Steinert's disease **37**, 359–361
Stellate cell **40**, 16–17, 40
Stereochemistry **14**, 318
Stereum, growth rate of **7**, 98
Steric interaction, emulsion stability **34**, 92–94
Sterility **41**, 131
Sterilization, during thermal process **2**, 58–60, 73, 85, 89, 104
–, –, effect of number of cells on **2**, 66
–, ground fish and meat **12**, 410–411
–, heat, preservation of concentrated foods by **3**, 455–457
–, high-temperature, short-time **3**, 441–443
–, IM meat **39**, 86
–, in canning **3**, 446
–, microwave heating **43**, 127–128
–, of juices by filtration **3**, 445
–, pilot process for **3**, 442
–, potato starch **12**, 411
–, tests **32**, 6, 14–15
–, with exclusion of oxygen **3**, 443–444
Sterilizing value, calculation of **23**, 88
–, –, computer program **23**, 93
Sterilmatic retort **32**, 60–65
Steritort **32**, 60–65, 75
Steroid hormone, effect on collagen formation **28**, 279
Steroidogenesis, cardiolipin **37**, 271
Steroids, dietary fiber and **31**, 159, 161, 169
–, endogenous proteolytic enzymes and **31**, 379
–, structure of **23**, 18, 19

Sterols, in olive oil **31**, 463, 466, 467, 473
–, in tea **11**, 226–227
Stevia, chocolate and **31**, 272
Sticky point **39**, 117
Stigmasterol, olive oil and **31**, 467, 473
Stigmasterol in molasses **2**, 277
Stokes–Einstein equation, diffusion coefficient **34**, 28–29
Stokes' equation, creaming rate **34**, 130
Stokes' law **22**, 315
Stomach, endogenous proteolytic enzymes and **31**, 344, 345
Storage **14**, 62, 256–257
–, controlled-atmosphere **12**, 97–98
–, –, fruits and vegetables **12**, 127–136
–, –, of apples **12**, 97–98
–, diseases of mango fruits **21**, 271–274
–, effects **13**, 289–311
–, – on fish lipid oxidation **33**, 289
–, – on whey proteins **33**, 373
–, food deterioration **13**, 315–316
–, hypobaric **21**, 340
–, IM meat **39**, 93
–, low temperature, average life **13**, 325
–, –, commercial **13**, 323–327
–, –, temperatures **13**, 323, 325–327
–, methods for mango fruits **21**, 274–285
–, of canned foods, effect on vitamin content **1**, 89–98
–, of fish sausage and ham **12**, 417–418
–, of food (*see also* Decomposition), insect damage to **4**, 281–348
–, of oils, effect on tocopherol content **33**, 163–164
–, of olive oil **31**, 461, 470, 471
–, of passion fruit **12**, 220–233
–, –, experiments **12**, 220–221
–, –, temperature and humidity **12**, 221–229
–, –, weight losses **12**, 222–223
–, –, wrappings **12**, 220
–, of potatoes, and glycoalkaloid formation **21**, 319–323
–, proteins **35**, 338–339
–, refrigerated **12**, 97–98
–, –, and common, passion fruit **12**, 220–223, 229
Storage modulus **39**, 22–23
Storage stability, predicting for low-moisture foods **11**, 313–314
–, sorption isotherms for predicting **11**, 313–314
Storage substance **41**, 4
Storage tissues **41**, 117
Stores, scrubbed **12**, 128–130
–, –, scrubbers **12**, 129
–, ventilated **12**, 127–128
–, –, control **12**, 128
Strain, Hencky rate **39**, 15
–, oscillatory **39**, 21–22
–, shear **39**, 10–12
Strain differences, lactic cultures **37**, 80–82
Strange attractor **40**, 327
Strawberries **15**, 121; **16**, 216
–, ascorbic acid content of, effect of sunlight on **1**, 301
–, –, influence of oxygen on deterioration of **1**, 341
–, canned, corrosiveness of in enameled cans **3**, 371
–, effect of acidity on **3**, 338
–, – of freezing on **2**, 335–336
–, – of plasmolysis on **2**, 308
–, – of temperature on **3**, 17
–, – of –, of freezing temperatures on micro-organisms in **3**, 448
–, – of –, of ozone on **3**, 466
–, firming agent **5**, 145
–, microbiology of **6**, 181
–, micro-organisms in frozen **6**, 179
–, ozone treatment **45**, 192
–, pH of **3**, 432
–, processing of **3**, 349
–, rate of respiration in **3**, 17
–, survival time of pathogenic bacteria in frozen **6**, 166
–, volatile composition of **2**, 269
–, with sulfur added **3**, 352
Strawberry, allergy **42**, 11
–, *Fragaria ananssa* **44**, 207
Strawberry jam, sulfite fate during production of **30**, 28
Strawberry juice, ascorbic acid loss in bottling **1**, 63
–, canned, use of ascorbic acid in **4**, 377–378
–, deterioration of **1**, 328, 333, 341
Strawberry preserves and jams, color of **5**, 328–330
–, darkening of **5**, 311
Strecker degradation **14**, 184–185, 235–237, 259
–, of amino acids **19**, 199–200
–, products **12**, 37–39
–, –, evolution of carbon dioxide **12**, 37–38
Strength, tensile **14**, 100–101
Streptococci, bacteriocidal substances production **43**, 14
–, chocolate and **31**, 218
–, inhibition by antitrypsin **1**, 385

–, probiotics **43**, 15
Streptococci mastitis, germicidal action of Phemerol on **2**, 155, 182
Streptococcus agalactiae, control of by Cetavlon **2**, 151, 176
Streptococcus cremoris, germicidal action of lauryldimethylbenzylammonium chloride **2**, 155
Streptococcus faecium, for biological synthesis of long-chain folates **33**, 11–12
Streptococcus hemolyticus, germicidal action of ADBACl **2**, 147, 148
–, – of CPCl **2**, 152
Streptococcus thermophilus, lactase **38**, 58
–, potential lactase sources **38**, 86
Streptococcus viridans, germicidal action of ADBACI **2**, 147, 148
–, – of CPCl **2**, 15
Streptomycin **44**, 322
–, in control of *Salmonella* infection **3**, 231
–, ion exchanger reactions with **2**, 32
–, sterilization by cathode rays **3**, 187
Stress, analysis of in proofing dough **11**, 401
–, compressive **39**, 7–8
–, oscillatory **39**, 21–23
–, shear **39**, 4–6, 24–33, 28
–, tensile **39**, 7–8, 16
–, yield **39**, 6, 46, 48
Stress coefficient **39**, 13, 23
Stress difference **39**, 13–14
Stress overshoot **39**, 17
Stress relaxation test **39**, 19–20, 58
Stripping **15**, 351
Stroma **9**, 3, 4
–, endogenous proteolytic enzymes and **31**, 372, 399
Strontium, in wines **8**, 139
Strontium-90 **17**, 218
Strontium hydroxide, use of to form pectic acid **1**, 406
Structural identifiability **40**, 313
Structure factor **42**, 143
Strychnine **44**, 324
Stunning, electrical **39**, 125
Sturgeon, anaerobic bacteria in **2**, 351
–, Caspian Sea, anaerobic bacteria in **2**, 351
Subcutaneous analysis, ultrafiltration **40**, 191–193
Suberin, dietary fiber and **31**, 119, 139, 140
–, in epidermal vegetable tissue **2**, 304
Sublimation, freeze-drying and **7**, 181–185, 186
Substrate (*see also* Membrane transport) **40**, 158, 244–245, 260–261
–, enzyme absorption **17**, 50
Subtilin, effect on flat sour bacteria spores **18**, 185
Subtilisin disulfide bonds **35**, 287–289
–, stability **35**, 252
–, –, thermal **35**, 255
Succimer **44**, 318
Succinamidopropyl derivative, enzyme immobilization **35**, 222
Succinate, acceleration of trimethylamine oxide reduction by **2**, 369
Succinic acid **16**, 190, 216
–, competitive interference in oxidation of **1**, 384
–, in corrosion **3**, 339, 340
Succinic acid dehydrogenase, competitive interference by malonic acid **1**, 384
–, in wheat germ **23**, 240
Succinylation, oat globulin and β-lactoglobulin effects **35**, 330
–, protein emulsifiers **34**, 151
–, protein stability **35**, 272
Succinylsulfathiazole, addition of Triton K-12 **2**, 137
Succulometer **9**, 106
Suchard conche, chocolate and **31**, 307
Sucralose, chocolate and **31**, 271
Sucrose, added to cocoa bean juice **8**, 245
–, chocolate and **31**, 330
–, –, cocoa bean chemistry **31**, 232, 233
–, –, emulsifiers **31**, 281
–, –, milk **31**, 255, 256, 258, 263
–, –, milk crumb **31**, 284–286, 295, 296
–, –, packaging **31**, 324, 325
–, –, processing **31**, 220
–, –, sweeteners **31**, 264–271, 274, 275
–, –, *Theobroma cacao* L. **31**, 326, 327
–, content of apples and pears **8**, 300
–, dental and nutritional properties of **25**, 142–143
–, effect in dried egg **1**, 173
–, effect on browning in potatoes during storage **1**, 269–270, 273–274
–, – on calcium absorption **33**, 127
–, gel rigidity and **7**, 297
–, in apples **8**, 317
–, in chocolate candies **6**, 44
–, –, dehydration products **6**, 16
–, –, effect on survival of bacteria **6**, 167
–, –, – on thiamine destruction **6**, 261
–, –, stability of thiamine **6**, 30
–, –, structure and simpler reactions of **6**, 4
–, in coffee **8**, 280

Sucrose (*cont'd*)
–, in coffee beans, pyrolysis during roasting **30**, 110
–, in diet of rats **1**, 112
–, in fermented cocoa bean, disappearance of **8**, 260, 262
–, in fresh cocoa bean juice **8**, 239
–, in ice cream mix **3**, 92
–, in olive oil **31**, 459
–, in wines **8**, 137
–, *N*-nitroso compounds and **31**, 80
–, permeability to gel aluminosilicate **2**, 4
–, production from sugar beet **2**, 25
–, removal from pineapple waste **2**, 19
–, solution, taste intensity effect of temperature on **2**, 246
–, sweetness of **2**, 261
–, synthesis **41**, 148–150
–, –, lactase usage **38**, 22
–, whey protein foaming properties **33**, 401, 403–404
–, xerophilic molds and **7**, 115
Sucrose polyester, chocolate and **31**, 274
Sucrose–sucrose fructosyltransferase **43**, 3
Sudangrass, ascorbic acid content of, effect of manganese on **1**, 308
Sudan III, staining fat globules by **3**, 51
Sugar, acid actions **14**, 227–234
–, aqueous solutions, viscosity temperature dependence **38**, 180–181
–, assimilation and fermentation **12**, 75–76
–, beet, composition of ion exchange treated juice **2**, 26
–, –, use of ion exchange in production **2**, 25–28
–, –, values of regenerant solutions **2**, 27
–, cane, composition of ion exchange treater juice **2**, 29–30
–, chemical reactions of **6**, 2
–, chocolate and **6**, 37; **31**, 330
–, –, alkalization **31**, 247, 248
–, –, cocoa butter **31**, 225, 226, 231–233, 235
–, –, conching **31**, 297, 307
–, –, emulsifiers **31**, 281
–, –, milk **31**, 255, 256, 258, 263
–, –, milk crumb **31**, 285–288, 291
–, –, processing **31**, 218, 221, 238, 242, 243
–, –, refining **31**, 292, 295
–, combination of milk solids and **6**, 2
–, content of cocoa bean juice **8**, 239
–, – of –, of frozen peas **8**, 102
–, corn, ion exchange treatment of **2**, 30
–, dental caries and **25**, 139
–, dietary fiber and, analysis **31**, 143, 145
–, –, components **31**, 122, 123, 141
–, –, dicotyledonous plants **31**, 126, 127, 130, 131
–, –, intestinal bacteria **31**, 175–177, 181, 186
–, effect of heat upon **6**, 16
–, effect on calcium absorption **33**, 127
–, – on discoloration **3**, 34–35
–, – on β-galactosidase stability **38**, 36
–, – on yeast survival **3**, 448
–, endogenous proteolytic enzymes and **31**, 410
–, fermentation data, analysis of variance **5**, 188
–, flat sour bacteria spores in **18**, 174–178
–, flavorful products from thermal treatment of **19**, 185
–, fragmentation products, in browning reaction **32**, 127–132
–, high intake, linkage to metabolic disorders **42**, 212
–, in abalone **23**, 162–163
–, in apples and pears **8**, 300, 312, 317
–, in candy making **6**, 15
–, in coffee **8**, 280
–, influence of concentration on bacterial resistance to heat **2**, 67
–, influence on milk powder solubility **3**, 101
–, in fruits **17**, 182–183
–, –, changes during browning **1**, 354–357
–, in honey **24**, 302–303
–, in kiwifruit, composition during ripening **29**, 295
–, –, during growth and ripening **29**, 291–292
–, –, fresh, frozen, canned **29**, 294
–, in meat curing **29**, 6–7
–, in olive oil **31**, 457, 479
–, in passion fruit **12**, 236
–, in peas, loss in processing **9**, 69–70
–, –, relation to maturity **9**, 68–69
–, in precooked frozen foods **6**, 199
–, in soy sauce **10**, 82
–, in tea **11**, 221–222; **17**, 231
–, in vegetables, effect of blanching on **1**, 68
–, invert, of fruits **17**, 177
–, in wheat germ **23**, 205–206, 230, 231
–, in wines **6**, 73, 84; **8**, 148
–, liberated from pectinic acids **11**, 13
–, loss of in blanched vegetables **8**, 68
–, malabsorption **38**, 2–4
–, mango fruits **21**, 238–239, 246, 259–260
–, manufacturing wastes **17**, 122–126
–, modification of properties **6**, 20

–, nitrogen in the ring **14**, 191–192
–, *N*-nitroso compounds and **31**, 55, 82, 84
–, plasticization and antiplasticization by **38**, 156–159
–, preference for, in relation to blood glucose **1**, 138
–, protection of bacteria during freezing by **6**, 169
–, protein stability effects **35**, 290–294
–, protein thermal behavior effects **35**, 327
–, reactions with amino acids **3**, 246, 249; **17**, 232–233
–, – with nitrogenous compounds **3**, 241–290
–, reactive fragments **14**, 188–189
–, reducing **17**, 232–233
–, –, effect on browning in potatoes **1**, 262–263, 268–271, 273–274, 277–278, 285
–, structures and simpler reactions of **6**, 4
–, ultraviolet radiation of **3**, 151
–, use in canning **3**, 350, 351
–, whiteness of **5**, 311–316
Sugar–amine model system, pyrazine formation **30**, 108
–, –, with various sugars **30**, 108
–, roasted food flavor and **30**, 108
Sugar beet, dicotyledonous plants **31**, 124, 130
–, dietary fiber and **31**, 146, 190
–, intestinal bacteria **31**, 176, 183, 185–187
Sugar–bisulfite addition compounds, analytical procedures **5**, 59
–, bleaching **5**, 104, 146
–, nature of **5**, 55
–, reaction equilibrium constant **5**, 63
–, reaction velocity constants **5**, 71
–, sulfitation **5**, 98
Sugarcane production, and ethanol production **32**, 191, 197–204, 211–215
Sugar–protein interaction **3**, 101–102
Sugary 1, characterization **41**, 110–111
–, debranching **41**, 154–155
–, effects **41**, 40
Sulfaguanidine, addition of Triton K-12 **2**, 137
Sulfamethoxazole **44**, 292
Sulfanilamide, fish preservation and **7**, 69–70
Sulfasalazine **44**, 300
Sulfates, alkyl-aryl **14**, 355
–, aryl alkyl polyether **14**, 352–353
–, in wines **8**, 137, 156, 164
Sulfathiazole, fish preservation and **7**, 69
Sulfation **14**, 252–253
Sulfenates **14**, 309
Sulfhydryl and disulfide groups, amperometric titration of **24**, 13–22
–, color reagents for **24**, 27
–, determination of **24**, 3–6
–, –, methods for meats **24**, 6–28
–, in meats **24**, 1–111
Sulfhydryl compounds as antioxidants **3**, 96
–, in heat treatment of milk **3**, 74, 75, 82
Sulfhydryl enzymes, poisons for **1**, 381–382
Sulfhydryl groups **15**, 68, 79
–, chlorine and **7**, 134, 156
–, estimation of **19**, 323
–, fish freshness and **7**, 62–63
–, in heated milk proteins **19**, 168
–, *N*-nitroso compounds and **31**, 73
–, role in enzymic food browning **19**, 100–102
Sulfide, in young wines **8**, 159, 160
Sulfite, freeze-dried citrus juices and **7**, 228
Sulfite-induced asthma **43**, 201
Sulfite oxidase, deficiency, asthmatic reaction to sulfites and **30**, 54
–, –, congenital, human **30**, 36
–, –, induced by high tungsten/molybdenum diet, rat **30**, 36–37
–, purification and properties **30**, 33
–, sulfite conversion to sulfates **30**, 33–35
Sulfites (*see also* Sulfiting agents) **14**, 169, 246–259
–, adverse reaction induction, anaphylactoid **30**, 47, 58
–, –, contact sensitivity **30**, 47, 58
–, –, hypotension **30**, 47, 58
–, –, urticaria **30**, 57–58
–, as dehydrated mashed potato additives **25**, 109–111
–, asthma induction (*see also* Asthma) 2-3 **30**, 47–57
–, bound **5**, 125
–, chemistry of **5**, 99
–, combined, metabolism, 3-deoxy-4-sulfohexosulose metabolism **30**, 37–38
–, –, sulfited proteins, conversion to sulfates **30**, 37
–, complexes with quinones **30**, 10
–, cytotoxicity in cell cultures **30**, 47
–, daily intake from various foods **30**, 3, 15–17, 31
–, effect on adhesive properties of pea coats **2**, 315
–, exposure assessments, from atmosphere **30**, 32
–, –, from drugs as antioxidants **30**, 31–32
–, –, from foods **30**, 30–31

Sulfites (*cont'd*)
–, fate in foods **30**, 22, 27–30
–, – in –, during strawberry jam production **30**, 28
–, – in –, in dehydrated vegetables **30**, 27–28
–, – in –, in hard sweet biscuit doughs **30**, 27
–, – in –, processing and **30**, 29
–, – in –, SO_2 absorption and **30**, 28–29
–, – in –, storage and **30**, 29
–, free, metabolism, diffusion-limited metabolism **30**, 34–35
–, –, –, oxidation to sulfates **30**, 33–35
–, –, –, sulfite oxidase deficiency and **30**, 36–37
–, –, products, urinary excretion rate **30**, 36
–, –, *S*-sulfonate nonenzymatic production **30**, 35–36
–, –, thiosulfate production, enzymatic reaction **30**, 35
–, future research **30**, 63–64
–, induced asthma **42**, 12–13
–, natural occurrence in alcoholic beverages, formation by yeast strains **30**, 6–7
–, – in –, limitations **30**, 6
–, – in –, residual SO_2 **30**, 7
–, reactions with anthocyanins **30**, 26
–, – with ascorbic acid **30**, 24
–, – with carbonyls **30**, 9, 22–23
–, – with β-carotene **30**, 25
–, – with enzyme-bound FAD, FMN, and NAD **30**, 25
–, – with fatty acids **30**, 27
–, – with hydroxycobalamin **30**, 24
–, – with nucleic acids **30**, 26
–, – with nucleotides **30**, 25–26
–, – with proteins and amino acids **30**, 23–24
–, – with reducing sugars **30**, 23
–, – with thiamine **30**, 24
–, – with vitamin K3 **30**, 24
–, residue analysis **30**, 2, 17–21, 27
–, –, aeration–oxidation method **30**, 27
–, –, critical evaluation **30**, 19–21
–, –, food processing and **30**, 30
–, –, free SO_2 **30**, 18–19, 27
–, –, radiolabeling **30**, 27
–, –, total SO_2 **30**, 19
–, sensitivity to, methods of evaluation **30**, 59–61
–, SO_2 liberation, pH and **30**, 21
–, toxicity, acute, of high doses **30**, 38
–, –, animal, acute, intraperitoneal and intravenous **30**, 39–40
–, –, antimutagenicity **30**, 46
–, –, human, absence by chronic administration **30**, 39
–, –, mutagenicity, absence in variety of systems **30**, 45–46
–, –, –, carcinogenicity, negative results **30**, 44–45
–, –, –, comutagenic with UV **30**, 46
–, –, –, in some *in vitro* systems **30**, 45
–, –, relative of free and combined sulfites **30**, 3–4
–, –, subchronic and chronic **30**, 39–44
–, –, –, with diets **30**, 41–44
–, –, –, with drinking water **30**, 41, 42
–, –, teratogenicity, negative results **30**, 46–47
Sulfite waste liquor, yeast production from, diagram **18**, 100
Sulfiting agents (*see also* Sulfites), CFR sections for use of **30**, 4, 5
–, food applications, as antimicrobial agents, pH and **30**, 11–12
–, –, –, selectivity **30**, 11–12
–, –, –, substitutes for **30**, 62
–, –, as antioxidants **30**, 12
–, –, –, substitutes for **30**, 62
–, –, as bleaching agents **30**, 13
–, –, –, substitutes for **30**, 63
–, –, as processing aids **30**, 13
–, –, enzymatic browning inhibition **30**, 10–11
–, –, –, substitutes for **30**, 61–62
–, –, history **30**, 7
–, –, mycotoxin degradation **30**, 17
–, –, *N*-nitrosodimethylamine formation inhibition in malt **30**, 17
–, –, nonenzymatic browning inhibition **30**, 9–10
–, –, –, substitutes for **30**, 62
–, –, secondary uses **30**, 13
–, GRAS (Generally Recognized as Safe), theoretical yield and solubility **30**, 4, 5
–, production in USA **30**, 8
Sulfiting potatoes, effect on browning after dehydration **1**, 266–268, 278–279, 285
Sulfocyanides, use in pectin extraction **1**, 403
Sulfonamides, competitive inhibition of enzymes by **1**, 394
–, control of in *Salmonella* infection **3**, 231
S-Sulfonate, sulfite nonenzymatic conversion to **30**, 35–36
Sulfonated coals, properties of **2**, 4
Sulfonic acid, adsorption of amino acids by exchanges **2**, 34
Sulfonic acid type cation exchanger **2**, 5
Sulfoxides **14**, 303–304

Sulfur **14**, 256–259
–, added in food canning **3**, 352–355
–, burners **5**, 100
–, chocolate and **31**, 235
–, elemental in wine **8**, 171
–, endogenous proteolytic enzymes and **31**, 382, 410
–, in potato oil **2**, 275
–, in radish **2**, 274
–, *N*-nitroso compounds and **31**, 90
–, organic in wine **8**, 171
Sulfur compounds (*see also* Hydrogen sulfide), biosynthesis **22**, 83–90
–, changes during blanching of vegetables **8**, 83
–, contribution to meat flavor **18**, 56–58
–, crushed **22**, 103–114
–, in *Allium* **22**, 74–83
–, in bread **16**, 363
–, in cheese **16**, 276
–, in dehydrated mashed potatoes **25**, 104–105
–, in dough **16**, 371, 380, 420
–, in peppergrass **2**, 275
–, in pineapple **2**, 268
–, in tea **2**, 287
Sulfur dioxide, analyses for **5**, 122
–, application **5**, 130, 134
–, as inactivator of polyphenoloxidase **19**, 106–107
–, as a preservative **5**, 123
–, as a sanitizing agent **5**, 123, 126
–, bleaching action **5**, 103
–, brining of cherries **5**, 143
–, chemistry of **5**, 99
–, distillation procedures for total **5**, 119
–, effect of variations in, on the equilibrium constant of glucose bisulfite **5**, 73
–, effect on ascorbic acid loss in orange juice **1**, 348–349, 362
–, – on browning of dehydrated potatoes **1**, 260–261, 266–268, 279
–, – on carbon dioxide production in dried fruit **1**, 347, 360
–, – on heat processing **5**, 126
–, – on pectin in apple pulp **1**, 401
–, – on wines **6**, 87
–, free **5**, 114
–, –, iodometric titration **30**, 18–19
–, freeze-dried fruits and **7**, 224
–, –, gelatin manufacture and **7**, 248
–, fumes **5**, 130
–, inactivation of disulfide enzymes by **1**, 382–383, 386
–, in atmosphere, estimation and national standards **30**, 32
–, in "barrelling" fruits **5**, 143
–, influence on browning in dried fruit **1**, 360–364
–, in food as stress factor **4**, 116
–, inhibition of enzymes by **1**, 386, 388
–, – of fermentation by **5**, 77
–, – of nonenzymatic browning by **5**, 54
–, in kiwifruit juice during vinification **29**, 303–305
–, in laboratory steeping **38**, 289
–, in transportation and storage of fruits **5**, 146
–, in wine **5**, 117
–, liquid, application **5**, 133
–, loss in dried apricots **1**, 330, 342–345, 360–362
–, measurement of browning in dried apricots **1**, 329
–, *N*-nitroso compounds and **31**, 90
–, preservation of fruits and vegetables with **5**, 53
–, recommended amount in wine making **6**, 89
–, role in corn wet milling **38**, 282–283, 285–286
–, total **5**, 119
–, –, Monier–Williams method **30**, 19
–, total and free, in wines **8**, 135, 157
–, treatment of grapes by **3**, 465
–, used in storage of wines **8**, 162
–, use in dried fruits and vegetables **5**, 141
–, – in fruit juices **9**, 254–257
Sulfur house, construction **5**, 142
–, operation **5**, 142
Sulfuric acid, in grape waste **2**, 16
–, use in regeneration of cation exchanger in pineapple industry **2**, 20
–, – in sugar beet industry **2**, 27
–, use to inhibit oxidation of ascorbic acid **1**, 293
Sulfurous acid, application **5**, 132
–, in food preservation **3**, 460–462
–, inhibition of enzymic browning by **3**, 30–32
–, in musts and wines **8**, 164
–, storage of fruit pulps with **1**, 401
–, used in storage of wines **8**, 162
Sulindac **44**, 297
Sumatriptan **44**, 297, 320
Sun-drying **39**, 73–74
Sunflower seed oil, reversion problems in **4**, 194

Sunflower seeds **16**, 12
–, phytate content **45**, 13
Sunlight, carcinogen risk assessment and **31**, 2, 3, 47
–, statistics **31**, 13, 15, 16
Supercooling **13**, 247–248, 264–266, 273, 311–313
Supercritical carbon dioxide extraction **42**, 253
Superoxide anion, control **33**, 302–303
–, formation **33**, 236
Superoxide dismutase, control of superoxide anion with **33**, 302
Superprecipitation test **19**, 325
Supersonic waves, destruction of microbial agents by **1**, 373
Supinine **45**, 73
Supplementation, methionine **40**, 161–162
Supplements, calcium, effects on calcium bioavailability **33**, 144–147
Surface-active agents, action on cell membrane by **1**, 378–379
Surface-active ions, affinity for proteins **1**, 379
Surface area-to-volume ratio **39**, 195
Surface hydrophobicity, heating effects **34**, 148–149
–, proteins **34**, 127–128
Surface pressure, charged protein film **34**, 40
–, desorption rates and **34**, 53–54
–, β-lactoglobulin **34**, 42–44, 53
–, proteins **34**, 16
–, –, as emulsifiers **34**, 112
–, steady-state, ionic strength and **34**, 43, 45
–, –, net charge and **34**, 42–43
–, –, salt effect **34**, 49, 51
–, time-dependent changes **34**, 22–23, 26–27, 42
–, time to **34**, 18
–, versus concentration **34**, 37–38, 41
Surface tension **34**, 3–4
–, salt solutions **35**, 296
Surface viscosity, proteins **34**, 124–125
Surfactant antiadhesive agents **43**, 353
Surfactants (*see also* Emulsifying agents) **34**, 2
–, adsorption kinetics **34**, 33–34
–, interfacial properties **34**, 104–106
Surimi **39**, 351
Suspensions, flow of **11**, 416
–, heat transfer to **11**, 422
–, role in fluid consistency **11**, 365
Sutures, surgical, sterilization of by cathode rays **3**, 163
Swedes, dehydrated, thiamine in **6**, 300
–, effect of blanching on **1**, 68
Sweet clover, toxic compound in **1**, 125
Sweet corn, effect of quality on sensory tests **2**, 230
Sweetener conversion **41**, 169
Sweetener-induced taste **42**, 211–236
–, gustducin/transducin involvement **42**, 227–229
–, multiple transduction pathways **42**, 233–234
–, proposed pathways **42**, 234–235
–, receptor-independent activation **42**, 230–232
–, transduction pathway, adenylyl cyclase cascade involvement **42**, 219–223
–, –, downstream components **42**, 219–227
–, –, phosphoinositide transduction pathway role **42**, 224–227
Sweeteners, amphipathic nonsugar, receptor-independent activation **42**, 230–232
–, chemical structures **42**, 216
–, multipoint attachment theory **42**, 215, 217
–, Nofre–Tinti model **42**, 217
–, recognition by taste-receptor cells **42**, 214–219
–, responses of mammalian species to **42**, 213
–, Shallenberger/Acree AH–B model **42**, 215
Sweetening agents, in meat curing **29**, 6–7
Sweet molecule, chemical aspects **42**, 215–217
Sweetness, age-related taste threshold **44**, 257, 258
Sweet potatoes **15**, 231
–, ascorbic oxidase activity in **3**, 16
–, blanching of **2**, 323, 324
–, carotenoid pigments in **2**, 306, 328
–, effect of killing on tissues of **2**, 309
–, expansion of lamellae in **2**, 319
–, tyrosinase in **3**, 15
–, F value for industrial processing of **2**, 102
–, wastes **17**, 86
Sweet products, from tropical fruit **17**, 195–196
Sweets, British term **6**, 6
Sweet-taste transduction, amiloride-sensitive **42**, 229–230
Sweet whey powder (SWP), amino acid composition of **19**, 158
–, lipids in **19**, 187
–, use in bakery and confectionery products **19**, 151

Swenson spray dryer, heat and materials balance of **2**, 512–513
–, operation of **2**, 414–420
–, secondary drying in **2**, 501
–, thermal efficiency of **2**, 506
Swimming cells **41**, 11
Swiss chard, total folate content, table **33**, 40
Swiss cheese, flavor **39**, 245
–, histamine poisoning **39**, 346
–, lactate **39**, 198, 200
–, lipolysis **39**, 201, 205
–, peptidases **39**, 224
–, peptides **39**, 231
–, proteolytic agents **39**, 211
–, ripening **39**, 255
–, texture **39**, 176
Swordfish, green discoloration of **7**, 55–57
–, jellied meat of **7**, 57
Sycamore cells, dietary fiber and **31**, 127, 128
Sympathomimetic drugs, smell sensation effects **44**, 323–324
–, taste sensation effects **44**, 313–314
Symphytine **45**, 75
Symphytum (comfrey) **45**, 74–76, 91
Symphytum uplandicum (Russian comfrey) **45**, 74–75
Symviridine **45**, 75
Synaptotagmin **45**, 30
Synbiotics **43**, 16, 17
Synchronizer, bioperiodicity **40**, 219–220
Syneresis **39**, 174, 185–186, 190–191; **41**, 166
Synthetases, in wheat germ **23**, 241
Syringaldehyde, in maple syrup **30**, 111
Syringic acid in molasses **2**, 277
Syrup added in canning **3**, 350, 351
– in –, ultraviolet radiation of **3**, 151
Syrup-packed product, convection in **32**, 52–54
Syrup production **41**, 163–164
SYSTAT software **40**, 221
Systemic lupus erythematosus, anti-cardiolipin antibodies **37**, 305
–, characterization **37**, 400
–, genetic basis **37**, 400
–, treatment **37**, 401
Systemic sclerosis **37**, 402

T cells, PGE_2 effects **35**, 100
T lymphocytes, activation by allergens **42**, 8
–, characterization **37**, 8
–, cytotoxic, gut-associated **37**, 19–21
–, effector functions **37**, 8
–, regulatory functions **37**, 8
–, splenic, aCLs binding **37**, 309–310
T_i-plasmid **41**, 126–128
Table wines, acidic components of **25**, 3–5
Takayanagi equations **34**, 272–274
Talin, chocolate and **31**, 271, 272
Tallow **43**, 296–297, 303, 305
Tallowiness in dry milk **3**, 93
TAL Pro-long **44**, 370
Tanako and Nikimoto's formulas **20**, 238
Tangerines **15**, 222
Tank installations **14**, 428
Tannic acid, as enzyme inhibitors **17**, 52
–, in fruits **17**, 177–179
Tannin extract, spherical formation during drying **2**, 472
Tannins (*see also* Chromogens) **27**, 191–208
–, analytical assay **13**, 191–195
–, animal toxicity of **27**, 195–204
–, bitterness in foods by **2**, 260
–, carcinogenesis and **27**, 206–208
–, chemical behavior **27**, 191–194
–, condensed **13**, 187–190, 200
–, –, catechin **13**, 189–190
–, content changes **13**, 196–205, 208
–, effect on bacteria in wine **6**, 87
–, formation of **17**, 223–225
–, hydrolyzable **13**, 187–189, 208
–, in apples and pears **8**, 300, 352, 353
–, in cocoa beans **8**, 267
–, in cocoa beans and nibs **6**, 38
–, in fermentation **17**, 265
–, in tea **2**, 284; **17**, 217, 220–227, 258–259
–, medical use **27**, 205–206
–, metabolism **27**, 203–204
–, microbial inhibition by **27**, 194
–, molecular size **13**, 208
–, origin **17**, 224
–, precipitation of, in cocoa bean juice **8**, 250
–, separation of **17**, 220–223
–, structure of **17**, 222–223
–, vegetable **13**, 186–190
Tansy ragwort (*Senecio jacobaea*) **45**, 70, 72
Tao's charts **20**, 239–246
Tapioca, expansion of lamellae of **2**, 319
–, gum drops produced with **6**, 34
Tapioca starch, gelatinization temperature of **2**, 319
Taraxacum officinalis (dandelion), inulin **43**, 3, 9, 39–40
"Target theory" **15**, 73
Tarichatoxin, isolation of **18**, 151
Taro, loss of thiamine on processing **6**, 290

Tartaric acid, effect on browning in fruit products **1**, 358
–, – on corrosion **3**, 338
–, – on saltiness **2**, 260
–, in fruit juices **9**, 262–264
–, method of removal from grape waste **2**, 15–17
Tartary buckwheat (*Fagopyrum tartaricum*) **44**, 396, 397, 406
–, nutritional function **44**, 409
–, processing **44**, 414
Tartness, of wine **25**, 3–4
Tartrate, precipitation of, during vinification **25**, 12–13, 16–23
Taste (*see also* Flavor), glycyrrhizin assay and **7**, 369
–, licorice and **7**, 353
–, loss of **32**, 245–246
–, sense of, and food preferences **32**, 243
–, temperature and **7**, 25–26
Taste buds **42**, 213–214; **44**, 250, 251
Taste cells **44**, 250, 251
–, apoptotic pathways **44**, 251
–, neural connections **44**, 252–253
Taste factors in meat **10**, 398–400
Taste panels **15**, 131
Taste perception, chemesthesis relationship **44**, 253
–, disease-related losses **44**, 264, 265–269
–, –, Alzheimer's disease **44**, 280–282
–, –, cancer **44**, 275–280
–, –, endocrine disease **44**, 267
–, –, local conditions **44**, 268
–, –, nervous disease **44**, 265
–, –, nutritional disease **44**, 266
–, elderly people **44**, 248–249, 256–262
–, –, suprathreshold perceptual losses **44**, 260–262
–, –, taste bud/tongue papillae changes **44**, 252
–, –, threshold recognition/detection elevation **44**, 256–260
–, –, trigeminal stimulants **44**, 257–258
–, for sweetness, depression of **1**, 138
–, learned associations **44**, 248
–, medication effects **44**, 248, 249, 283–284, 285–318, 319
–, neural pathway **44**, 252–253
–, physiology **44**, 250–253
–, –, age-related changes **44**, 252
–, role in food intake/digestion **44**, 248
–, thermal taste **44**, 253
–, transduction pathways **44**, 252
Taste-receptor cell, recognition stage **42**, 214–219
Tasters, expert, function of **7**, 6
Taste tests, classification of **7**, 11
TATA box **36**, 97
–, 7S globulins **36**, 105
Taurine, in abalone **23**, 156–157
Tauri's disease **37**, 378–379
Tazobactam **44**, 292
TBA, *see* 2-Thiobarbituric acid
TCA, *see* Trichloroacetic acid
TCA-cycle intermediates, benzoic and salicylic acids effects on micro-organism oxidation of **11**, 342–343
Tea **24**, 229–286
–, acids **11**, 216–217
–, aldehydes **17**, 239
–, –, formation **11**, 220
–, alkaloids **17**, 234–236
–, amides **11**, 218–219
–, amino acids **11**, 218–219; **17**, 236–241; **24**, 240–241
–, ammonia formation **11**, 220
–, analyses of commercial teas **11**, 249
–, analysis by grades **11**, 246
–, aroma **11**, 228–231; **17**, 233
–, aroma development **24**, 256–257
–, biochemistry **17**, 260–272
–, biological value **17**, 278–279
–, black tea **24**, 251–261
–, caffeine **17**, 234; **24**, 241–243
–, –, in plant **11**, 232
–, caffeine and other purines **11**, 217–218
–, carbohydrates **17**, 231–233; **24**, 243
–, carbon dioxide formation **11**, 220
–, catechin mixture **11**, 212
–, catechins (flavanols) **5**, 292; **11**, 210–214
–, –, formulae **11**, 210–211
–, chemical changes in fermentation **11**, 234–241
–, chemical constituents **17**, 219–260
–, chemical evaluation **11**, 245–248
–, chemistry **17**, 215–292
–, –, leaves **11**, 207–232
–, –, plant other than leaves **11**, 232–233
–, –, pollen **11**, 232
–, chemistry and manufacturing **11**, 201–262
–, chlorophyll and carotenoids **24**, 245–246
–, chromatograms, flavanol fractions **11**, 212, 213
–, –, flavonols **11**, 214
–, clinical effects **24**, 269–271
–, comparison of dialysis of green and black **2**, 286

–, – of quercetin and catechins of **2**, 284–285
–, composition **24**, 232–251
–, –, after fermenting **11**, 234
–, –, changes in processing **11**, 233
–, –, chemical and biochemical components **24**, 233–249
–, –, distillate of black tea **2**, 286–287
–, –, factors affecting **24**, 248–249
–, –, leaves **11**, 207
–, –, seisin-oolong tea oil **2**, 287
–, crude fiber **11**, 224
–, depsides **11**, 216–217
–, dyes from **17**, 219
–, enzymes **17**, 217; **24**, 233–236
–, –, in leaves **11**, 231
–, enzyme-substrate studies **11**, 234–237
–, essential oils **11**, 228–231; **17**, 251
–, evaluation of quality **11**, 241–250
–, fermentation **5**, 293; **24**, 253–260
–, flavan molecule **11**, 209
–, flavanols (catechins) **5**, 292; **11**, 210–214
–, –, formulae **11**, 210–211
–, flavones **5**, 292
–, –, structure **11**, 209
–, flavonols, in brew **11**, 214–215
–, –, in plant **11**, 232
–, –, structural formulae **11**, 214
–, flavor constituents **2**, 284
–, freeze-drying **7**, 231
–, general analyses **11**, 207, 208
–, glossary of tasting terms **11**, 242–244
–, green tea **24**, 261–263
–, history **24**, 229–230
–, host plant–pest relationships **24**, 271
–, influence of light on constituents **11**, 233
–, initiation of fermentation **11**, 233
–, instant **17**, 219, 278–279; **24**, 272–273
–, isotope use in research **11**, 250
–, Legg cutter **11**, 206
–, leucoanthocyanins **11**, 215
–, –, structural formulae **11**, 215
–, lipids **11**, 226–227; **24**, 243–244
–, manufacture **17**, 216–219
–, –, in India **11**, 204
–, –, in Russia **11**, 205
–, methods of processing **11**, 203–207
–, minerals **24**, 246–248
–, nitrogenous substances **11**, 218–221
–, non-phenolic substances **11**, 217–228
–, nutrients **11**, 224–226
–, optical rotations of extractable fractions **2**, 286
–, organic acids **11**, 223–224
–, organoleptic evaluation **11**, 248–250
–, organoleptic properties **24**, 263–267
–, oxidation in fermentation **11**, 240, 241
–, oxidation of gallocatechins **11**, 235–236
–, pectins **11**, 222–223
–, phenolic substances **11**, 208–217
–, phosphate esters, nucleotides, and caffeine **24**, 241–243
–, pigments **11**, 226–227
–, polyphenols **8**, 267; **24**, 236–240
–, –, and enzymic browning **19**, 109–112
–, polysaccharides **11**, 221–222
–, potential by-products **24**, 268–269
–, precursors of aroma **8**, 279, 281
–, processing changes **24**, 248–263
–, proteins **11**, 218–221
–, purines **11**, 217–218
–, relation of flavonoids to quality **5**, 293
–, research needs **11**, 251; **24**, 273
–, resinous substances **17**, 244–245
–, standards on Indian tea **11**, 247
–, steps in manufacture **11**, 204–207
–, sterols **11**, 226–227
–, storage **24**, 266–268
–, sugars **11**, 221–222
–, table of essential oil compounds **11**, 229
–, tasting and terms used **11**, 241–245
–, taxonomy **11**, 202
–, theanine **11**, 218–219
–, thearubigen formation **11**, 238–241
–, trace substances **11**, 237–238
–, triterpenoids **24**, 244–245
–, types and grades **2**, 284; **11**, 203; **17**, 215
–, vitamins **11**, 224–226
–, volatile compounds **11**, 228–231; **24**, 248
–, waxes **11**, 226–227
–, withering process **11**, 233
TEAE-cellulose, for monoglutamyl folate separations **33**, 26
Tea leaves, fermentation in **3**, 16
–, respiration in **3**, 14
Tea lignans **44**, 207
TEE, *see* Total energy expenditure
Teenagers, food attitudes **32**, 247–248
–, meal patterns **32**, 250–251
Teeth, xylitol effects on **25**, 137–180
Teleosts, marine, autolysis in **7**, 49
–, oxide content of **2**, 368
Tempeh, as fermented food **22**, 200
–, fermentation organisms **44**, 213
–, isoflavones **44**, 212, 213
–, phytic acid content **28**, 60
Temperature (*see also* Heating), cardiolipin fatty acyl composition **37**, 299
–, center-line in fluids in tubes **11**, 420–422

Temperature (*cont'd*)
–, chlorination and **7**, 151–152
–, chocolate and, alkalization **31**, 247
–, –, conching **31**, 296–298, 302, 303
–, –, milk **31**, 260
–, –, milk crumb **31**, 287, 289, 290
–, –, packaging **31**, 317, 318
–, –, processing **31**, 215, 217, 218, 222, 223, 239–243
–, –, refining **31**, 294
–, –, sweeteners **31**, 264, 266, 2689 269
–, –, tempering **31**, 308–312
–, –, *Theobroma cacao* L. **31**, 322
–, cold shortening effect in meat **21**, 161–170, 182–191
–, creaming action **39**, 276–277
–, Δ^6-desaturase, regulation **35**, 47
–, determination **13**, 350–355
–, –, by extrapolation **13**, 351–352, 355
–, –, reported for bacteria **13**, 353–354
–, dietary fiber and **31**, 129, 143, 164
–, distribution for plug flow **11**, 422
–, effects (*see also* Heat effects), in breadmaking **16**, 383
–, –, in food dehydration **15**, 335
–, –, in irradiated fungi **15**, 169
–, –, on binding of flavor compounds to whey proteins **33**, 411–412
–, –, on cardiolipin content **37**, 300
–, –, on carotenoids **15**, 231, 257
–, –, on enzymic reactions in low-moisture foods **11**, 314–316
–, –, on fish lipid oxidation **33**, 288
–, –, on mango **21**, 255
–, –, on phenol formation in curing smoke **29**, 124–125, 140
–, endogenous proteolytic enzymes and **31**, 395, 397, 398, 400, 403
–, energy costs **39**, 144
–, environmental factors **13**, 370–378
–, –, cultural conditions **13**, 377–378
–, –, explanation **13**, 378–381
–, –, humidity **13**, 376–377
–, –, incomplete freezing **13**, 370–371
–, –, solutes **13**, 371–375
–, –, supercooled substrates **13**, 375
–, flavor **39**, 131–132
–, flavor testing and **7**, 25–26
–, for enzyme inactivation in low-moisture foods **11**, 314–316
–, freshness **39**, 349–350
–, gelation **39**, 192
–, glass transition **39**, 117–118, 134–135, 150
–, glycoalkaloid formation in potato **21**, 319–323
–, high-temperature conditioning of meat **21**, 197–198
–, histamine poisoning **39**, 348
–, lactase selection and **38**, 33–35
–, lowest recorded **13**, 355–358
–, meat quality and animal stress **21**, 74–79, 132
–, microbial control **39**, 119–121
–, microbial growth during meat conditioning **21**, 199–206
–, minimum growth **13**, 349–396
–, *N*-nitroso compounds and, indirect contamination **31**, 94
–, –, nitrite/nitrate addition **31**, 76–78, 81, 82
–, –, processing **31**, 87, 89–91
–, olive oil and **31**, 466, 470
–, on meat emulsion **16**, 115ff, 143, 150
–, optima for low-moisture foods as affected by humidity **11**, 314–316
–, perception by oral cavity **29**, 168–169
–, physics of meat chilling **21**, 206–213
–, processing hams **21**, 124–128
–, process optimization **39**, 139, 140
–, quality factor **39**, 187–188, 253–254
–, reaction time and, lactase **38**, 70–76
–, ripening **39**, 253–254, 256–257
–, role in corn wet milling **38**, 286–287
–, thaw shortening in meat **21**, 170–173, 182–185
–, ultrasonic sensing **45**, 132–133
–, water requirements and **7**, 109
Temperature processes, cold storage **2**, 334
–, frozen foods **2**, 335
–, winter hardening **2**, 334
Temperature profile **32**, 50, 52, 54–56
Tempering, chocolate and **31**, 308–313
Tenderay process **14**, 69
Tenderization, aging **31**, 394, 395, 397–399, 401, 402
–, endogenous proteolytic enzymes and **31**, 345, 346, 411–413
–, enzymology **31**, 404, 407, 408
–, methods **26**, 142–146
Tenderizers, commercial **9**, 38–40
–, distribution of in meat **9**, 41
–, enzymes used **9**, 38–39
–, histological effects **9**, 41–44
–, liquid **14**, 51
–, producers of **9**, 38
Tenderness (*see also* Meat tenderness) **10**, 400–401; **14**, 42–43
–, IM meat **39**, 91

–, meat texture **14**, 33–165
–, –, slice **14**, 81–83
–, paired eating **14**, 131–132
–, scale **14**, 131
Tenderometer **9**, 63, 67, 74, 87, 101, 103, 105, 116
–, MIT denture **14**, 90–92
–, Swift's **14**, 97–98
–, Volodkevich bite **14**, 87–89
Tensile forces, acting on dough **11**, 398
Tensile strength, of fluids **11**, 399
Tensile stress **39**, 7–8, 16
Tensile test, for seal integrity in flexible packaging **23**, 350–351
Terbinafine **44**, 283, 318
Terbutaline **44**, 302
Terfenadine **44**, 289, 319
Tergitol 7, effect on influenza virus **2**, 138
Termamyl, dietary fiber and **31**, 143, 144
Termination, olive oil and **31**, 472
Terpene compounds, in black tea oil **2**, 287, 288
–, in onion oil **2**, 273
–, in strawberries **2**, 270
Terpenes **14**, 308–309
–, shoyu flavor and **30**, 283
d-Terpineol in orange peel oil **2**, 265
dl-Terpineol in strawberries **2**, 270
Terpin in strawberries **2**, 270
Tertiary butyl alcohol, solubility of DDT in **2**, 204
Testes, desaturase and elongate activity **35**, 81–82
–, linoleic acid deficiency **35**, 129
–, vitamin A **40**, 9, 11
Testosterone, effects on cardiolipin content **37**, 300
Tetanus toxin, effect of X-rays on **3**, 159
Tetracaine **44**, 320
Tetrachloroethane, solubility of DDT in **2**, 203
Tetrachloroethylene, carcinogen risk assessment and **31**, 26
Tetrachlorophenol, fish preservation and **7**, 67
Tetracyclines **44**, 292
n-Tetradecyldimethylallylammonium bromide, germicidal activity of **2**, 137
n-Tetradecyldimethylbenzylammonium chloride, germicidal activity of **2**, 137
n-Tetradecyltrimethylammonium bromide, germicidal activity of **2**, 137
5,6,7,8-Tetrahydrofolate, energy of activation for degradation in aqueous solution, table **33**, 50
–, oxidative degradation by air **33**, 44
–, preparation, 6-ambo form, chemical reduction of 7,8-H_2folate **33**, 8
–, –, –, electrochemical method **33**, 9
–, –, –, folic acid–sodium dithionite method **33**, 8
–, –, –, hydrogenation of folic acid in glacial acetic acid **33**, 8
–, –, 6S form, enzymatic reduction with dihydrofolate reductases **33**, 9
–, –, –, labeling at C-6 with tritium or deuterium **33**, 11
Tetrahydrofolic acid, oxidative degradation mechanism **33**, 42–43
Tetrahydronaphthalene, solubility of DDT in **2**, 203
Tetralin, solubility of DDT in **2**, 203
Tetraodon, *see* Puffer poisoning
Tetra-Pak unit **32**, 17–19
Tetrodotoxin, properties and pharmacology of **18**, 147–151
–, structure of **18**, 150
Texture **15**, 80
–, factors **14**, 38–65
–, measurement **14**, 64–136
–, –, chemical **14**, 114–125
–, –, histological **14**, 125–129
–, –, physical **14**, 65–114
–, –, sensory **14**, 129–136
–, of abalone **23**, 174
–, of cheese, *see* Cheese, texture
–, of foods, advances in research on **19**, 229–231
–, of freeze-dried foods **13**, 76–77
–, of IM meat **39**, 124–126
–, of meat **14**, 33–165
–, ultrasonic sensing **45**, 142–148
–, viscosity measurements **45**, 147–148, 149
Textured vegetable protein (TVP), isoflavone content **44**, 214–215
Texturized cheese **39**, 261
Texturometer **9**, 102–103
–, Christel **14**, 81
–, General Foods **14**, 93–95
Thai bamee noodles (*see also* Oriental noodles) **43**, 148
–, quality evaluation **43**, 171, 175, 180, 181
Thallium, in fermenting musts **8**, 137
Thaumatin, chocolate and **31**, 271, 272
Thawing **13**, 272–274
–, commercial processes **13**, 327–329

Thawing (*cont'd*)
–, effects on food **13**, 289–311, 317
–, of foods, heat transfer of **20**, 217–256
–, –, time estimation of **20**, 235–251
–, rates **13**, 278–287
Thaw rigor (*see also* Rigor mortis) **9**, 11, 23–26
Theaflavin **17**, 269–271
–, structure and role in tea fermentation **19**, 111–112
Theanine, in tea **11**, 218–219; **17**, 238
Thearubigens, formation in tea **11**, 238–241
–, formation of **17**, 269–271
Theobroma cacao L. **31**, 320, 328, 329
–, embryonic axis **31**, 326, 327
–, flushing **31**, 327
–, lipid metabolism **31**, 324, 325
–, plant pathology **31**, 328
–, secondary metabolism **31**, 325, 326
–, shoot organogenesis **31**, 322
–, somatic embryogenesis **31**, 322–324
Theobromine, added to alcoholic extract of cocoa **8**, 280
–, chocolate and **31**, 247
–, diffusion of, during fermentation of cocoa beans **8**, 263
–, in cocoa beans and nibs **6**, 38
–, in cocoa bean shell and pulp **8**, 260
–, in tea **17**, 235
Theophylline, in tea **17**, 236
Therapeutic drugs, antifolate effects **33**, 70–71
Thermal analysis, chemical modification **35**, 329–331
–, differential scanning calorimetry **35**, 319–320
–, kinetic studies, denaturation studies **35**, 344–345
–, –, methodology **35**, 343–344
–, protein–protein interactions **35**, 331–333
–, proteins **35**, 317–358
–, scanning microcalorimetric studies **35**, 321–322
–, thermodynamic studies **35**, 320–322
–, thermogravimetry **35**, 348–350
Thermal analyzer, schematic diagram **35**, 318
Thermal behavior, proteins, pH effects **35**, 323–325
–, –, salts effects **35**, 325–326
–, –, structure modifying agents **35**, 327–329
–, –, sugars and polyols **35**, 327
Thermal death time (TDT), curves, calculation **23**, 77, 79
–, –, errors in data **2**, 82–86
–, –, improvements in methods **2**, 86–88
–, –, interpretation of data **2**, 70–76
–, –, slope **2**, 52–53
–, –, use in measuring resistance of bacteria in foods **2**, 68–69
–, –, – in processes **2**, 50–58
–, F value **44**, 177
Thermal degradation, inositol phosphates **45**, 16
Thermal denaturation, proteins **35**, 244
Thermal efficiency of spray dryers **2**, 503
Thermal energy, *see* Energy
Thermal energy analyzer, *N*-nitroso compounds and **31**, 57, 67–69
Thermal impulse sealing of retort pouches **23**, 358–359
Thermally irreversible gels **34**, 221
–, dynamic versus isothermal conditions **34**, 238, 240
–, gelation **34**, 241–242
–, reasons for irreversibility **34**, 237–239
–, soluble and insoluble aggregates **34**, 241
–, thermal denaturation **34**, 240–241
Thermal polymers **10**, 199–200
Thermal processes, basic principles of **23**, 76–83
–, computerized estimation of **23**, 91–97
–, –, parametric values for **23**, 91–97
–, –, programs for **23**, 110–138
–, –, terminology for **23**, 108–109
–, –, without manual calculations **23**, 97–104
–, data required for **23**, 76–82
–, evaluations of **2**, 49
–, general method **2**, 49–51
–, improvements in **2**, 61
–, mathematical estimation of **2**, 51–61; **23**, 75–141
–, –, research needs for **23**, 104–106
–, procedures for determination of **23**, 83–91
–, thermal death time in **23**, 76–80
Thermal processing (*see also* Heat effects), current USA regulations **44**, 148–152
–, –, food service/retail operations **44**, 149
–, –, home cooking **44**, 149
–, –, meat processors **44**, 149–152
–, endpoint cooking temperature indicators **44**, 169–176
–, –, enzymatic methods **44**, 170–173
–, –, immunoassays **44**, 173–175
–, –, physical methods **44**, 175–176
–, –, USDA tests **44**, 170
–, folate stability during **33**, 47–51
–, meat/poultry products **44**, 147–186
–, microbial pathogens inactivation **44**, 152

–, –, kinetic parameters determination **44**, 163–166
–, –, kinetics **44**, 153–162
–, –, mathematical models **44**, 164–165
–, –, microbial survival curves **44**, 163–164
–, –, sample parameters **44**, 166
–, –, *D* values **44**, 152
–, –, *z* values **44**, 152
–, time–temperature integrators **44**, 176–185
–, verification of adequacy **44**, 166–185
–, – of –, color determination **44**, 167–169
–, – of –, thermocouples **44**, 166–167
–, – of –, thermometers **44**, 166–167
Thermal resistance of bacteria in foods **2**, 65
– of – in –, anaerobic bacteria in canned peas **2**, 71
– of – in –, effect of heat suspension medium on bacteria **2**, 67–68
– of – in –, – of nature of growing medium of bacteria on **2**, 66–67
– of – in –, – of number of cells on **2**, 66–70
– of – in –, method of measuring **2**, 68
Thermal sanitization, ozone sequential procedures **45**, 202
Thermal scanning, rigidity monitor **35**, 351
Thermal scanning rheological analysis, comminuted meat systems **35**, 352, 354–355
–, muscle proteins **35**, 351–353
–, nonmuscle proteins **35**, 354–357
–, protein gels **35**, 350–357
–, sinusoidal oscillatory tests **35**, 351
–, zig-zag oscillatory tests **35**, 351
Thermal separation, whey proteins **33**, 361–362
Thermal taste **44**, 253
Thermal treatment, mechanism of **17**, 273
–, of tea **17**, 272–278
Thermal unfolding, protein digestibility **35**, 189
–, reversible, proteins **35**, 240–246
–, –, theory **35**, 242
–, –, thermodynamic parameters **35**, 242
–, ribonuclease **35**, 188
Thermitase, thermal stability **35**, 255
Thermocouple probes, microwave temperature measurements **43**, 83
Thermodynamics of enzyme inactivation **17**, 37–39
Thermodynamic studies, proteins **35**, 320–322
Thermodynamic theory, emulsion stability **34**, 86–88
Thermogravimetry, proteins **35**, 348–350
Thermolysin, thermal stability **35**, 254
Thermometers/thermocouple probes, meat cooking adequacy **44**, 166–167
Thermomycolase, thermal stability **35**, 255
Thermoprocessed foods, filling of **23**, 364–369
–, flexible packaging for **23**, 305–428
–, microwave processing of **23**, 397–398
–, process determination for **23**, 380–386
Thermosetting, amorphous polymers **38**, 212–226
Thermovac Company **32**, 10
Thermovac Sterilpac Drum Filling System **32**, 11–13
Thiamine (*see also* Vitamin B) **15**, 127
–, effect of cathode rays on **3**, 168
–, freeze-dried pork and **7**, 218
–, in wheat germ **23**, 208, 209
–, loss in vegetables during blanching **8**, 74
–, retention of, in electronic cooking **3**, 139, 140, 142
–, –, in wheat germ **3**, 146
–, ultraviolet examination for **3**, 153
Thiamine content, deficiency **1**, 113, 117, 131
–, destruction in potatoes by sulfiting **1**, 261
–, of apples and pears **8**, 368
–, of canned citrus juices, effect of storage on **1**, 92
–, of eggs **1**, 153
–, of foods **1**, 41–46, 50
–, –, effect of can size on **1**, 86, 88
–, –, – of heat sterilization on **1**, 84–89
–, –, – of storage on **1**, 92–98
–, of plants, effect of climate on **1**, 306–307
–, of vegetables, effect of blanching on **1**, 79–81
–, requirements of rat **1**, 116–117
Thiamine disulfide method in determining reducing capacity of milk **3**, 75–78
Thiaminepyrophosphate, mitochondrial activity during avocado ripening and **30**, 173–174
Thiazoles, in potato products **25**, 105
Thiazolidine, *N*-nitroso compounds and **31**, 82, 83
Thickening, shear **39**, 5–6
Thienyl mercaptans in coffee **2**, 281
Thin-layer chromatography of histamine **24**, 134–135
Thinning, shear **39**, 5–6
Thioaldehyde in onion oil **2**, 273
Thiobarbituric acid, gelatin and **7**, 271
2-Thiobarbituric acid **17**, 21
–, in rancidity tests **17**, 33
Thioctic acid **16**, 366

Thioctic acid (*cont'd*)
–, in wheat germ **23**, 237
Thiocyanates **14**, 304–315
–, gelatin sols and **7**, 279
–, *N*-nitroso compounds and **31**, 60
Thiocyanic acid, in onion oil **2**, 273
Thiodipropionic acid, effect on growth **3**, 204
–, – on mortality of rats **3**, 205
–, pathologic effects of **3**, 207
–, toxicity of as an antioxidant **3**, 200
Thiolation, whey protein modification by **33**, 420–421
Thiol enzymes, endogenous proteolytic enzymes and **31**, 347
Thiol groups, effect on, gill lipoxygenase **33**, 296–297
–, whey protein gels **33**, 388–389
Thiol protease, endogenous proteolytic enzymes and **31**, 382
Thiol proteinase, endogenous proteolytic enzymes and **31**, 413
–, endopeptidases **31**, 352, 355–360
–, exopeptidases **31**, 348
–, nonmuscle cathepsins **31**, 364–366
–, proteinase activity **31**, 384
Thiols **14**, 169, 260–262, 268
β-Thiols, meat mutagen modulation **34**, 431
5-Thiomethylfurfural, in meaty aroma **18**, 58–59
Thionitrite esters, *N*-nitroso compounds and **31**, 61
Thiophene carboxy-2-aldehyde, in meaty aroma **18**, 59
Thiopropanal *S*-oxide, structure of **22**, 97
5-Thiopyridoxine **44**, 297
Thiosulfate, in inhibition of corrosion **3**, 342
–, sulfite enzymatic conversion to **30**, 35
Thiouracil **44**, 299
Thiourea, in browning control in frozen fruits **3**, 32
–, in darkening of apple juice **3**, 24
–, in inhibition of corrosion **3**, 343
–, in tallowiness of dried milk **3**, 96
–, oxidation products of **3**, 32
Thirst, licorice and **7**, 353
Thixotropic fluids **11**, 393; **32**, 46
Thixotropy **9**, 178–179
–, in fluid consistency **11**, 367
Thomsen's disease **37**, 383–384
Thoral, use in brewing industry **2**, 175
Thornton Canning Company **32**, 10
Thouet conche, chocolate and **31**, 304
Threonine **16**, 247
Thrombosis, anti-cardiolipin antibodies **37**, 304–305
–, dietary fat effects **37**, 181–185
Thromboxane **35**, 97–98
Thyme, antioxidant activity **42**, 248–249
–, health implications **42**, 264–267
–, monterpenes **42**, 250
Thymectomy treatment, for myasthenia gravis **37**, 367–368
Thymol **42**, 249–250
Thyroidectomy, effect on rats **1**, 124
Thyroid hormones, Δ^6-desaturase, regulation effects **35**, 45
–, in porcine stress syndrome **28**, 189–190
Thyroxine, effect of feeding to animals **1**, 130
Ticarcillin **44**, 293, 322
Tides, and shellfish poisoning **10**, 140–141
Tien and Geiger method, for study of heat conduction problems **20**, 229–230
Tilsit cheese **39**, 287
Time and motion studies, *see* Work methods design and simplification
Time-dependent flow behavior **32**, 45–46
Time domain spectroscopy, dielectric properties measurement **43**, 82
Time-independent flow behavior **32**, 45–46, 47
Time-intensity, flavor profile and **7**, 32–33
Time–temperature integrators, chemical **44**, 182–183
–, definition **44**, 177
–, enzymatic **44**, 180–182
–, ideal properties **44**, 177
–, meat/poultry products thermal processing adequacy evaluation **44**, 176–185
–, microbiological **44**, 179–180
–, phycoerythrin **44**, 184–185
–, physical **44**, 182–183
–, theoretical aspects **44**, 176–179
–, thermal death time (F value) **44**, 177
–, triose phosphate isomerase **44**, 183–184
–, types **44**, 179
Time–temperature scaling parameter, WLF plots **38**, 189–190
Time–temperature transformation reaction diagram **38**, 212–213
Timing, food intake **40**, 225–226
Tin, in wine **8**, 138, 198
Tin plate, cans, enameled **3**, 371–374
–, coating, porosity of **3**, 360–363
–, containers, corrosion studies with **3**, 376
–, –, headspace in **3**, 347, 348
–, –, processing in **3**, 348, 349

–, –, relation of to corrosion **3**, 356
–, –, steel base for **3**, 363–366
–, –, storage temperatures in **3**, 349–350
–, –, trace elements added to foods in **3**, 352–356
–, –, vacuum in **3**, 347
–, effect of acidity on **3**, 337–340
–, – of oxygen on **3**, 345, 346
–, electrolytic **3**, 374–377
–, inhibitors of corrosion in **3**, 342–344
–, manufacture of **3**, 329–334
–, measurements of corrosiveness of **3**, 344
–, mechanism of corrosion in **3**, 334–336
–, packaging and storage in **3**, 344–345
–, reactivity of foods in **3**, 340–342
–, testing of **3**, 366–371
–, weight of **3**, 356–360
Tin uptake, in peas **9**, 78
Tissue, adipose **14**, 37
–, connective **14**, 37, 39–43
–, –, determination **14**, 114–120
–, –, histological analysis **14**, 125–127
–, fat **14**, 37–38
Tissue-specific expression **41**, 128–129
Titanium, in wines **8**, 137, 198
Titin, endogenous proteolytic enzymes and **31**, 400, 401, 406, 408
Titration method for determining quaternary ammonium compounds **2**, 170
Titration test for quality of fish **2**, 382
Titron, solubility of DDT in **2**, 203
TLC, *see* Chromatography
TMAOase, *see* Trimethylamine oxidase
Tobacco, amino acids formed in **8**, 281
–, blended for aroma **8**, 284
–, licorice and **7**, 350–351
–, nitrosamines in **22**, 53–55
–, *N*-nitroso compounds and **31**, 72, 95, 97, 98
Tobacco mosaic virus, destruction of by supersonic vibrations **3**, 130
Tocainide **44**, 307, 321
α-Tocopherol (*see also* Tocopherols *and* Vitamin E) **17**, 31
–, antioxidant, chain-breaking **33**, 310
–, –, effectiveness, heat stability **42**, 258–263
–, –, function in membranes **33**, 207–211
–, –, in dried egg **1**, 181
–, binding to membranes **33**, 196–199
–, bioavailability, bran effects **33**, 172–173
–, –, fish oil effects **33**, 173
–, concentration, in membranes **33**, 212–214
–, –, in vegetable oils, table **33**, 161
–, content of vegetable oils, heat effects **33**, 164–165
–, deficiency **1**, 119
–, destruction by rancid fats **1**, 125
–, deuterated, incorporation into lipoproteins **33**, 176–177
–, distribution in plasma lipoproteins **33**, 174
–, diurnal/seasonal changes in plasma concentrations **33**, 176
–, exchange between lipoprotein classes **33**, 174–175
–, exchange rate across bilayers **33**, 214
–, form in vegetable oils **33**, 159
–, inhibition of lipid oxidation by microsomes **33**, 306
–, – of membrane peroxidation **33**, 210
–, – of *N*-nitrosamine formation in cured meat **29**, 60–61
–, in membranes, hemolysis inhibition in human erythrocytes **33**, 219
–, –, in phospholipid vesicles **33**, 217
–, –, permeability to ions or small molecules **33**, 218–219
–, –, physical effects, acyl chain order of phospholipid bilayers **33**, 216
–, –, platelet membrane fluidity **33**, 217–218
–, –, platelet phospholipase A, activity **33**, 219–220
–, –, stabilization **33**, 214–215
–, –, thermotropic behavior **33**, 215–216
–, in milk (human) **33**, 179
–, in ocular tissues **33**, 180
–, intakes **33**, 166–167
–, interactions with γ-tocopherol **33**, 206–207
–, intestinal absorption **33**, 168–170
–, linoleic acid sources and **33**, 167–168
–, measurement for vitamin E status **33**, 189
–, metabolism, biliary metabolites **33**, 199–202
–, –, polar metabolites **33**, 200–202
–, –, quinone derivative **33**, 199–201
–, –, urinary metabolites **33**, 202–204
–, mobility in membranes **33**, 212–214
–, *N*-nitroso compounds and **31**, 80, 81
–, olive oil and **31**, 467
–, phenoxyl radical formation **33**, 208–201
–, postprandial changes in lipoprotein fractions **33**, 176
–, protection and repair of membrane proteins **33**, 210–211
–, quenching, of reactive oxygen species **33**, 210
–, –, of singlet oxygen **33**, 210, 303
–, radical quenching capability **33**, 208–201

α-Tocopherol (*cont'd*)
–, regeneration from α-tocopheroxyl radical **33**, 211–212
–, removal from tissue, role of plasma lipoproteins **33**, 185
–, *RRR* and *SRR* forms **33**, 187–188
–, structure **33**, 159
–, tissue levels **33**, 178–179
–, tissue mobilization and turnover **33**, 186–189
–, transfer between tocopherol-deficient and tocopherol-sufficient erythrocytes **33**, 185
–, transfer factors, between dipalmitoyl-phosphatidylcholine liposomes and rat liver microsomes **33**, 195
–, –, from liposomes to human erythrocyte ghosts **33**, 195–196
–, –, from phosphatidylcholine liposomes to rat liver mitochondria **33**, 194
–, –, δ-tocopherol effects **33**, 195
β-Tocopherol (*see also* Tocopherols), antioxidant function in membranes **33**, 207
–, in vegetable oils **33**, 159–160
γ-Tocopherol (*see also* Tocopherols), antioxidant function in membranes **33**, 207
–, bioavailability, wheat bran effects **33**, 173
–, concentration in vegetable oils, table **33**, 161
–, content of soybean oil, heat effects **33**, 165
–, effect on α-tocopherol transfer **33**, 195
–, form of, in vegetable oils **33**, 159
–, in milk (human) **33**, 179
–, intakes **33**, 166
–, interactions with α-tocopherol **33**, 206–207
–, intestinal absorption **33**, 170–171
–, lipoprotein lipase-mediated transfer to fibroblasts **33**, 183
–, metabolism **33**, 205–206
–, structure **33**, 159
–, tissue levels **33**, 179
δ-Tocopherol (*see also* Tocopherols), antioxidant function in membranes **33**, 207
–, concentration in vegetable oils, table **33**, 161
–, effects on α-tocopherol transfer **33**, 195
–, metabolism **33**, 195
–, structure **33**, 159
–, tissue levels **33**, 179
α-Tocopherol-binding protein **33**, 191–194
α-Tocopherol hydroquinone, metabolism **33**, 201
α-Tocopherol quinone, formation and distribution **33**, 200–201
Tocopherols (*see also specific forms*) **10**, 199
–, antioxidant function in membranes **33**, 207–211
–, binding factors **33**, 191–194
–, binding to membranes **33**, 196–199
–, bioavailability, diet composition effects **33**, 171–173
–, –, fiber effects **33**, 171–173
–, –, pectin effects **33**, 171–172
–, –, wheat bran effects **33**, 172–173
–, dietary intake **33**, 166–168
–, food processing/preparation effects **33**, 164–166
–, in animal fats **33**, 164
–, in chocolate **31**, 251–253
–, in fats and oils **33**, 159–164
–, in Finnish oils **33**, 162
–, in fish and fish oils **33**, 164
–, in olive oil **31**, 466, 467
–, in plasma lipoproteins **33**, 174–177
–, –, exchanges between **33**, 174–175
–, –, isotopically labeled, incorporation over time **33**, 176–177
–, intestinal absorption, effects of gastric or intestinal destruction **33**, 169–170
–, –, efficiency **33**, 168–171
–, –, mechanism **33**, 168–171
–, –, via lymphatic system **33**, 168–169
–, in tissues, human **33**, 178–179
–, –, ocular **33**, 280
–, in wheat germ **23**, 236
–, losses due to processing **33**, 160
–, – to –, extraction method **33**, 162
–, – to –, hydrogenation effects **33**, 163
–, – to –, steam refining **33**, 160, 162
–, – to –, storage effects **33**, 163–164
–, metabolism, regulation **33**, 206–207
–, –, α-tocopherol **33**, 199–205
–, –, γ-tocopherol **33**, 205–206
–, –, δ-tocopherol **33**, 205–206
–, mobilization and turnover in tissues **33**, 186–189
–, multicomponent film incorporation **44**, 384
–, *N*-nitroso compounds and **31**, 63, 64, 80, 81
–, physical effects in membranes **33**, 214–220
–, plasma concentration, diurnal and seasonal variations **33**, 176
–, postprandial changes **33**, 176
–, recommended daily intake **33**, 166
–, removal from tissues **33**, 185
–, sources **33**, 167
–, status assessment in humans **33**, 189–191
–, transfer factors **33**, 194–196
–, transport in blood **33**, 174–177

–, uptake by tissues **33**, 180–186
–, – by –, biphasic patterns of disappearance and accumulation **33**, 184–185
–, – by –, chylomicron role **33**, 183–184
–, – by –, donation from formed elements of blood **33**, 185–186
–, – by –, HDL-mediated transfer **33**, 183
–, – by –, lipoprotein lipase-mediated transfer **33**, 183–184
–, – by –, receptor-mediated LDL internalization **33**, 180–182
–, – by –, tissue LDL clearance and **33**, 182
–, – by –, VLDL-mediated transfer **33**, 183
–, vitamers in vegetable oils, table **33**, 161
Tocopheronic acid, structure **33**, 203
Tocopheronolactone, structure **33**, 203
Tocopheronolactone glucuronide, structure **33**, 203
Tocotrienols, in Finnish oils **33**, 162
–, in vegetable oils **33**, 160
Tofu isoflavones **44**, 212, 213, 215
–, low-fat products **44**, 216–217
To-fu-pi **44**, 374
Toluene, solubility of DDT in **2**, 203
Toluene distillation method for dried milk **3**, 59
p-Toluidides in raspberries **2**, 269
Tomatine, isolation of **17**, 99
Tomatoes **15**, 231; **16**, 216
–, ascorbic acid content **4**, 380
–, –, effect of fertilizers on **1**, 307–309
–, –, – of location and season on **1**, 296–298
–, –, – of sunlight on **1**, 300–301
–, –, – of temperature on **1**, 303
–, *Bacillus thermoacidurans* in **3**, 437
–, –, destruction of **3**, 441–442
–, canned, corrosion characteristics of **3**, 336
–, –, effect of storage on vitamin content of **1**, 94–96
–, –, nutrients in **1**, 43, 46–50
–, carotene content of, effect of sunlight on **1**, 305
–, carotenoid pigments in **2**, 328
–, color specifications **5**, 321–326
–, effect of copper equipment on **3**, 355
–, firmness in **2**, 316
–, grading of **5**, 345
–, iodine wrapping for **3**, 465
–, juice, ascorbic acid content of **1**, 56
–, –, canned, ascorbic acid content of **1**, 56–63
–, –, –, carotene content of **1**, 57
–, –, effect of headspace on shelf-life of **3**, 348
–, –, time–temperature relationship in sterilizing of **3**, 438
–, loss of thiamine on processing **6**, 290, 296
–, ozone treatment **45**, 191
–, particulate, processing of **32**, 30–31
–, pectic enzymes in **8**, 86
–, pH of **3**, 432
–, plants, copper deficiency in **3**, 16
–, polyphenols and enzymic browning in **19**, 120
–, redness of **5**, 307–311
–, treatment with ammonia **3**, 465
–, use in establishing processing specifications **2**, 81
–, B vitamins in **1**, 42, 44, 45
–, washing water-related salmonellosis outbreaks **45**, 169
–, wastes **17**, 81–85, 103–104
Tomato juice, canned, ascorbic acid content **4**, 373–375, 380
–, –, effect of oxygen on **1**, 58–60
–, –, – of storage on **1**, 93–97
–, –, – of –, vitamin content of **1**, 93–95, 97
–, –, niacin content of **1**, 58, 57
–, –, nutrients in **1**, 43, 46–49
–, –, riboflavin content of **1**, 56, 57
–, –, thiamine content of **1**, 56, 57
–, –, tin vs. glass containers for **1**, 98–99
–, –, use of ascorbic acid in **4**, 368
–, color specifications **5**, 321
–, comparative composition of **5**, 171
–, flat sour spoilage of **18**, 167–168
–, in canning plant **18**, 187–188
–, pectase from **1**, 411
–, sampling for **18**, 191
–, spray-drying **2**, 486
–, thiamine destruction in **6**, 258, 297
Tomato leaves, ascorbic acid content of, effect of sunlight on **1**, 302
Tomato paste **32**, 10–13, 21, 23, 34
–, color specifications for **5**, 321
Tomato pulp (puree), color specifications **5**, 321
–, spray-drying **2**, 496, 500
Tomato sauce, ultrasonic Doppler velocimetry **45**, 148, 149
Tongue, age-related changes **44**, 252
–, sensory papillae **44**, 251
Toppings **12**, 328
–, alginates in **11**, 151
–, carrageenan in **11**, 133, 136
Torsion tests, gels **34**, 218
Tortenguss, furcellaran in **11**, 160
Torula, heat destruction of **3**, 435

Torula (*cont'd*)
–, in bacon **3**, 308
–, in dates **3**, 452
–, in pork **3**, 293
–, survival at low temperatures **3**, 446
Torulopsis utilis, growth in molasses **17**, 124
Total energy expenditure **40**, 171–180
Total interaction energy, emulsion stability **34**, 95–97
Total parenteral nutrition, safflower oil-based **35**, 113–114
Total residual chlorine, definition of **7**, 143
Touch pressure, oral cavity sensitivity to **29**, 166–167
Townsend, C.T. **32**, 6
Toxic factors, in wheat germ **23**, 255–258
Toxicity, chemical assay **10**, 170–172
–, in food **15**, 39; **16**, 32
–, measurement in shellfish **10**, 164–173
–, mouse bioassay **10**, 164–170
–, *N*-nitroso compounds and **31**, 54, 64
–, of quaternary ammonium compounds **2**, 130
–, tests for quaternary ammonium compounds **2**, 158
Toxicology, 2-amino-3-methylimidazo-[4,5-*f*]quinoline and IQ-like compounds **34**, 405–408
–, in relation to food science **10**, 13
Toxic substances, in fruits **17**, 185
Toxic Substances Control Act, carcinogen risk assessment and **31**, 2, 3, 6, 12, 41, 47
Toxins, from *Clostridium botulinum* **22**, 151–153
Toyo Seikan Kaisha, Ltd, flexible-package durability of **23**, 403
TPNH diphorase, in wheat germ **23**, 240
TPNH oxidase, in wheat germ **23**, 240
Trace elements (*see also* Milk, specific elements) **36**, 210
–, effects on fruit composition **9**, 300
–, metals, effect on folate bioavailability **33**, 79–80
Trace nutrients **10**, 12
Tracer (*see also* Radioactive tracer *and* Stable isotope tracer), carbon-13 **40**, 64–75, 171–172
–, extraction **40**, 256–257
–, modeled **40**, 245–251, 255–257
–, washout rate **40**, 249–250
Tracer method, by vitamin B6 **40**, 137–140
–, β-carotene **40**, 26, 30–31, 42–43, 63–75
–, energy expenditure **40**, 175–176
–, folate **40**, 86–90
–, for vitamin B6 **40**, 114–116
–, glycogen phosphorylase **40**, 137–140
–, membrane transport **40**, 249–250, 255–257
–, membrane vesicles **40**, 200, 203
–, transthyretin metabolism **40**, 150–152
–, vitamin A **40**, 5, 7–8
Tracheids, composition and types of **2**, 299, 301, 331
Training, food science **39**, 119
Transaminases **16**, 248, 303
–, in wheat germ **23**, 240
Transcarboxylase, in wheat germ **23**, 240
Transducin, involvement in sweetener-induced taste **42**, 227–229
Transduction pathways, smell perception **44**, 254
–, taste perception **44**, 252
Transelimination, dietary fiber and **31**, 129, 165
Trans fatty acids **36**, 304–305
Transfection, genetic **40**, 95, 96–101, 105
Transfer, atmospheric freeze-drying **13**, 38–42
–, –, economics **13**, 42–43
–, –, governing equations **13**, 40
–, –, process variables **13**, 41–42
–, –, solid foods **13**, 41–42
–, conduction **13**, 11
–, driving forces **13**, 34–35
–, drying time vs thickness **13**, 32–34
–, equation for rate **13**, 34–36
–, gas sweep **13**, 36
–, heat **13**, 11–32
–, inside food **13**, 12–19
–, –, chamber pressures **13**, 16–17
–, –, desorption **13**, 12
–, –, drying time **13**, 17–19
–, –, thermal conductivity **13**, 14–16
–, mass **13**, 23–43
–, radio-frequency energy **13**, 27–32
–, –, dielectric properties **13**, 28–29
–, –, heating effects **13**, 27–28
–, –, microwave range **13**, 27–28
–, to food surface **13**, 19–27
–, –, contact freeze-drying **13**, 19–20
–, –, evaporation rate **13**, 23
–, –, platen temperature **13**, 21–23, 25, 27, 39
–, –, pressure **13**, 23–26
–, –, product loading **13**, 21–23
–, to product slab **13**, 65–66
–, vacuum importance **13**, 38–40
Transferases, in wheat germ **23**, 240

Transfer coefficient, fractional **40**, 31, 40–43, 267–268, 312
Transfer factors, α-tocopherol **33**, 194–196
Transfer function, identifiability **40**, 316–317
Transformations, unimolecular **14**, 285–324
Transgalactosylase activity, *see* Lactase
Transgalactosylation, versus reverse hydrolysis **38**, 61–64
Transgene **41**, 126
Transgenic foods, concerns regarding allergenicity **42**, 64
Transgenic plants, seed storage proteins, proteins **36**, 163–172
Transgenic wheat, breadmaking quality differences **45**, 262–265
–, transformation system **45**, 253–254
Transglutaminase, polymerization by, protein emulsifier modification **34**, 160
Transient flow **39**, 17
Transient gels **34**, 206
Transition metals, initiation of lipid oxidation **33**, 238
–, oxidation of fish lipids **33**, 289–291
Transition mutation **34**, 390
Transition state theory **14**, 291–292
Transition temperature peak **35**, 320
Translational diffusion **38**, 196–197
Transmissible mink encephalopathy (TME) **43**, 279–280
Transmission electron microscopy (TEM) **22**, 206
–, comparison to scanning electron microscopy **22**, 210–211
Transpeptidase, endogenous proteolytic enzymes and **31**, 358
Transport, Bell–Coleman **12**, 149
–, –, carbon dioxide **12**, 149
–, –, use of brine **12**, 149
–, history **12**, 147–201
–, mechanical **12**, 148–149
–, –, ammonia-vapor **12**, 149
–, refrigerated on ships **12**, 147–201
–, temperature control **12**, 166–167
–, –, inertia of cargo **12**, 167
–, –, thermostats **12**, 167
–, tocopherols in blood **33**, 174–177
Transport equations for fluids **32**, 42–43
Transporting organelles **41**, 143–144
Transport values, K_m folates **33**, 53
Transthyretin metabolism **40**, 4, 13–14, 149–155
–, human subject **40**, 150–154
–, MET30 **40**, 150–155
–, modeling **40**, 151–154
–, tracer methods **40**, 150–152
Transversion mutation **34**, 390
Trays, for retorting **23**, 388–390
Trazodone **44**, 312
Trees, ascorbic acid as spray for **18**, 295–296
Trehalose, C'_g value **38**, 168
Triacontane distillate from apples **2**, 262
Triamine-oxidase, study of in fish **2**, 309
Triamterene **44**, 307
Triangle sensory difference tests **2**, 222–224
Triazolam **44**, 308
Tributyrinase in eggs **1**, 183
Trichinella spiralis in pork **2**, 82
Trichlorethylene, carcinogen risk assessment and **31**, 20, 26
Trichloroacetic acid **41**, 108
Trichoderma lignorum **15**, 177
Trichodesmine **45**, 67, 78, 80
Trichomonas vaginalis, germicidal action of CPCl on **2**, 152
Trichophyton interdigitale, germicidal action of ADBACl on **2**, 147
Trichophyton mentagrophytes, germicidal action of CPCl on **2**, 152
Trichophyton tonsurans, treatment by Phemerol **2**, 182
2,4,6-Tri-(3′,5′-di-*tert*-butyl-4′-hydroxybenzyl)-mesitylene **15**, 6
2,4,6-Tri-(3′,5′-di-*tert*-butyl-4′-hydroxybenzyl)-phenol **15**, 6
Triethylaminoethyl-cellulose, for monoglutamyl folate separations **33**, 26
Trifluoperazine **44**, 312
2,2,2-Trifluoroethanol **42**, 96
Triglycerides **40**, 62–63
–, acyl differences in cardiolipin **37**, 298–299
–, chocolate and, cocoa bean chemistry **31**, 229, 230
–, –, cocoa butter **31**, 250, 251, 275–280
–, –, milk **31**, 254, 264
–, –, milk crumb **31**, 291
–, –, packaging **31**, 324
–, –, tempering **31**, 309, 310
–, –, *Theobroma cacao* L. **31**, 325
–, digestion **35**, 21–22
–, fatty acid changes **35**, 56–58
–, in milkfat **37**, 148–149
–, olive oil and **31**, 458, 464, 465, 473
–, serum, effects of lactic acid cultures **37**, 93–96
–, structure, in dietary fats **37**, 185–188
–, structure, **23**, 5–9, 10
–, ultrasonic phase transition monitoring **45**, 141

Trigonelline in coffee **2**, 280
Trihydroxybenzene in oxidation of catechol **3**, 21
Trimethamine **44**, 296
Trimethoprim **44**, 292
–, effects on folate absorption and metabolism **33**, 70
Trimethylamine **16**, 178
–, estimation of **7**, 59–61
–, fish **3**, 185, 186, 341
–, –, pH **7**, 48–49
–, –, spoilage **7**, 43, 44, 46, 51–52
–, from abalone spoilage **23**, 164
–, in coffee gases **2**, 280
–, *N*-nitroso compounds and **31**, 55, 78, 90
–, shark flesh and **7**, 53–54
–, test for spoilage, fish **2**, 375–381
–, –, –, cod **2**, 368–369
Trimethylamine oxidase (TMAOase), distribution in fish **26**, 298–300
–, enzymatic activity in frozen fish **26**, 298–304
–, formaldehyde, effect and mode of action **26**, 301–302
–, properties of **26**, 302–304
Trimethylamine oxide, cause of spoilage in fish **2**, 368, 378, 381
–, effect of bacterial enzymes on **2**, 369
–, number of organisms in fish reducing **2**, 355
Trimethylammonium, permeability to gel aluminosilicates **2**, 4
2,4,5-Trimethyloxazoline, in meaty aroma **18**, 60
Trimethylpicene, glycyrrhizin and **7**, 361
2,4,6-Trinitrobenzene sulfonate, reactive lysine measurement **35**, 192–193
Triolein, in cocoa fat **6**, 39
Triose phosphate, formation during rigor mortis **1**, 5
Triose phosphate isomerase **41**, 120, 122
–, endpoint cooking temperature indicator **44**, 172
–, time–temperature integrator **44**, 183–184
Tripe, yellow color **5**, 270
Tripeptides, with physiological activity **36**, 180–181
Triphosphate, adenosine **14**, 122–123
Tripipramine maleate **44**, 313
Tripolyphosphate, *N*-nitroso compounds and **31**, 80
Tristearin **14**, 398–401, 417–418
Trisulfide in garlic oil **2**, 272
Triterpene alcohols, olive oil and **31**, 466, 467
Triticale **41**, 38
Triticins, genetic control **36**, 35
–, wheat proteins **36**, 24, 26
Triticum dicoccoides **45**, 253
Triticum monococcum, ssp. *boeoticum* **45**, 226
–, ssp. *monococcum* **45**, 226
Triticum timopheevi **45**, 228
Triticum tsudchii **45**, 228
Triticum turgidum ssp. *dicoccoides* **45**, 226
Triticum urartu **45**, 226
Tritium–hydrogen isotope exchange measurement **35**, 274
Triton, solubility of DDT in **2**, 203
Triton K-12, effect of pH on germicidal power **2**, 134
–, use of **2**, 136
Triton W-30, effect on influenza virus **2**, 138
Tritordeum, transformation **45**, 255–256
–, transgenic line breadmaking qualities **45**, 263
Tropacocaine **44**, 287
Tropical fruit, anthocyanins in **17**, 174
–, origin of **17**, 161–163
–, technology of **17**, 153–214
Tropocollagen, endogenous proteolytic enzymes and **31**, 365, 372
Tropomyosin **9**, 7–8
–, endogenous proteolytic enzymes and, meat technology **31**, 399, 400, 404, 407, 409
–, molecular weight **9**, 8
–, muscle physiology **31**, 370, 374
–, native type **19**, 312
–, properties **9**, 8
–, properties and structure of **19**, 308–312
–, SH groups in **24**, 36
–, –, function **24**, 39–40
Tropomyosin B, preparation of **19**, 334–337
Troponin, endogenous proteolytic enzymes and, meat technology **31**, 398, 399
–, muscle physiology **31**, 370, 374
–, preparation of **19**, 332–334
–, properties and structure of **19**, 312–313
–, SH groups in **24**, 36
–, –, function **24**, 39–40
Troponin-T, endogenous proteolytic enzymes and **31**, 398–400, 404, 406, 409
Trout (*see also* Rainbow trout) **39**, 349
–, aerobic bacterial flora of **2**, 350
Trypsin, dietary fiber and **31**, 170, 171
–, endogenous proteolytic enzymes and **31**, 345, 354

–, regeneration of **17**, 53
–, stabilization **35**, 331
Trypsin inhibitor, effect on biosynthesis of crypsinogen **28**, 140
–, effects on microbiological agents **1**, 385
–, from beans **28**, 131–133
–, in Leguminosae **28**, 138
–, –, lima bean, amino acid sequence **28**, 134
–, in relation to aging of poultry meat **1**, 210
Tryptophan **16**, 195
–, carcinogen risk assessment and **31**, 28
–, chlorine and **7**, 143
–, deficiency of **17**, 117
–, effect in diet of rat **1**, 115
–, effect on browning in orange juice **1**, 354
–, *N*-nitroso compounds and **31**, 91
Tryptophan synthase, site-directed mutagenesis **35**, 281–282
–, α-subunit, Gibbs free energy **35**, 262–263
TTR, *see* Transthyretin metabolism
Tube method of testing germicidal action of quaternary ammonium compounds **2**, 162
Tubercle bacilli, effect of Zephiran on **2**, 148
Tubers **15**, 179; **41**, 3
Tubes, Bingham plastic flowing in **11**, 413
Tube viscometers **11**, 384–393
Tubulaine spray dryer, operation of **2**, 423, 425–426, 470
Tubular heat exchanger **32**, 15
Tumbling, IM meat **39**, 103
Tumor cells, cardiolipin content **37**, 302
Tumor growth, effects of lactic cultures **37**, 103–107, 119–120
Tumorigenesis, *n*-3 PUFA effects **35**, 144
Tumor initiation, inhibition by rosemary **42**, 264–266
Tumors, carcinogen risk assessment and **31**, 43, 44, 47
–, –, laboratory data **31**, 25, 26, 28–32, 35, 36
–, –, statistics **31**, 15, 22
–, *N*-nitroso compounds and **31**, 64–66
Tuna fish **39**, 337, 338, 350
–, acid formation in decomposition **2**, 371
–, chromatography **39**, 353–354, 355
–, quality control **39**, 351–352
Tung oil, solubility of DDT in **2**, 203
Tung seed meal **17**, 107
Tungsten carbide, use in nozzle of spray dryer **2**, 450
Tungsten/molybdenum ratio, high dietary, sulfite oxidase deficiency and **30**, 36–37
Turbidity, coalescence measurement **34**, 177–179
–, reduced **34**, 172
–, theory of light scattering **34**, 178–179
Turbo pica, ciguatera from **18**, 143
Turbulence, estimating onset in pseudo-plastic fluids **11**, 413–416
Turgidity **15**, 120
Turkey (country), IM meat **39**, 74–75
Turkeys, fatty acid **5**, 5
–, monocarbonyl compounds in fat **5**, 11
–, peroxides in fat **5**, 11
–, salmonellae on skin of **6**, 194
–, stability of eviscerated **5**, 6, 7
–, thiamine loss in **6**, 280
–, thiamine retention in frozen **6**, 294
–, tocopherol in tissue **5**, 7
–, use of antioxidants **5**, 27
Turku sugar studies, dental caries and **25**, 139–147
Turmeric/curcumin **43**, 196, 209
–, adverse reactions **43**, 210
Turnips, carotene content of, effect of fertilizers on **1**, 309
–, gelatinization of starch in **2**, 232
–, greens, ascorbic acid content, effect of light **1**, 302
–, –, –, – of location and season **1**, 296, 298–299
–, –, –, – of rainfall **1**, 304
–, –, –, – of temperature **1**, 303
–, –, calcium content, effect of fertilizers **1**, 310–311
–, –, canned, nutrients in **1**, 43, 46–49
–, –, carotene content, effect of location **1**, 306
–, –, –, – of moisture **1**, 306
–, –, –, – of season **1**, 305–306
–, –, iron content, effect of fertilizers **1**, 314
–, –, phosphorus content, effect of fertilizers **1**, 313
–, inositol phosphates content **45**, 23
–, leaves, ascorbic acid and moisture content **5**, 184
–, loss of moisture **5**, 231
–, – of thiamine on processing **6**, 290
–, moisture content and size of **5**, 248
Turnover, folates **40**, 83–85, 89–90
–, –, *in vivo* kinetics **33**, 57–58
–, glycogen phosphorylase **40**, 124, 137–140, 142
–, tocopherols **33**, 186–189
–, vitamin A **40**, 12–13, 14, 19, 21
–, vitamin B6 **40**, 114–127
–, water **40**, 173

Tussilago farfara (coltsfoot; coughwort) **45**, 76, 91
Two-stage methods, population analysis **40**, 273–274
Tylosin, effect on flat sour bacteria spores **18**, 186
Tyralbumines, *see* Caseoglutines
Tyramine, fish spoilage and **7**, 46, 47
Tyramine poisoning **39**, 290, 291–292
Tyrocaseines, *see* Caseoglutines
Tyrocidine, damage to cell membrane by **1**, 378, 379
Tyrosinase (*see also* Oxidase, *o*-diphenol), in respiration of plants **3**, 14, 15
–, oxidation of tyrosine by **3**, 23
Tyrosine, chlorine and **7**, 143
–, color test for proteolysis in fish **2**, 371, 382
–, conversion of into melanin **3**, 23
–, dietary fiber and **31**, 132
–, gelatin and **7**, 264
–, in bacon discoloration **3**, 315
–, in cocoa bean, oxidation of **8**, 259
–, inhibition of oxidation of **3**, 20
"Tyrosine" value, fish spoilage and **7**, 49
Tyrothricin **44**, 293, 322

Ubiquinones **17**, 60
UDP-glucose, regulation **41**, 125
–, role **41**, 35–36, 39–40
UDPglucose:protein transglucosylase **41**, 109–110
UDP-D-glucuronic acid decarboxylase, in wheat germ **23**, 240
Ulcerative colitis **37**, 31–32
–, inulin effects **43**, 18, 43
Ulcers, antipeptic ulcer factors in cabbage **10**, 241
–, licorice and **7**, 353, 355–356
–, treatment by anion exchangers **2**, 32
Ultradian rhythm (*see also* Bioperiodicity) **40**, 219
Ultrafiltration **40**, 183–193, 195
–, bioprocess reactors, lactose hydrolysis **38**, 47, 50, 52–56
–, cheese **39**, 193–195
–, enzyme bioreactor, modified localized **38**, 52, 54
–, lactase immobilization **38**, 18–20
–, whey protein preparation with **33**, 361
Ultrahigh temperature milk **32**, 20
Ultrahigh temperature pasteurization of milk, effect on folate activity **33**, 51
Ultramarine, volume per oxygen atom in **2**, 3
Ultrasonic composition sensors **45**, 133–139
–, application to animal carcasses **45**, 138–139
Ultrasonic conching, chocolate and **31**, 308
Ultrasonic flow meters **45**, 130–132
–, Doppler flowmeters **45**, 131–132
–, transit-time mode **45**, 130–131
–, vortex shedding **45**, 132
Ultrasonic imaging **45**, 153–157
–, carcass grading **45**, 154
–, high-resolution **45**, 156–157
–, limitations **45**, 155
–, noncontact methodology **45**, 155
–, protein gels **34**, 284
–, scanning acoustic microscopy **45**, 156
Ultrasonic measurement systems **45**, 121–129
–, air–transducer impedance barrier **45**, 124
–, digitizer **45**, 122–123
–, guided wave sensors **45**, 128
–, Love wave sensors **45**, 128–129
–, noncontact measurements **45**, 124–126
–, pulsed modes **45**, 123–124
–, –, pathlength measurement **45**, 124
–, reflectance methods **45**, 127–128
–, resonance methods **45**, 126–127
–, –, resonance cell losses (*Q*-factor) **45**, 127
–, signal generator **45**, 122
–, ultrasonic transducers **45**, 122
Ultrasonic phase transition monitoring **45**, 139–142
–, isothermal scanning **45**, 139–140
–, temperature scanning **45**, 140–142
Ultrasonic sealing, of retort pouches **23**, 359
Ultrasonic sensors **45**, 101–158
–, advantages/disadvantages **45**, 157–158
–, applications **45**, 129–157
–, –, composition **45**, 133–139
–, –, dispersed systems **45**, 148, 150–151
–, –, fluid flow **45**, 130–132
–, –, imaging **45**, 153–157
–, –, level sensors **45**, 129–130
–, –, phase transitions **45**, 139–142
–, –, polymeric systems **45**, 151–153
–, –, rheological properties (texture) **45**, 142–148
–, –, temperature **45**, 132–133
–, –, viscosity measurements **45**, 147–148
–, nondestructive testing **45**, 104
–, theoretical aspects **45**, 103–121
Ultrasonic thermometry **45**, 132–133
Ultrasonic transducers **45**, 122
Ultrasonic wave propagation **45**, 103–104
–, attenuation **45**, 105, 109–111

–, –, coefficient **45**, 105–106
–, –, overestimation **45**, 120
–, –, relaxation **45**, 111
–, diffraction **45**, 120–121
–, homogeneous materials **45**, 105–111
–, –, adiabatic elastic modulus **45**, 106
–, –, properties of materials **45**, 106, 107–108
–, inhomogeneous media **45**, 112–117
–, –, emulsions **45**, 112, 114–116
–, –, flocculated emulsions **45**, 116–117
–, –, multiple scattering theory **45**, 113–116
–, –, particle sizing **45**, 115–116
–, –, scattering interactions **45**, 112–113
–, interfaces **45**, 117–120
–, –, acoustic impedance **45**, 117–118
–, –, reflection coefficient **45**, 118, 119
–, –, refractive index **45**, 118–119
–, –, transmission coefficient **45**, 118, 119
–, longitudinal (compression) waves **45**, 104–106, 109
–, –, critical angle interactions at boundaries **45**, 119–120
–, near-field/far-field regions **45**, 121
–, shear (transverse) waves **45**, 104, 105, 109
–, surface waves **45**, 104–105
–, –, Love **45**, 104
–, –, Raleigh **45**, 104–105
–, velocity **45**, 105, 106, 109
–, –, adiabatic compressibility calculation **45**, 151
–, –, gases **45**, 106, 109
–, –, liquids **45**, 109
–, –, solids **45**, 109
–, wave characterisitcs **45**, 103–105
Ultrasound, for muscle cross-sectional area **37**, 346
–, wheat proteins solubilization **36**, 15–17
Ultraviolet (UV) radiation, absorbance, detection of eluted folates with **33**, 28
–, comutagenicity with sulfites **30**, 46
–, effect on flat sour bacteria spores **18**, 186–187
–, explanation of **3**, 127
–, gelatin sterility and **7**, 250
–, germicidal action of **3**, 147–152
–, in destruction of bacteria, molds, and yeasts **3**, 149
–, in egg industry **3**, 154
–, in food analysis **3**, 153
–, ozone combined sanitization procedures **45**, 202–203
–, uses of **3**, 147–155
–, –, sterilization **32**, 5
Unbound moisture, definition **39**, 97–98
Unfolding, reversible thermal, proteins **35**, 240–246
Uniaxial extension **39**, 14–16
a,B-Unsaturated acids in rye bread **2**, 276
Unsaturated fatty acids **35**, 24
–, Δ^6-desaturase, desaturation and elongation **35**, 35–36
–, –, diet effects on activity **35**, 35–37
–, –, fat type effects **35**, 40–41
–, –, feedback inhibitors **35**, 43
–, –, inhibition **35**, 39–40
–, –, *in vitro* studies **35**, 43
–, –, linolenate and linoleate effects **35**, 38–39
–, –, protein effects **35**, 44
–, –, regulation **35**, 35–44
–, desaturation **35**, 24, 27–29
–, elongation **35**, 24–27
–, extent of desaturation of oleic, linoleic, and linolenic acids **35**, 31, 33
–, isomers **35**, 24–25
–, metabolism **35**, 22
–, oxidation rates **35**, 23
–, rates of desaturation and elongation **35**, 31–33
Uplandicine **45**, 72
UPTG, *see* UDPglucose:protein transglucosylase
Uracil, reactions with sulfites **30**, 25
Uranium, carcinogen risk assessment and **31**, 15
Urbanization, and food selection **32**, 263–265
Urea, as dispersing agent **6**, 24
–, effect on oat globulin thermal characteristics **35**, 327–328
–, gelatin manufacture and **7**, 240, 241
–, gel–sol state and **7**, 279, 297, 303
–, shark flesh and **7**, 53
–, ultrafiltration **40**, 192–193
Urease **16**, 308
Uridine, reactions with sulfites **30**, 25–26
Urine, calcium, balance measurements and **33**, 108
–, –, diet effects **33**, 120
–, distribution of DDT in **2**, 210–211, 217
–, α-tocopherol metabolites **33**, 202–204
–, γ-tocopherol metabolites **33**, 205–206
–, δ-tocopherol metabolites **33**, 205–206
Uronic acid, dietary fiber and, analysis **31**, 148, 153
–, –, dicotyledonous plants **31**, 126
–, –, intestinal bacteria **31**, 175
–, –, properties **31**, 164–166
Uronic acid cycle, xylitol in **25**, 161

Uronides, in pectins **11**, 58
Uroporphyrinogen III cosynthetase, in wheat germ **23**, 241
Ursodiol **44**, 318
Urticaria, reaction to sulfites **30**, 57–58
USA, annual agricultural and forestry harvest **32**, 193
–, annual biomass production **32**, 192
–, biomass energy used **32**, 191
–, biomass resources **32**, 189–190
–, consumption of commercial energy **32**, 190
–, ethanol production **32**, 197–202, 215–216
–, food selection in **32**, 240–267
–, forest utilization **32**, 194
–, gross national product **32**, 189
–, household composition **32**, 241–242
–, land distribution by use **32**, 190
–, soil erosion in **32**, 216–221
USC*PACL software **40**, 276
Utensils, choice of **7**, 27
–, flavor testing and **7**, 22
Uterine cancer, carcinogen risk assessment and **31**, 15, 17
Uterotrophic assay **44**, 197

Vaccinium corymbosum (blueberry) **44**, 211
Vaccinium oxycoccos, *see* Cranberry
Vaccinium vitusidea (lingonberry) **44**, 207, 211
Vacuole in vegetable tissue, composition of **2**, 306
– in –, effect of osmosis on **2**, 306
Vacutainer **40**, 185, 190
Vacuum, freeze-drying and **7**, 176–177
Vacuum chambers, for package air removal **23**, 371–372
Vacuum cooking **15**, 309
Vacuum equipment **16**, 129
Vacuum evaporator **15**, 310
Vacuum flash cooling **32**, 11
Vacuum pumps **15**, 315
Vaginal cornification assay **44**, 197
Vaginitis, effects of lactic cultures **37**, 111–114
Valeric acid **16**, 186
–, fish spoilage and **7**, 48
–, in apples **2**, 263
–, in cocoa **2**, 283
–, in coffee **2**, 280
–, in peaches **2**, 265
–, in tea **2**, 285
Valve homogenizers **34**, 168
Valves and fittings, equivalent lengths **11**, 411
Vanadium, inositol phosphate interactions **45**, 36
–, in wines **8**, 137, 198
Van der Waals interaction, emulsion stability **34**, 88–90
Vanillic acid, in wheat germ **23**, 237
Vanillic acid esters in preservation of fruit juices **3**, 460
Vanillin, flavor and **30**, 78
–, glycyrrhetic acid assay and **7**, 371
–, in maple syrup **30**, 111
Vanillone in coffee **2**, 282
Vapor, diffusion through dried meat **7**, 195–196
–, transport, freeze-drying and **7**, 187–188
–, –, pressure and **7**, 196–198
Vapor–liquid equilibria, in food drying **20**, 10–19
Vapor pressure **39**, 97–98
Vapor pressure–moisture content curves for milk products **3**, 56, 57, 58
Variant Creutzfeldt–Jakob disease (vCJD) **43**, 266, 283–284, 289–290, 292–293
–, prion susceptibility polymorphism **43**, 293
Variotin, from *Byssochlamys* spp. **25**, 276–277
Vascular bundles in vegetable matter, lignification of **2**, 304
Vasodilators, taste sensation effects **44**, 314
Vegetable juices, ascorbic acid added to **18**, 227
–, ascorbic acid content **4**, 373
–, in American dietary **4**, 371–372
–, phase transition temperature of **27**, 339
–, use of ascorbic acid in **4**, 371–381
Vegetable oils, ascorbic acid protection of **18**, 248
–, autoxidation of **17**, 28–29
–, emulsification of **16**, 119
–, tocopherols, hydrogenation **33**, 163
–, –, losses due to, extraction method **33**, 162
–, –, processing **33**, 160
–, –, steam refining **33**, 160, 162
–, –, storage **33**, 163–164
–, vitamers in, table **33**, 161
Vegetable-oxidation systems **17**, 1–76
Vegetable-processing wastes **17**, 80–88
Vegetable products **14**, 238–241
Vegetable proteins, compositional analysis **35**, 341–343
Vegetables **15**, 57ff, 147ff
–, anaerobic deterioration of **17**, 5–6

–, analysis **31**, 146–148, 150, 152
–, atmospheric conditions in storage of **3**, 467–470
–, blanching of **8**, 63
–, boundary temperatures for freeze-drying **27**, 336
–, canned, factors controlling mineral and vitamin content of **1**, 291–292
–, –, use of ascorbic acid in **4**, 368
–, canning, effect of storage on **1**, 64–65
–, –, – of time of harvest on **1**, 64–65
–, carotenoids in **15**, 216
–, chlorine treatment **45**, 188
–, chlorophyll-containing, greenness of **5**, 326
–, components **31**, 120, 140
–, dehydrated **5**, 142; **6**, 300, 315, 367; **15**, 288
–, –, sulfite fate **30**, 27–28
–, dicotyledonous plants **31**, 126, 128
–, dietary fiber and **31**, 119, 190, 191
–, discoloration prevention by ascorbic acid **18**, 255–256
–, dried, enzymic changes during storage **11**, 285–289
–, –, protection of by packing **3**, 457
–, –, sorption isotherms of **3**, 456
–, fiber, effect on calcium bioavailability **33**, 139–141
–, flat sour spoilage and contamination by **18**, 188–189
–, flexible packaging for **23**, 325–326
–, folate bioavailability **33**, 75
–, freeze-drying of **7**, 204, 228–229
–, freezing of **8**, 64
–, frozen **6**, 174; **25**, 181–235
–, –, bacterial flora in **6**, 183, 185, 187
–, –, danger of botulism in **6**, 185
–, –, freezing effects on **25**, 214–218
–, –, ice formation in **25**, 183–193
–, –, off-flavors in unblanched **8**, 103
–, –, problems in **25**, 229–230
–, –, steps prior to freezing **25**, 219–221
–, –, storage changes in **25**, 227–228
–, –, thawing of **6**, 206
–, –, treatment for micro-organisms in **3**, 449–450
–, fungicidal treatment of **3**, 463–466
–, greenness in **5**, 311
–, Indian, thiamine destruction in **6**, 292
–, inositol phosphates **45**, 22–23
–, in-plant contamination **45**, 194
–, intestinal bacteria **31**, 171, 172, 176–178, 180–182, 186
–, irradiation of **24**, 183
–, loss of nutrients during blanching of **8**, 74, 76
–, – of thiamine **6**, 296
–, – of –, during processing **6**, 285
–, measuring tenderness **8**, 17
–, oils in **15**, 237
–, ozone treatment **45**, 190, 191, 192, 194, 195–196
–, –, pesticide residues reduction **45**, 199
–, pH of **3**, 432
–, prefreezing **13**, 320
–, preservation of at low temperatures **3**, 446–450
–, – of –, by chemicals **3**, 458–463
–, – of –, by lactic acid fermentation **3**, 457–458
–, properties **31**, 155, 157, 160, 163–165
–, quality of **16**, 203ff
–, quality–price survey of **3**, 421
–, radurization of **24**, 194–196
–, sanitary handling of **3**, 470–471
–, sanitization methods **45**, 170
–, selenium in **32**, 95
–, shredded **5**, 146
–, sterilization of by heat **3**, 433–443
–, sulfiting **5**, 143
–, supercooling **27**, 307–315
–, –, cryoscopic temperature of **27**, 310–315
–, survival of *Salmonella* in **3**, 219, 220
–, texture, ultrasonic sensing **45**, 142
Vegetable wastes, as leaf meals **17**, 98–99
–, as source of protein **17**, 100–104
Vegetative cells **41**, 11
Velocity profiles, and convection currents **32**, 50–54
Velocity vectors, resolution of along a curved streamline **11**, 369
Venlafaxine **44**, 313
Very-low-density lipoproteins, *see* Lipoproteins, very-low-density
Vessel segments, *see* Tracheids
Vibrio, found in fresh fish **2**, 350
–, growth rate of **7**, 105
–, salt requirement of **7**, 112
Vibrio cholerae **45**, 180
Vibrio costicolus in bacon **3**, 308
Vibrio halonitrificans in bacon **3**, 308
Vibrio parahaemolyticus **45**, 180
Vicia faba legumin **36**, 119
–, food protein engineering **36**, 184–185
–, gelation **36**, 128, 131
Vicilin, expression in micro-organisms **36**, 161

Vicilin (*cont'd*)
–, pea **36**, 114
Vincristine **44**, 294
Vinegar, production of **17**, 93, 96
–, use of SO_2 **5**, 136, 141
Viners, pea **9**, 123–126
Vinification, of kiwifruit juice, chemical changes during **29**, 303–305
p-Vinyl catechol in coffee **2**, 282
Vinyl chloride, carcinogen risk assessment and **31**, 33, 39, 41, 47
Vinylguaiacol in coffee **2**, 281–282
p-Vinyl guaiacol in coffee **2**, 282
Viral agents, gastroenteritis-producing **37**, 38
Viral infections, smell perception effects **44**, 274, 275
Viral myocarditis **37**, 33
Viruses, carcinogen risk assessment and **31**, 13, 15
–, food-borne, radiation effects on **24**, 186
Viscoelasticity **39**, 9–12
–, biopolymetric materials **39**, 48–53
–, definition **39**, 9
–, emulsions **39**, 56–57
–, gels **34**, 212–214
–, linear **39**, 10, 18–23
–, whey protein films **33**, 394
Viscoelastic liquid **32**, 47
Viscoelastic liquid and solid, response to applied stress **34**, 212–213
Viscometers **39**, 26, 30
–, cone-and-plate **11**, 377
–, narrow-gap coaxial **11**, 374–377
–, parallel-plate **11**, 371, 374
–, rotational, fluid with a yield stress in **11**, 381–384
–, tube **11**, 384–393
–, wide-gap rotational **11**, 378–381
Viscosin **43**, 323
Viscosity **41**, 165, 167
–, apparent **39**, 5–6, 25, 274
–, as function of reduced temperature for glassy and partially crystalline polymers **38**, 108–109
–, chocolate and, conching **31**, 300
–, –, dietary fiber and **31**, 142, 166–170, 182
–, –, emulsifiers **31**, 281–283
–, –, processing **31**, 242, 243, 245
–, –, refining **31**, 294
–, –, sweeteners **31**, 266, 269
–, coefficient **39**, 4–5
–, complex **39**, 23
–, definition **39**, 4
–, dynamic **39**, 4–5
–, extensional **39**, 16, 17
–, Eyring theory of coefficient of in liquid structure **11**, 358–362
–, fish freshness and **7**, 63
–, glass transition **39**, 117
–, intrinsic **39**, 116
–, local **38**, 198
–, measurement methods **7**, 249; **19**, 323–324; **32**, 47–48
–, –, empirical **32**, 48
–, –, fundamental **32**, 47–48
–, –, imitative **32**, 48
–, Newtonian **39**, 5
–, of agar **11**, 118
–, of alginates **11**, 118
–, of carrageenan **11**, 118
–, of cheese **39**, 189
–, of food **9**, 175–187
–, –, absolute **9**, 180
–, –, apparent **9**, 180–181
–, –, formula for **9**, 180
–, –, measurement of **9**, 181–187
–, –, relative **9**, 181
–, of furcellaran **11**, 118
–, of guar gum **11**, 118
–, of gum arabic **11**, 118
–, of gum karaya **11**, 118
–, of gum tragacanth **11**, 118
–, of locust bean gum **11**, 118
–, of pectins as affected by arabinose **11**, 77
–, polymeric proteins **36**, 41–43
–, rework **39**, 274
–, rheological instrumentation **39**, 24–33
–, selected foods **39**, 44–46
–, temperature dependence, aqueous solutions **38**, 180–181
–, transient **39**, 17
–, ultrasonic measurement **45**, 147–148, 149
–, von Kármán vortex street **45**, 132
Viscosity function **32**, 45, 50, 79
Viscosity method, coalescence measurement **34**, 180–181
Viscous drag **39**, 24
Viscous flow **39**, 4–6
–, fundamental rate process in **11**, 359
Viscous friction, as element of consistency **11**, 358
Visual examination, for seal integrity in flexible packaging **23**, 351–352
Visual function, *n*-3 PUFA **35**, 117–120
Visual guide, modeling **40**, 282, 283
Vitamin A (*see also* Vitamins) **15**, 209, 248
–, carcinogen risk assessment and **31**, 21, 22
–, chocolate and **31**, 274

–, concentrate **34**, 165
–, deficiency **1**, 111, 119
–, effect of spray-drying on **2**, 401
–, in canning **15**, 239
–, in eggs, dried, loss during storage **1**, 174, 181
–, –, effect of hen's diet on **1**, 153
–, in tropical fruits **17**, 174–175
–, metabolism (*see also* β-Carotene metabolism, Retinol, Retinol-binding protein, Retinyl ester) **40**, 3–24
–, –, background information **40**, 3–5
–, –, catabolic rate **40**, 7, 13
–, –, chylomicrons **40**, 4, 16
–, –, compartmental analysis **40**, 9–21
–, –, –, empirical **40**, 11–14
–, –, –, model **40**, 14–21
–, –, disposal rate **40**, 4–5, 7, 12, 21–22
–, –, experimental design **40**, 5–7
–, –, organs (*see also* Liver) **40**, 4, 9, 11, 19–21
–, –, tracer **40**, 5, 7–8
–, –, turnover **40**, 12–13, 14, 19, 21
–, –, whole-body models **40**, 8–11
–, oxidation of **17**, 29
–, ultraviolet measurement of **3**, 153
Vitamin B (*see also* Thiamine *and* Vitamins) **17**, 246
–, carcinogen risk assessment and **31**, 22
–, in fruits **17**, 181
–, Vitamin B-complex, effect of cathode rays on **3**, 170
Vitamin B_1 (*see also* Thiamine *and* Vitamins), form of the vitamin **6**, 261
–, in baked products **6**, 271
–, in breads **6**, 265
–, in dehydrated products **6**, 299
–, loss, in canned products **6**, 296
–, –, in dairy products **6**, 293
–, –, in meats **6**, 275
–, –, in processing vegetables **6**, 285
–, pharmaceuticals containing **6**, 301
–, thermal destruction in foods **6**, 257, 294
Vitamin B_2, *see* Riboflavin
Vitamin B6 (*see also* Vitamins), metabolism (*see also* Glycogen phosphorylase metabolism) **40**, 107–132
–, –, brain **40**, 112
–, –, clearance values **40**, 110–111
–, –, compartmental modeling **40**, 114–116
–, –, conservation effect **40**, 117, 120–121, 127
–, –, dietary factors **40**, 117
–, –, doses **40**, 117–118, 119–120
–, –, equilibration **40**, 126
–, –, erythrocytes **40**, 111
–, –, flushing effect **40**, 122, 127
–, –, glycogen phosphorylase **40**, 115–116, 118, 121
–, –, human subject **40**, 115, 121, 145
–, –, intestines **40**, 109–110, 115, 121
–, –, kidneys **40**, 201
–, –, kinetics **40**, 113–127, 137–140
–, –, –, growth requirements **40**, 116–117
–, –, –, tracers, radioactive **40**, 114–116
–, –, –, –, stable isotope **40**, 116
–, –, lactation **40**, 112–113
–, –, liver **40**, 108, 110–111, 112, 115, 121
–, –, McArdle's disease **40**, 142–145
–, –, membrane vesicles **40**, 201
–, –, metabolic pathways **40**, 107–110
–, –, model refinement **40**, 117–127
–, –, –, dosing protocols **40**, 119–120
–, –, –, fasting **40**, 120–121
–, –, –, form comparisons **40**, 121–122, 123
–, –, –, microgravity **40**, 121
–, –, –, physiological observations **40**, 118–119
–, –, –, protein-binding **40**, 122–127
–, –, muscle **40**, 115–116, 120–121
–, –, oral versus intravenous intake **40**, 115, 127
–, –, plasma **40**, 110–111
–, –, pregnancy **40**, 112–113
–, –, protein binding **40**, 117, 122–127
–, –, protein intake **40**, 117
–, –, tissue distribution **40**, 112
–, –, turnover **40**, 114–127
Vitamin B_{12} (*see also* Vitamins), deficiency, effects on folate bioavailability **33**, 79
–, protection from asthmatic reaction to sulfites **30**, 54
Vitamin C (*see also* Ascorbic acid *and* Vitamins) **15**, 124; **17**, 200, 246
–, carcinogen risk assessment and **31**, 22, 24
–, chocolate and **31**, 268
–, content of plants, influence of climate on **1**, 295–307
–, – of –, – of fertilizers on **1**, 307–310
–, – of tropical fruits **17**, 180–181
–, in dehydrated mashed potatoes **25**, 96–102
–, in radiowave treatment **3**, 144
–, *N*-nitroso compounds and **31**, 62
–, oxidation of **17**, 18
–, pulsed electric field (PEF) processed fruit juice, apple **44**, 20–21
–, –, orange **44**, 17–20
–, retention in blanched foods **3**, 136

Vitamin C, retention (*cont'd*)
–, – in potatoes **6**, 249
Vitamin D (*see also* Vitamins), and calcium intake, effects on calcium absorption **33**, 115–116
–, content of shells of sundried cocoa beans **8**, 263
–, deficiency **1**, 119
–, –, in eggs as affected by hen's diet **1**, 153
–, –, utilization of phosphorus induced by **1**, 132
–, effect of spray-drying on **2**, 401
–, ultraviolet measurement of **3**, 153
–, Vitamin D/calcitriol **44**, 318
–, Vitamin D–parathyroid hormone system, regulation of plasma calcium concentrations **33**, 113–114
–, Vitamin D status **40**, 197, 198, 201–202
Vitamin E (*see also* α-Tocopherol *and* Vitamins) **15**, 49, 215
–, as antioxidant **17**, 59–60
–, carcinogen risk assessment and **31**, 22
–, chocolate and **31**, 274
–, endogenous proteolytic enzymes and **31**, 384–386, 389
–, from wheat germ **23**, 285–286
–, *N*-nitroso compounds and **31**, 63
–, olive oil and **31**, 467, 477
–, status assessment in humans **33**, 189–191
Vitamin K (*see also* Vitamins) **17**, 59–60, 246
–, counteracting hemorrhagic tendencies **1**, 125
–, deficiency **1**, 119
–, –, effect on appetite **1**, 116–119
–, factors influencing stability of **1**, 53
–, in canned foods **1**, 39–100
–, –, distribution between solid and liquid portions **1**, 44–49
–, –, effect of blanching **1**, 66–82
–, –, – of canning **1**, 52–89
–, –, – of grading and cutting **1**, 66
–, –, – of preparation **1**, 49–52
–, –, – of storage **1**, 89–98
–, –, – of type of container **1**, 98–100
Vitamin K^1 (*see also* Vitamins), Vitamin K^1/ phytonadione **44**, 318
Vitamin K_3 (*see also* Vitamins), reaction with sulfites **30**, 24
Vitamin P (*see also* Vitamins) **17**, 245–246
–, content of black tea **17**, 271–278
–, in tea, activity **17**, 218, 231, 278–279
–, –, capillary-strengthening effect **17**, 218
–, licorice and **7**, 355
–, therapeutic effects in tea **17**, 218
Vitamin concentrates from wheat germ **23**, 285–286
Vitamin deficiency as nutritional stress factor **4**, 109
Vitamins (*see also* specific vitamins) **14**, 313–314; **39**, 280–281
–, bifidobacteria synthesis **43**, 34
–, chocolate and **31**, 274, 314, 327
–, in cheese ripening **16**, 279ff
–, in citrus fruits, ascorbic acid **9**, 310–311
–, –, others **9**, 311–312
–, in fish sauce **4**, 216–217
–, in mango fruit **21**, 268–269, 293
–, in milk powders **19**, 192–195
–, in passion fruit, enzymes **12**, 244–245
–, –, minerals **12**, 245
–, –, niacin **12**, 243
–, –, pantothenic acid **12**, 243
–, –, riboflavin **12**, 243
–, –, vitamin A **12**, 242
–, –, vitamin C **12**, 243–244
–, –, vitamin B: thiamine **12**, 242–243
–, in peas **9**, 78–91
–, –, ascorbic acid **9**, 86–90
–, –, biotin **9**, 85–86
–, –, carotene **9**, 78–80
–, –, folic acid **9**, 85–86
–, –, inositol **9**, 85–86
–, –, miscellaneous **9**, 91
–, –, niacin **9**, 84–85
–, –, pantothenic acid **9**, 85–86
–, –, pyridoxine **9**, 85–86
–, –, riboflavin **9**, 83–84
–, –, thiamine **9**, 80–83
–, –, vitamin A **9**, 78–80
–, in tea **11**, 224–226; **17**, 245–247
–, in wheat germ **23**, 208–209, 235–236, 271
–, meat mutagen modulation **34**, 430–431
–, microwave exposure effects **43**, 92, 93
Vitamin transport, membrane vesicle **40**, 201–202, 203, 204
Vitellin in egg yolk **1**, 150, 169
VLDL, *see* Lipoprotein, very-low-density
Vocabulary, flavor profile and **7**, 27–28
Vogel–Tammann–Fulcher equation **38**, 194
Volatile carbonyl compounds **17**, 29
Volatile compounds, bread **30**, 101
–, browning flavors, characteristics **30**, 113, 114–119, 120
–, cocoa beans **30**, 97–100
–, –, classes of **30**, 99
–, –, fraction A, compounds **30**, 98, 99
–, –, identification of constituents **30**, 97–98

–, coffee **30**, 109, 110
–, cooked meat **30**, 104–106
–, flavor compounds from lipid oxidation, in biological tissues, table **33**, 274
–, – from –, in fish tissues, table **33**, 275
–, from acyl hydroperoxides **33**, 273–275
–, generation in fish **33**, 298–302
–, in cured meat, nitrite effect **29**, 64–70
–, in food **33**, 280–281
–, koikuchi shoyu **30**, 261–287
–, shoyu **30**, 305–313
Volatile constituents in citrus fruit, in juices **9**, 333–340
– in –, in peels **9**, 332–333
Volatile flavor components **17**, 6
Volatile flavoring, of passion fruit juice **27**, 269–281
Volatiles, *see* Volatile compounds
Volatility, chocolate and, cocoa bean chemistry **31**, 234, 235
–, –, conching **31**, 298, 299, 307
–, –, processing **31**, 244, 246
–, *N*-nitroso compounds and **31**, 97–100
–, –, fundamentals **31**, 66, 69, 70, 72, 74
–, –, indirect contamination **31**, 94–96
–, –, nitrite/nitrate addition **31**, 85
–, –, processing **31**, 91, 92
Volodkevich apparatus **14**, 41
Volume changes, in freezing **13**, 272–274
–, tissue sample **40**, 186–187
Vomitoxin, effects on gastrointestinal immunity **37**, 35, 40
Von Gierke's disease **37**, 374–377
Vortex shedding **45**, 132

Walnuts **16**, 16
–, enzymic changes in **11**, 309
–, leuco-anthocyanins **5**, 288
Warburg's formula **10**, 321
"Warmed-over" flavor (WOF) **23**, 1–74
–, development **23**, 46–57
–, effects of antioxidants **23**, 57–58
–, – of chelating **23**, 57–58
–, – of chopping and emulsifying **23**, 53
–, – of curing **23**, 54–57
–, – of deboning of meat **23**, 47–48
–, – of heating **23**, 48–53
–, – of retorting or overheating **23**, 50–51
–, occurrence **23**, 2
–, practical aspects **23**, 59
–, prevention **23**, 57–59
–, reducing conditions and **23**, 58
–, research needs **23**, 59–61
–, species differences in **23**, 46–47
Warner–Bratzler machine **21**, 167
Warner–Bratzler shear **14**, 66–77, 82–83, 96–97, 129, 132–133
Wash columns, for aroma recovery in freeze concentration **20**, 44–45
Waste, asparagus **17**, 85–86
–, potato **17**, 87–88
–, sweet potato **17**, 86–87
–, tomato **17**, 81–85
–, utilization as food **17**, 76–152
Water, absorptionally bound **27**, 304
–, addition to wheat flour, effect on baking **29**, 205
–, amphiphile retention at interface **34**, 9
–, and ice **13**, 221–235, 238–244
–, as crystallizing plasticizer **38**, 161
–, as plasticizer **38**, 150–159
–, –, breakfast cereals, crispness and **38**, 185
–, –, distinguished from presence of water **38**, 156–157
–, –, food and biological materials **38**, 120–123
–, –, independent mechanical aspect **38**, 187–188
–, –, mechanical relaxation kinetics **38**, 186–187
–, –, unfreezability **38**, 170
–, bound **14**, 77, 123
–, –, and unbound **39**, 97–98, 265
–, –, in foods **13**, 4–10, 234–235, 273
–, –, in plants **13**, 308
–, capacity for holding, heat effects on **20**, 295–297
–, –, in meat **20**, 277–281
–, capillary-bound **27**, 305
–, chemically bound **27**, 304
–, chlorination of **7**, 130–131
–, competition for **7**, 87–88
–, conductivity, thermal **13**, 241–242
–, content, of plant tissue **27**, 299
–, density **13**, 239–240
–, diffusion coefficient **39**, 132, 135, 142
–, diffusion in aqueous food glasses **38**, 169–177
–, diffusivity, thermal **13**, 242–244
–, doubly labeled, *see* Doubly labeled water method
–, dynamics **38**, 127, 129–133, 160
–, effect on enzymes **17**, 48
–, – on protein structure **13**, 232–234
–, flat sour bacteria spores in **18**, 169–173
–, freezing point **13**, 238–239
–, –, depression by solutes **13**, 238–239

Water (*cont'd*)
–, holding capacity **39**, 100, 125–126
–, ice, structure **27**, 301–302
–, latent heat of fusion **13**, 240–241
–, mobility, in glassy materials **38**, 169–170
–, moisture distribution in plants **27**, 303–307
–, molecular structure of **11**, 362–365
–, osmotically retained moisture **27**, 305–307
–, phase diagram **27**, 302–307
–, physical characteristics **27**, 302
–, pollution **32**, 221–223
–, potential energy of dimer as function of hydrogen acceptor bond **34**, 8
–, protection of foods against absorption **3**, 457
–, protein foods, from **20**, 189–216
–, pure, phase diagram **13**, 236–238
–, removal **7**, 177–181
–, –, from foods **3**, 450–457
–, –, –, processes for **20**, 3
–, requirements **7**, 88–117
–, –, adaptation and **7**, 110–111
–, –, factors affecting **7**, 107–117, 122
–, –, food preservation and **7**, 117–122
–, –, general relationships **7**, 106
–, –, inhibitors and **7**, 110
–, –, pH and **7**, 109–110
–, –, research problems and **7**, 122–123
–, –, special groups and **7**, 111–117
–, –, temperature and **7**, 109
–, –, viable counts and **7**, 106
–, reused, chlorination of **7**, 159–160
–, *Salmonella* in **3**, 229
–, sausage fermentation **39**, 109–110
–, seawater, demineralization **13**, 232
–, shortage **32**, 188
–, sorption isotherms **7**, 92–93
–, specific heat **13**, 240
–, structure **7**, 85; **13**, 221–235; **27**, 299–300; **34**, 7–13
–, –, alterations using ionic and nonionic additives **34**, 47–48
–, –, clathrate structure formation **34**, 8–9
–, –, dimers in ice **34**, 7–8
–, –, effect of solutes **13**, 228–229
–, –, – of temperature **13**, 228
–, –, icelike clusters in **13**, 226–228
–, –, role in adsorption **34**, 47–52
–, supercooling in foods **27**, 307–315
–, – in –, cryoscopic temperatures **27**, 310–315
–, – in –, nucleation and growth of crystals **27**, 308–310
–, tetrahedral coordination of molecules in ice **11**, 363, 364
–, vapor pressure **39**, 97–98
Water activity (a_w), cheese ripening **39**, 178
–, concept **38**, 229–230
–, definition **39**, 98
–, degree of Maillard reaction **35**, 195–196
–, IM meat, *see* Dehydration control, IM meat
Water adsorption **39**, 100
Water-binding agents, IQ-like compounds and **34**, 435
Waterbloom poisoning **10**, 137
Water-cook system, for retorting **23**, 390–392
Water cress, composition of oil of **2**, 275
Water–food structure interactions (*see also* Food polymer science *and* Glass transition temperature) **38**, 103–233
–, studies **38**, 104–105
Water-holding capacity **39**, 100, 125–126
–, dietary fiber and **31**, 157–159
Water–hydrocarbon interfacial tensions **34**, 5–6
Watermelon, rind, bleaching **5**, 98
Water solubles, in wheat flours, breadmaking and **29**, 261
–, –, fractionation **29**, 226–227
–, –, interchanging between two samples **29**, 228–230
–, –, separation **29**, 222–224
Water temperature, and shellfish poisoning **10**, 140
Water turnover **40**, 173
Waveguide measurement method **43**, 79–80, 81
Waxes, dietary fiber and **31**, 139, 140
–, in tea **11**, 226–227
Waxy gene **41**, 81–82, 84–85
Weakness, muscle **37**, 341–342
Weber number **32**, 80
Web-fed bags **32**, 34
Weeds, effect on milk and meat flavor **23**, 37–38
Weight control, relationship to low-fat diets **37**, 226–229
Weight gain, bioperiodicity **40**, 220–226
Weight loss, IM meat **39**, 101
Welan, molecular shapes and interactions **42**, 191–194
Westphal's solution, of heat conduction problems **20**, 226
Wet heat **39**, 120
Wetting **14**, 334–338
–, acid agents **14**, 442
–, adhesive **14**, 338–339

–, immersion **14**, 339
–, processes **14**, 339–343
Wetting agent, used in removal of fats, proteins, and phosphorus from zeolite **2**, 23
Whalemeat, bacterial flora in **6**, 191
Whale muscle, rigor in **9**, 22
WHC, *see* Water-holding capacity
Wheat **15**, 235; **16**, 7
–, analysis **31**, 148, 150, 152, 153
–, and erosion **32**, 218
–, as source of protein **17**, 114
–, best consistency of **8**, 10
–, breeding **41**, 131
–, –, for flour baking quality **29**, 211–213
–, characterization **41**, 6–7
–, destruction of insects in **3**, 135
–, dicotyledonous plants **31**, 127, 133
–, dietary fiber and **31**, 120, 190
–, effect of moist heat on nutritive value of **4**, 254
–, – of storage on biological value of protein in **4**, 268
–, gelatinization temperature of **2**, 319
–, gene families **41**, 59
–, glutenin **45**, 219–290
–, glycemic response **41**, 159
–, hard red spring, moisture content **5**, 222
–, inositol phosphates **45**, 12, 13, 16, 20
–, –, degradation during digestion **45**, 24
–, –, degradation during processing **45**, 21
–, insect species infesting **8**, 111
–, in soy sauce **10**, 76, 105, 107, 109
–, intestinal bacteria **31**, 177, 179, 182–185, 187
–, iron, biological value of **28**, 35
–, modification **41**, 130–131
–, monocotyledonous plants **31**, 135–138
–, oriental noodles, *see* Oriental noodles
–, phytase **45**, 11
–, –, activity **28**, 62
–, projection separation of insects **8**, 124
–, properties **31**, 158, 160, 165, 169–171
–, roasting **30**, 217–219
–, –, starch and protein digestibility **30**, 218–219
–, selenium in **32**, 92, 93–94
–, shoyu preparation, in mixture with soybeans, browning reactions during brewing **30**, 248–249
–, –, koji cultivation **30**, 224
–, starch synthesis **41**, 121
–, storage proteins **45**, 220
–, swelling of **2**, 319
–, transformation system **45**, 253–254
–, varieties, gliadin composition in flours **29**, 268
–, world production of **23**, 189
Wheat and wheat products, flat sour bacteria spores in **18**, 179
Wheat bran, action of intestinal bacteria on **1**, 135
–, calcium content of, effect of fertilizers on **1**, 312
–, effects on calcium absorption **33**, 137–138
–, – on tocopherol bioavailability **33**, 172–173
–, germ oil in diet of rats **1**, 112
–, monoferric phytate, purification **28**, 34
–, phosphorus content of, effect of fertilizers on **1**, 313
–, thiamine content of, effect of location on **1**, 306–307
Wheat dough **39**, 53–55, 58–59
–, properties **43**, 228–229
Wheat flours **16**, 335ff
–, baking quality **29**, 201–271
–, –, approaches to research **29**, 214–216
–, –, breeding for **29**, 211–213
–, –, component interchanging between two samples **29**, 228–230
–, –, conclusions and future research **29**, 269–271
–, –, evaluation **29**, 204–216
–, –, gliadin composition and **29**, 268
–, –, gluten amidation and **29**, 265–267
–, –, glutenin subunits and **29**, 268–269
–, –, gluten molecular weight distribution and **29**, 265
–, –, limiting variables **29**, 204–206
–, –, protein–lipid interaction and **29**, 263–264
–, –, sulfur-containing amino acids in gluten and **29**, 267–268
–, calcium bioavailability **45**, 35
–, carbohydrates **16**, 382ff
–, defatted, functionality **29**, 220–221
–, effect of environment on **16**, 344, 365, 383, 397
–, – of plant age on **16**, 344, 382
–, fatty acids **16**, 426
–, gluten, fractionation and reconstitution **29**, 224–226
–, –, separation **29**, 222–224
–, glycolipid interaction with, in baking **20**, 153–188
–, iron absorption influence **45**, 33–34
–, lipids (*see also* Lipids) **16**, 397
–, –, breadmaking and **29**, 251–258

Wheat flours, lipids (*cont'd*)
–, –, cake quality and **29**, 260–261
–, –, cookie quality and **29**, 259–260
–, –, extraction and properties **29**, 217–222
–, maturation **16**, 343ff, 367ff
–, mechanism **20**, 166–167
–, milling of **2**, 321–322
–, ozone treatment **45**, 192
–, proteins **16**, 343ff
–, starch, breadmaking and **29**, 262
–, –, fractionation **29**, 227–228
–, –, separation **29**, 222–224
–, storage **16**, 425
–, water solubles, breadmaking and **29**, 261
–, –, fractionation **29**, 226–227
–, –, separation **29**, 222–224
–, zinc absorption influence **45**, 33
Wheat germ **23**, 187–304
–, air classification of **23**, 201–204
–, amino acids in, nutritive aspects **23**, 242–243
–, –, of mill germ **23**, 216–220
–, –, processing effects on **23**, 203, 251
–, amino acid supplementation of **23**, 253–254
–, antioxidants for **23**, 268
–, as cereal supplement **23**, 284–285
–, carbohydrates in, of mill germ **23**, 230–232
–, –, processing effects on **23**, 204
–, chemical composition **23**, 204–241
–, –, of dissected germ **23**, 205–211
–, –, of mill germ **23**, 211–241
–, definition of **23**, 193
–, deoiling of **23**, 268
–, drying of **23**, 268–269
–, embryonic axis of **23**, 194
–, enzymes in, of dissected germ **23**, 209–211
–, –, of mill germ **23**, 237–241
–, epiblast of **23**, 195
–, epoxy compound treatment of **23**, 267
–, ethylene dichloride treatment of **23**, 267
–, fatty acids in **23**, 225–228
–, fermented **23**, 275–276
–, flaked, separation of **23**, 199–200
–, food uses of **23**, 282–287
–, freshness evaluation in **23**, 262–263
–, heat processing of **23**, 264–267
–, in animal feeds **23**, 286
–, in bakery and pastry products **23**, 282–284
–, in breadmaking **23**, 273–281
–, in fermented foods **23**, 285
–, infrared radiation of **23**, 267
–, infrared treatment of **3**, 146
–, lipids in **23**, 220–230
–, –, characteristics **23**, 227–228
–, –, composition **23**, 221–223
–, –, effect on baking quality **23**, 280–281
–, –, of dissected germ **23**, 206–207
–, –, variety effects **23**, 221
–, minerals in, of dissected germ **23**, 207–208
–, –, of mill germ **23**, 232–235
–, –, processing effects on **23**, 204
–, moisture effects on **23**, 260–261
–, nucleic acids of **23**, 220
–, nutritive value of **23**, 242–258
–, –, by biological method **23**, 244–246
–, –, by chemical methods **23**, 242–244
–, –, processing effects on **23**, 249–253
–, –, storage effects on **23**, 270–272
–, –, supplementary value **23**, 246–249
–, physical characteristics **23**, 200–201
–, pigments in **23**, 237
–, processed **23**, 277–280
–, proteins in, of dissected germ **23**, 205
–, –, of mill germ **23**, 213–216
–, –, processing effects on **23**, 203
–, research needs for **23**, 287–289
–, scutellum of **23**, 194–195
–, separation of **23**, 197–204
–, sieve analysis of **23**, 201
–, spoilage causes in **23**, 261–262
–, steeping of **23**, 276–277
–, storage and stabilization of **23**, 258–273
–, –, effect on nutrients **23**, 270–272
–, structural components of **23**, 190
–, –, composition **23**, 197
–, –, diagram **23**, 195
–, –, quantitative determination **23**, 196
–, –, separation methods **23**, 195–196
–, sugars in, of dissected germ **23**, 205–206
–, –, of mill germ **23**, 230, 231
–, –, storage effects on **23**, 232
–, temperature effects on **23**, 259–260
–, tocopherols in **23**, 237
–, toxic factors in **23**, 255–258
–, vacuum packaging of **23**, 259
–, vitamin concentrates from **23**, 285–286
–, Vitamin B_1 in **6**, 263, 296
–, vitamins in, of dissected germ **23**, 208–209
–, –, of mill germ **23**, 235–236
–, –, storage effects on **23**, 271
Wheat germ oil, analysis of **23**, 225
–, constants of **23**, 228–229
–, stability of **23**, 229–230
–, uses of **23**, 285
Wheat gluten **40**, 231–232, 238–240; **45**, 220–221
–, amino acid sequences **42**, 85–87

–, as cryostabilizer **35**, 347–348
–, polymorphisms **45**, 221, 222
–, proteins **45**, 221–224
Wheat gluten–lipid films, oxygen barrier properties **44**, 378
–, –, relative humidity effects **44**, 381
–, water barrier properties **44**, 373–374
Wheat kernel, structural diagram of **23**, 191
–, transections of **23**, 192
Wheat-mill feeds **17**, 114
Wheat milling products, composition **17**, 114
Wheat proteins **10**, 61–63; **36**, 1–79
–, amino acid composition **36**, 37
–, breeding strategies **36**, 3, 70–76
–, –, alien gene incorporation **36**, 70–73
–, –, chromosomal and genetic engineering techniques **36**, 75–76
–, –, excessive dough-mixing requirements **36**, 73–74
–, –, future directions **36**, 79
–, –, increasing protein content **36**, 75
–, –, lack of extensibility **36**, 74–75
–, chromosomal structure **36**, 30–32
–, classification **36**, 17–28
–, –, molecular-size-based **36**, 20–22
–, –, monomeric proteins **36**, 27–28
–, –, polymeric proteins **36**, 22–27
–, –, solubility-based **36**, 17–19
–, composition/functionality relationships **36**, 44–60
–, –, addition of fractions **36**, 45–48
–, –, biotypes **36**, 60
–, –, environmental effects **36**, 55–56
–, –, future directions **36**, 78–79
–, –, genetic variants **36**, 56–60
–, –, HMW null lines **36**, 56–57
–, –, interchange experiments **36**, 49
–, –, qualitative relationships **36**, 50–51, 51–55
–, –, reconstitution methods **36**, 45–49
–, disulfide–sulhydryl interchange reactions **36**, 64
–, extensigraph parameters **36**, 65
–, –, application **36**, 67–68
–, –, extensibility **36**, 68–69
–, –, high polymer studies **36**, 65–67
–, food protein engineering **36**, 186
–, genetic control **36**, 28, 30–37
–, –, albumins/globulins **36**, 36–37
–, –, gliadins **36**, 36
–, –, HMW albumins **36**, 35–36
–, –, HMW glutenin subunits **36**, 32–33
–, –, LMW glutenin subunits **36**, 33–35
–, –, monomeric proteins **36**, 36–37
–, –, polymeric proteins **36**, 32–36
–, –, triticins **36**, 35
–, glutenin structure, future directions **36**, 77–78
–, new research materials **36**, 76–77
–, processes in dough mixing **36**, 61–64
–, – in –, macroscopic level **36**, 61
–, – in –, molecular level **36**, 62–64
–, prolamins **36**, 95
–, solubility properties **36**, 4–17
–, –, application **36**, 11–14
–, –, average hydrophobicity **36**, 9–10
–, –, charged group frequency **36**, 8
–, –, fundamental aspects **36**, 6–7
–, –, general **36**, 4–7
–, –, hydrophobic effect **36**, 7
–, –, increase by dough mixing **36**, 14–15
–, –, neutral salt effects **36**, 12–14
–, –, nonpolar side chain frequency **36**, 8
–, –, polarity ratio **36**, 8
–, –, residue accessibility **36**, 10–11
–, solubilization of highest molecular weight glutenin **36**, 14–17
–, – of –, sonication **36**, 15–17
–, – of –, structural parameters and **36**, 7–11
–, – of –, surface hydrophobicities **36**, 11–12
–, structure, gliadins **36**, 38–39
–, –, HMW glutenin subunits **36**, 37–38
–, –, LMW glutenin subunits **36**, 38–39
–, –, physical studies of glutenin subunits **36**, 39
–, –, polymeric proteins in native state **36**, 39–44
–, thermal characteristics **35**, 342
Wheat starch, aging gels of **6**, 12
–, effect of diastatic activity on **2**, 322
Whey, chocolate and **31**, 254, 255, 257, 258, 261–263
–, dried, lactose content of **3**, 57
–, drying of **3**, 84, 89–91
–, β-galactosidase stability in **38**, 36
–, half-life in column reaction **38**, 47, 50
–, hydrolysis, immobilized lactase reactors **38**, 46–47
–, lactose syrup production **38**, 21–22
–, uses **17**, 132–133
–, waste utilization **38**, 20–21
Whey products, demineralized delactosed whey **33**, 347
–, dry sweet whey **33**, 347
–, powder (WP), as replacement for nonfat dry milk **33**, 348
–, –, composition of **19**, 154
–, –, flow diagram **19**, 153

Whey products, powder (WP) (*cont'd*)
–, –, minerals and salts in **19**, 194
–, –, preparation of **19**, 152–153
–, –, types used in food, table **33**, 348
–, –, upgrading and refining **33**, 348–349
–, –, uses, table **33**, 346
–, –, vitamins in **19**, 192
–, susceptibility to denaturation **33**, 347
–, use of **33**, 347
–, whey protein concentrate **33**, 347
Whey protein concentrates and isolates, elasticity with cooling and reheating **34**, 245–246
–, gelation mechanisms **34**, 244–247
–, gel properties **34**, 247–249
–, gel strength **34**, 337–344
–, –, cysteine effect **34**, 339–340
–, –, presence of NaCl and $CaCl_2$ **34**, 338–339
–, –, protein–protein interactions **34**, 340–341
–, –, transition from viscous to viscoelastic structure **34**, 245–246
–, –, variation with added cosolute **34**, 337–340
–, –, – with protein concentrate **34**, 340–344
Whey protein isolate–lipid films, applications **44**, 382
–, oxygen barrier properties **44**, 378
–, water barrier properties **44**, 376–378
–, –, relative humidity effects **44**, 381
Whey protein nitrogen index, whey protein denaturation **33**, 372
Whey proteins, adsorption **33**, 391–393
–, and flavors, interactions **33**, 415–416
–, as gelling ingredients **33**, 389–391
–, composition and distribution of **19**, 155
–, composition of concentrates and isolates **34**, 243
–, concentrate **35**, 195–196, 354
–, definition and classification **34**, 242–243
–, emulsifying properties, characterization **33**, 405–406
–, –, factors affecting **33**, 408
–, –, protein conformation and **33**, 406–408
–, –, surface hydrophobicity and **33**, 406–408
–, films **33**, 395–396
–, –, effects of aging **33**, 394
–, –, pH and ionic strength effects **33**, 394
–, –, protein structure and **33**, 393–395
–, –, stability **33**, 394
–, –, viscoelastic behavior **33**, 394–395
–, flavor binding **33**, 410–413
–, –, thermodynamic representation **33**, 412
–, foaming properties **33**, 402–404
–, foams **33**, 400–402
–, functional properties **33**, 364–365
–, –, effects of variability in protein preparations **33**, 370–373
–, –, factors affecting, extrinsic **33**, 369–370
–, –, –, intrinsic **33**, 365–369
–, –, –, table **33**, 367
–, –, requirements in food products, table **33**, 366
–, gelation **33**, 381–385
–, –, factors affecting gel composition and properties **33**, 385–389
–, –, forces in gel formation and stabilization, table **33**, 384
–, –, gel structure **33**, 383–384
–, gel strength **34**, 247
–, heated **35**, 220
–, hydration **33**, 373–374
–, hydrophobic properties **34**, 248
–, infant formula **33**, 422–423
–, in milk **10**, 48–50, 51–52
–, β-lactoglobulin **34**, 243–244
–, lipid binding **33**, 408–409
–, modification, chemical **33**, 417–418
–, –, –, acylation **33**, 418–419
–, –, –, amidation and esterification **33**, 419–420
–, –, –, glycosylation **33**, 421–422
–, –, –, phosphorylation **33**, 419
–, –, –, reductive alkylation **33**, 421
–, –, –, thiolation **33**, 420–421
–, –, enzymatic **33**, 416–417
–, nutritional aspects **33**, 422–423
–, preparation and isolation, chromatographic methods **33**, 361
–, –, combined reverse osmosis–ultrafiltration **33**, 361
–, –, compositions of derived proteins, table **33**, 363
–, –, conventional methods **33**, 360–361
–, –, denaturation assessment methods **33**, 363
–, –, reverse osmosis **33**, 361
–, –, thermal separation **33**, 361–362
–, –, ultrafiltration **33**, 361
–, research needs **33**, 424–425
–, role in breadmaking **19**, 177–179
–, solubility **33**, 374–375
–, structure, amino acid compositions, table **33**, 350
–, –, bovine serum albumin **33**, 357
–, –, emulsifying properties and **33**, 406–408
–, –, film-forming properties and **33**, 393–395
–, –, foam stability and **33**, 398–400

–, –, immunoglobulins **33**, 357–358
–, –, α-lactalbumin **33**, 354–357
–, –, lactoferrin **33**, 358–359
–, –, β-lactoglobulin **33**, 350–354
–, –, lysozyme **33**, 359
–, –, physicochemical characteristics, table **33**, 349
–, –, proteose–peptones **33**, 358
–, surface activity **33**, 391–397
–, thermal properties **33**, 376
–, –, casein effect **35**, 332–333
–, –, heat denaturation **33**, 378–379
–, –, heat denaturation temperatures and enthalpies, table **33**, 377
–, –, heat effects on conformation **33**, 376–378
–, –, pH effects **35**, 324–325
–, ultrasonic analysis **45**, 152, 153
–, water-holding ability **34**, 247–248
White blood cells, tocopherol association with **33**, 177
White muscle, *see* Muscle
Whiting, aerobic bacteria in **2**, 350
–, formation of dimethylamine in stored **2**, 371
–, gurnard, aerobic bacteria in **2**, 350
–, organoleptic spoilage of **2**, 377
–, rigor mortis in **2**, 363, 366
–, tests for quality of **2**, 381
Whole-body model, folate **40**, 83
–, membrane transport **40**, 259–260
–, vitamin A **40**, 8–11
–, vitamin B6 **40**, 116–117
Whole grain, phytic acid content **28**, 14
Wide-gap rotational viscometers **11**, 378–381
Wiener conche, chocolate and **31**, 304, 305
Wieners, thermal scanning rheological analysis **35**, 354–355
Willia in dates **3**, 452
Williams–Landel–Ferry free-volume theory **38**, 135, 177
Wiltshire bacon, *see* Bacon
Winemaking, sulfites as antimicrobial agents **30**, 11–12
Winery equipment, ozone treatment **45**, 192
Winery wastes **17**, 131–132
Wines **17**, 196–197
–, acetal **5**, 385
–, acetaldehyde **5**, 382, 384
–, acetone **5**, 385
–, acetylmethylcarbinol in various types **5**, 382
–, acidic components **25**, 3–10
–, –, changes during vinification **25**, 10–13
–, –, recommended levels **25**, 4–5
–, acids **5**, 386, 388
–, –, changes during storage **5**, 397
–, acrolein **5**, 386
–, aging **5**, 393, 444
–, alcohols and related compounds **5**, 358
–, aldehydes and related compounds **5**, 382
–, alginates in clarification **11**, 153
–, aromatic constituents **5**, 454, 460
–, ascorbic acid **5**, 457
–, –, as reducing agent **18**, 283–287
–, bacteria in California **6**, 90
–, benzaldehyde **5**, 385
–, buffer capacity **5**, 417
–, carbohydrates **5**, 418
–, chemical abnormalities induced by bacteria **6**, 76
–, chromatography of **5**, 357
–, citric acid **5**, 397, 401
–, color **5**, 330, 441
–, constituents in white and port **5**, 358
–, content of 2,3-butylene glycol **5**, 381
–, Danish fruit **6**, 82
–, deacidification **25**, 1–53
–, –, biological methods for **25**, 25–42
–, –, physicochemical methods **25**, 13–25
–, determination of total SO_2 **5**, 422, 123
–, effect of air on **6**, 89
–, enzymes **5**, 454
–, esters **5**, 430, 435
–, extract **5**, 428
–, fermentation, acids produced during **25**, 10–11
–, fining **5**, 444
–, from kiwifruit juice **29**, 302–306
–, growth of bacteria **6**, 82
–, hexosis **5**, 419
–, hydroxymethylfurfural **5**, 385
–, inorganic constituents of **8**, 135
–, lactic acid **5**, 403, 405
–, malic acid **5**, 395, 398
–, mannitol **5**, 425
–, methods of analyses **5**, 356
–, microbiology of **6**, 67
–, nicotinic acid **5**, 460
–, nitrogenous compounds **5**, 448, 449, 452, 454–456
–, –, in clouding **5**, 451
–, organic constituents **5**, 353
–, oversulfiting **5**, 140
–, pantothenic acid **5**, 460
–, pentoses and related compounds **5**, 423
–, pH of **5**, 416
–, polyhydroxyphenols **5**, 435

Wines (*cont'd*)
–, polyphenols and enzymic browning **19**, 117–118
–, problems in Germany **5**, 355
–, – in Hungary **5**, 355
–, pyridoxine **5**, 460
–, radio-frequency waves in pasteurization of **3**, 133
–, riboflavin **5**, 459
–, slimy or ropy **6**, 82
–, sophistication, detection **5**, 494
–, spoilage caused by bacteria **6**, 75, 76
–, storage temperature **6**, 89
–, suceinic acid **5**, 402, 403
–, sucrose **5**, 424
–, sulfur dioxide **8**, 135, 157, 162
–, tannins **5**, 436, 437, 439, 440
–, tartaric acid **5**, 391, 394, 415
–, tartness of **25**, 3–4
–, thiamin **5**, 458
–, titratable acidity **5**, 390
–, ultrasonic alcohol determination **45**, 138
–, use of ascorbic acid **4**, 406
–, – of SO_2 **5**, 136, 137
–, vitamins **5**, 454, 456, 462
–, volatile acidity **5**, 407, 412
–, yeast, temperature–time relationship for destruction of **3**, 436
Winkler device **14**, 89–90
Winnowing, chocolate and **31**, 241, 243, 244
Wisconsin system, meat quality judging **21**, 73
Witch, rigor mortis in **2**, 366
Withering process, in tea manufacture **17**, 261–263, 272
WLF behavior, compared to Arrhenius behavior **38**, 188–200
–, effect on kinetics of diffusion-limited relaxation processes **38**, 208–209
–, relaxation times **38**, 189–191
WLF coefficients, intuitive implications **38**, 200
WLF equation **38**, 160, 177–188
–, analogy with Michaelis–Menten equation **38**, 200–204
–, application **38**, 178, 230
–, aqueous food–polymer systems, viscoelastic behavior **38**, 183–188
–, correct glass transition temperature reference state **38**, 230–231
–, crystallization kinetics **38**, 181–182, 210–212
–, explicit reference temperature **38**, 207
–, mobility definition **38**, 179
WLF kinetics **38**, 135, 176
–, contrast with Arrhenius kinetics **38**, 204–212
WLF shift factor **38**, 189–190
Wofatit C, preparation of **2**, 5
WOF (warmed-over flavor), *see* Meat, cooked, warmed-over flavor development
Women, employed outside home **32**, 242
–, food preferences and attitudes **32**, 255–258
Wood, dietary fiber and **31**, 126, 151
Wood materials, dry distillation products **29**, 93–94
–, for curing smoke generation **29**, 90–92
–, –, effect on food flavoring **29**, 139–140
–, –, main constituents **29**, 90–91
–, –, pyrolysis during **29**, 93–98
–, –, smoldering **29**, 92–95
–, smoke compounds from various species **29**, 107–108
Work methods, analysis and development of operations **4**, 67–90
–, – of processes **4**, 51–66
–, description of methods **4**, 44–48
–, design and simplification **4**, 37–104
–, development of methods **4**, 48–50
–, simplification of work **4**, 91–96
Workplace exposure, carcinogen risk assessment and **31**, 2, 3, 5
–, –, epidemiology **31**, 38
–, –, laboratory data **31**, 37
–, –, statistics **31**, 13, 18
–, *N*-nitroso compounds and **31**, 98
World, food situation in **18**, 85–86
World Health Organization, recommended dietary allowances for calcium, table **33**, 109
World Wide Web, semiparametric tools **40**, 275
Wurster spray dryer, use in manufacture of soap powder **2**, 431–432
Wyman-linkage theory **35**, 299

X-protein **9**, 4
Xanthan, molecular shapes and interactions **42**, 196–199
Xanthan gum, creaming and **34**, 133–135
Xanthates **14**, 311–312
Xanthine, chocolate and **31**, 326
Xanthine derivatives, meat mutagen modulation **34**, 433
Xanthophylls **15**, 217
Xeromyces, growth rate of **7**, 98–99
X-ray analysis cap **41**, 167

X-ray diffraction, polysaccharides **42**, 133–146
X-ray diffraction of **3**, 158
X-ray fluoroscopy **3**, 158, 159
X-ray microanalysis in scanning electron microscopy **22**, 216, 219
X-rays **15**, 71
–, carcinogen risk assessment and **31**, 2, 3
–, destruction of toxins by **3**, 159
–, effect on vitamins **3**, 157, 158
–, explanation of **3**, 127, 128
–, germicidal action of **3**, 156, 157
–, relative penetration of **3**, 128
–, uses of **3**, 156–160
Xylan, chocolate and **31**, 269
–, dietary fiber and, analysis **31**, 146, 148
–, –, dicotyledonous plants **31**, 127, 129, 133, 135
–, –, intestinal bacteria **31**, 177, 181, 183, 185, 187
–, –, properties **31**, 170, 171
Xylem, desirability of in foods **2**, 304, 305
–, dietary fiber and **31**, 122
Xylene, solubility of DDT in **2**, 203
Xylitol **25**, 137–180
–, adverse effects of **25**, 171–174
–, boiling point **28**, 384
–, browning reactions **28**, 389
–, caloric value **28**, 389
–, carcinogenicity studies on **25**, 173–174
–, chocolate and **31**, 269, 274, 275
–, confectionery uses **28**, 392–395
–, crystallization **28**, 382–383
–, density **28**, 387
–, dental and nutritional properties of **25**, 142–143
–, dental caries and **25**, 139–147
–, effects on renal and cerebral function **25**, 173
–, enzyme stability **35**, 247
–, exocrine glands and **25**, 149–152
–, fermentation **28**, 389–390
–, food applications **28**, 392–399
–, foods containing lowered cariogenicity **25**, 139
–, food technological properties **28**, 389–392
–, heat of solution **28**, 385–386
–, history **28**, 375–378
–, hygroscopicity **28**, 387–388
–, in chewing gum **28**, 392–393
–, in chocolate **28**, 395
–, in coatings **28**, 395
–, in compressed tablets **28**, 394–395
–, in confectionery jellies **28**, 394
–, in drinks **28**, 398–399
–, in gum drops **28**, 394
–, in hard candy **28**, 393–394
–, in ice cream **28**, 395–396
–, in jams **28**, 396–398
–, in jellies **28**, 396–398
–, in marmalades **28**, 396–398
–, in yogurt **28**, 396
–, large scale production **28**, 378–382
–, –, hydrogenation **28**, 381
–, –, hydrolysis **28**, 380
–, –, purification **28**, 381–382
–, –, xylose purification **28**, 380
–, mechanism of action of **25**, 153–156
–, metabolism of **25**, 160–161
–, –, hepatic **25**, 164–165
–, –, intermediary **25**, 163–164
–, –, intestinal absorption **25**, 162–163
–, microbiological aspects of **25**, 147
–, occurrence, in fruit **28**, 376–377
–, –, in nature **28**, 374–375
–, periodontal disease and **25**, 152–153
–, physicochemical properties **28**, 382–388
–, plaque studies on **25**, 149
–, research needs **25**, 176; **28**, 399–400
–, sialomacromolecules and **25**, 150–152
–, solubility **28**, 385
–, specific heat **28**, 384–385
–, structure **28**, 382
–, sweetness **28**, 390–392
–, –, chemical basis **28**, 390
–, –, in water and acid solutions **28**, 391
–, –, synergistic effects **28**, 391–392
–, therapeutic use of **25**, 167–170
–, –, for diabetics **25**, 168–169
–, –, for hemolytic anemia **25**, 169–170
–, –, in parenteral nutrition **25**, 167–168
–, toxicology of **25**, 170–174
–, viscosity **28**, 386
Xyloglucans, dietary fiber and, dicotyledonous plants **31**, 126–129, 135
–, intestinal bacteria **31**, 172, 177, 179, 187
–, monocotyledonous plants **31**, 137
–, pectin-bound **30**, 151
–, physiological role **30**, 179
–, plant cell wall, cellulose-bound **30**, 150–151
Xylose, addition to dough, aroma and **30**, 100–101
–, chocolate and **31**, 269
–, dietary fiber and, analysis **31**, 146, 148
–, –, dicotyledonous plants **31**, 126, 133, 135
–, –, intestinal bacteria **31**, 175, 177, 181, 185, 187, 188

Xylose, dietary fiber and (*cont'd*)
–, –, monocotyledonous plants **31**, 137
–, in apples and pears **8**, 313
–, utilization by shoyu, color formation and **30**, 245–246
L-Xylosone **14**, 233
D-Xylulokinase, in wheat germ **23**, 240

Yacon, inulin **43**, 6, 8, 9
Yeasts (*see also individual organisms*) **32**, 15
–, action of epoxides on **1**, 389
–, – of formaldehyde on **1**, 389
–, – of sulfur dioxide on **1**, 388
–, amino acid composition **18**, 109
–, as sources of protein **18**, 88–116
–, – of –, nutritional value **18**, 107–116
–, – of –, propagation methods **18**, 91–107
–, – of –, useful species **18**, 90–91
–, behavior toward salts **12**, 64
–, Brewers **17**, 130–132
–, cell membranes **12**, 64–69
–, chocolate and **31**, 218, 256
–, cloned gene expression **36**, 150
–, copper as a poison in wine **8**, 179
–, destruction by supersonic vibrations **3**, 131
–, – by ultraviolet light **3**, 149
–, destruction of cells by ether **1**, 377
–, dried stabilizer in candy **6**, 13
–, ecological aspects **12**, 83–84
–, effect of pH on growth **3**, 431
–, – of – on salt tolerance **3**, 453
–, – of radio waves on growth **3**, 144
–, effect on malic acid **9**, 267–268
–, extract, thiamine destruction in **6**, 294, 304
–, folate bioavailability **33**, 73–74
–, from shoyu mash, ferulic acid conversion into 4-ethylguaiacol **30**, 278, 280
–, from sulfite waste liquor, diagram **18**, 100
–, growth and fermentation **12**, 69–76
–, –, assimilation of sugars **12**, 75–76
–, –, balances of products **12**, 76
–, –, culture temperature **12**, 73–75
–, –, hydrogen ion concentration **12**, 72–73
–, –, in high concentrations of sodium chloride **12**, 70
–, –, nitrogen sources **12**, 69–71
–, –, vitamins **12**, 71–72
–, growth curve in presence of sulfur dioxide **3**, 502
–, inactivation, pulsed electric field (PEF) processing **44**, 13, 14–15
–, in brines **12**, 55–56
–, in cocoa bean pulp **8**, 263
–, in diet of rats **1**, 112, 114
–, in fermenting cocoa beans **8**, 232, 252
–, in food spoilage **12**, 85–86
–, in grape juice **9**, 231–234
–, in noncitrus fruit juices **9**, 228–234
–, –, in apple juice **9**, 229–230
–, –, in concentrates **9**, 230–231
–, in olive oil **31**, 461, 471
–, in soy sauce and mash **10**, 113–115, 119–121
–, in substrates with high sugar content **12**, 54–55
–, in sugar solution **3**, 448–449
–, intake by depancreatinized rats **1**, 123
–, intestinal overgrowth **43**, 20–21
–, miso **12**, 56–58
–, Na- **12**, 64, 67
–, obligate **12**, 59
–, on refrigerated meats **6**, 139
–, osmophilism and **7**, 113–115; **12**, 53–94
–, palatability of **18**, 115–116
–, pH and **7**, 109–110
–, photomicrographs of spray-dried **2**, 516
–, physiological adaptation and training **12**, 59–62
–, –, depressed viability **12**, 59–60
–, –, reversibility of salt tolerance **12**, 60–61
–, practical applications **12**, 84–85
–, problems **12**, 86
–, proteins of **16**, 18, 24
–, recovery of **17**, 131
–, reduction of growth rate by mustard gas **1**, 378
–, salt-tolerant **12**, 78–79
–, soy **12**, 56–58
–, sugar and salt tolerance **12**, 58–59
–, –, difference in same species **12**, 63–64
–, –, osmotic effects **12**, 58
–, sulfite formation by various strains **30**, 6–7
–, temperature and **7**, 109
–, thiamine in **6**, 262
–, *Torula*, growth of **17**, 94
–, toxicity **18**, 112–115
–, use of Bishop spray dryer for **2**, 410
–, water requirements **7**, 100–101
–, wine **6**, 87
Yellow tail, spoilage of **7**, 51–52
Yersinia, attachment to meat tissue **43**, 336
Yield stress **39**, 6, 46, 48
Yogurt **39**, 187, 189
–, allolactose and galactobiose in **38**, 84
–, ascorbic acid fortification of **18**, 294
–, lactose content **38**, 14–16

–, ultrasonic sol–gel transition monitoring **45**, 147
Young's modulus **39**, 7, 254
Yuba **44**, 374
YX-proteinase, lyotropic salt effect **35**, 296–298

Z-disk protein, endogenous proteolytic enzymes and **31**, 398, 399, 404, 407
Z value, of enzymes **17**, 44–45
–, thermal inactivation **17**, 39, 42
z values **44**, 15252
–, *Escherichia coli* O157:H7 **44**, 158, 159, 160, 161, 163, 16565
–, *Listeria monocytogenes* **44**, 16060
–, *Salmonella* **44**, 153, 154, 155, 156, 157, 163, 164, 16565
–, time–temperature integrators, chemical **44**, 18282
–, –, peroxidase **44**, 18080
–, –, phycoerythrin **44**, 18585
–, –, triose phosphate isomerase **44**, 18383
Z*Coat **44**, 381
Zahn spray dryer **2**, 430
Zalcitabine **44**, 285, 320
Zea mays, *see* Corn
Zearalenones **44**, 196
Zeaxanthin **15**, 218
Zein-extracted gluten **17**, 121
Zeins **36**, 101–103; **38**, 275, 277
–, acid hydrolysis of **3**, 272
–, consensus sequence **36**, 101
–, expression in micro-organisms **36**, 163
–, food protein engineering **36**, 185–186
–, transgenic plants **36**, 169–170
α-Zeins, structural model **36**, 101–102
β-Zeins **36**, 101
γ-Zeins **36**, 101, 103
δ-Zeins **36**, 103
Zenker's waxy degeneration **13**, 114–115
Zeo-Karb, adsorption of polypeptide fraction by **2**, 12
–, use as catalyst **2**, 36
–, use in pectin extraction **2**, 21
–, – in reducing lead in maple syrup **2**, 37
Zeolite, regeneration of **2**, 24
Zeolite treatment, on cow's milk **2**, 21–24
Zeo-Rex, adsorption of polypeptide fraction by **2**, 12
Zephiran, effect of pH on germicidal power **2**, 134
–, effect on influenza virus **2**, 138, 183
–, – on tubercle bacilli **2**, 148
–, film formation of **2**, 144
–, neutralization by anionic agent **2**, 132
–, structure of **2**, 120
–, therapeutic action of **2**, 143
–, toxicity of **2**, 130, 131
–, use on sewage **2**, 183
Zephirol, concentration to destroy staphylococci **2**, 135
–, structure of **2**, 120, 146
–, toxicity of **2**, 130
Zero flow, extrapolation **40**, 189
Zeta potential, coalescence rate constant variation with **34**, 138
Zidovudine **44**, 285
Zig-zag oscillatory tests **35**, 351
Zinc **36**, 225
–, absorption, inositol phosphates influence **45**, 32, 33, 35, 36, 42
–, –, inulin effects **43**, 33
–, bioavailability **36**, 227–228
–, –, effect of autoclaving **28**, 40
–, –, in foodstuffs **28**, 39–41
–, content of apples and pears **8**, 371
–, – of plants, effect of fertilizers on **1**, 314
–, deficiency **1**, 121; **36**, 225
–, –, in apples **8**, 378
–, effect on ascorbic acid content of tomatoes **1**, 308
–, endogenous proteolytic enzymes and **31**, 347
–, in milk **36**, 225–228
–, in musts and wines **8**, 137, 138, 198
–, RDAs **36**, 226
–, soy protein effects on absorption and metabolism, human **30**, 369–379
Zinc–folate interactions, effects on folate bioavailability **33**, 79–80
Zirconium, in fermenting musts **8**, 137
Zizinia spray dryer, operation of **2**, 407–408
Zolpidem **44**, 308
Zoplicone **44**, 308
Zousoon **39**, 76, 137
–, color **39**, 128–129
–, energy costs **39**, 145–146, 147
–, flavor **39**, 132, 133, 136
–, microbial control **39**, 124
–, osmosis **39**, 111–113
–, prerigor treatment **39**, 93, 147
–, process improvement **39**, 89–90
–, texture **39**, 125
Zucca melon, bleaching **5**, 98
Zygosaccharomyces, growth inhibition by SO_2 **5**, 125
–, in dates **3**, 452

Zygosaccharomyces (*cont'd*)
–, in glycerol production **12**, 76–77
–, toleration of moisture by **3**, 451, 452
Zygosaccharomyces bailii **45**, 197
Zygosaccharomyces barkeri **3**, 452
Zygosaccharomyces cerevisiae **3**, 452
Zygosaccharomyces ellipsoideus **3**, 452
Zygosaccharomyces japonicus **12**, 56
Zygosaccharomyces nussbaumeri **12**, 54–55
Zygosaccharomyces salsus **12**, 56
Zygosaccharomyces soya **12**, 56

ISBN 0-12-016446-9
9 780120 164462